DIABETES & HYPOGLYCEMIA

Topical and Important Articles from the

AMERICAN DIABETES ASSOCIATION

SCHOLARLY JOURNALS

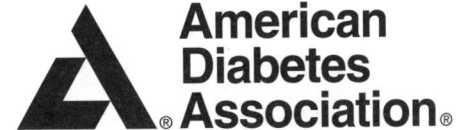

American Diabetes Association®

DIABETES & HYPOGLYCEMIA

Printed in the United States of America
1 3 5 7 9 10 8 6 4 2

The suggestions and information contained in this publication are generally consistent with the *Clinical Practice Recommendations* and other policies of the American Diabetes Association, but they do not represent the policy or position of the Association or any of its boards or committees. Reasonable steps have been taken to ensure the accuracy of the information presented. However, the American Diabetes Association cannot ensure the safety or efficacy of any product or service described in this publication. Individuals are advised to consult a physician or other appropriate health care professional before undertaking any diet or exercise program or taking any medication referred to in this publication. Professionals must use and apply their own professional judgment, experience, and training and should not rely solely on the information contained in this publication before prescribing any diet, exercise, or medication. The American Diabetes Association—its officers, directors, employees, volunteers, and members—assumes no responsibility or liability for personal or other injury, loss, or damage that may result from the suggestions or information in this publication.

♾ The paper in this publication meets the requirements of the ANSI Standard Z39.48-1992 (permanence of paper).

ADA titles may be purchased for business or promotional use or for special sales. To purchase more than 50 copies of this book at a discount, or for custom editions of this book with your logo, contact the American Diabetes Association at the address below, at booksales@diabetes.org, or by calling 703-299-2046.

American Diabetes Association
1701 North Beauregard Street
Alexandria, Virginia 22311

DOI: 10.2337/9781580404648

DIABETES AND HYPOGLYCEMIA

Recurrent Moderate Hypoglycemia Ameliorates Brain Damage and Cognitive Dysfunction Induced by Severe Hypoglycemia

Erwin C. Puente,[1] Julie Silverstein,[1] Adam J. Bree,[1] Daniel R. Musikantow,[1] David F. Wozniak,[2] Susan Maloney,[2] Dorit Daphna-Iken,[1] and Simon J. Fisher[1,3]

OBJECTIVE—Although intensive glycemic control achieved with insulin therapy increases the incidence of both moderate and severe hypoglycemia, clinical reports of cognitive impairment due to severe hypoglycemia have been highly variable. It was hypothesized that recurrent moderate hypoglycemia preconditions the brain and protects against damage caused by severe hypoglycemia.

RESEARCH DESIGN AND METHODS—Nine-week-old male Sprague-Dawley rats were subjected to either 3 consecutive days of recurrent moderate (25–40 mg/dl) hypoglycemia (RH) or saline injections. On the fourth day, rats were subjected to a hyperinsulinemic (0.2 units $\cdot$ kg^{-1} $\cdot$ min^{-1}) severe hypoglycemic (~11 mg/dl) clamp for 60 or 90 min. Neuronal damage was subsequently assessed by hematoxylin-eosin and Fluoro-Jade B staining. The functional significance of severe hypoglycemia–induced brain damage was evaluated by motor and cognitive testing.

RESULTS—Severe hypoglycemia induced brain damage and striking deficits in spatial learning and memory. Rats subjected to recurrent moderate hypoglycemia had 62–74% less brain cell death and were protected from most of these cognitive disturbances.

CONCLUSIONS—Antecedent recurrent moderate hypoglycemia preconditioned the brain and markedly limited both the extent of severe hypoglycemia–induced neuronal damage and associated cognitive impairment. In conclusion, changes brought about by recurrent moderate hypoglycemia can be viewed, paradoxically, as providing a beneficial adaptive response in that there is mitigation against severe hypoglycemia–induced brain damage and cognitive dysfunction. *Diabetes* 59:1055–1062, 2010

From the [1]Division of Endocrinology, Metabolism, and Lipid Research, Department of Medicine, Washington University, St. Louis, Missouri; the [2]Department of Psychiatry, Washington University, St. Louis, Missouri; and the [3]Department of Cell Biology and Physiology, Washington University, St. Louis, Missouri.

Corresponding author: Simon Fisher, sfisher@dom.wustl.edu.

Received 8 October 2009 and accepted 6 January 2010. Published ahead of print at http://diabetes.diabetesjournals.org on 19 January 2010. DOI: 10.2337/db09-1495.

Hypoglycemia is the major obstacle in achieving tight glycemic control in people with diabetes (1). Intensive insulin therapy increases the risk of iatrogenic hypoglycemia (2). Episodes of both moderate and severe hypoglycemia have long-term clinical consequences. Recurrent moderate hypoglycemia induces a maladaptive response that limits symptoms of hypoglycemia (hypoglycemia unawareness), limits the counterregulatory response to subsequent hypoglycemia (hypoglycemia-associated autonomic failure), and thus jeopardizes patient safety (1). By depriving the brain of glucose, more severe hypoglycemia causes brain damage in animal studies and leads to long-term impairments in learning and memory (3,4). However, studies examining the effect of severe hypoglycemia in humans are conflicting. Severe hypoglycemia has been shown to alter brain structure (5–7) and cause significant cognitive damage in many (5,7–12) but not all (13–16) studies. Reasons for the discrepancy between human and animal studies are unknown, but a major contributing factor may be the extent of glycemia control (including recurrent hypoglycemia) prior to the episode of severe hypoglycemia.

In other models of brain damage, such as ischemic stroke, brief, mild episodes of antecedent brain ischemia has been shown to cause a beneficial adaptation that protects the brain against a subsequent episode of more severe ischemia (a phenomena known as ischemic preconditioning) (17). In a similar fashion, antecedent, recurrent episodes of moderate hypoglycemia were hypothesized to protect the brain against damage caused by a subsequent episode of more severe hypoglycemia.

To investigate this hypothesis, recurrent moderately hypoglycemic (25–40 mg/dl) rats (RH rats) and control saline-injected rats (CON rats) were subjected to hyperinsulinemic, severe hypoglycemic clamps (10–15 mg/dl). One group of rats was killed 1 week after severe hypoglycemia to quantify brain damage, while a second group of rats was evaluated by behavioral and cognitive tests 6–8 weeks after the severe hypoglycemia. The results demonstrated that recurrent antecedent moderate hypoglycemia preconditioned the brain and protected it against neurological damage and cognitive defects induced by an episode of severe hypoglycemia.

RESEARCH DESIGN AND METHODS

Nine-week-old male Sprague-Dawley rats (Charles River Laboratories) were individually housed in a temperature- and light-controlled environment maintaining the animal's diurnal cycle (12 h light and 12 h dark) with an ad libitum standard rat chow diet. All studies were done in accordance with the Animal Studies Committee at the Washington University School of Medicine.

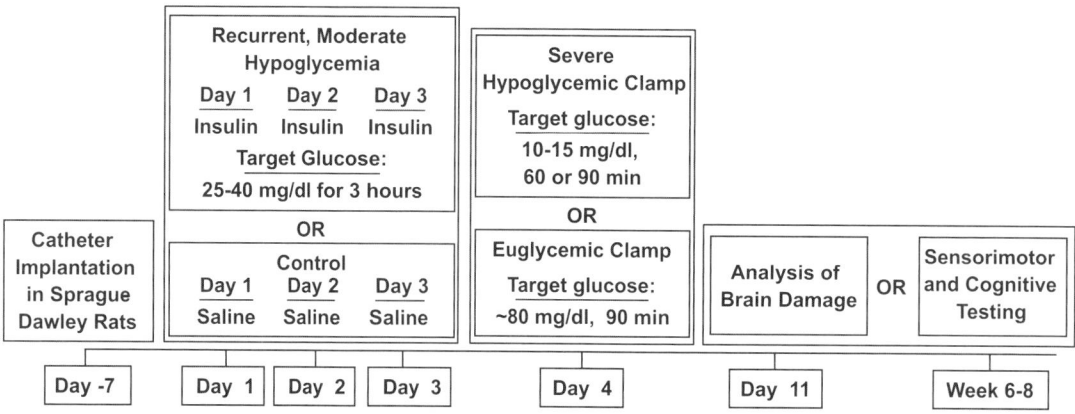

FIG. 1. Experimental protocol. Arterial and venous catheters were implanted into 9-week-old Sprague-Dawley rats. After 1 week of recovery, animals were either given an insulin injection daily for 3 consecutive days to induce moderate hypoglycemia (25–40 mg/dl) or they were given saline injections as a control. On the fourth day, rats underwent a severe hypoglycemic (10–15 mg/dl) hyperinsulinemic (0.2 units $\cdot$ kg^{-1} $\cdot$ min^{-1}) clamp for either 60 or 90 min or, alternatively, underwent a 90-min euglycemic ($\sim$80 mg/dl) hyperinsulinemic (0.2 units $\cdot$ kg^{-1} $\cdot$ min^{-1}) clamp. Animals were either killed 1 week later to assess neuronal damage by H-E and Fluoro-Jade B staining or underwent sensorimotor and cognitive testing 6–8 weeks following the clamp.

Implantation of arterial and venous catheters. Micro-renathane (Braintree Scientific) catheters were inserted into the left carotid artery and into the right jugular vein of anesthetized rats (40–80 mg/kg ketamine with 5–8 mg/kg xylazine). To maintain patency, catheters were filled with 40% polyvinylpyrrolidone (Sigma) in heparin (1,000 units/ml; USP) (Baxter Healthcare Corporation).

Recurrent moderate hypoglycemia (hypoglycemic preconditioning). One week after catheter implantation, recurrent moderate hypoglycemia was induced in nonfasted rats with injections of subcutaneous regular human insulin (Lilly) (6 units/kg on day 1, 5 units/kg on day 2, and 4 units/kg on day 3), while CON rats were given equal-volume saline injections for 3 consecutive days. Food was withheld, and tail-vein blood glucose values were measured hourly. For insulin-treated rats, recurrent hypoglycemia resulted in blood glucose levels of 25–40 mg/dl for 3 h. To terminate moderate hypoglycemia, rats were given a subcutaneous injection of dextrose (Hospira) and were allowed free access to food.

Hyperinsulinemic-severe hypoglycemia clamp. Animals were fasted overnight after the third day of injections and the following morning were subjected to a hyperinsulinemic (0.2 units $\cdot$ kg^{-1} $\cdot$ min^{-1}) severe hypoglycemic clamp (Fig. 1). Rats were awake, unrestrained, and had free access to water. Arterial blood glucose was measured every 15 min with Ascensia Contour glucose monitors (Bayer HealthCare), which are reported to have accurate blood glucose readings in the hypoglycemia range, although accuracy in the severe hypoglycemia range has not been reported. Insulin and glucose were coinfused intravenously to lower blood glucose to 10–15 mg/dl, as this level of severe hypoglycemia was necessary to induce neuronal damage (3,18). Severe hypoglycemia (SH rats) was maintained between 10 and 15 mg/dl for either 60 min (CON-SH60, $n = 6$; RH-SH60, $n = 10$) or 90 min (CON-SH90, $n = 20$; RH-SH90, $n = 18$) for the CON and RH-treated rats, respectively. To terminate hypoglycemia, insulin infusion was stopped and infusions of dextrose were given until animals could maintain euglycemia. Additional blood samples were obtained during the basal period and 2 h into the hyperinsulinemic clamp when severe hypoglycemia had been reached for 30 min for epinephrine measurements, as determined by the single-isotope derivative method (19).

Tonic-clonic seizure-like behavior was visually noted by characteristic brief (5–10 s) neck extensions, tonic stretching, uncontrolled limb movements, and spontaneous spinning (18,20). The number of episodes of seizure-like behavior during the clamp was quantified for each rat and was later correlated with histological and cognitive findings.

Two other groups of rats were made either recurrently hypoglycemic or given saline injections as described above and, on the fourth day, underwent a 90-min hyperinsulinemic-euglycemic (0.2 units $\cdot$ kg^{-1} $\cdot$ min^{-1}) clamp (CON-euglycemic [EUG], $n = 9$; RH-EUG, $n = 11$). These two additional groups served as euglycemic control rats treated in the same fashion except that they were not exposed to severe hypoglycemia.

The first grouping of rats that underwent hyperinsulinemic severe hypoglycemic clamps or hyperinsulinemic-euglycemic clamps was analyzed for brain damage. The second grouping of rats was subjected to the same hyperinsulinemic clamp protocols except that they underwent sensorimotor and behavioral testing (Fig. 1).

Histology. One week after the severe hypoglycemic or euglycemic clamps, anesthetized rats were intracardially perfused with 0.01 mol/l PBS (Sigma) followed by 4% paraformaldehyde (Electron Microscopy Sciences, Hatfield, PA). Brains were immersed in 4% paraformaldehyde overnight and then cryoprotected in 30% sucrose. Beginning at 2.8 mm posterior to the bregma, coronal cryostat sections (20 μm) were collected on Superfrost coated slides (VWR). Four coronal sections, 120 μm apart, were analyzed for neuronal damage by Fluoro-Jade B (Chemicon International) and hematoxylin-eosin (H-E) (Sigma) staining according to the manufacturer's protocol. Fluoro-Jade B is a well-characterized stain for degenerating neurons (21). Fluorescent cells (Fluoro-Jade–positive cells) were quantified in both hemispheres of the cortex and of the hippocampal structures CA1 and dentate gyrus. For each region of interest, data are expressed as the average number of Fluoro-Jade B–positive (FJB$^+$) cells per section. (CON-SH90, $n = 9$; RH-SH90, $n = 8$).

Behavioral testing. Consistent with other protocol designs (4,22,23), histopathological outcomes were assessed 1 week following the hypoglycemic neuronal insult, while cognitive studies were performed 6–8 weeks later in a separate group of similarly treated rats. This later assessment of cognitive function is a more useful measure of clinical outcome and a better functional index of neuroprotection because it allows for a complete and integrated evaluation of ongoing damage and possible recovery (24). Because the Morris water maze test is a measure of hippocampal-dependent spatial learning/memory and because the rats that underwent 60 min of severe hypoglycemia had little damage in the hippocampus, cognitive testing was not performed in this group. Cognitive testing was performed in the rats that underwent 90 min of severe hypoglycemia because these animals had marked damage in the hippocampus. After a 6- to 8-week recovery from the severe hypoglycemic (CON-SH90, $n = 11$; RH-SH90, $n = 9$) and euglycemic (CON-EUG, $n = 7$; RH-EUG, $n = 9$) clamps, rats were transferred to the behavioral testing facility and allowed 1 week to acclimate before locomotor activity, sensorimotor measures, and Morris maze tests were performed under euglycemic conditions.

One-hour locomotor activity test and sensorimotor battery. General locomotor activity and exploratory behavior were evaluated for 1 h using a computerized system (MotorMonitor; Kinder Scientific) of photobeam pairs to quantify ambulations (whole body movements) and rearing frequency. As previously described (25), the ledge, platform, 90°-inclined screen, and walking initiation tests were conducted to measure balance, strength, coordination, and initiation of movement.

Water maze cognitive testing. Spatial learning and memory were assessed using the Morris water maze test similarly to previously published methods (25). Briefly, a computerized tracking program (Polytrack; San Diego Instruments) recorded the swim-path lengths and time required to find the platform. For the cued trials, rats were trained to swim to the submerged platform (1.5 cm below the surface) marked (cued) by a visible pole. Spatial learning capabilities of the rats were tested during the place trials. In the place trials, rats were trained to learn the position of a submerged and nonvisible platform that remained in the same location across all trials. To evaluate memory retention of the platform location, a probe trial was conducted 1 h after the last place trial, which involved removing the platform from the pool and

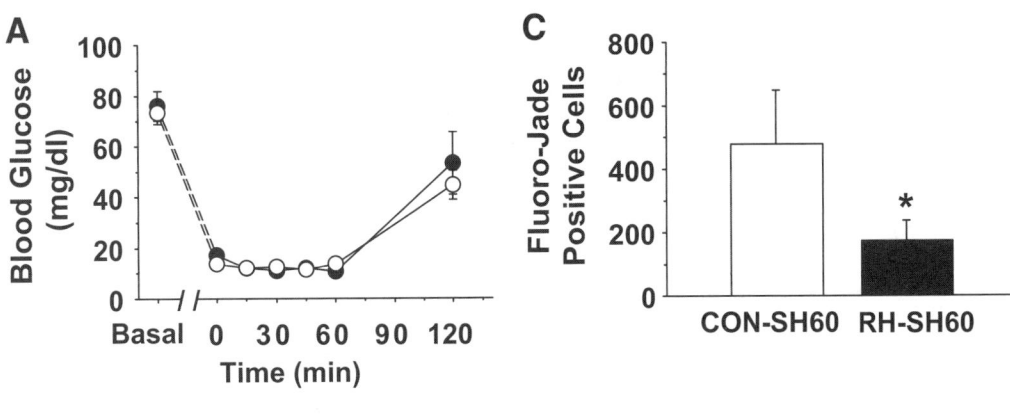

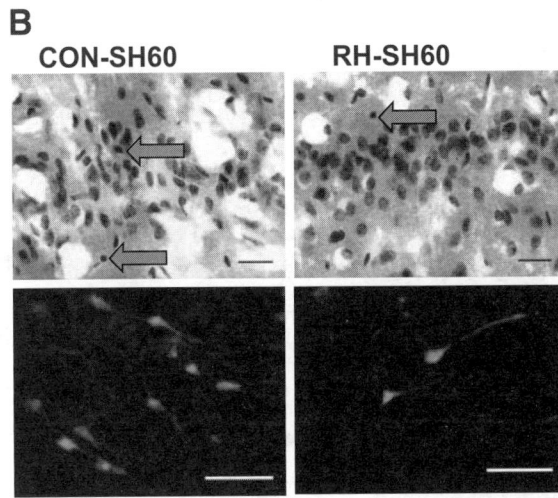

FIG. 2. Recurrent hypoglycemia attenuates brain damage after 60 min of severe hypoglycemia. *A*: Blood glucose levels are shown in rats subjected to a 60-min severe hypoglycemic (10–15 mg/dl) hyperinsulinemic (0.2 units · kg^{-1} · min^{-1}) clamp. Blood glucose was not significantly different between CON-SH6 (open circles) (*n* = 6) and RH-SH60 (closed circles) (*n* = 10) rats during 60 min of severe hypoglycemia. *B*: Representative H-E (*top panel*) and Fluoro-Jade B–positive (*bottom panel*) staining of the cortex of CON-SH60 and RH-SH60 rats 1 week following 60 min of severe hypoglycemia. Neuronal damage is indicated by pyknotic cells (H-E staining; green arrows) or with Fluoro-Jade B–positive cells (green fluorescence). Scale bar = 100 μm. *C*: Quantification of Fluoro-Jade B staining in CON-SH60 (white bar) (*n* = 6) and RH-SH60 (black bar) (*n* = 10) rats. Following severe hypoglycemia, RH rats had significantly fewer degenerating cells in the cortex than CON rats (*P < 0.05, by Student's *t* test). (A high-quality digital representation of this figure is available in the online issue.)

quantifying rats' search behaviors for 30 s. Probe trial performance indexes included the following: the number of times a rat passed directly over the platform location (platform crossings), the time spent in the target quadrant versus the time spent in each of the other pool quadrants (spatial bias), and average proximity (distance to the platform location sampled and averaged across 1-s epochs throughout the trial).

Statistical analysis. All data are expressed as means ± SEM. Statistical analyses were performed by either Student's *t* tests or ANOVA. Quantification of brain damage and behavioral assessments were made by investigators blinded to treatment conditions.

RESULTS

Recurrent hypoglycemia reduced cortical brain damage induced by 60 min of severe hypoglycemia. No significant differences in blood glucose were observed before, during, or after the 60-min severe hypoglycemic clamps between RH and CON rats (Fig. 2*A*). As expected, RH-SH60 rats had an attenuated epinephrine response to hypoglycemia compared with CON-SH60 rats (2001 ± 241 and 3,487 ± 474 pg/ml; *P* < 0.01) (supplementary Fig. 1, available in an online appendix at http://diabetes. diabetesjournals.org/cgi/content/full/db09-1495/DC1). Importantly, RH-SH60 rats had 64% less neuronal damage, as assessed by the number of FJB$^+$ cells, in the cortex than CON-SH60 rats (173 ± 64 vs. 479 ± 170 cells; *P* < 0.05) (Fig. 2*B* and *C*). Of note, 60 min of severe hypoglycemia did not induce significant damage in the hippocampus in either RH-SH60 or CON-SH60 rats.

Recurrent hypoglycemia attenuated cortical and hippocampal brain injury after 90 min of severe hypoglycemia. To consistently induce hypoglycemic brain damage in the hippocampus, the above experiments were

repeated except that the duration of severe hypoglycemia was extended to 90 min. The average blood glucose during 90 min of severe hypoglycemia was 10.9 ± 0.2 vs. 11.0 ± 0.3 mg/dl in the CON-SH90 and RH-SH90 rats, respectively (*P* = NS) (Fig. 3*C*). As an additional set of experimental controls, euglycemic-hyperinsulinemic clamps were also performed in RH-EUG (*n* = 2) or CON-EUG (*n* = 2) rats. Blood glucose was maintained at 76 ± 5 and 84 ± 6 mg/dl in the CON-EUG and RH-EUG rats, respectively (*P* = NS) (Fig. 3*C*).

Again validating the model of hypoglycemia-associated autonomic failure, RH reduced the epinephrine response to hypoglycemia (CON-SH90 3,175 ± 516 mg/dl and RH-SH90 2077 ± 426 pg/ml; *P* < 0.05) (supplementary Fig. 1). Severe hypoglycemia of 90 min induced significant cellular damage in the cortex, as evidenced by the presence of pyknotic cells observed with H-E staining (Fig. 3*A*) and the marked number of fluorescent cells with Fluoro-Jade B staining (Fig. 3*B*). Interestingly, 90 min of severe hypoglycemia induced sixfold-greater cortical neuronal damage than 60 min of severe hypoglycemia (Figs. 2*C* and 3*D*). Recurrent antecedent moderate hypoglycemia decreased cortical brain damage induced by 90 min of severe hypoglycemia by 62% (RH-SH90 1,107 ± 428 FJB$^+$ cells and CON-SH90 2,918 ± 615 FJB$^+$ cells; *P* < 0.05). Unlike 60 min of severe hypoglycemia, 90 min of severe hypoglycemia did induce hippocampal brain damage (Fig. 3). Recurrent antecedent hypoglycemia resulted in less hippocampal brain damage following 90 min of severe hypoglycemia compared with that in CON-SH90 rats (Fig. 3).

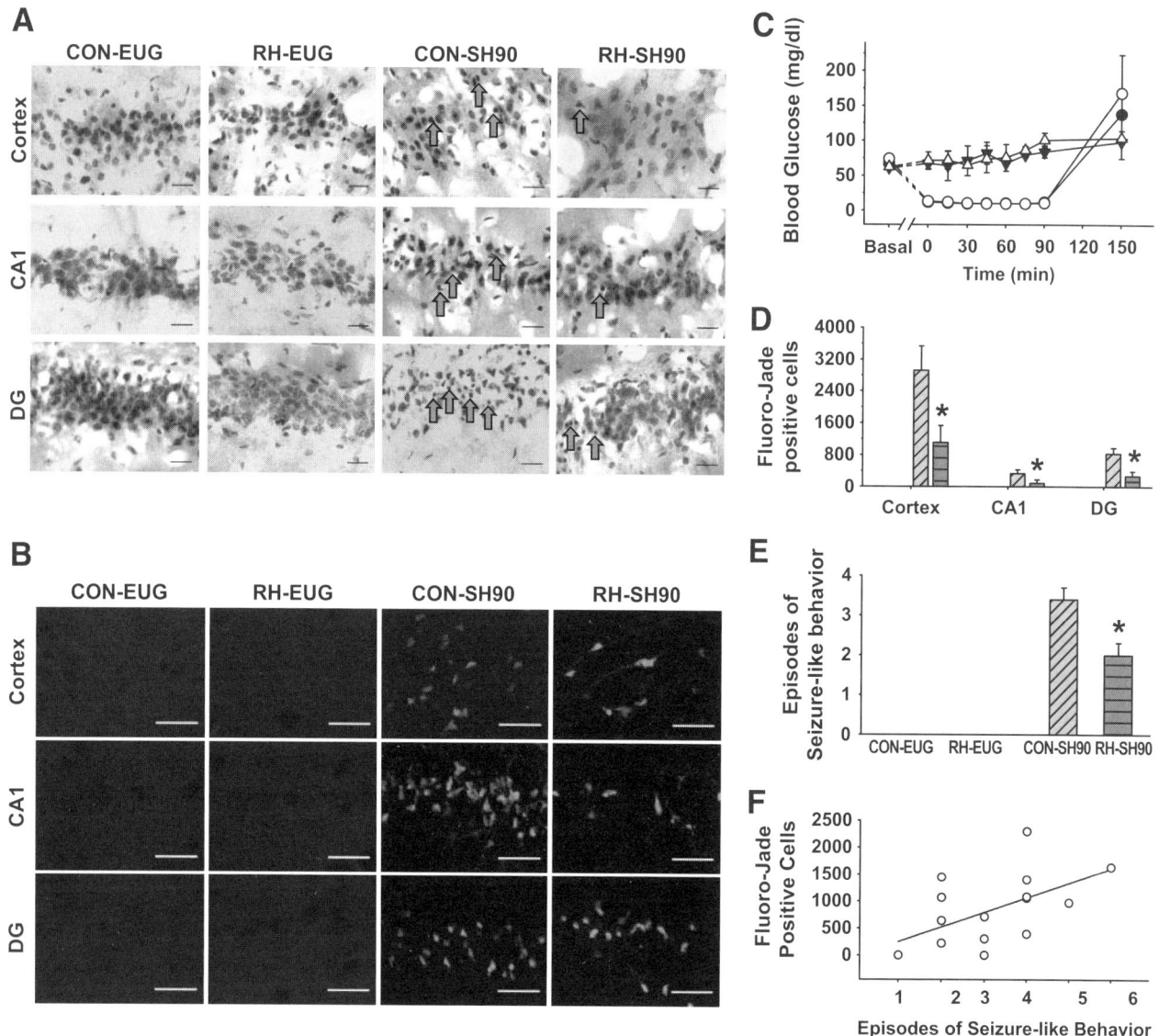

FIG. 3. Recurrent hypoglycemia limits brain cell death 1 week following 90 min of severe hypoglycemia. *A*: Representative H-E staining of the cortex and hippocampal structures, CA1, and the dentate gyrus (DG), 1 week following 90-min severe hypoglycemic or euglycemic clamps in RH-SH90, RH-EUG, CON-SH90, and CON-EUG rats. Rats that underwent severe hypoglycemia had damaged neurons characterized by pyknotic nuclei (green arrows). Scale bar = 100 μm. *B*: Fluoro-Jade B–positive cells (green fluorescence) in the cortex, hippocampal CA1 region, and dentate gyrus of the same four treatment groups. Scale bar = 100 μm. *C*: Blood glucose was not significantly different between CON-SH90 (open circles) (*n* = 9) and RH-SH90 (closed circles) (*n* = 8) rats during 90 min of severe hypoglycemia. Blood glucose was clamped at equal levels of euglycemia in CON-EUG (open triangles) (*n* = 9) and RH-EUG (closed triangles) (*n* = 11) rats for 90 min. *D*: Following 90 min of severe hypoglycemia, the markedly increased number of FJB$^+$ cells in the cortex, CA1, and dentate gyrus observed in the CON-SH90 rats (diagonal hatch) was significantly (*$P < 0.05$) reduced in RH-SH90 rats (gray horizontal hatch). Bars representing Fluoro-Jade B–positive cells in CON-EUG and RH-EUG groups are not visible in this figure because no appreciable brain damage was observed in euglycemic rats not exposed to severe hypoglycemia. *E*: CON-EUG and RH-EUG rats experienced no seizure-like behavior. Rats exposed to 90 min severe hypoglycemia exhibited seizure-like behavior, although RH-SH90 rats had significantly less seizure-like behavior than CON-SH90 rats (*$P < 0.01$). *F*: In rats that experienced severe hypoglycemia (RH-SH90 and CON-SH90), seizure-like behaviors positively correlated with the amount of Fluoro-Jade B cells in the hippocampus (*$R = 0.572$; $P < 0.05$*). (A high-quality digital representation of this figure is available in the online issue.)

Specifically, RH-SH90 rats had decreased FJB$^+$ cells in the CA1 region by 74% (RH-SH90 88 ± 56 cells vs. CON-SH90 334 ± 91 cells; $P < 0.05$) and by 67% in the dentate gyrus (RH-SH90 274 ± 119 cells vs. CON-SH90 833 ± 148 cells; $P < 0.05$) compared with CON-SH90 (Fig. 3*D*). No damage was observed in the hypothalamus in either CON-SH90 or RH-SH90 rats (supplementary Fig. 2).

Interestingly, recurrent hypoglycemia also reduced the episodes of seizure-like behavior observed during severe hypoglycemia (RH-SH90 2.0 ± 0.3 vs. CON-SH90 3.4 ± 0.3; $P < 0.01$) (Fig. 3*E*). There was a significant corre-

lation between the number of episodes of seizure-like behavior and number of FJB$^+$ cells ($R = 0.572$; $P < 0.05$) (Fig. 3*F*).

In the absence of severe hypoglycemia, virtually no Fluoro-Jade–positive cells or pyknotic cells (H-E) were observed in the cortex or hippocampus of either the CON-EUG or RH-EUG groups (Fig. 3).

Preserved cognitive function in recurrently hypoglycemic rats. General activity was not different between groups (supplementary Fig. 3). The severe hypoglycemic groups (both CON-SH90 and RH-SH90) exhibited signifi-

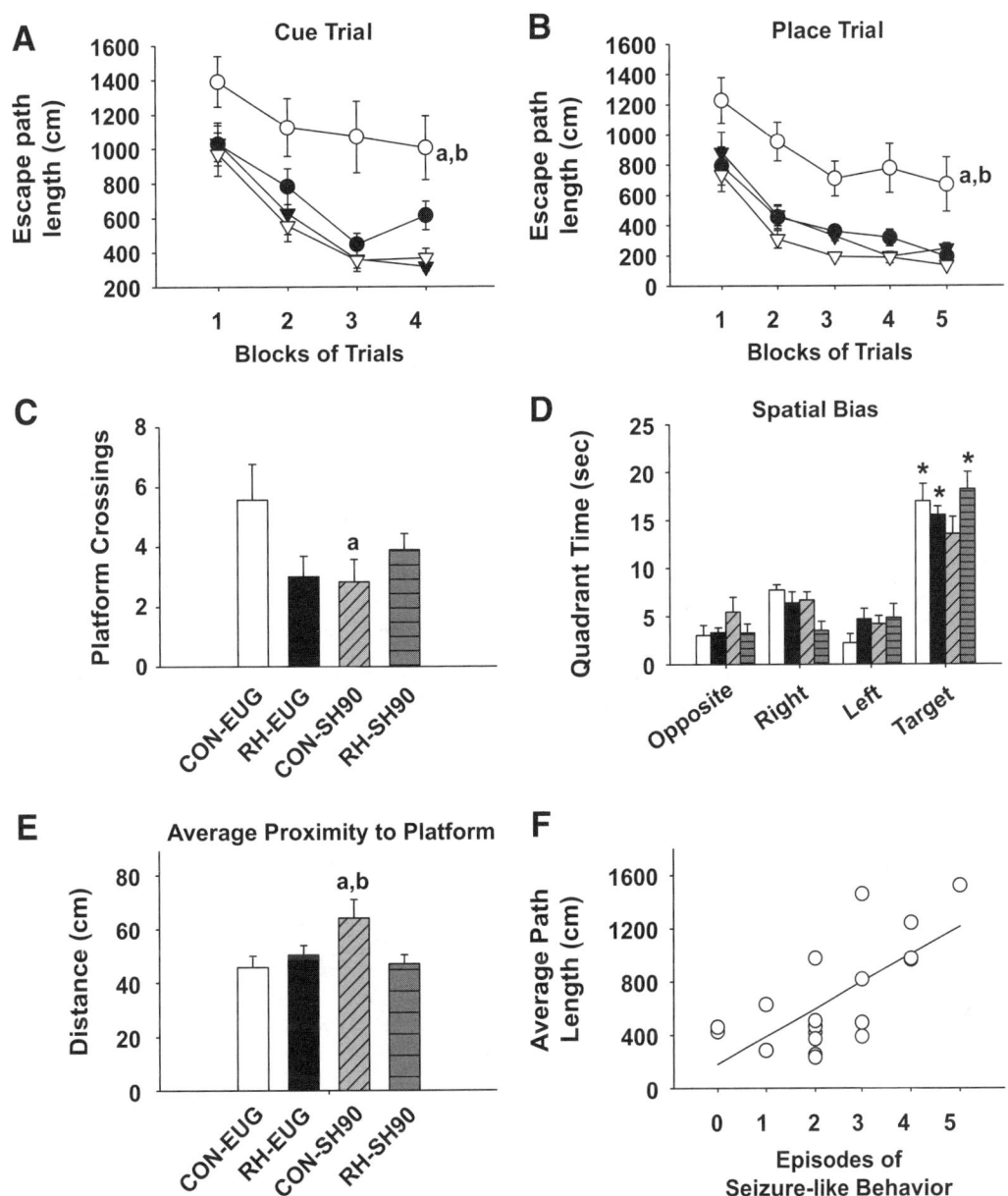

FIG. 4. Antecedent recurrent hypoglycemia mitigated cognitive dysfunction induced by severe hypoglycemia. Morris water maze testing was performed 6–8 weeks following severe hypoglycemic or euglycemic clamps. *A*: During the cue trial, CON-SH90 rats (open circles) (*n* = 11) performed worse as evidenced by longer escape-path lengths than those of CON-EUG rats (open triangles) (*n* = 7) ([a]*P* = 0.002). Notably, rats exposed to recurrent moderate hypoglycemia before severe hypoglycemia (RH-SH90, *n* = 9 (closed circles) had shorter escape-path lengths than CON-SH90 rats ([b]*P* = 0.0025) and performed similarly to CON-EUG and RH-EUG rats (closed triangles) (*n* = 9). *B*: A similar pattern was observed during the place trials, where CON-SH90 rats had significantly higher escape-path lengths than CON-EUG ([c]*P* = 0.0001) and RH-SH90 ([d]*P* = 0.0006) rats. *C*: During the probe trial, CON-SH90 rats (diagonal hatch) had significantly fewer platform crossings than CON-EUG rats (white bar) ([e]*P* = 0.014). No significant differences were observed between CON-SH90 and RH-SH90 rats (gray horizontal hatch) or between CON-EUG and RH-EUG rats (black bar). *D*: RH-SH90, CON-EUG, and RH-EUG rats had a spatial bias toward the target quadrant while CON-SH90 rats did not (*P < 0.0025). *E*: During the probe trial, CON-SH90 rats showed an average proximity to the platform location that was significantly farther away than that of the CON-EUG rats ([f]*P* = 0.014). RH-SH90 rats swam significantly closer to the platform location than CON-SH90 rats ([g]*P* = 0.014)—similar to euglycemic controls. *F*: The number of episodes of seizure-like behaviors observed during severe hypoglycemia 6–8 weeks prior positively correlated with average path length during the place trials (*R* = 0.685; *P* < 0.001; *n* = 20).

cantly (*P* = 0.02) more rearings than the two groups of EUG rats (supplementary Fig. 3*B*). Data from the walking initiation, ledge, platform, and 90°-inclined screen were not significantly different between groups (supplementary Fig. 3*C–F*).

During the cue (Fig. 4*A*) and place (Fig. 4*B*) trials, the CON-SH90 rats performed worse than the other three groups in spite of having normal swimming speeds (sup-

plementary Fig. 4). In the cue trials, CON-SH90 rats had significantly longer path lengths across the blocks of trials than the CON-EUG rats (*P* = 0.0002). Importantly, RH-SH90 rats had significantly shorter path lengths relative to the CON-SH90 rats (*P* = 0.0025), while no differences were observed between RH-SH90 and CON-EUG or between the two EUG control groups.

During the place (spatial learning) trials, the CON-SH90

rats again showed significant performance deficits. CON-SH90 rats had significantly ($P = 0.0001$) longer path lengths across the blocks of trials than the CON-EUG rats (Fig. 4B). Notably, RH-SH90 rats had significantly shorter path lengths than CON-SH90 rats ($P = 0.0006$) (Fig. 4B). Again, no differences were observed between RH-SH90 and CON-EUG rats or between the two euglycemic groups.

During the probe trial, CON-SH90 rats made significantly fewer platform crossings relative to the CON-EUG rats ($P = 0.014$), though no differences in platform crossings between CON-SH90 and RH-SH90 rats were observed (Fig. 4C). However, with regard to spatial bias and average proximity to the platform location, RH-SH90 rats did have improved performance compared with CON-SH90 rats. In spatial bias analysis, RH-SH90, CON-EUG, and RH-EUG rats all exhibited spatial bias for the target quadrant; each group spent significantly more time in the target quadrant compared with the other pool quadrants ($P < 0.0025$). CON-SH90 rats did not show significant spatial bias (Fig. 4D). Further, CON-SH90 rats had significantly higher average proximity scores than CON-EUG ($P = 0.014$) and RH-SH90 ($P = 0.014$) rats. RH-SH90 rats performed similarly to CON-EUG rats (Fig. 4E). In summary, during the probe trial, severe hypoglycemia (CON-SH90 rats) significantly impaired all three tests of memory retention, and antecedent recurrent moderate hypoglycemia pretreatment (RH-SH90 rats) significantly improved memory performance on two out of three measures.

Interestingly, the number of episodes of seizure-like behavior during severe hypoglycemia positively correlated with performance during Morris water maze testing (Fig. 3F). Specifically, increases in the number of episodes of seizure-like behavior were associated with longer average path lengths ($R = 0.685$; $P < 0.001$) (Fig. 3F).

DISCUSSION

Given that severe hypoglycemia affects 40% of insulin-treated people with diabetes (26), concern regarding the hazardous potential for severe hypoglycemia to cause "brain damage" continues to be a very real barrier for realizing the full benefits of intensive glycemic control (27). Patients with the highest incidence of severe hypoglycemia are most often those who maintain intensive glycemic control and, hence, are likely to have had recurrent bouts of moderate hypoglycemia. In this study, recurrent moderate hypoglycemia preconditioned the brain and protected it against brain damage and cognitive dysfunction induced by severe hypoglycemia.

In these experiments, severe hypoglycemic brain injury was consistently induced with hyperinsulinemic-hypoglycemic (<15 mg/dl) clamps that carefully controlled the depth and duration of severe hypoglycemia and avoided the confounding effects of anesthesia (28–31). The amount and distribution of neuronal damage was markedly different between the 60- and 90-min clamp studies (Figs. 2 and 4). In spite of similar degrees of hypoglycemia (10–15 mg/dl), the extra 30 min of severe hypoglycemia induced a sixfold increase in cortical brain damage and markedly increased hippocampal brain damage (which was minimal in the 60-min clamp). These findings emphasize the importance of the duration of severe hypoglycemia, and not hypoglycemic nadir alone, as a critically important component in determining the extent of brain damage and cognitive dysfunction (22). Of note, the lack of brain-damaged cells in the euglycemic controls indicated that

experimental conditions other than severe hypoglycemia (i.e., catheter implantation surgery, recurrent moderate hypoglycemia, hyperinsulinemic clamp, and glucose infusion) did not cause significant brain damage.

The most notable findings were that rats exposed to 3 days of recurrent moderate hypoglycemia had less brain injury associated with severe hypoglycemia in both the cortex and hippocampus. Thus, as with ischemic preconditioning (17), hypoglycemic preconditioning attenuated brain damage by 62–74%. Although hypoglycemia-induced neuronal damage in the hypothalamus has been noted (32), other studies (33) as well as this study observed no severe hypoglycemia-induced neuronal injury in the hypothalamus.

In spite of the marked degree of cortical neuronal damage induced by severe hypoglycemia, the rats had no meaningful deficit in sensorimotor function as measured by the locomotor activity and sensorimotor tests. Further supporting the absence of gross motor deficits following severe hypoglycemia was the observation of no differences between groups in swimming speeds (supplementary Fig. 4). Importantly, rats exposed to severe hypoglycemia showed no signs of sensorimotor impairments that could have affected interpretation of cognitive function as measured during the Morris water maze.

Cognitive assessment with water maze testing documented severe cognitive performance deficits induced by severe hypoglycemia, and these impairments were prevented by antecedent recurrent moderate hypoglycemia. Specifically, analysis of the escape path–length data showed that severe hypoglycemia significantly impaired performance relative to that of euglycemic controls during both the cued and place trials and that recurrent hypoglycemia completely prevented the impaired performance induced by severe hypoglycemia (Fig. 4). For the probe trial, three measures of memory performance were evaluated: platform crossings, spatial bias toward the target quadrant, and average proximity (Fig. 4). Severe hypoglycemia again induced significant memory impairment in all three measures. Antecedent recurrent hypoglycemia prevented these impairments in two of those measures (spatial bias and average proximity). Regarding platform crossings, recurrent hypoglycemia tended to improve performance but not significantly (RH-SH90 vs. CON-SH90 rats), indicating that recurrent hypoglycemia was unable to completely reverse the retention deficits concerning the exact location of the platform. However, analysis of the spatial bias and average proximity data demonstrated that recurrent hypoglycemia did preserve retention of a more general platform location. Specifically, RH-SH90 rats exhibited a spatial bias for the target quadrant, whereas CON-SH90 rats did not, and CON-SH90 rats had an average proximity that was farther away from the platform location than RH-SH90 rats and the euglycemic controls. These findings indicate that memory retention was impaired as a result of severe hypoglycemia relative to euglycemic controls in all probe trial variables and that recurrent hypoglycemia prevented severe hypoglycemia–induced impairments in two of three probe trial indexes.

Consistent with the notion that recurrent hypoglycemia induces an adaptive brain response is the observation that RH-SH90 rats had less seizure-like behavior during severe hypoglycemia (Fig. 3E), suggesting that the RH-treated brain better tolerated severe hypoglycemia. A novel finding of this study is that the number of episodes of seizure-like behavior observed during severe hypoglycemia also correlated with cognitive performance (Fig. 4F). As in the real-world setting, witnessed hypoglycemic seizures were defined clinically. In the absence of electroencephalogram monitoring, the effect of subclinical seizures (i.e., seizures not associated with noticeable motor activity) on brain damage and cognition could not be assessed. Nonetheless, in these experimental conditions, observable instances of seizure-like behavior correlated with the extent of neuronal damage and long-term cognitive function, and while not causative, the number of seizures during hypoglycemia was a marker for the extent of neuronal injury and was prognostic of long-term cognitive outcomes. Indeed, clinical studies support these findings because the presence of hypoglycemic seizures, even more than severe hypoglycemia per se, correlate more closely with impaired cognitive function (10,12).

Independent of episodes of severe hypoglycemia, previous studies have shown that recurrent moderate hypoglycemia can alter cognitive function. Recurrent moderate hypoglycemia did not cause neuronal damage in the hippocampus (as confirmed in this study) but has been shown to impair hippocampal long-term potentiation, a cellular mechanism believed to be involved in learning and memory (34). Conversely, recurrent hypoglycemia improved cognitive ability in rats tested in an euglycemic state (35,36). In the current study, recurrent moderate hypoglycemia-treated control rats not exposed to severe hypoglycemia did not have impaired or improved cognitive ability during Morris water maze testing. Since 2–3 weeks of scrupulous avoidance of hypoglycemia reverses the hypoglycemia unawareness associated with recurrent hypoglycemia (37,38), it is presumed that any effect of antecedent recurrent hypoglycemia on cognition may have dissipated during the 6–8 weeks' recovery prior to cognitive testing.

Although recurrent moderate hypoglycemia leads to maladaptive responses resulting in hypoglycemia unawareness and hypoglycemia-associated autonomic failure, the mechanism(s) by which recurrent hypoglycemia leads to these adaptations remains elusive. Similarly, the current experiments do not identify the mechanisms by which recurrent moderate hypoglycemia *1)* protected against severe hypoglycemia–induced neuronal damage, *2)* limited severe hypoglycemia–induced neurocognitive dysfunction, or *3)* increased thresholds for hypoglycemic seizures. Putative mechanisms for these beneficial adaptations could include glycogen supercompensation (increased brain glycogen content above prehypoglycemic levels) (39–43). By keeping a higher level of stored fuel units, increased brain glycogen content has been shown to reduce hypoglycemic neuronal injury by maintaining brain electrical activity and forestalling electroencephalogram isoelectricity (44). Enhanced nutrient transport may also contribute to the neuroprotective effects of recurrent hypoglycemia (45,46). Monocarboxylate acid transport is increased during hypoglycemia in patients with well-controlled type 1 diabetes (45,46). Increased transport of monocarboxylate acids (e.g., lactate) could provide an alternative energy source that maintains neuronal function (4). Other possibilities that could account for the observed neuroprotective effect of recurrent hypoglycemia could be altered brain metabolism or neuronal activity (39,47–49). Recurrent hypoglycemia enhances the inhibitory neurotransmitter, γ-aminobutyric acid, which could reduce neuronal activity and limit excitotoxic damage (48). Further

studies on the precise mechanisms of how recurrent hypoglycemia exerts its neuroprotective effects are warranted.

These studies demonstrate that recurrent moderate hypoglycemia preconditions and protects the brain against severe hypoglycemia–induced neuronal damage and its associated cognitive deficits. These intriguing findings suggest that recurrent bouts of moderate hypoglycemia that occur with intensive glycemic control might, paradoxically, render an individual more prone but less vulnerable to an episode of severe hypoglycemia. If the current data indicating a neuroprotective preconditioning effect of recurrent moderate hypoglycemia were to be extrapolated to the clinical setting, it could explain the apparent divergent findings between animal and clinical studies and may also explain the seemingly incongruous clinical findings that intensively treated patients who experience recurrent moderate and severe hypoglycemia may be paradoxically protected from severe hypoglycemia–induced brain damage and may not suffer from associated long-term cognitive damage (13,50).

ACKNOWLEDGMENTS

Research support from the National Institutes of Health (DK073683) and the Juvenile Diabetes Research Foundation (CDA 2-2004-541) and core grant support from Washington University's Diabetes Research and Training Center (DK020579), Clinical Nutrition Research Unit (DK056341), and Neuroscience Blueprint Center (NS057105) are gratefully acknowledged.

No potential conflicts of interest relevant to this article were reported.

Parts of this study were presented in abstract form at the 68th Scientific Sessions of the American Diabetes Association, San Francisco, California, 6–10 June 2008.

The authors thank the laboratory of Dr. P. Cryer for performing the catecholamine determinations and Dr. K. Yamada for assistance with Fluoro-Jade staining.

REFERENCES

1. Cryer PE. Diverse causes of hypoglycemia-associated autonomic failure in diabetes. *N Engl J Med* 2004;350:2272–2279
2. The Diabetes Control and Complications Trial Research Group. Hypoglycemia in the Diabetes Control and Complications Trial. Diabetes 1997;46: 271–286
3. Auer RN. Hypoglycemic brain damage. Metab Brain Dis 2004;19:169–175
4. Suh SW, Aoyama K, Matsumori Y, Liu J, Swanson RA. Pyruvate administered after severe hypoglycemia reduces neuronal death and cognitive impairment. Diabetes 2005;54:1452–1458
5. Northam EA, Rankins D, Lin A, Wellard RM, Pell GS, Finch SJ, Werther GA, Cameron FJ. Central nervous system function in youth with type 1 diabetes 12 years after disease onset. Diabetes Care 2009;32:445–450
6. Perantie DC, Wu J, Koller JM, Lim A, Warren SL, Black KJ, Sadler M, White NH, Hershey T. Regional brain volume differences associated with hyperglycemia and severe hypoglycemia in youth with type 1 diabetes. Diabetes Care 2007;30:2331–2337
7. Musen G, Lyoo IK, Sparks CR, Weinger K, Hwang J, Ryan CM, Jimerson DC, Hennen J, Renshaw PF, Jacobson AM. Effects of type 1 diabetes on gray matter density as measured by voxel-based morphometry. Diabetes 2006;55:326–333
8. Bjørgaas M, Gimse R, Vik T, Sand T. Cognitive function in type 1 diabetic children with and without episodes of severe hypoglycaemia. Acta Paediatr 1997;86:148–153
9. Hershey T, Lillie R, Sadler M, White NH. Severe hypoglycemia and long-term spatial memory in children with type 1 diabetes mellitus: a retrospective study. J Int Neuropsychol Soc 2003;9:740–750
10. Kaufman FR, Epport K, Engilman R, Halvorson M. Neurocognitive functioning in children diagnosed with diabetes before age 10 years. J Diabetes Complications 1999;13:31–38
11. Langan SJ, Deary IJ, Hepburn DA, Frier BM. Cumulative cognitive impair-

ment following recurrent severe hypoglycaemia in adult patients with insulin-treated diabetes mellitus. Diabetologia 1991;34:337–344

12. Rovet JF, Ehrlich RM. The effect of hypoglycemic seizures on cognitive function in children with diabetes: a 7-year prospective study. J Pediatr 1999;134:503–506

13. Jacobson AM, Musen G, Ryan CM, Silvers N, Cleary P, Waberski B, Burwood A, Weinger K, Bayless M, Dahms W, Harth J. Long-term effect of diabetes and its treatment on cognitive function. N Engl J Med 2007;356: 1842–1852

14. Kramer L, Fasching P, Madl C, Schneider B, Damjancic P, Waldhausl W, Irsigler K, Grimm G. Previous episodes of hypoglycemic coma are not associated with permanent cognitive brain dysfunction in IDDM patients on intensive insulin treatment. Diabetes 1998;47:1909–1914

15. Strudwick SK, Carne C, Gardiner J, Foster JK, Davis EA, Jones TW. Cognitive functioning in children with early onset type 1 diabetes and severe hypoglycemia. J Pediatr 2005;147:680–685

16. Wysocki T, Harris MA, Mauras N, Fox L, Taylor A, Jackson SC, White NH. Absence of adverse effects of severe hypoglycemia on cognitive function in school-aged children with diabetes over 18 months. Diabetes Care 2003; 26:1100–1105

17. Gidday JM. Cerebral preconditioning and ischaemic tolerance. Nat Rev Neurosci 2006;7:437–448

18. Bree AJ, Puente EC, Daphna-Iken D, Fisher SJ. Diabetes increases brain damage caused by severe hypoglycemia. Am J Physiol Endocrinol Metab 2009;297:E194–E201

19. Shah SD, Clutter WE, Cryer PE. External and internal standards in the single-isotope derivative (radioenzymatic) measurement of plasma norepinephrine and epinephrine. J Lab Clin Med 1985;106:624–629

20. Del Campo M, Abdelmalik PA, Wu CP, Carlen PL, Zhang L. Seizure-like activity in the hypoglycemic rat: lack of correlation with the electroencephalogram of free-moving animals. Epilepsy Res 2009;83:243–248

21. Schmued LC, Hopkins KJ. Fluoro-Jade B: a high affinity fluorescent marker for the localization of neuronal degeneration. Brain Res 2000;874:123–130

22. Suh SW, Aoyama K, Chen Y, Garnier P, Matsumori Y, Gum E, Liu J, Swanson RA. Hypoglycemic neuronal death and cognitive impairment are prevented by poly(ADP-ribose) polymerase inhibitors administered after hypoglycemia. J Neurosci 2003;23:10681–10690

23. Suh SW, Gum ET, Hamby AM, Chan PH, Swanson RA. Hypoglycemic neuronal death is triggered by glucose reperfusion and activation of neuronal NADPH oxidase. J Clin Invest 2007;117:910–918

24. Corbett D, Nurse S. The problem of assessing effective neuroprotection in experimental cerebral ischemia. Prog Neurobiol 1998;54:531–548

25. Wong M, Wozniak DF, Yamada KA. An animal model of generalized nonconvulsive status epilepticus: immediate characteristics and long-term effects. Exp Neurol 2003;183:87–99

26. ter Braak EW, Appelman AM, van de LM, Stolk RP, van Haeften TW, Erkelens DW. Clinical characteristics of type 1 diabetic patients with and without severe hypoglycemia. Diabetes Care 2000;23:1467–1471

27. Cox DJ, Irvine A, Gonder-Frederick L, Nowacek G, Butterfield J. Fear of hypoglycemia: quantification, validation, and utilization. Diabetes Care 1987;10:617–621

28. Alkire MT, Pomfrett CJ, Haier RJ, Gianzero MV, Chan CM, Jacobsen BP, Fallon JH. Functional brain imaging during anesthesia in humans: effects of halothane on global and regional cerebral glucose metabolism. Anesthesiology 1999;90:701–709

29. Canabal DD, Potian JG, Duran RG, McArdle JJ, Routh VH. Hyperglycemia impairs glucose and insulin regulation of nitric oxide production in glucose-inhibited neurons in the ventromedial hypothalamus. Am J Physiol Regul Integr Comp Physiol 2007;293:R592–R600

30. Jeong YB, Kim JS, Jeong SM, Park JW, Choi IC. Comparison of the effects of sevoflurane and propofol anaesthesia on regional cerebral glucose metabolism in humans using positron emission tomography. J Int Med Res 2006;34:374–384

31. Nakao Y, Itoh Y, Kuang TY, Cook M, Jehle J, Sokoloff L. Effects of

32. Tkacs NC, Pan Y, Raghupathi R, Dunn-Meynell AA, Levin BE. Cortical Fluoro-Jade staining and blunted adrenomedullary response to hypoglycemia after noncoma hypoglycemia in rats. J Cereb Blood Flow Metab 2005;25:1645–1655

33. Tkacs NC, Dunn-Meynell AA, Levin BE. Presumed apoptosis and reduced arcuate nucleus neuropeptide Y and pro-opiomelanocortin mRNA in non-coma hypoglycemia. Diabetes 2000;49:820–826

34. Yamada KA, Rensing N, Izumi Y, De Erausquin GA, Gazit V, Dorsey DA, Herrera DG. Repetitive hypoglycemia in young rats impairs hippocampal long-term potentiation. Pediatr Res 2004;55:372–379

35. McNay EC, Sherwin RS. Effect of recurrent hypoglycemia on spatial cognition and cognitive metabolism in normal and diabetic rats. Diabetes 2004;53:418–425

36. McNay EC, Williamson A, McCrimmon RJ, Sherwin RS. Cognitive and neural hippocampal effects of long-term moderate recurrent hypoglycemia. Diabetes 2006;55:1088–1095

37. Dagogo-Jack S, Rattarasarn C, Cryer PE. Reversal of hypoglycemia unawareness, but not defective glucose counterregulation, in IDDM. Diabetes 1994;43:1426–1434

38. Fanelli CG, Epifano L, Rambotti AM, Pampanelli S, Di Vincenzo A, Modarelli F, Lepore M, Annibale B, Ciofetta M, Bottini P. Meticulous prevention of hypoglycemia normalizes the glycemic thresholds and magnitude of most of neuroendocrine responses to, symptoms of, and cognitive function during hypoglycemia in intensively treated patients with short-term IDDM. Diabetes 1993;42:1683–1689

39. Alquier T, Kawashima J, Tsuji Y, Kahn BB. Role of hypothalamic adenosine 5'-monophosphate-activated protein kinase in the impaired counterregulatory response induced by repetitive neuroglucopenia. Endocrinology 2007;148:1367–1375

40. Brown AM, Sickmann HM, Fosgerau K, Lund TM, Schousboe A, Waagepetersen HS, Ransom BR. Astrocyte glycogen metabolism is required for neural activity during aglycemia or intense stimulation in mouse white matter. J Neurosci Res 2005;79:74–80

41. Brucklacher RM, Vannucci RC, Vannucci SJ. Hypoxic preconditioning increases brain glycogen and delays energy depletion from hypoxiaischemia in the immature rat. Dev Neurosci 2002;24:411–417

42. Choi IY, Seaquist ER, Gruetter R. Effect of hypoglycemia on brain glycogen metabolism in vivo. J Neurosci Res 2003;72:25–32

43. Wender R, Brown AM, Fern R, Swanson RA, Farrell K, Ransom BR. Astrocytic glycogen influences axon function and survival during glucose deprivation in central white matter. J Neurosci 2000;20:6804–6810

44. Suh SW, Hamby AM, Swanson RA. Hypoglycemia, brain energetics, and hypoglycemic neuronal death. Glia 2007;55:1280–1286

45. Boyle PJ, Kempers SF, O'Connor AM, Nagy RJ. Brain glucose uptake and unawareness of hypoglycemia in patients with insulin-dependent diabetes mellitus. N Engl J Med 1995;333:1726–1731

46. Mason GF, Petersen KF, Levon V, Rothman DL, Shulman GI. Increased brain monocarboxylic acid transport and utilization in type 1 diabetes. Diabetes 2006;55:929–934

47. Chan O, Lawson M, Zhu W, Beverly JL, Sherwin RS. ATP-sensitive K(+) channels regulate the release of GABA in the ventromedial hypothalamus during hypoglycemia. Diabetes 2007;56:1120–1126

48. Chan O, Cheng H, Herzog R, Czyzyk D, Zhu W, Wang A, McCrimmon RJ, Seashore MR, Sherwin RS. Increased GABAergic tone in the ventromedial hypothalamus contributes to suppression of counterregulatory responses after antecedent hypoglycemia. Diabetes 2008;57:1363–1370

49. Dunn-Meynell AA, Routh VH, Kang L, Gaspers L, Levin BE. Glucokinase is the likely mediator of glucosensing in both glucose-excited and glucoseinhibited central neurons. Diabetes 2002;51:2056–2065

50. Amiel SA. Hypoglycaemia in diabetes mellitus–protecting the brain. Diabetologia 1997;40(Suppl. 2):S62–S68

anesthesia on functional activation of cerebral blood flow and metabolism. Proc Natl Acad Sci U S A 2001;98:7593–7598

Insulin Pump Therapy With Automated Insulin Suspension in Response to Hypoglycemia

Reduction in nocturnal hypoglycemia in those at greatest risk

PRATIK CHOUDHARY, MD[1]
JOHN SHIN, PHD[2]
YONGYIN WANG, PHD[2]
MARK L. EVANS, MD[3]
PETER J. HAMMOND, FRCP[4]

DAVID KERR, FRCPE[5]
JAMES A.M. SHAW, PHD[6]
JOHN C. PICKUP, FRCPATH[1]
STEPHANIE A. AMIEL, FRCP[1]

OBJECTIVE—To evaluate a sensor-augmented insulin pump with a low glucose suspend (LGS) feature that automatically suspends basal insulin delivery for up to 2 h in response to sensor-detected hypoglycemia.

RESEARCH DESIGN AND METHODS—The LGS feature of the Paradigm Veo insulin pump (Medtronic, Inc., Northridge, CA) was tested for 3 weeks in 31 adults with type 1 diabetes.

RESULTS—There were 166 episodes of LGS: 66% of daytime LGS episodes were terminated within 10 min, and 20 episodes lasted the maximum 2 h. LGS use was associated with reduced nocturnal duration ≤2.2 mmol/L in those in the highest quartile of nocturnal hypoglycemia at baseline (median 46.2 vs. 1.8 min/day, P = 0.02 [LGS-OFF vs. LGS-ON]). Median sensor glucose was 3.9 mmol/L after 2-h LGS and 8.2 mmol/L at 2 h after basal restart.

CONCLUSIONS—Use of an insulin pump with LGS was associated with reduced nocturnal hypoglycemia in those at greatest risk and was well accepted by patients.

Diabetes Care 34:2023–2025, 2011

Continuous glucose monitoring (CGM) can reduce HbA$_{1c}$ in type 1 diabetes (1–3). Despite the use of hypoglycemia alarms, most studies have not demonstrated a significant reduction in hypoglycemia, and prolonged nocturnal hypoglycemia occurs frequently (4). This may be because patients sleep through many of the alarms (5) and insulin delivery continues during hypoglycemia.

We report a user evaluation of the Paradigm Veo insulin pump (Medtronic, Inc., Northridge, CA), which can automatically suspend basal insulin delivery for up to 2 h in the event of CGM-detected hypoglycemia, thus reducing the duration of hypoglycemia.

RESEARCH DESIGN AND METHODS

—The Veo was evaluated by 31 patients (10 men) with type 1 diabetes (mean age, 41.9 ± 10.6 years) from six U.K. centers. Regional ethics committees approved the study, and patients provided informed consent. The Veo system has alarms for hypoglycemia, predicted hypoglycemia, rate-of-change of glucose, and, uniquely, a low glucose suspend (LGS) feature that is activated when sensor glucose reaches a glucose threshold set by the user. An alarm sounds, and if the user does not respond, basal insulin delivery is suspended for a maximum of 2 h, after which basal insulin delivery is resumed at the programmed rate. The patient may resume basal insulin delivery at any point.

During a 2-week run-in, CGM was used with only predictive, rate-of-change, high and low alerts active (LGS-OFF). LGS was then activated for 3 weeks (LGS-ON). We evaluated the response to LGS and compared hypoglycemia exposure and mean blood glucose during LGS-OFF and LGS-ON. Patients were divided into four equal groups (quartiles) by the duration of hypoglycemia during the run-in period, because we wished to test the hypothesis that those with the most hypoglycemia at baseline (without LGS) would have the greatest benefit with LGS. Hypoglycemia was defined as the lower limit of detection of the sensor (2.2 mmol/L) (6). The glucose threshold to trigger LGS was individualized (median 2.4 [range 2.2–3.5] mmol/L). Night was defined as 0000–0800 h. Treatment satisfaction questionnaires were completed at study end.

Data were compared using the Student *t* test, except for skewed data (hypoglycemia duration), which were compared with the Wilcoxon test. Values are mean ± SD or median (range).

RESULTS—Two subjects withdrew during run-in due to difficulties using sensors, and one subject failed to activate the LGS. There were 166 LGS episodes in 25 of 28 (89%) completers (mean 1.9 LGS events/week), of which 76% occurred during daytime, and 55% were terminated within 10 min. LGS continued for the maximum 2 h in 20 episodes (12%), 75% of which were nocturnal. Of 20 completed 2-h suspends, 7 (35%) had no patient response throughout. In the remaining 13 (65%), patients responded to the alarm but elected to continue LGS for 2 h. Mean response time to the LGS alarm was longer at night compared with day (63.2 ± 8.2 vs. 17.4 ± 2.7 min, P < 0.001).

From the ¹Department of Diabetes, King's College London School of Medicine, London, U.K.; ²Medtronic, Inc., Northridge, California; the ³Institute of Metabolic Science, Addenbrooke's Hospital, University of Cambridge, Cambridge, U.K.; the ⁴Harrogate District Hospital, Harrogate, U.K.; the ⁵Bournemouth Diabetes and Endocrine Centre, Bournemouth District General Hospital, Bournemouth, U.K.; and the ⁶Institute of Cellular Medicine, Newcastle University, Newcastle upon Tyne, U.K.
Corresponding author: Pratik Choudhary, pratik.choudhary@kcl.ac.uk.
Received 6 January 2011 and accepted 13 May 2011.
DOI: 10.2337/dc10-2411. Clinical trial reg. no. NCT01267175, clinicaltrials.gov.
See accompanying editorial, p. 2136.

LGS use was associated with significant reduction in the duration of nocturnal hypoglycemia (≤2.2 mmol/L) in those in the highest quartile of hypoglycemia duration at baseline: median 46.2 (36.6–191.4) vs. 1.8 (0.0–45) min/day ($P = 0.02$; LGS-OFF vs. LGS-ON) (Fig. 1) and mean 75.1 ± 54 vs. 10.2 ± 18 min/day ($P = 0.02$). Mean sensor glucose was not different with LGS-OFF or LGS-ON (6.4 ± 1.3 vs. 6.6 ± 1.1 mmol/L, $P = 0.26$). After the 20 complete 2-h LGS episodes, median sensor glucose was 3.9 (2.4–14.2) mmol/L at the restart of basal insulin and was 8.2 (3.3–17.3) mmol/L 2 h after restart. Carbohydrate ingestion was not recorded.

Concomitant (within 15 min of LGS) capillary glucose values were available for 43 of 166 episodes (25.9%) of LGS. These were >5 mmol/L in 13 episodes and >10 mmol/L in 4, although we do not know if any carbohydrate was ingested before testing. LGS was terminated within 2 min in all four episodes with capillary glucose >10 mmol/L, with sensor error alerts in two of these.

All subjects reported finding LGS "useful," and 93% reported feeling more secure at night, with reduced anxiety, and wanted to continue using it.

CONCLUSIONS—These data suggest that LGS has the potential to reduce nocturnal hypoglycemia in patients with type 1 diabetes at the highest risk. This is similar to results with insulin pump therapy providing the greatest reduction in hypoglycemia in those with the most hypoglycemia at baseline (7).

The risk of ketosis and hyperglycemia after the 2-h suspension of insulin delivery is low (8,9). In our study, median sensor glucose after 2 h of LGS was 3.9 (2.4–14.2) mmol/L. We could not determine if carbohydrate had been consumed during the LGS. There was no evidence of deterioration of overall glucose control with LGS activated.

Patients took longer to respond to the LGS alarm at night, and 75% of completed 2-h LGS events occurred overnight. This may relate to the combined effects of sleep and hypoglycemia on alertness/ arousability, and reduced counter-regulatory responses during sleep (10). Most daytime LGS episodes were terminated by users within 10 min.

The sensor may under-report glucose, particularly during nocturnal hypoglycemia and in view of the lag between interstitial and capillary glucose (11). Although the lowest displayed sensor value is 2.2 mmol/L, the Veo algorithm has improved hypoglycemia detection compared with previous algorithms, with a mean absolute relative difference between 2.2 and 4.4 mmol/L reduced from 24.8 to 19.5% (12). We set the LGS threshold low (mean, 2.4 mmol/L), and a higher threshold may have led to greater reduction in hypoglycemia. Our study could not determine rates of false-positive LGS: 4 of 43 LGS had a capillary glucose reading within 15 min >10 mmol/L, and

2 of these were preceded by sensor error alerts. However, these capillary readings may be biased toward episodes when the patient thought the LGS was erroneous.

LGS reduces anxiety about nocturnal hypoglycemia. Randomized controlled trials that evaluate hypoglycemia and quality-of-life in type 1 diabetes using LGS pumps compared with insulin pump therapy alone, with or without CGM, are now needed. This is the first system that modulates insulin delivery in response to glucose levels without human intervention and is an important step toward clinically available closed-loop systems.

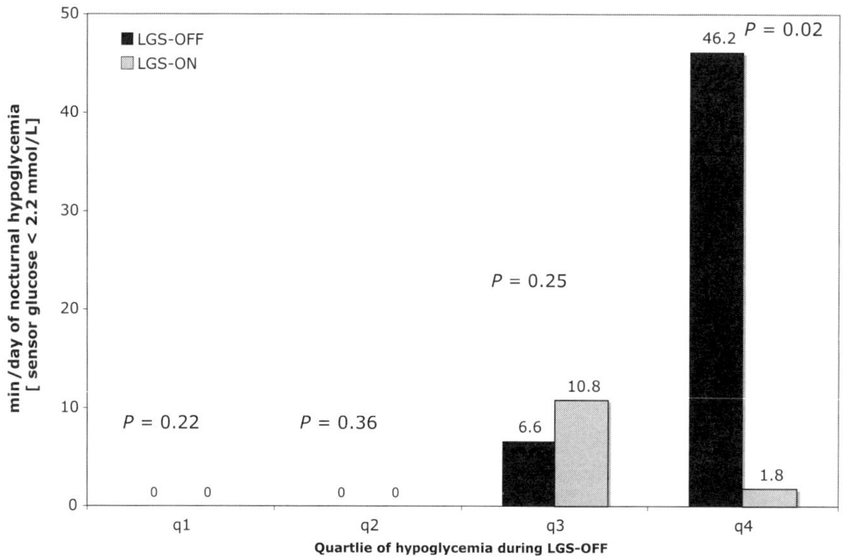

Acknowledgments—This study was funded by Medtronic, Inc. (Northridge, CA). P.C., M.L.E., P.J.H., D.K., J.A.M.S., J.C.P., and S.A. A. have received speaker fees and/or travel support and/or serve on advisory boards from or for Medtronic, Inc. J.S. and Y.W. are employees of Medtronic, Inc. No other potential conflicts of interest relevant to this article were reported.

P.C. collected data, completed the analyses, wrote the manuscript, and reviewed the manuscript. J.S. and Y.W. completed the analyses. M.L.E., P.J.H., D.K., and J.A.M.S. collected data and reviewed the manuscript. J.C.P. and S.A.A. collected data and reviewed the manuscript.

The authors acknowledge the help of Dr. Reman McDonagh and Brenda Perry of Medtronic Diabetes, Ltd., in conducting this study and the help of the research and clinical teams at each of the centers.

Figure 1—*Duration of nocturnal hypoglycemia (sensor glucose < 2.2 mmol/L) with and without LGS. The bars show median duration of hypoglycemia at night with LGS-OFF (black bars) and LGS-ON (gray bars) by quartile (q) of nocturnal hypoglycemia exposure at baseline.*

References
1. Juvenile Diabetes Research Foundation Continuous Glucose Monitoring Study Group, Tamborlane WV, Beck RW, Bode BW, et al. Continuous glucose monitoring and intensive treatment of type 1 diabetes. N Engl J Med 2008;359:1464–1476
2. Raccah D, Sulmont V, Reznik Y, et al. Incremental value of continuous glucose monitoring when starting pump therapy in patients with poorly controlled type 1 diabetes: The RealTrend study. Diabetes Care 2009;32:2245–2250
3. O'Connell MA, Donath S, O'Neal DN, et al. Glycaemic impact of patient-led use of sensor-guided pump therapy in type 1 diabetes: a randomised controlled trial. Diabetologia 2009;52:1250–1257
4. Juvenile Diabetes Research Foundation Continuous Glucose Monitoring Study Group. Prolonged nocturnal hypoglycemia is common during 12 months of continuous glucose monitoring in children and adults with type 1 diabetes. Diabetes Care 2010;35:1004–1008
5. Buckingham B, Block J, Burdick J, et al.; Diabetes Research in Children Network. Response to nocturnal alarms using a

real-time glucose sensor. Diabetes Technol Ther 2005;7:440–447

6. UK Hypoglycaemia Study Group. Risk of hypoglycaemia in types 1 and 2 diabetes: effects of treatment modalities and their duration. Diabetologia 2007;50:1140–1147

7. Pickup JC, Sutton AJ. Severe hypoglycaemia and glycaemic control in type 1 diabetes: meta-analysis of multiple daily insulin injections compared with continuous subcutaneous insulin infusion. Diabet Med 2008;25:765–774

8. Guerci B, Meyer L, Sallé A, et al. Comparison of metabolic deterioration between insulin analog and regular insulin after a 5-hour interruption of a continuous subcutaneous insulin infusion in type 1 diabetic patients. J Clin Endocrinol Metab 1999;84:2673–2678

9. Pickup JC, Viberti GC, Bilous RW, et al. Safety of continuous subcutaneous insulin infusion: metabolic deterioration and glycaemic autoregulation after deliberate cessation of infusion. Diabetologia 1982;22:175–179

10. Jones TW, Porter P, Sherwin RS, et al. Decreased epinephrine responses to hypoglycemia during sleep. N Engl J Med 1998;338:1657–1662

11. Monsod TP, Flanagan DE, Rife F, et al. Do sensor glucose levels accurately predict plasma glucose concentrations during hypoglycemia and hyperinsulinemia? Diabetes Care 2002;25:889–893

12. Keenan DB, Cartaya R, Mastrototaro JJ. Accuracy of a new real-time continuous glucose monitoring algorithm. J Diabetes Sci Technol 2010;4:111–118

Naloxone, but Not Valsartan, Preserves Responses to Hypoglycemia After Antecedent Hypoglycemia

Role of Metabolic Reprogramming in Counterregulatory Failure

Michal M. Poplawski,[1] Jason W. Mastaitis,[2] and Charles V. Mobbs[1]

OBJECTIVE—Hypoglycemia-associated autonomic failure (HAAF) constitutes one of the main clinical obstacles to optimum treatment of type 1 diabetes. Neurons in the ventromedial hypothalamus are thought to mediate counterregulatory responses to hypoglycemia. We have previously hypothesized that hypoglycemia-induced hypothalamic angiotensin might contribute to HAAF, suggesting that the angiotensin blocker valsartan might prevent HAAF. On the other hand, clinical studies have demonstrated that the opioid receptor blocker naloxone ameliorates HAAF. The goal of this study was to generate novel hypothalamic markers of hypoglycemia and use them to assess mechanisms mediating HAAF and its reversal.

RESEARCH DESIGN AND METHODS—Quantitative PCR was used to validate a novel panel of hypothalamic genes regulated by hypoglycemia. Mice were exposed to one or five episodes of insulin-induced hypoglycemia, with or without concurrent exposure to valsartan or naloxone. Corticosterone, glucagon, epinephrine, and hypothalamic gene expression were assessed after the final episode of hypoglycemia.

RESULTS—A subset of hypothalamic genes regulated acutely by hypoglycemia failed to respond after repetitive hypoglycemia. Responsiveness of a subset of these genes was preserved by naloxone but not valsartan. Notably, hypothalamic expression of four genes, including pyruvate dehydrogenase kinase 4 and glycerol 3-phosphate dehydrogenase 1, was acutely induced by a single episode of hypoglycemia, but not after antecedent hypoglycemia; naloxone treatment prevented this failure. Similarly, carnitine palmitoyltransferase-1 was inhibited after repetitive hypoglycemia, and this inhibition was prevented by naloxone. Repetitive hypoglycemia also caused a loss of hypoglycemia-induced elevation of glucocorticoid secretion, a failure prevented by naloxone but not valsartan.

CONCLUSIONS—Based on these observations we speculate that acute hypoglycemia induces reprogramming of hypothalamic metabolism away from glycolysis toward β-oxidation, HAAF is associated with a reversal of this reprogramming, and naloxone preserves some responses to hypoglycemia by preventing this reversal. *Diabetes* **60:39–46, 2011**

From the [1]Fishberg Center for Neurobiology, Mount Sinai School of Medicine, New York, New York; and the [2]Department of Internal Medicine, The Anlyan Center, Yale University School of Medicine, New Haven, Connecticut.
Corresponding author: Charles V. Mobbs, charles.mobbs@mssm.edu.
Received 4 March 2010 and accepted 26 August 2010. Published ahead of print at http://diabetes.diabetesjournals.org on 14 September 2010. DOI: 10.2337/db10-0326.

See accompanying commentary, p. 24.

Hypoglycemia-associated autonomic failure (HAAF) is thought to constitute one of the main obstacles to optimum treatment of type 1 diabetes (1). The causes of HAAF are not known, but counterregulatory responses appear to be mediated by glucose-sensing neurons in the ventromedial hypothalamus (2–6). We have reported that acute hypoglycemia induces hypothalamic expression of angiotensinogen (7). Furthermore, inhibition of ACE activity appears to reduce the risk of hypoglycemia episodes (8,9), suggesting that angiotensin receptor blockers might prevent or even reverse HAAF. On the other hand, the angiotensin receptor blocker losartan is reported to attenuate counterregulatory responses to hypoglycemia (10), though it is not clear if losartan crosses the blood-brain barrier. In contrast, clinical studies have demonstrated that naloxone improves counterregulatory responses (11) and prevents HAAF (12) in humans. In this study we therefore assessed the effects of treatment with valsartan, an angiotensin receptor blocker that crosses the blood-brain barrier, or naloxone on counterregulatory and molecular responses to hypoglycemia after antecedent hypoglycemia.

RESEARCH DESIGN AND METHODS

All studies were approved by the appropriate institutional animal review board (Institutional Animal Care and Use Committee). Twelve-week-old male C57BL/6J mice were obtained from The Jackson Laboratory (Bar Harbor, ME) and housed five per cage with free access to food and water under 12:12-h light-dark cycle (lights on at 7:00 A.M.).

Drugs. This study was designed to assess if blocking angiotensin receptors would prevent counterregulatory failure based on our observation that hypoglycemia induces expression of angiotensin (7). Acute inhibition of angiotensin II production by an ACE inhibitor attenuates acute sympathetic responses to hypoglycemia in humans (13), but specific blockade of the angiotensin receptor A1 subtype does not block responses to hypoglycemia in humans (14), suggesting that the AT2 receptor may mediate acute counterregulatory responses. Furthermore, in a wide variety of circumstances, the AT1 receptor antagonizes effects of the AT2 receptor. For example, the AT1 receptor inhibits effects of the AT2 receptor on vasodilation (15), which is consistent with opposing effects of these receptors in a variety of systems (16). Furthermore, activation of the AT1 receptor increases glucose uptake (17), suggesting that activation of the AT1 receptor would reduce sensitivity to hypoglycemia and thus lead to counterregulatory failure. Therefore, valsartan was chosen for the present studies because it primarily blocks AT1 receptors, and it is the optimum protocol for oral delivery to produce protective effects in the mouse brain without producing hypotension, which has been exhaustively characterized by Wang et al. (18). We therefore administered valsartan orally as described in that article.

Naloxone hydrochloride dihydrate (Sigma Chemical, St. Louis, MO) was dissolved in sterile saline and injected intraperitoneally at a dose of 2 mg/kg in a volume of 0.1 ml/10 g of body weight.

A

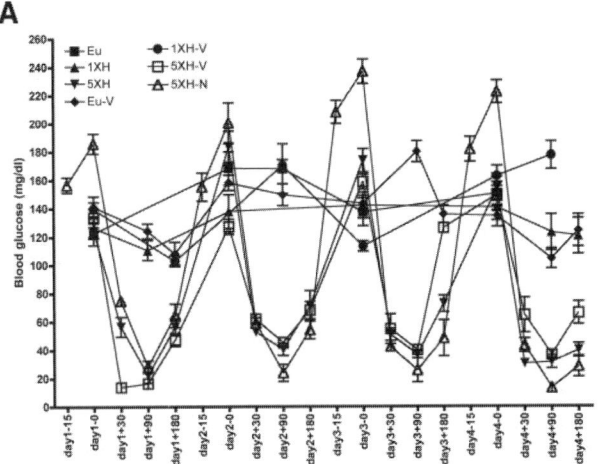

B

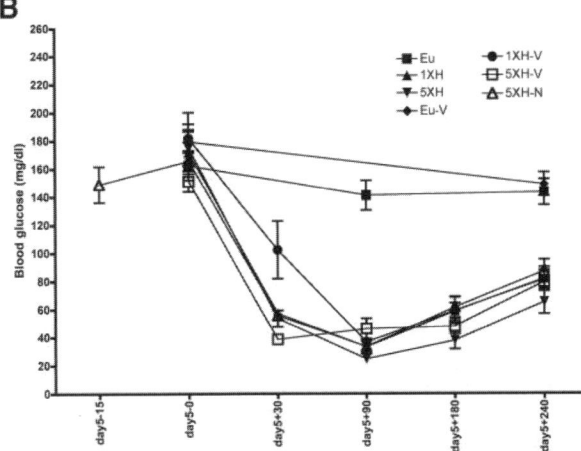

FIG. 1. Blood glucose concentration throughout the study for all experimental groups: Eu, 1XH, 5XH, Eu-V, 1XH-V, 5XH-V, 5XH-N. The *x*-axis indicates the day and time points of the study (with insulin or saline injected at time 0, and for the 5XH-N group, naloxone was injected 15 min prior). Data are means ± SE (*n* = 10 for all groups).

Insulin-induced hypoglycemia. Hypoglycemia was produced by insulin (2.5 units/kg body weight) injected intraperitoneally into mice previously fasted for 3 h, a protocol that produced blood glucose <40 mg/dl when measured at 90 min after injection and without producing unconsciousness, seizures, or death. We previously used a similar protocol to study hypothalamic gene expression following hypoglycemia (7). The insulin dose was tested and optimized prior to the experiments on age-matched C57Bl6/J mice. Blood glucose was measured before insulin injection and after 30, 90, and 180 min via tail prick. For antecedent hypoglycemia episodes, mice were placed in cages without food for 3 h after the insulin injection and then moved back into home cages with food 3 h after the insulin injection. The euglycemic experimental group was similarly denied food access after the saline injection concurrently with the hypoglycemia groups. On the final day of hypoglycemia, blood glucose was additionally measured over 240 min, at which time the animals were killed.

Experimental design. Animals were randomly assigned to one of seven groups (*n* = 10), designated in Figure 1: Eu (saline-injected euglycemic), 1XH (acute insulin-induced hypoglycemia without antecedent hypoglycemia), 5XH (acute hypoglycemia with four antecedent days of hypoglycemia), Eu-V (euglycemic group with oral valsartan 40 mg/kg/day), 1XH-V (acute hypoglycemia with oral valsartan), 5XH-V (acute hypoglycemia with four antecedent days of hypoglycemia maintained on oral valsartan), 5XH-N (acute hypoglycemia with four antecedent days of hypoglycemia with 2 mg/kg naloxone injected intraperitoneally 15 min before every insulin injection). Antecedent hypoglycemia (5XH) consisted of four consecutive days of insulin-induced hypoglycemia (3 h), followed on the 5th day with the final episode of acute hypoglycemia and the animals killed 4 h after insulin injection. The group exposed to acute insulin–induced hypoglycemia without antecedent hypoglycemia (1XH) received physiological saline injections for 4 days, followed by

acute hypoglycemia on the 5th day. The euglycemic group (Eu) received saline injections for five consecutive days. The valsartan groups (1XH-V, 5XH-V) ingested 40 mg/kg/day oral valsartan starting 5 days prior to commencing the 5-day injection protocol and continued on oral valsartan throughout the study. Before the 40-mg/kg/day dose, the valsartan groups received a 20-mg/kg/day dose for a 2-day adjustment period. The naloxone group (5XH-N) received an injection of naloxone (2 mg/kg, intraperitoneally) 15 min before every insulin injection. Therefore, the 5XH-N group received a total of 5 days of insulin injections preceded on each day by an injection of naloxone.

In all cases, mice were killed 4 h after the injection of insulin (or saline for euglycemic mice). Mice were killed following a balanced design at the start of the light period (10:00 A.M. to 2:00 P.M.). Mice were killed by decapitation after a brief exposure to carbon dioxide. Hypothalamic and cortical areas, along with peripheral tissues, were quickly removed, frozen on dry ice, and stored at −70°C until extraction of RNA. Trunk blood was collected for analysis of corticosterone levels.

Blood chemistry. Blood chemistry was carried out in all mice (*n* = 10, 7 groups). Blood glucose was measured by a Contour glucose meter (Bayer, Mountain View, CA). Blood corticosterone levels were measured using an enzyme-linked immunosorbent assay (ELISA) from Assay Designs (Ann Arbor, MI). Blood glucagon was measured using an ELISA from Wako Chemicals USA (Richmond, VA), and epinephrine was measured using an ELISA from Rocky Mountain Diagnostics (Colorado Springs, CO).

Extraction of hypothalamic RNA and cDNA synthesis. Gene expression was assessed for six mice per group based on the quality of the RNA. To obtain the RNA for gene expression analysis by real-time RT-PCR, hypothalamic tissue was homogenized in tubes containing RLT buffer (Qiagen, Valencia, CA) supplemented with 2-ME, and total RNA was extracted using an RNeasy Mini Kit (Qiagen). The quality of the total RNA was assessed using the Biophotometer (Eppendorf, Hauppauge, NY). Due to the capacity limitations of the PCR array plates, six out of ten samples from each experimental group were selected (based on superior RNA quality) and were subjected to reverse transcription. One μg of high-quality total RNA was used for cDNA synthesis using RT₂ First Strand Kit (SABiosciences, Frederick, MD). All procedures were performed according to the manufacturers' protocols.

RT-PCR with custom RT² profiler PCR arrays. RT² Profiler PCR Array (SABiosciences) technology for gene expression analysis entails a synthesis between the profiling capabilities of DNA microarray and the quantitative reliability and sensitivity of quantitative PCR (qPCR). The results are highly reproducible within the same assay run or between different assay runs. RT² Profiler Custom PCR Arrays were used to simultaneously examine the mRNA levels of 187 genes, including 7 housekeeping genes in 384-well plates according to the protocol of the manufacturer (SuperArray Bioscience). The genes were chosen based on prior DNA microarray studies as described in the RESULTS section. The qPCR reactions were carried out using an ABI Prism 7900 thermocycler. Six of the seven housekeeping genes on the array were used to normalize the gene expression by the ΔΔCt method. Data were analyzed using a web-based software program provided by the manufacturer with additional analysis using GraphPad Prism 4 for Macintosh.

Data analysis. All data are presented as mean ± SEM. Statistical analysis was performed using GraphPad Prism 4.0 by one-way ANOVA followed by Dunnett post hoc test. *P* < 0.05 indicates statistical significance.

RESULTS

Novel hypothalamic hypoglycemia–induced genes. As shown in Fig. 1, similar levels of hypoglycemia were achieved in all insulin-injected groups.

One purpose of this study was to expand the panel of hypothalamic genes regulated by hypoglycemia (7) to facilitate assessing mechanisms of HAAF. Toward this end, a series of DNA microarray studies were undertaken to discover genes that are regulated by hypoglycemia and fasting. From these microarrays, a set of genes was chosen that were significantly (by uncorrected *t* test) regulated in the same direction by both hypoglycemia and fasting. The expression of a subset of these genes was assessed in the present study using a custom-designed qPCR array (SABiosciences). This array is now commercially available from SABiosciences and constitutes a powerful resource for the scientific community. After qPCR, expression of these genes was statistically assessed by one-way ANOVA followed by Dunnett post hoc test. Only genes for which the overall ANOVA was significant (*P* < 0.05) and an effect

TABLE 1
Gene nomenclature and regulation by acute insulin–induced hypoglycemia

Gene symbol	Gene name	Reference sequence no.	Fold change (mean ± SE)	P
Angptl4	Angiopoietin-like 4	NM_020581	2.13 ± 0.15	0.00003
Cdkn1a	Cyclin-dependent kinase inhibitor 1A (p21)	NM_007669	5.67 ± 0.44	0.000001
Cpt1a	Carnitine palmitoyltransferase 1a	NM_013495	1.10 ± 0.11	0.53285
Cxcl14	Chemokine (C-X-C motif) ligand 14	NM_019568	0.82 ± 0.03	0.00133
GLUT1	facilitated glucose transporter, member 1	NM_011400	1.91 ± 0.32	0.01853
Gpd1	Glycerol 3-phosphate dehydrogenase 1 (soluble)	NM_010271	1.67 ± 0.16	0.00708
Gpd2	Glycerol 3-phosphate dehydrogenase 2 (mitocho)	NM_010274	0.94 ± 0.01	0.03812
Hif3α	Hypoxia inducible factor 3, α subunit	NM_016868	2.06 ± 0.27	0.00575
Pdk4	Pyruvate dehydrogenase kinase, isoenzyme 4	NM_013743	1.77 ± 0.23	0.01009
Pnpla2	Patatin-like phospholipase domain containing 2	NM_025802	1.64 ± 0.13	0.00084
S3-12	Perilipin 4	NM_020568	3.04 ± 0.21	0.00007
Sox17	SRY-box containing gene 17	NM_011441	1.46 ± 0.12	0.00565
Ucp2	Uncoupling protein 2	NM_011671	1.98 ± 0.28	0.01186

of either acute or repetitive hypoglycemia was significant by post hoc test, which were also significantly regulated by fasting in a separate study, are presented in this article (Table 1).

Hypoglycemia-induced elevation of plasma corticosterone fails after antecedent hypoglycemia: prevention of failure by naloxone, but not valsartan. In the present study, mice were killed 4 h after insulin injection to allow examination of hypothalamic molecular responses to gene expression (7). However, this time point is not optimum for the assessment of the failure of hormonal responses, which in mice are usually measured 120 min after the induction of hypoglycemia (19,20), similar to studies in rats (4,21) and humans (22). Thus, although we measured all three counterregulatory hormones, any conclusions based on hormone levels at this late time point must be interpreted with caution. As observed in humans (23), a single acute exposure to hypoglycemia caused a significant elevation of plasma corticosterone, a response completely prevented by antecedent hypoglycemia (Fig. 2A). This counterregulatory failure was not prevented by treatment with valsartan, but was completely prevented by treatment with naloxone. Similarly, a single exposure to hypoglycemia caused a significant elevation of plasma glucagon, and this induction was completely prevented by antecedent hypoglycemia (Fig. 2B). Furthermore, the failure of glucagon to respond to hypoglycemia was not rescued by either drug treatment (Fig. 2B). Finally, plasma epinephrine was also induced by a single episode of hypoglycemia, but this induction was not blocked at this time point by antecedent hypoglycemia (Fig. 2C). However, the induction appears to have been attenuated by valsartan and naloxone (Fig. 2C). Subject to the caveat concerning the late time point, these results do not support that valsartan will prevent counterregulatory failure and may in fact worsen failure. Furthermore, naloxone, while possibly protective for activation of the hypothalmic-adrenal-pituitary axis, may not protect against failure in glucagon and epinephrine secretion after antecedent hypoglycemia.

Hif3α, S3-12, and GLUT1 are induced after acute and repetitive hypoglycemia. As shown in Table 1 and Fig. 3, Hif3α (hypoxia-induced factor 3α), S3-12 (perilipin 4), and GLUT1 (facilitative GLUT isoform 1) were induced by acute hypoglycemia. Induction by hypogly-

cemia was not influenced by antecedent hypoglycemia, valsartan, or naloxone. Thus, the induction of these genes did not correlate with HAAF or its reversal by naloxone. Furthermore, the induction of these genes appears not to be dependent on hypoglycemia-induced angiotensin since valsartan did not influence the expression of these genes. It should be noted that in this study the induction of angiotensin by hypoglycemia did not reach statistical significance, so these results are not presented here.

Induction of Pdk4, Gpd1, Angptl4, and Cdkn1a by acute hypoglycemia fails after antecedent hypoglycemia: prevention of failure by naloxone, not valsartan. Another set of genes was induced by acute hypoglycemia but not after antecedent hypoglycemia: Pdk4 (pyruvate dehydrogenase kinase 4), Gpd1 (glycerol 3-phosphate dehydrogenase isoform 1), Angptl4 (also known as fasting-induced adipose factor), and Cdkn1a (also known as p21) (Fig. 4). The failure of these genes to respond to hypoglycemia after antecedent hypoglycemia was prevented by treatment with naloxone, but not by treatment with valsartan (Fig. 4).

Naloxone prevents the regulation of Gpd2, Cxcl14, and Sox17 by hypoglycemia. A different pattern of expression was observed for the genes in Fig. 5: the regulation of these genes by hypoglycemia was not impaired by antecedent hypoglycemia but was prevented by naloxone, though not by valsartan. In contrast to Gpd2 (glycerol 3-phosphate dehydrogenase isoform 2) and Cxcl14 (chemokine [C-X-C] motif ligand14), which were inhibited by hypoglycemia, Sox17 (SRY-box containing gene 17) was induced by hypoglycemia.

Naloxone prevents the inhibition of Cpt1a by repetitive hypoglycemia. The only gene in our panel that was significantly regulated by repetitive hypoglycemia but not acute hypoglycemia was Cpt1a. This inhibition was prevented by naloxone (Fig. 6).

Induction of Ucp2 and Pnpla2 by acute hypoglycemia fails after repetitive hypoglycemia, and failure is not reversed by naloxone or valsartan. Finally, Fig. 7 depicts the genes whose induction by acute hypoglycemia failed after antecedent hypoglycemia and whose failure was not prevented by naloxone. These genes were Ucp2 (Uncoupling Protein 2) and Pnpla2 (also known as adipose triglyceride lipase).

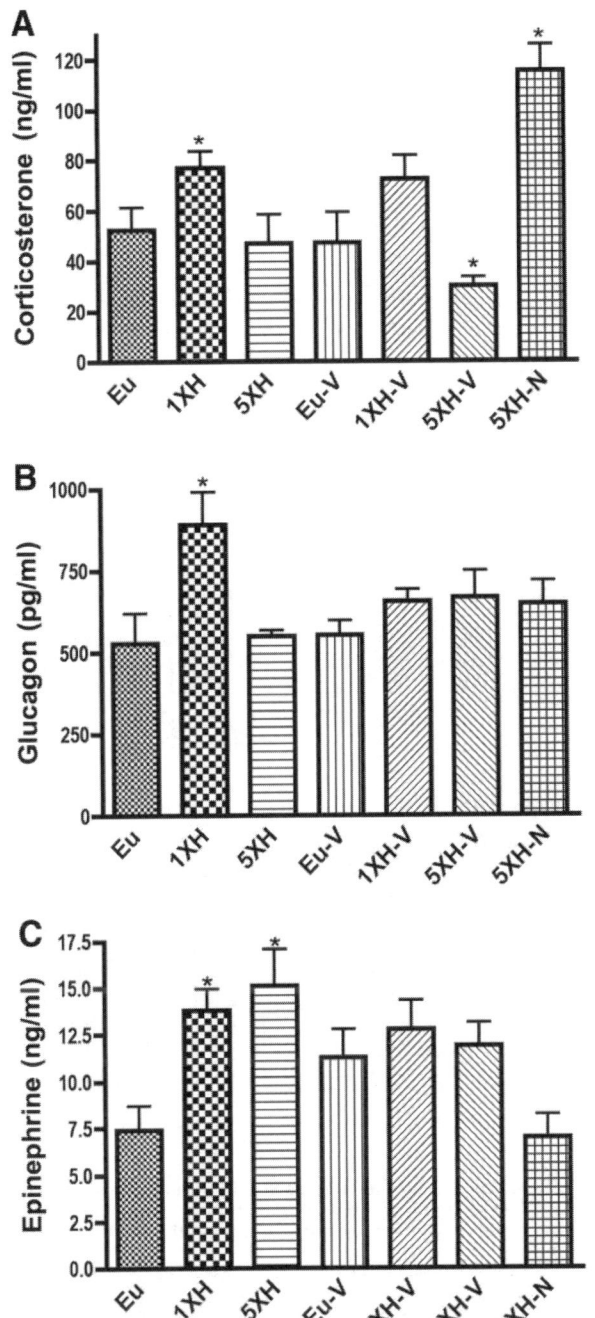

FIG. 2. Counterregulatory hormones in mice exposed to antecedent hypoglycemia and naloxone (2 mg/kg) or valsartan (40 mg/kg/day). Trunk blood was collected at the time the animals were killed, 4 h after final insulin or saline injection. Hormone levels were measured by ELISA in the same groups as described in Fig. 1. Data are means ± SE (n = 10 for all groups). *P < 0.05 as compared with the euglycemic group (Dunnett test).

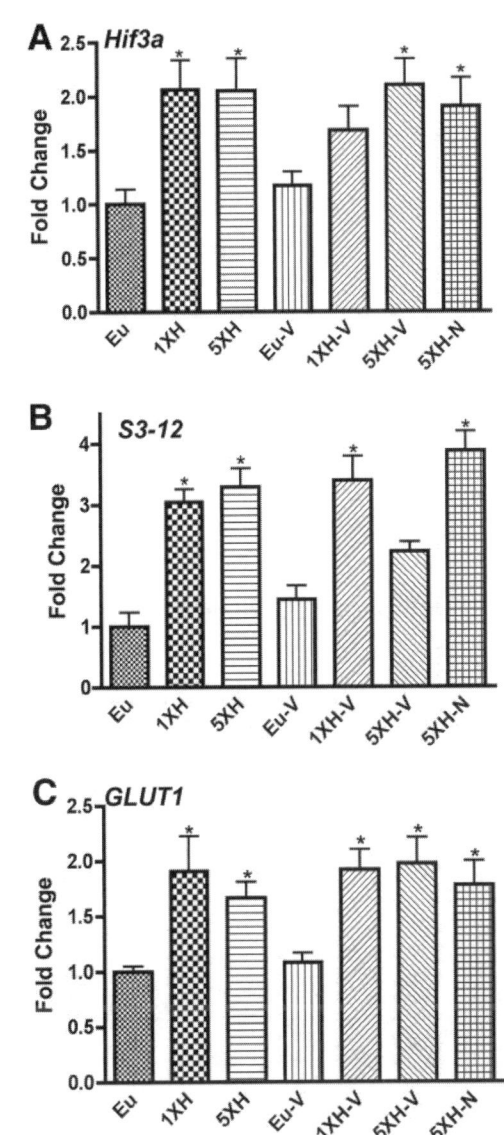

FIG. 3. Real-time qPCR data for murine hypothalamic genes that do not correlate with counterregulatory failure or its reversal by naloxone or valsartan. Relative expression levels of (A) Hif3a, (B) S3-12, and (C) GLUT1 were assessed using custom PCR arrays in the same groups described in Fig. 1. Animals were killed 4 h after the final insulin or saline injection. Data for each gene were normalized to a panel of housekeeping transcripts and expressed as fold change compared with the saline-injected (euglycemic) group. Data are means ± SE (n = 6 for all groups). *P < 0.05 as compared with the euglycemic group (Dunnett test).

DISCUSSION

In these studies, we observed that 4 days of antecedent hypoglycemia in mice completely prevented the elevation of corticosterone produced by acute hypoglycemia (Fig. 2A) and glucagon (Fig. 2B) but not epinephrine (Fig. 2C) when measured 240 min after the injection of insulin. The counterregulatory failure to increase corticosterone was prevented by naloxone, but not valsartan, and the coun-terregulatory failure of glucagon was not prevented by either treatment.

The pattern of gene expression in these studies suggests a metabolic basis for HAAF and its prevention by nalox-one. (We conclude that the effects of insulin-induced hypoglycemia on gene expression are due to hypoglyce-mia, not insulin, since in every case the effects of insulin-induced hypoglycemia were in the same direction as produced by fasting, a condition characterized by reduced glucose and reduced insulin.) First, it should be noted that acute hypoglycemia–induced Pdk4 (Fig. 4), which inhibits pyruvate dehydrogenase, constitutes a classic mechanism to shift metabolic economy away from glycolysis and toward β-oxidation (24). Such a shift would be expected to

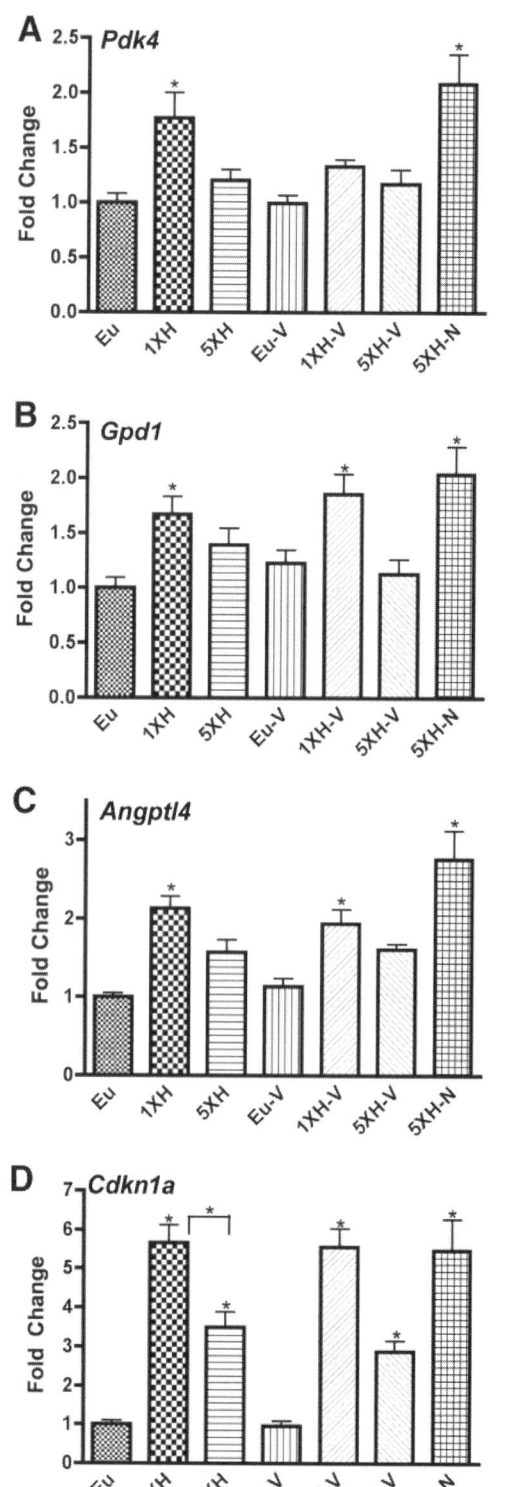

FIG. 4. Real-time qPCR data for murine hypothalamic genes that fail to respond after antecedent hypoglycemia, and the failure was prevented by naloxone, but not valsartan. Relative expression levels of (A) Pdk4, (B) Gpd1, (C) Angptl4, and (D) Cdkn1a were assessed using custom PCR arrays from SABiosciences in the same groups described in Fig. 1. Animals were killed 4 h after the final insulin or saline injection. Data for each gene were normalized to a panel of housekeeping transcripts and expressed as fold change compared with the saline-injected (euglycemic) group. Data are means ± SE (n = 6 for all groups). *P < 0.05 as compared with the euglycemic group (Dunnett test).

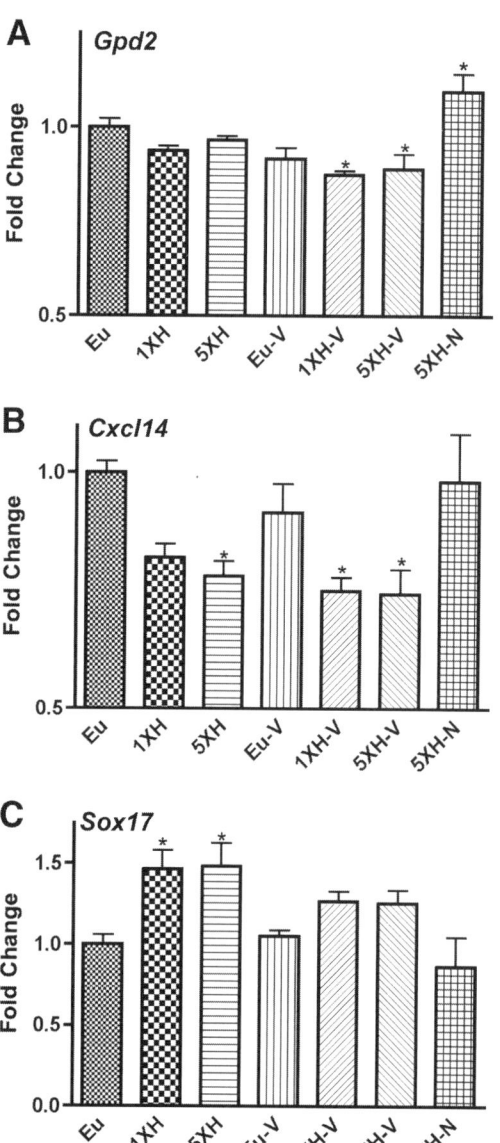

FIG. 5. Real-time qPCR data for murine hypothalamic genes whose regulation by hypoglycemia were not impaired by antecedent hypoglycemia but were prevented by naloxone, though not by valsartan. Relative expression levels of (A) Gpd2 (glycerol 3-phosphate dehydrogenase 2, mitochondrial), (B) Cxcl14, and (C) Sox17 were assessed using custom PCR arrays from SABiosciences in the same groups described in Fig. 1. Animals were killed 4 h after the final insulin or saline injection. Data for each gene were normalized to a panel of housekeeping transcripts and expressed as fold change compared with the saline-injected (euglycemic) group. Data are means ± SE (n = 6 for all groups). *P < 0.05 as compared with the euglycemic group (Dunnett test).

enhance sensitivity to hypoglycemia by reducing glucose metabolism. However, the induction of *Pdk4* was reversed after antecedent hypoglycemia and was prevented by valsartan, conditions in which glucocorticoid induction was impaired. Most important, naloxone treatment maintained the induction of *Pdk4* by hypoglycemia in association with the maintenance of the glucocorticoid response. We have previously reported that estradiol, which impairs counterregulatory responses in humans (25) and rats (26), inhibits hypothalamic *Pdk4* in association with impaired hypothalamic responses to hypoglycemia (27). Similarly, Jiang et al. (28) demonstrated with the use of metabolic

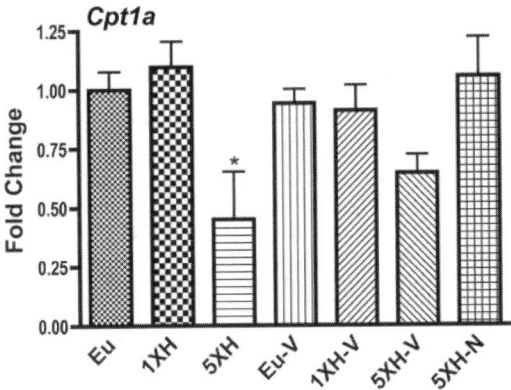

FIG. 6. Hypothalamic expression of *Cpt1a* was significantly regulated by repetitive hypoglycemia but not acute hypoglycemia, and this inhibition was prevented by naloxone. Relative expression level of *Cpt1a* (carnitine palmitoyltransferease 1a, liver) was assessed with custom PCR arrays from SABiosciences in the same groups described in Fig. 1. Animals were killed 4 h after the final insulin or saline injection. Data for each gene were normalized to a panel of housekeeping transcripts and expressed as fold change compared with the saline-injected (euglycemic) group. Data are means ± SE ($n = 6$ for all groups). *$P < 0.05$ as compared with the euglycemic group (Dunnett test).

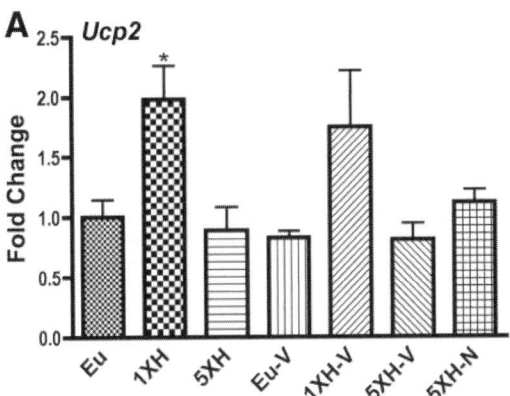

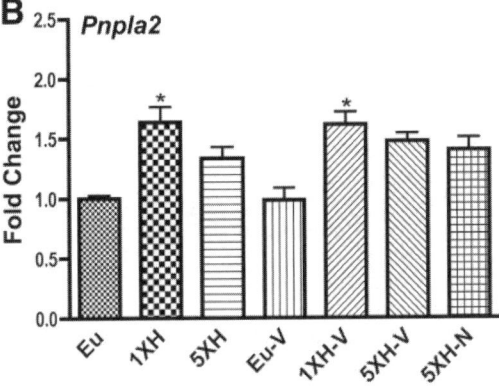

FIG. 7. Hypothalamic expression of genes whose induction by acute hypoglycemia was prevented by antecedent hypoglycemia but not maintained by exposure to naloxone. Relative expression levels of (*A*) *Ucp2* (uncoupling protein 2) and (*B*) *Pnpla2* (patatin-like phospholipase domain containing 2) were assessed with custom PCR arrays from SABiosciences in the same groups described in Fig. 1. Animals were killed 4 h after the final insulin or saline injection. Data for each gene were normalized to a panel of housekeeping transcripts and expressed as fold change compared with the saline-injected (euglycemic) group. Data are means ± SE ($n = 6$ for all groups). *$P < 0.05$ as compared with the euglycemic group (Dunnett test).

tracers that recurrent antecedent hypoglycemia caused a robust increase in neuronal, but not glial, pyruvate dehydrogenase activity in association with counterregulatory failure, consistent with a decrease in *Pdk4* activity. This set of observations suggests that HAAF is caused by a failure to maintain the shift away from glycolysis toward alternate fuel use in neurons, and that naloxone prevents HAAF by maintaining this shift.

The pattern of expression of other genes supports this metabolic shift hypothesis. For example, like *Pdk4*, the induction of *Angptl4* by hypoglycemia fails after antecedent hypoglycemia, and this failure is prevented by naloxone. *Angptl4* stimulates β-oxidation and uncoupling (29), directly supporting that acute hypoglycemia reprograms hypothalamic metabolism away from glycolysis and toward alternate fuel use (β-oxidation), that HAAF is associated with the failure of this reprogramming, and that naloxone prevents HAAF by preventing this failure. Similarly, hypothalamic *Ucp2* has recently been shown to mediate an induction of β-oxidation (23). Similarly, repetitive hypoglycemia inhibited *Cpt1a* (Fig. 6), an effect prevented by naloxone. β-Oxidation mediated by *Cpt1* constitutes a key element by which hypothalamic neurons sense nutritional state, plausibly by reducing nutrient flux through pathways that metabolize glucose (23,30). Therefore the reduction in β-oxidation produced by repetitive hypoglycemia would be expected to increase nutrient flux through pathways that metabolize glucose, thus increasing sensitivity to glucose and reducing sensitivity to hypoglycemia. The prevention of this effect by naloxone also supports that HAAF is caused by the failure to produce alternative metabolic pathways to glucose utilization.

Furthermore, the induction of *Gpd1* by hypoglycemia (Fig. 4) fails after antecedent hypoglycemia, a failure prevented by naloxone but not valsartan. *Gpd1* catalyzes the interconversion of glycerol and dihydrooxyacetone (DHA). DHA is converted to glycerol as part of the glycerol NADH shuttle mechanism. However, this shuttle requires the activity of *Gpd2*, and in this study we observed that hypoglycemia inhibited *Gpd2* (Fig. 5), an effect that was prevented by naloxone but not valsartan. Thus, inhibition of the glycerol shuttle activity (which is active during glycolysis) correlated with the failure of the counterregulatory elevation of corticosterone. This suggests that the key metabolic effect of *Gpd1* induction by hypoglycemia is to catalyze conversion of glycerol to DHA, providing an alternative to glucose for fuel; that failure in this conversion is associated with counterregulatory failure; and that naloxone prevents counterregulatory failure by maintaining this alternative metabolic pathway.

The other gene most prominently implicated in HAAF and its reversal by naloxone is *Cdnk1a*, more commonly known as p21, a major inhibitor of cell division. However, the functional significance of *Cdnk1a* in counterregulation and its failure is unclear. It is plausible that *Cdnk1a* expression is a reflection, rather than a cause, of counterregulatory failure since this gene is induced by glucocortiocoids (31). Interestingly, *Cxc114* appears to produce insulin resistance (32), so its inhibition by hypoglycemia might enhance the inhibitory effect of insulin on the counterregulatory response (33), and reversal of this inhibition might mediate part of the reversal of impairments by naloxone. Finally, *Sox17* is the canonical inhibitor of the Wnt signaling pathway (34), and some evidence suggests that the Wnt pathway promotes glycolysis at the expense of β-oxidation (35). Thus, *Sox17* may contribute to the apparent switch away from glycolysis produced by hypoglycemia as indicated above, but since the induction continues even after antecedent hypoglycemia, counterregulatory failure is probably not attributable to the *Sox17/Wnt* pathway.

It should also be noted that many of the genes associated here with impaired counterregulatory elevation of corticosterone are induced by the metabolic transcription factor *Ppar-α*, including *Pdk4*, *Cpt1a*, *Ucp2* (36), and *Gpd1* (36,37). Indeed, a major function of Ppar-α is to activate the uptake and oxidation of free fatty acids (36) and glycerol metabolism (37). Furthermore, *Ppar-α* knockout exhibit hypoglycemia during fasting (38), a phenomenon plausibly similar to HAAF. Of particular interest, wholebody glucose use is reduced by infusing an activator of *Ppar-α* into the third ventricle (38). We therefore speculate that counterregulatory responses are enhanced by hypothalamic activation of *Ppar-α*, that this action fails after repetitive hypoglycemia, that this failure is reversed by naloxone, and that *Ppar-α* activators such as WY13643 might also be useful in reversing counterregulatory failure. It must be emphasized however that this speculation has not been directly tested.

To the extent that naloxone prevented the loss of responsiveness to hypoglycemia by antecedent hypoglycemia (e.g., corticosterone, *Pdk4*, *Angptl4*, and *Cdkn1a/p21*), the precise mechanism mediating these effects remains unclear. It seems very likely that these effects of naloxone are mediated by blockade of μ-opioid receptors since these are the main known mechanisms of action of naloxone (39). One of the most prominent responses to hypoglycemia is the release of the natural μ-opioid agonist β-endorphin into the plasma from the anterior pituitary (40). Conversely, infusion of β-endorphin into the hypothalamus inhibits some hypothalamic responses to hypoglycemia (41), which would have the effect of amplifying glucocorticoid responses to hypoglycemia as observed in this study. However, it remains to be determined if β-endorphin released from the pituitary exerts these effects in the hypothalamus or if other sources of opioids within the central nervous system mediate these effects.

Several major caveats apply to the present studies. Firstly, the counterregulatory hormones were measured 240 min after insulin injection, well after the more typical time point of around 120 min (19,20). Since those studies demonstrated counterregulatory failure of epinephrine after only a single antecedent exposure to hypoglycemia, which is similar to the results in humans (42), further analysis will be required to determine if the protocol used in the present studies is in fact an adequate model for human HAAF. Replicating these studies with glucose clamps and sampling blood earlier will clarify this issue, and the use of different doses of insulin could improve the similarity to human HAAF. Secondly, drug levels were not measured, so failure to produce protective effects could be due to low drug levels in the blood. However, the doses of valsartan were chosen based on previous doses that produced neuroprotection without reducing blood pressure (18). Thirdly, valsartan did in fact appear to impair several responses to hypoglycemia, including glucagon and *Pdk4*, suggesting that the drug was in fact having effects at the dose used. Similarly naloxone clearly produced several effects on hormonal and molecular responses to hypoglycemia. Whether other doses would have produced a better outcome remains to be determined. Another concern is that the magnitudes of the

effects on gene expression were rather small. However the results were reliable because in most cases they were observed in more than one condition, and we have corroborated that fasting similarly and significantly regulates every gene described in this study. A more telling concern is whether the effects observed here could functionally account for counterregulation or its failure given the small magnitude of the effects. With respect to this concern, we anticipate that the most important mode of regulation of these gene products is at the allosteric level (e.g., of *Cpt1a* by malonyl-CoA) and that the regulation of expression functions mainly as a clue to which gene products are involved in various processes. Nevertheless, as always with studies of gene expression, any conclusions must be considered provisional until corroborated by more direct assessment of function; in this case by analysis of metabolic fluxes.

In conclusion we describe here that naloxone, but not valsartan, prevents counterregulatory failure after antecedent hypoglycemia in mice as in humans (11,12). Preservation of counterregulatory responses was associated with the preservation of responsiveness to hypoglycemia of a subset of hypoglycemia-regulated genes reported here for the first time. The pattern of responses of these genes in relation to counterregulatory failure and its prevention by naloxone suggests that naloxone preserves counterregulatory responses by maintaining a metabolic profile in which alternate fuels are used instead of glucose. Nevertheless, since this study did not include groups in which naloxone was only given once or not on the last day, it remains to be determined if the effect of naloxone was to prevent the failure of hypoglycemia-induced responses or to directly induce corticostereone secretion and related changes in hypothalamic gene expression. In contrast, valsartan did not prevent or reverse loss of responsiveness to hypoglycemia of these genes. Nevertheless, the dose of valsartan used is neuroprotective (18) and did block some responses to hypoglycemia, suggesting that the hypothesis that elevated angiotensin produces HAAF is probably incorrect. Further analysis with mice in which either the AT1 or the AT2 receptor has been ablated may clarify this issue. Taken together, these studies suggest that manipulations causing reprogramming of hypothalamic metabolic processes away from glycolysis and toward alternate fuel use might be useful in preventing or reversing HAAF.

ACKNOWLEDGMENTS

These studies were supported by the Juvenile Diabetes Research Foundation.

No potential conflicts of interest relevant to this article were reported.

M.M.P. designed the studies, carried out the animal work and the qPCR and hormone analysis, and wrote the manuscript. J.W.M. carried out the microarray studies and reviewed the manuscript. C.V.M. conceived the studies and wrote the manuscript.

REFERENCES

1. Cryer PE. Hypoglycemia-associated autonomic failure in diabetes. Am J Physiol Endocrinol Metab 2001;281:E1115–E1121
2. Borg MA, Tamborlane WV, Shulman GI, Sherwin RS. Local lactate perfusion of the ventromedial hypothalamus suppresses hypoglycemic counterregulation. Diabetes 2003;52:663–666
3. Borg MA, Borg WP, Tamborlane WV, Brines ML, Shulman GI, Sherwin RS. Chronic hypoglycemia and diabetes impair counterregulation induced by

localized 2-deoxy-glucose perfusion of the ventromedial hypothalamus in rats. Diabetes 1999;48:584–587

4. Borg MA, Sherwin RS, Borg WP, Tamborlane WV, Shulman GI. Local ventromedial hypothalamus glucose perfusion decreases counterregulation during systemic hypoglycemia in awake rats. J Clin Invest 1997;99:361–365

5. Borg WP, Sherwin RS, During MJ, Borg MA, Shulman GI. Local ventromedial hypothalamus glucopenia triggers counterregulatory hormone release. Diabetes 1995;44:180–184

6. Borg WP, During MJ, Sherwin RS, Borg MA, Brines ML, Shulman GI. Ventromedial hypothalamic lesions in rats suppress counterregulatory responses to hypoglycemia. J Clin Invest 1994;93:1677–1682

7. Mastaitis JW, Wurmbach E, Cheng H, Sealfon SC, Mobbs CV. Acute induction of gene expression in brain and liver by insulin-induced hypoglycemia. Diabetes 2005;54:952–958

8. Pedersen-Bjergaard U, Agerholm-Larsen B, Pramming S, Hougaard P, Thorsteinsson B. Prediction of severe hypoglycaemia by angiotensin-converting enzyme activity and genotype in type 1 diabetes. Diabetologia 2003;46:89–96

9. Pedersen-Bjergaard U, Agerholm-Larsen B, Pramming S, Hougaard P, Thorsteinsson B. Activity of angiotensin-converting enzyme and risk of severe hypoglycaemia in type 1 diabetes mellitus. Lancet 2001;357:1248–1253

10. Deininger E, Oltmanns KM, Wellhoener P, Fruehwald-Schultes B, Kern W, Heuer B, Dominiak P, Born J, Fehm HL, Peters A. Losartan attenuates symptomatic and hormonal responses to hypoglycemia in humans. Clin Pharmacol Ther 2001;70:362–369

11. Caprio S, Gerety G, Tamborlane WV, Jones T, Diamond M, Jacob R, Sherwin RS. Opiate blockade enhances hypoglycemic counterregulation in normal and insulin-dependent diabetic subjects. Am J Physiol 1991;260: E852–E858

12. Leu J, Cui MH, Shamoon H, Gabriely I. Hypoglycemia-associated autonomic failure is prevented by opioid receptor blockade. J Clin Endocrinol Metab 2009;94:3372–3380

13. Madsen BK, Hølmer P, Ibsen H, Christensen NJ. The influence of captopril on the epinephrine response to insulin-induced hypoglycemia in humans. The interaction between the renin-angiotensin system and the sympathetic nervous system. Am J Hypertens 1992;5:361–365

14. Worck RH, Frandsen E, Ibsen H, Petersen JS. AT1 and AT2 receptor blockade and epinephrine release during insulin-induced hypoglycemia. Hypertension 1998;31:384–390

15. Li XC, Widdop RE. AT2 receptor-mediated vasodilatation is unmasked by AT1 receptor blockade in conscious SHR. Br J Pharmacol 2004;142:821–830

16. de Gasparo M, Catt KJ, Inagami T, Wright JW, Unger T. International union of pharmacology. XXIII. The angiotensin II receptors. Pharmacol Rev 2000;52:415–472

17. Han HJ, Heo JS, Lee YJ. ANG II increases 2-deoxyglucose uptake in mouse embryonic stem cells. Life Sci 2005;77:1916–1933

18. Wang J, Ho L, Chen L, Zhao Z, Zhao W, Qian X, Humala N, Seror I, Bartholomew S, Rosendorff C, Pasinetti GM. Valsartan lowers brain beta-amyloid protein levels and improves spatial learning in a mouse model of Alzheimer disease. J Clin Invest 2007;117:3393–3402

19. Jacobson L, Ansari T, Potts J, McGuinness OP. Glucocorticoid-deficient corticotropin-releasing hormone knockout mice maintain glucose requirements but not autonomic responses during repeated hypoglycemia. Am J Physiol Endocrinol Metab 2006;291:E15–E22

20. Jacobson L, Ansari T, McGuinness OP. Counterregulatory deficits occur within 24 h of a single hypoglycemic episode in conscious, unrestrained, chronically cannulated mice. Am J Physiol Endocrinol Metab 2006;290: E678–E684

21. Levin BE, Becker TC, Eiki J, Zhang BB, Dunn-Meynell AA. Ventromedial hypothalamic glucokinase is an important mediator of the counterregulatory response to insulin-induced hypoglycemia. Diabetes 2008;57:1371–1379

22. Kerr D, Sherwin RS, Pavalkis F, Fayad PB, Sikorski L, Rife F, Tamborlane WV, During MJ. Effect of caffeine on the recognition of and responses to hypoglycemia in humans. Ann Intern Med 1993;119:799–804

23. Andrews ZB, Liu ZW, Walllingford N, Erion DM, Borok E, Friedman JM, Tschöp MH, Shanabrough M, Cline G, Shulman GI, Coppola A, Gao XB, Horvath TL, Diano S. *UCP2* mediates ghrelin's action on NPY/AgRP neurons by lowering free radicals. Nature 2008;454:846–851

24. Mobbs CV, Mastaitis JW, Zhang M, Isoda F, Cheng H, Yen K. Secrets of the lac operon. Glucose hysteresis as a mechanism in dietary restriction, aging and disease. Interdiscip Top Gerontol 2007;35:39–68

25. Sandoval DA, Ertl AC, Richardson MA, Tate DB, Davis SN. Estrogen blunts neuroendocrine and metabolic responses to hypoglycemia. Diabetes 2003; 52:1749–1755

26. Adams JM, Legan SJ, Ott CE, Jackson BA. Modulation of hypoglycemia-induced increases in plasma epinephrine by estrogen in the female rat. J Neurosci Res 2005;79:360–367

27. Cheng H, Isoda F, Mobbs CV. Estradiol impairs hypothalamic molecular responses to hypoglycemia. Brain Res 2009;1280:77–83

28. Jiang L, Herzog RI, Mason GF, de Graaf RA, Rothman DL, Sherwin RS, Behar KL. Recurrent antecedent hypoglycemia alters neuronal oxidative metabolism in vivo. Diabetes 2009;58:1266–1274

29. Mandard S, Zandbergen F, van Straten E, Wahli W, Kuipers F, Müller M, Kersten S. The fasting-induced adipose factor/angiopoietin-like protein 4 is physically associated with lipoproteins and governs plasma lipid levels and adiposity. J Biol Chem 2006;281:934–944

30. Pocai A, Lam TK, Obici S, Gutierrez-Juarez R, Muse ED, Arduini A, Rossetti L. Restoration of hypothalamic lipid sensing normalizes energy and glucose homeostasis in overfed rats. J Clin Invest 2006;116:1081–1091

31. Harms C, Albrecht K, Harms U, Seidel K, Hauck L, Baldinger T, Hübner D, Kronenberg G, An J, Ruscher K, Meisel A, Dirnagl U, von Harsdorf R, Endres M, Hörtnagl H. Phosphatidylinositol 3-Akt-kinase-dependent phosphorylation of p21(Waf1/Cip1) as a novel mechanism of neuroprotection by glucocorticoids. J Neurosci 2007;27:4562–4571

32. Hara T, Nakayama Y. *CXCL14* and insulin action. Vitam Horm 2009;80: 107–123

33. Paranjape SA, Chan O, Zhu W, Horblitt AM, McNay EC, Cresswell JA, Bogan JS, McCrimmon RJ, Sherwin RS. Influence of insulin in the ventromedial hypothalamus on pancreatic glucagon secretion in vivo. Diabetes 2010;59:1521–1527

34. Fu DY, Wang ZM, Li-Chen, Wang BL, Shen ZZ, Huang W, Shao ZM. *Sox17*, the canonical Wnt antagonist, is epigenetically inactivated by promoter methylation in human breast cancer. Breast Cancer Res Treat 2010;119: 601–612

35. Chafey P, Finzi L, Boisgard R, Caïuzac M, Clary G, Broussard C, Pégorier JP, Guillonneau F, Mayeux P, Camoin L, Tavitian B, Colnot S, Perret C. Proteomic analysis of beta-catenin activation in mouse liver by DIGE analysis identifies glucose metabolism as a new target of the Wnt pathway. Proteomics 2009;9:3889–3900

36. Mandard S, Müller M, Kersten S. Peroxisome proliferator-activated receptor alpha target genes. Cell Mol Life Sci 2004;61:393–416

37. Patsouris D, Mandard S, Voshol PJ, Escher P, Tan NS, Havekes LM, Koenig W, März W, Tafuri S, Wahli W, Müller M, Kersten S. PPARalpha governs glycerol metabolism. J Clin Invest 2004;114:94–103

38. Knauf C, Rieusset J, Foretz M, Cani PD, Uldry M, Hosokawa M, Martinez E, Bringart M, Waget A, Kersten S, Desvergne B, Gremlich S, Wahli W, Seydoux J, Delzenne NM, Thorens B, Burcelin R. Peroxisome proliferator-activated receptor-alpha-null mice have increased white adipose tissue glucose utilization, GLUT4, and fat mass: role in liver and brain. Endocrinology 2006;147:4067–4078

39. Goodman AJ, Le Bourdonnec B, Dolle RE. Mu opioid receptor antagonists: recent developments. ChemMedChem 2007;2:1552–1570

40. Nakao K, Nakai Y, Jingami H, Oki S, Fukata J, Imura H. Substantial rise of plasma beta-endorphin levels after insulin-induced hypoglycemia in human subjects. J Clin Endocrinol Metab 1979;49:838–841

41. Suda T, Sato Y, Sumitomo T, Nakano Y, Tozawa F, Iwai I, Yamada M, Demura H. Beta-endorphin inhibits hypoglycemia-induced gene expression of corticotropin-releasing factor in the rat hypothalamus. Endocrinology 1992;130:1325–1330

42. Hvidberg A, Fanelli CG, Hershey T, Terkamp C, Craft S, Cryer PE. Impact of recent antecedent hypoglycemia on hypoglycemic cognitive dysfunction in nondiabetic humans. Diabetes 1996;45:1030–1036

Effects of Intensive Therapy and Antecedent Hypoglycemia on Counterregulatory Responses to Hypoglycemia in Type 2 Diabetes

Stephen N. Davis,[1,2] Stephanie Mann,[1] Vanessa J. Briscoe,[1] Andrew C. Ertl,[1] and Donna B. Tate[1]

OBJECTIVE—The physiology of counterregulatory responses during hypoglycemia in intensively treated type 2 diabetic subjects is largely unknown. Therefore, the specific aims of the study tested the hypothesis that *1*) 6 months of intensive therapy to lower A1C <7.0% would blunt autonomic nervous system (ANS) responses to hypoglycemia, and *2*) antecedent hypoglycemia will result in counterregulatory failure during subsequent hypoglycemia in patients with suboptimal and good glycemic control.

RESEARCH DESIGN AND METHODS—Fifteen type 2 diabetic patients (8 men/7 women) underwent 6-month combination therapy of metformin, glipizide XL, and acarbose to lower A1C to 6.7% and 2-day repeated hypoglycemic clamp studies before and after intensive therapy. A control group of eight nondiabetic subjects participated in a single 2-day repeated hypoglycemic clamp study.

RESULTS—Six-month therapy reduced A1C from 10.2 ± 0.5 to 6.7 ± 0.3%. Rates of hypoglycemia increased to 3.2 episodes per patient/month by study end. Hypoglycemia (3.3 ± 0.1 mmol/l) and insulinemia (1,722 ± 198 pmol/l) were similar during all clamp studies. Intensive therapy reduced ($P < 0.05$) ANS and metabolic counterregulatory responses during hypoglycemia. Antecedent hypoglycemia produced widespread blunting ($P < 0.05$) of neuroendocrine, ANS, and metabolic counterregulatory responses during subsequent hypoglycemia before and after intensive therapy in type 2 diabetic patients and in nondiabetic control subjects.

CONCLUSIONS—Intensive oral combination therapy and antecedent hypoglycemia both blunt physiological defenses against subsequent hypoglycemia in type 2 diabetes. Prior hypoglycemia of only 3.3 ± 0.1 mmol/l can result in counterregulatory failure in type 2 diabetic patients with suboptimal control and can further impair physiological defenses against hypoglycemia in intensively treated type 2 diabetes. *Diabetes* **58:701–709, 2009**

Large randomized controlled multicenter clinical trials have demonstrated the benefit of improved glycemic control on microvascular complications in both type 1 and type 2 diabetes (1,2). These compelling data have produced a paradigm shift in the treatment of diabetes (particularly type 2 diabetes) striving for A1C values <7.0% (3). The major drawbacks of tight metabolic control in patients with type 1 diabetes are well documented and include increased hypoglycemia and weight gain (4–8).

Recently, three large studies have investigated the effects of rigorous metabolic control (A1C <7.0%) on the prevalence of macrovascular disease in type 2 diabetes (9–11). The overall conclusion of these studies was that A1C values <7.0% did not produce a statistically significant reduction in macrovascular events but did produce a marked increase in hypoglycemia in type 2 diabetes. The effects of intensive therapy on physiological counterregulatory responses during hypoglycemia in type 2 diabetes have not been thoroughly investigated. Burge et al. (12) demonstrated that improving glycemic control during an 8-day in-patient admission could lower symptom responses and plasma glucose levels for activation of epinephrine during hypoglycemia. Levy et al. (13), using a cross-sectional study design, also concluded that improved glycemic control in type 2 diabetes shifts the thresholds for counterregulatory hormone release to lower plasma glucose concentrations during hypoglycemia. Korzon-Burakowska et al. (14) improved A1C from 11.3 ± 1.1 to 8.1 ± 0.9% during a 4-month period. Thresholds (i.e., plasma glucose values) for counterregulatory hormone release and epinephrine and cortisol responses were lowered by improved glycemic control. Spyer et al. (15), investigating a group of seven type 2 diabetic patients with an A1C of 7.4%, also found that the glycemic thresholds for counterregulatory hormone release were reduced from elevated to normal physiological glucose levels. However, similar to some (13,16) but not all studies (17), there was no difference in values of the key counterregulatory hormones, epinephrine and glucagon, during hypoglycemia when compared with nondiabetic control subjects. Studies investigating the mechanisms regulating counterregulatory responses during hypoglycemia in type 2 diabetes are even fewer. Segel et al. (16) determined that antecedent hypoglycemia in a group of type 2 diabetic patients with an A1C of 8.1% resulted in hypoglycemia-associated autonomic failure similar to patients with type 1 diabetes. Despite the above data, two questions remain unanswered: *1*) What are the effects of a period of rigorous glycemic control to reduce A1C <7.0% on counterregulatory responses in type 2 diabetes, and *2*) what are the effects of antecedent hypoglycemia on autonomic nervous system (ANS), neuroendocrine, and metabolic counterregulatory mechanisms before and after a period of rigorous metabolic control in type 2 diabetes? In the present study, we tested the hypothesis that 6-month intensive therapy to lower A1C <7.0% would impair counterregulatory response to hypoglycemia and that antecedent hypoglycemia would further impair key homeo-

From the [1]Department of Medicine, Vanderbilt University, Nashville, Tennessee; and [2]Veterans Affairs, Nashville, Tennessee.

Corresponding author: Stephen N. Davis, steve.davis@vanderbilt.edu.

Received 4 September 2008 and accepted 26 November 2008.

Published ahead of print at http://diabetes.diabetesjournals.org on 10 December 2008. DOI: 10.2337/db08-1230. Clinical trial registry no. NCT00732862, clinicaltrials.org.

See accompanying commentary, p. 515.

static counterregulatory mechanisms during subsequent hypoglycemia in type 2 diabetes.

RESEARCH DESIGN AND METHODS

Fifteen patients (8 men/7 women) with type 2 diabetes (age 47 ± 2 years), BMI of 33 ± 2 kg/m^2, glycosylated hemoglobin of $10.2 \pm 0.5\%$ (normal range 4–6.5%), anti-GAD and anti–islet cell antibody negative, and disease duration of 6 ± 2 years were studied. Patients were receiving diet and exercise ($n = 2$) or oral agent monotherapy [metformin (mean 750 mg/day, $n = 10$) or sulfonylurea (glyburide or glipizide mean 5 mg/day, $n = 3$)]. Eight nondiabetic control subjects (4 men/4 women), aged 48 ± 3 years, BMI 30 ± 2 kg/m^2, and A1C $5.1 \pm 0.2\%$ were also studied. Each subject had a normal blood count, plasma electrolytes, and liver and renal function. All gave written informed consent. Studies were approved by the Vanderbilt University Human Subjects Institutional Review Board.

Type 2 diabetic subjects. Fifteen participated in two 2-day hypoglycemia experiments separated by 6 months. Subjects were asked to avoid any exercise and consume their usual weight-maintaining diet for 3 days before each study. Two days before a study, sulfonylurea and metformin tablets were omitted. After 6 months when the patients were in good metabolic control, these medications were replaced with injections of regular insulin before each meal. The dose of regular insulin was carefully adjusted so that hypoglycemia (<3.9 mmol/l) and hyperglycemia (>11.1 mmol/l) were avoided in the 2 days before a study. Each subject was admitted to the Vanderbilt General Clinical Research Center (GCRC) at 5:00 P.M. on the evening before an experiment. At this time, two intravenous cannulae were inserted under 1% lidocaine local anesthesia. One cannula was placed in a retrograde fashion into a vein on the back of the hand. This hand would be placed in a heated box (55–60°C) during the study so that arterialized blood could be obtained (18). The other cannula was placed in the contralateral arm for infusions. Patients then received a standardized evening meal, and a continuous low-dose infusion of insulin was started to normalize plasma glucose. The insulin infusion was adjusted overnight to maintain blood glucose between 4.4 and 7.2 mmol/l.

Hypoglycemia experiments. After an overnight 10-h fast at 0 min, a primed (18 μCi) continuous infusion (0.18 μCi/min) of high-performance liquid chromatography (HPLC)-purified [3-^{3}H]glucose (11.5 mCi · mmol^{-1} · l^{-1}; Perkin Elmer Life Sciences, Boston, MA) was administered via a precalibrated infusion pump (Harvard Apparatus, South Natick, MA). A period of 90 min was allowed to elapse followed by a 30-min basal control period. Plasma glucose was maintained at euglycemia during this period by continuing the overnight basal insulin. At time 120 min, a primed constant (15.0 pmol · kg^{-1} · min^{-1}) infusion of insulin (Human Regular Insulin; Eli Lilly, Indianapolis, IN) was started and continued until 240 min. The rate of fall of glucose was controlled (0.07 mmol/min), and the hypoglycemic nadir (3.3 mmol/l) was achieved using a modification of the glucose clamp technique (19). During the clamp period, plasma glucose was measured every 5 min, and a 20% dextrose infusion was adjusted so that plasma glucose levels were held constant at 3.3 ± 0.1 mmol/l (20). Potassium chloride (20 mmol/l) was infused during the clamp to reduce insulin-induced hypokalemia. After completion of the 2-h test period, the insulin infusion was turned down to the basal rate, and the plasma glucose was rapidly restored to euglycemia with 20% dextrose. In the afternoon after a 2-h period of euglycemia, a second 2-h hypoglycemic clamp of 3.3 mmol/l was performed similar to the morning study. No tritiated glucose was infused during the afternoon studies. After completion of the afternoon hypoglycemic clamp, a basal insulin infusion was restarted and a standardized evening meal and snack was given. Similar to the previous night, a variable low-dose infusion was used to maintain glucose levels (4.4–7.2 mmol/l) overnight. The next morning after a 10-h overnight fast, an identical (including a tritiated glucose infusion) 2-h hypoglycemic clamp at 3.3 ± 0.1 mmol/l was performed as described for day 1.

Study medication. After completion of the first 2-day clamp studies, patients were started on triple oral combination therapy. Metformin and acarbose were increased to 1 g twice a day and 50 mg three times a day over a 4-week period, respectively. Glipizide XL was increased to 10 mg once or twice a day over a period of 3 weeks. All patients performed intensive self-reported blood glucose monitoring before main meals, snacks, and at bedtime or any time that they felt low glucose or a second individual thought they had a low glucose. Thus, study subjects tested their glucose levels between four to seven times per day. Patients were contacted by study nurses twice a week and by a dietitian weekly to adjust diet, exercise, and medication and to discuss any treatment side effects. Patients were seen by S.N.D., study nurses, and/or a dietitian monthly. Patient adherence to protocol was assessed at monthly visits and found to be excellent. One patient moved out of state during the 6-month treatment period and was lost to follow-up. After completion of the 6-month intensive treatment period, patients were readmitted to the Vander-

bilt GCRC for an identical 2-day hypoglycemic clamp protocol as described above. The nondiabetic control subjects underwent a single 2-day in-patient hypoglycemic clamp protocol similar (without overnight glucose control) to the type 2 diabetic patients.

Direct measurement of muscle sympathetic nerve activity. Muscle sympathetic nerve activity (MSNA) was recorded from the peroneal nerve at the level of the fibular head and popliteal fossa (21,22). The approximate location of this nerve was determined by transdermal electrical stimulation (10–60 V, 0.01-ms duration). This stimulation produced painless muscle contraction of the foot. After this, a reference stainless steel microelectrode with a shaft diameter of 200 μm was placed subcutaneously. A similar tungsten electrode, with an uninsulated tip (1–5 μm), was inserted into the nerve and used for recording of MSNA.

Criteria for acceptable MSNA recordings were *1*) electrical stimulation produced muscle twitches but not paresthesia, *2*) nerve activity increased during phase II of the Valsalva maneuver (hypotensive phase) and was suppressed during phase IV (blood pressure overshoot), and *3*) nerve activity increased in response to held expiration.

Tracer calculations. Rates of glucose appearance (R_a), endogenous glucose production (EGP), and glucose utilization were calculated according to the methods of Wall et al. (23). EGP was calculated by determining the total R_a (this comprises both EGP and any exogenous glucose infused to maintain the desired hypoglycemia) and subtracting it from the amount of exogenous glucose infused. It is now recognized that this approach is not fully quantitative, because underestimates of total R_a and rate of glucose disposal (R_d) can be obtained. The use of a highly purified tracer and taking measurements under steady-state conditions (i.e., constant specific activity) in the presence of low glucose flux eliminates most, if not all, of the problems. In addition, to maintain a constant specific activity, isotope delivery was increased commensurate with increases in exogenous glucose infusion. During these studies, only glucose flux results from the steady-state basal and the final 30-min periods of the hypoglycemic clamps are reported.

Analytical methods. Plasma glucose concentrations were measured in triplicate using the glucose oxidase method with a glucose analyzer (Beckman, Fullerton, CA). Glucagon was measured according to a modification of the method of Aguilar-Parada et al. (24) with an interassay coefficient of variation (CV) of 12%. Insulin was measured as previously described (25) with an interassay CV of 9%. Catecholamines were determined by HPLC (26) with an interassay CV of 12% for epinephrine and 8% for norepinephrine. Two modifications to the procedure for catecholamine determination were made: *1*) a five-point rather than a one-point standard calibration curve was used, and *2*) the initial and final samples of plasma were spiked with known amounts of epinephrine and norepinephrine so that accurate identification of the relevant respective catecholamine peaks could be made. Cortisol was assayed using the Clinical Assays Gamma Coat Radioimmunoassay (RIA) kit with an interassay CV of 6%. Growth hormone was determined by RIA (27) with a CV of 8.6%. Pancreatic polypeptide was measured by RIA using the method of Hagopian et al. (28) with an interassay CV of 8%. Lactate, glycerol, alanine, and β-hydroxybutyrate were measured in deproteinized whole blood using the method of Lloyd et al. (29). Nonesterified fatty acids (NEFAs) were measured using the WAKO kit adopted for use on a centrifugal analyzer (30).

Blood for hormones and intermediary metabolites were drawn twice during the control period and every 15 min during the experimental period. Cardiovascular parameters (pulse, systolic, diastolic, and mean arterial pressure) were measured noninvasively by a Dinamap (Critikon, Tampa, FL) every 10 min throughout each study starting at 80 min.

Hypoglycemic symptoms were quantified using a previously validated semiquantitative questionnaire (31). Each individual was asked to rate his or her experience of the symptoms twice during the control period and every 15 min during experimental periods. Symptoms measured included sweaty, tremor/shaky, hot, thirsty/dry mouth, agitation/irritability, palpitations, tired/fatigued, confusion, dizzy, difficulty thinking, blurriness of vision, and sleepy. The ratings of the first six symptoms were summed to get the autonomic score, whereas the ratings from the last six symptoms provide a neuroglycopenic symptom score.

Statistical analysis. Data are expressed as mean $\pm$ SE and were analyzed using standard, parametric, one- and two-way ANOVA, and repeated measures where appropriate (SigmaStat; SPSS Science, Chicago). Tukey's post hoc analysis was used to delineate statistical significance across time within each group and for each group compared with day 1 of the preintensive therapy group. A P value of <0.05 was accepted as statistically significant. The baseline and final 30 min of hypoglycemia were compared for most parameters, because steady-state glucose levels, insulin levels, and glucose infusion rates were achieved by this time.

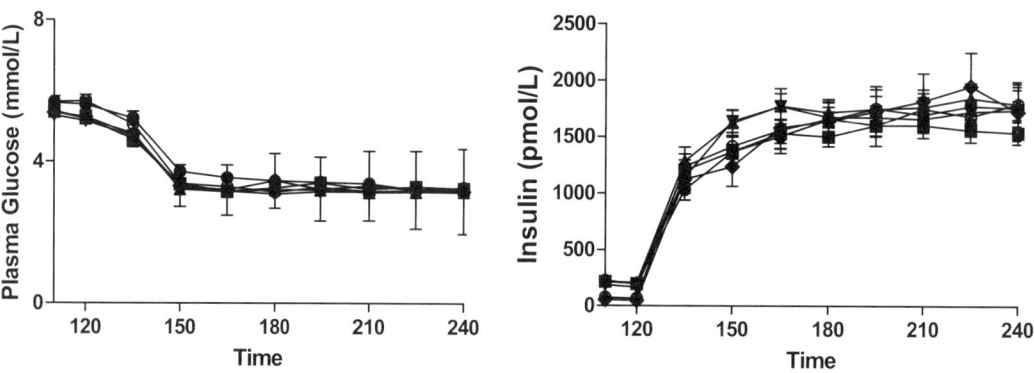

FIG. 1. Plasma glucose and insulin levels during repeated 2-day hyperinsulinemic-hypoglycemic clamps in overnight-fasted individuals with type 2 diabetes and healthy control subjects. Type 2 diabetic patients are studied before (pre) and after (post) 6 months of intensive triple oral combination anti-diabetes therapy. ●, Day 1 pre; ■, day 2 pre; ▲, day 1 post; ▽, day 2 post; ◆, day 1 controls; ○, day 2 controls.

RESULTS

Effects of 6-month intensive therapy on counterregulatory responses to hypoglycemia, insulin, glucose, and A1C levels. A1C levels were reduced from 10.2 ± 0.5 to $6.7 \pm 0.3\%$ during the 6 months of intensive therapy. Body weight remained stable throughout 6 months of intensive therapy (97.6 ± 7 to 96.1 ± 6 kg). Plasma glucose levels were controlled overnight and were similar at the start of the preintensive therapy and postintensive therapy

(5.6 ± 0.3 and 5.3 ± 0.2 mmol/l, respectively). Basal plasma glucose levels in the control group were also equivalent at 5.3 ± 0.2 mmol/l. Plasma glucose levels (3.3 ± 0.1 mmol/l) were equivalent during preintensive therapy, postintensive therapy, and control hypoglycemic clamps (Fig. 1).

Basal insulin levels were 198 ± 36, 210 ± 30, and 66 ± 18 pmol/l in the preintensive therapy, postintensive therapy, and control groups, respectively. Insulin levels during

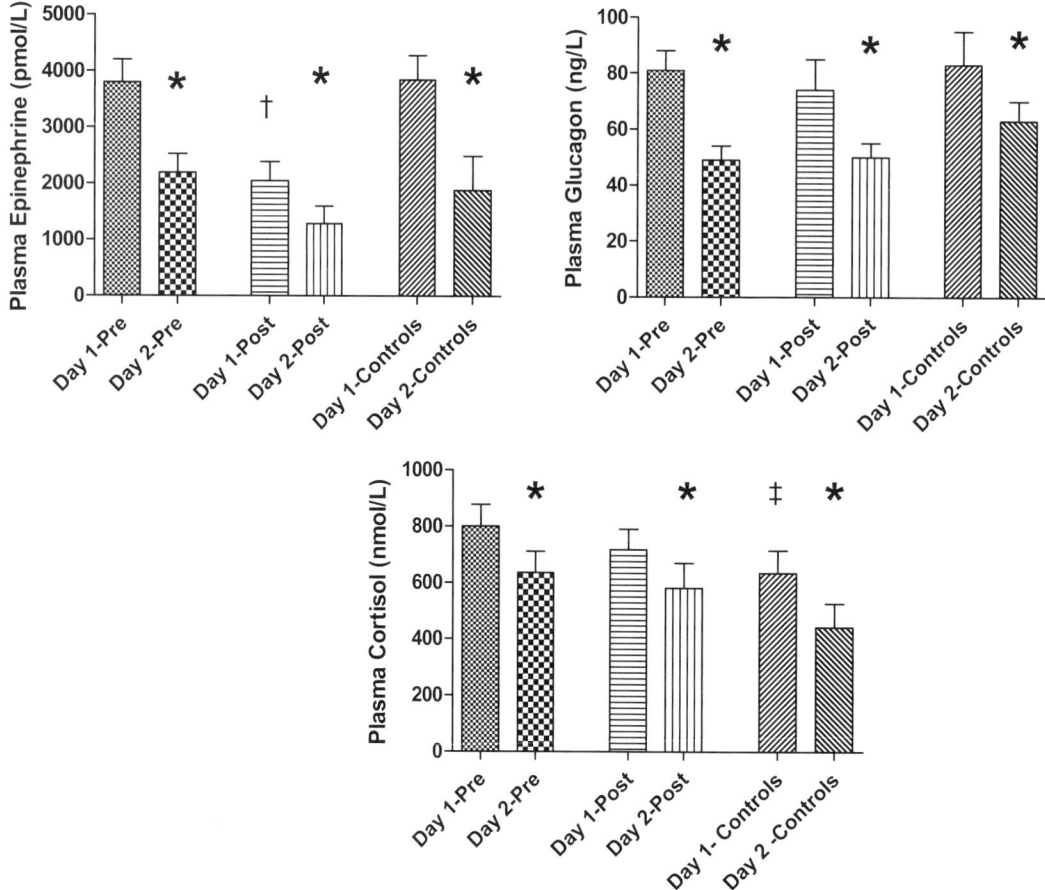

FIG. 2. Plasma epinephrine, glucagon, and cortisol levels in the final 30 min of hypoglycemia during repeated 2-day hyperinsulinemic-hypoglycemic clamps in overnight-fasted individuals with type 2 diabetes and healthy control subjects. *Plasma epinephrine, glucagon, and cortisol levels are significantly reduced ($P < 0.05$) after day 1 hypoglycemia in healthy control subjects and patients with type 2 diabetes both before (pre) and after (post) 6-month intensive triple oral combination anti-diabetes therapy. †Plasma epinephrine levels are significantly reduced ($P < 0.05$) after 6-month intensive triple oral combination anti-diabetes therapy. ‡Plasma cortisol levels are significantly reduced ($P < 0.05$) in healthy control subjects compared with type 2 diabetic patients before intensive therapy.

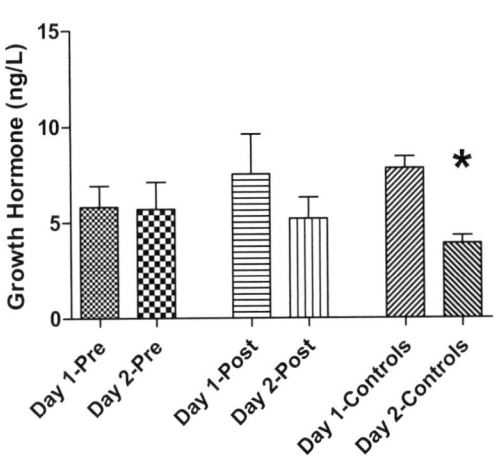
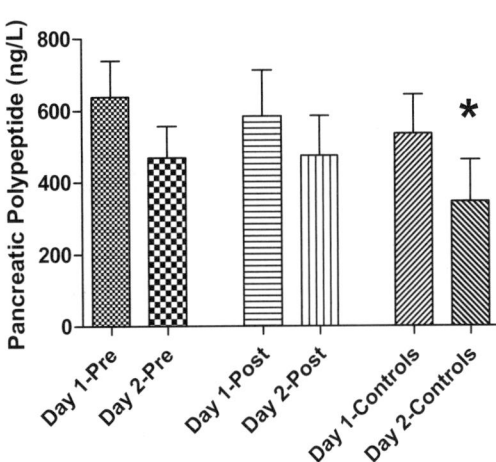

FIG. 3. Plasma growth hormone and pancreatic polypeptide levels in the final 30 min of hypoglycemia during repeated 2-day hyperinsulinemic-hypoglycemic clamps in overnight-fasted individuals with type 2 diabetes and healthy control subjects. *Plasma growth hormone and pancreatic polypeptide levels are significantly reduced ($P < 0.05$) after day 1 hypoglycemia in healthy control subjects.

the clamp studies were similar among groups ($1,722 \pm 198$ pmol/l). C-peptide levels decreased from 0.75 ± 0.12 to 0.17 ± 0.02 ng/l during hypoglycemia in preintensive therapy. After intensive therapy, basal C-peptide levels were increased (1.2 ± 0.2 ng/ml; $P < 0.05$) and were higher during postintensive therapy clamps (0.3 ± 0.03 ng/l; $P < 0.05$) compared with preintensive therapy.

Neuroendocrine responses. After 6-month intensive therapy, epinephrine responses were significantly blunted in postintensive therapy compared with preintensive therapy and control values ($2,033 \pm 343$ vs. $3,788 \pm 414$ and $3,837 \pm 441$ pmol/l, respectively; $P < 0.05$) (Fig. 2). Intensive therapy had no effect on other neuroendocrine (glucagon, growth hormone, cortisol, norepinephrine, or pancreatic polypeptide) responses to hypoglycemia (Fig. 3). Cortisol levels were higher ($P < 0.05$) in preintensive therapy compared with control subjects (801 ± 77 vs. 635 ± 80 nmol/l).

Glucose kinetics and intermediary metabolism. Basal EGP was similar in all three groups (preintensive therapy, 9.9 ± 1.1; postintensive therapy, 9.5 ± 1.1; control, 9.4 ± 1.1 μmol $\cdot$ kg^{-1} $\cdot$ min^{-1}). EGP declined significantly in all three groups ($P < 0.01$). However, EGP was higher ($P < 0.01$) during hypoglycemia in preintensive therapy (6.6 ± 1.1 μmol $\cdot$ kg^{-1} $\cdot$ min^{-1}) compared with postintensive therapy and control values where there was no measurable EGP. Rates of glucose infusion were significantly greater ($P < 0.01$) in postintensive therapy (10.5 ± 3.3 μmol $\cdot$ kg^{-1} $\cdot$ min^{-1}) and control (16.5 ± 3.9 μmol $\cdot$ kg^{-1} $\cdot$ min^{-1}) compared with preintensive therapy (2.2 μmol $\cdot$ kg^{-1} $\cdot$ min^{-1}).

Intermediary metabolism. NEFAs (193 ± 22 vs. 303 ± 38 μmol/l), lactate (1.52 ± 0.17 vs. 1.96 ± 0.18 mmol/l), and glycerol (49 ± 7 vs. 69 ± 9 μmol/l) were significantly blunted ($P < 0.05$) during postintensive therapy compared with preintensive therapy, respectively (Fig. 4). Plasma lactate, glycerol, and blood NEFA levels were higher ($P < 0.05$) during preintensive therapy versus control.

MSNA. Basal rates of MSNA were similar in preintensive therapy (34 ± 3 bursts/min), postintensive therapy (31 ± 4 bursts/min), and control (38 ± 6 bursts/min). MSNA increased by 17 ± 3 bursts/min during preintensive therapy, which was increased ($P < 0.05$) compared with the responses during postintensive therapy (5 ± 3 bursts/min) and control clamps (8 ± 2 bursts/min) (Fig. 5).

Hypoglycemic symptom scores. Total hypoglycemic scores increased by 33 ± 6 during hypoglycemia in preintensive therapy, which was increased ($P < 0.01$) compared with the response during postintensive therapy (19 ± 4). Symptom responses were lower ($P < 0.01$) in control (12 ± 2) compared with both preintensive therapy and postintensive therapy studies (Fig. 5). Intensive treatment blunted autonomic symptom responses (preintensive therapy, 18 ± 3, vs. postintensive therapy, 10 ± 4; $P < 0.05$) and neuroglycopenic symptom responses to hypoglycemia (15 ± 3 vs. 9 ± 3; $P < 0.05$).

Cardiovascular responses. Intensive therapy significantly blunted cardiovascular responses to hypoglycemia. Systolic blood pressure increased from 120 ± 6 to 129 ± 6 mmHg ($P < 0.05$) during hypoglycemia in preintensive therapy but remained similar to baseline (129 ± 6 to 130 ± 7 mmHg) in postintensive therapy. Heart rate also increased during hypoglycemia in preintensive therapy (74 ± 5 to 85 ± 6 beats/min; $P < 0.05$) but remained similar to baseline (70 ± 4 to 73 ± 4 beats/min) in postintensive therapy. Systolic blood pressure increased by a nonsignificant amount in control subjects (119 ± 5 to 125 ± 4 mmHg), but heart rate increased significantly (62 ± 4 to 72 ± 4 beats/min; $P < 0.05$).

Hypoglycemic events during intensive treatment. Self-reported blood glucose readings <3.9 mmol/l are shown in Table 1. No patient experienced any hypoglycemia in the month before the start of the study. During the study, all patients experienced hypoglycemic readings between 3.3 and 3.9 mmol/l. Thirteen patients had readings between 2.8 and 3.3 mmol/l, and frequency of hypoglycemia increased to 3.2 episodes per patient per month by the end of the 6-month study. No major episodes of hypoglycemia occurred during the study. Four patients documented hypoglycemic readings <2.8 mmol/l.

Effects of antecedent hypoglycemia on counterregulatory responses to hypoglycemia before and after 6-month intensive therapy

Insulin, C-peptide, and glucose levels. Insulin levels were similar during the morning of day 1 and day 2 clamp studies in all three groups ($1,534 \pm 174$ to $1,890 \pm 222$ pmol/l). Plasma glucose levels were equivalent during morning day 1 and day 2 studies (3.3 ± 0.1 mmol/l) in all groups. Antecedent hypoglycemia attenuated the fall in C-peptide during day 2 in both preintensive therapy (day 1,

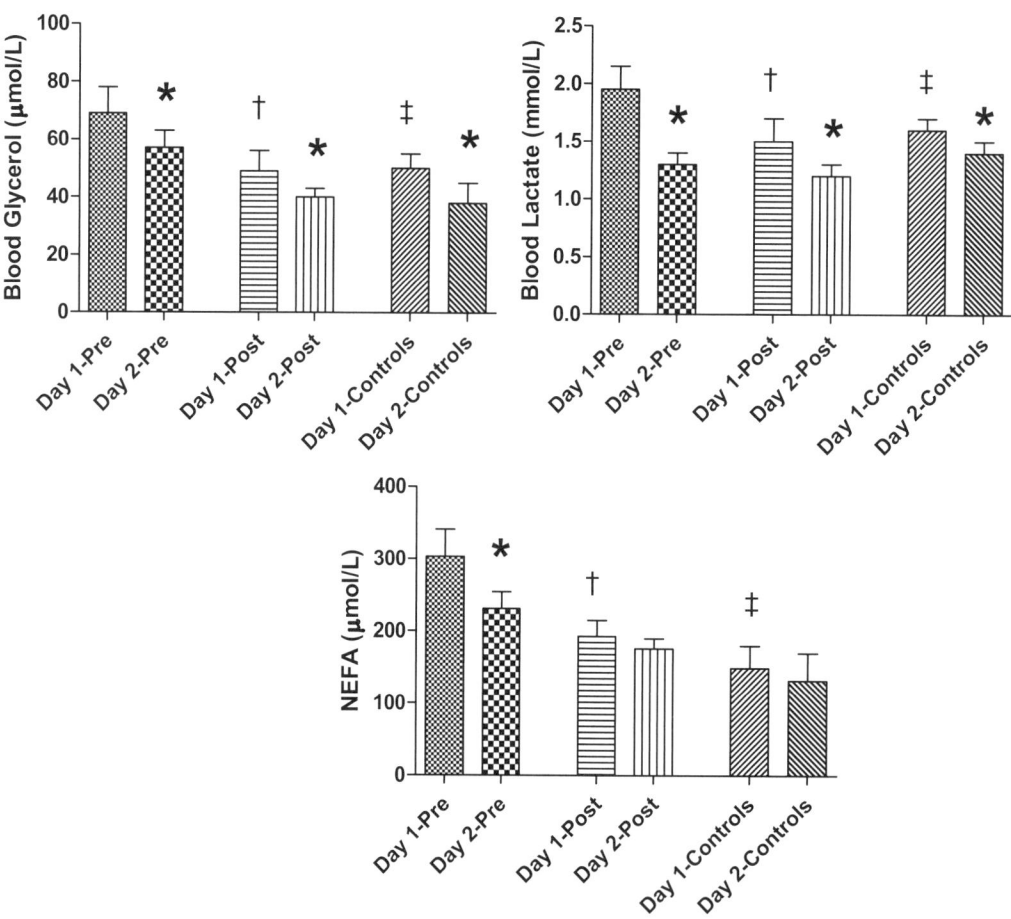

FIG. 4. Blood glycerol, lactate, and plasma NEFA levels in the final 30 min of hypoglycemia during repeated 2-day hyperinsulinemic-hypoglycemic clamps in overnight-fasted individuals with type 2 diabetes and healthy control subjects. *Blood glycerol, lactate, and plasma NEFA levels are significantly reduced ($P < 0.05$) in healthy control subjects and patients with type 2 diabetes both before (pre) and after (post) 6-month intensive triple oral combination anti-diabetes therapy. †Blood glycerol, lactate, and plasma NEFA levels are reduced ($P < 0.05$) after 6-month intensive therapy in type 2 diabetes. ‡Blood glycerol, lactate, and plasma NEFAs are significantly reduced ($P < 0.05$) in healthy control subjects compared with type 2 diabetes before intensive therapy.

-0.58 ± 0.08 vs. day 2, -0.39 ± 0.11 ng/l) and postintensive therapy studies (day 1, -0.98 ± 0.15, vs. day 2, -0.61 ± 0.11 ng/l; $P < 0.05$).

Neuroendocrine levels. Baseline neuroendocrine hormone levels were similar at the start of preintensive therapy, postintensive therapy, and control studies (Table

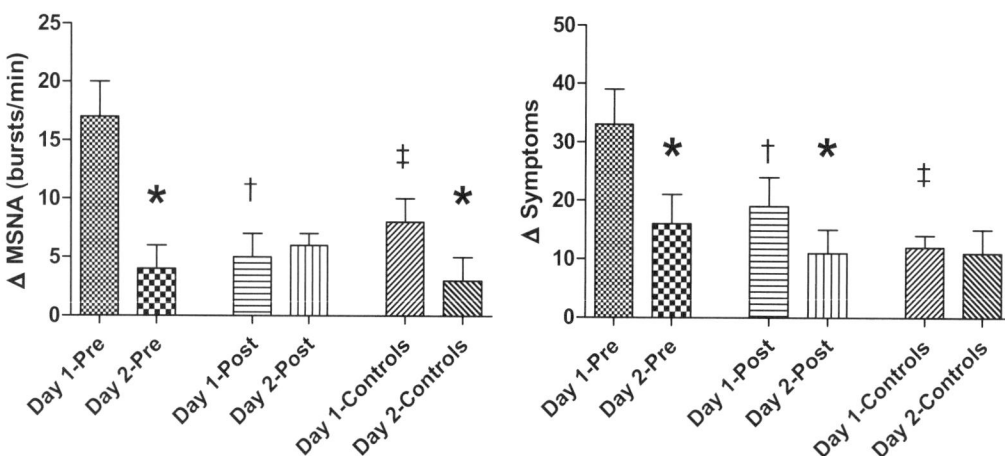

FIG. 5. Δ responses from baseline in MSNA and hypoglycemic symptom scores in the final 30 min of hypoglycemia during repeated 2-day hyperinsulinemic-hypoglycemic clamps in overnight-fasted individuals with type 2 diabetes and healthy control subjects. *Δ MSNA and symptom responses are significantly reduced ($P < 0.05$) in type 2 diabetic patients and healthy control subjects. †Δ MSNA and symptom responses are significantly reduced ($P < 0.05$) in type 2 diabetes after 6-month intensive triple oral combination anti-diabetic therapy. ‡Δ MSNA and symptom responses are significantly reduced ($P < 0.05$) in healthy control subjects compared with type 2 diabetes before intensive therapy (PRE).

TABLE 1
Self-reported blood glucose readings (<3.9 mmol/l) by patients
during 6-month intensive treatment period

	Month						Total readings <3.9 mmol/l
	1	2	3	4	5	6	
Level of hypoglycemia							
<3.3–3.9 mmol/l	12	26	27	33	26	34	158
<2.9–3.3 mmol/l	5	8	6	6	12	13	50
<2.9 mmol/l			7	3	2	2	1	15
Total episodes recorded	17	41	36	41	40	48	
Frequency per patient/month	1.1	2.7	2.4	2.7	2.7	3.2	

All 15 patients recorded episodes of hypoglycemia (<3.9 mmol/l)
during the 6-month intensive treatment period.

2). Despite equivalent glucose and insulin levels, antecedent hypoglycemia significantly blunted day 2 epinephrine
levels in preintensive therapy (day 1, 3,788 ± 414, vs. day
2, 2,191 ± 332 pmol/l; $P < 0.01$), postintensive therapy (day
1, 2,033 ± 343, vs. day 2, 1,281 ± 316 pmol/l; $P < 0.05$), and
control groups (day 1, 3,837 ± 441, vs. day 2, 1,880 ± 611
pmol/l; $P < 0.05$). Plasma glucagon levels were also
significantly blunted by antecedent hypoglycemia in preintensive therapy (day 1, 81 ± 7, vs. day 2, 49 ± 5 ng/l; $P <$
0.05), postintensive therapy (day 1, 74 ± 11, vs. day 2, 50 ±
5.2 ng/l; $P < 0.05$), and control groups (day 1, 83 ± 12, vs.
63 ± 7 ng/l; $P < 0.05$). Similarly, cortisol levels were
blunted by antecedent hypoglycemia in preintensive therapy (day 1, 801 ± 77 vs. 635 ± 75 nmol/l; $P < 0.05$),
postintensive therapy (day 1, 718 ± 72, vs. day 2, 582 ± 88
nmol/l; $P < 0.05$), and control groups (day 1, 635 ± 80, vs.
day 2, 492 ± 86 nmol/l; $P < 0.05$). Antecedent hypoglycemia did not significantly blunt day 2 growth hormone,
pancreatic polypeptide, or norepinephrine responses in
the preintensive therapy or postintensive therapy patient
studies. However, growth hormone (day 1, 7.8 ± 0.6, vs.
day 2, 3.9 ± 0.4 ng/l; $P < 0.05$) and pancreatic polypeptide
(day 1, 128 ± 26, vs. day 2, 83 ± 28 ng/l; $P < 0.05$) levels
were significantly blunted by antecedent hypoglycemia in
the control group.
Glucose kinetics. Glucose specific activity was in a
steady state at the start and final 30 min of each hypoglycemic clamp (Table 3). Antecedent hypoglycemia significantly reduced EGP during preintensive therapy (day 1,
6.6 ± 0.6, vs. day 2, 0.6 ± 1.1 μmol · kg^{-1} · min^{-1}; $P < 0.01$).
EGP was not measurable during both days of postinten-

sive therapy and control studies. Antecedent hypoglycemia resulted in greater glucose infusion rates to maintain
target glucose in preintensive therapy (day 1, 2.2 ± 1.1, vs.
day 2, 8.8 ± 1.6 μmol · kg^{-1} · min^{-1}; $P < 0.05$), postintensive
therapy (day 1, 10.5 ± 3.3, vs. day 2, 15.4 ±
2.7 μmol · kg^{-1} · min^{-1}; $P < 0.05$), and control (day 1,
16.5 ± 3.3, vs. day 2, 23.1 ± 3.9 μmol · kg^{-1} · min^{-1}; $P < 0.05$).
Intermediary metabolism. Plasma glycerol responses
were blunted ($P < 0.05$) by antecedent hypoglycemia in
preintensive therapy (day 1, 13 ± 3, vs. day 2, 3 ± 1
μmol/l), postintensive therapy (day 1, −2 ± 1, vs. day 2,
−18 ± 3 μmol/l), and control studies (day 1, −22 ± 3, vs.
day 2, −41 ± 4 μmol/l). Similarly, plasma lactate levels
were also blunted ($P < 0.05$) by day 1 hypoglycemia in
preintensive therapy (day 1, 1.95 ± 0.2, vs. day 2, 1.31 ±
0.2 mmol/l), postintensive therapy (day 1, 1.5 ± 0.22, vs.
day 2, 1.2 ± 0.1 mmol/l), and control (day 1, 1.6 ± 0.1, vs.
day 2, 1.4 ± 0.1 mmol/l).
MSNA. Day 1 hypoglycemia reduced MSNA responses
during day 2 hypoglycemia in preintensive therapy (17 ± 3
vs. 4 ± 2 bursts/min; $P < 0.05$) and in control (8 ± 2 vs. 3 ±
2 bursts/min; $P < 0.05$, respectively). MSNA responses
during day 1 hypoglycemia in postintensive therapy were
significantly blunted by intensive treatment and did not
decline further during day 2 hypoglycemia (5 ± 2 vs. 6 ±
1 bursts/min).
Hypoglycemia symptoms. Day 1 hypoglycemia reduced
symptom responses ($P < 0.05$) during day 2 hypoglycemia
in preintensive therapy 33 ± 6 vs. 16 ± 5) and postintensive therapy (19 ± 4 vs. 10 ± 3). Symptoms were unchanged during day 1 and day 2 hypoglycemia in control
(12 ± 2 vs. 11 ± 4). Day 1 hypoglycemia blunted ($P < 0.05$)
both autonomic (18 ± 3 vs. 9 ± 4) and neuroglycopenic
(15 ± 4 vs. 7 ± 2) scores during day 2 hypoglycemia in
preintensive therapy. In postintensive therapy, day 1 hypoglycemia predominantly blunted day 2 neuroglycopenic
symptoms (7 ± 2 vs. 3 ± 2).
Cardiovascular responses. Blood pressure and heart
rate responses were similar during day 1 and day 2
hypoglycemia in all groups.

DISCUSSION

This study has prospectively determined the effects of
6-month intensive triple combination oral therapy with
improvement of A1C to 6.7% on integrated counterregulatory responses during repeated hypoglycemia in a group of
patients with type 2 diabetes. Our results demonstrate that
intensive treatment with oral combination therapy substantially reduces ANS and metabolic (EGP, lipolysis)

TABLE 2
Baseline neuroendocrine hormone levels at the start of day 1 and day 2 hyperinsulinemic-hypoglycemic clamps in healthy individuals
(control) and patients with type 2 diabetes preintensive therapy and postintensive therapy

	Type 2 diabetes				Healthy individuals	
	Preintensive therapy		Postintensive therapy		Control	
	Day 1	Day 2	Day 1	Day 2	Day 1	Day 2
Epinephrine (pg/ml)	278 ± 82	180 ± 38	202 ± 44	218 ± 33	223 ± 48	184 ± 48
Norepinephrine (pg/ml)	1.07 ± 0.15	1.0 ± 0.14	0.9 ± 0.2	0.9 ± 0.18	0.7 ± 0.2	1.17 ± 0.26
Glucagon (ng/l)	54 ± 5	45 ± 5	48 ± 3	46 ± 4	48 ± 8	47 ± 6
Growth hormone (μg/l)	2 ± 1	2 ± 0.5	1 ± 0.5	1.5 ± 0.5	1 ± 0.3	1 ± 0.2
Cortisol (pmol/l)	345 ± 61	248 ± 69	248 ± 55	237 ± 44	254 ± 43	235 ± 58
Pancreatic polypeptide (pmol/l)	48 ± 19	31 ± 9	30 ± 9	29 ± 8	28 ± 8	25 ± 7

Data are means ± SE.

TABLE 3
Glucose specific activity (dpm/mmol) during the basal period and the final 30 min of day 1 and day 2 hyperinsulinemic-hypoglycemic clamps in healthy individuals (control) and patients with type 2 diabetes preintensive therapy and postintensive therapy

	100 min	110 min	120 min	210 min	225 min	240 min
Preintensive therapy type 2 diabetes						
Day 1	286 ± 33	283 ± 31	279 ± 27	310 ± 27	314 ± 26	306 ± 25
Day 2	299 ± 40	300 ± 35	305 ± 36	303 ± 21	295 ± 21	304 ± 22
Postintensive therapy type 2 diabetes						
Day 1	257 ± 51	266 ± 51	265 ± 50	290 ± 41	288 ± 43	290 ± 42
Day 2	330 ± 27	329 ± 26	325 ± 26	332 ± 20	336 ± 20	326 ± 20
Control						
Day 1	373 ± 30	374 ± 30	374 ± 29	306 ± 26	320 ± 29	312 ± 33
Day 2	370 ± 30	375 ± 36	363 ± 33	308 ± 34	295 ± 39	294 ± 38

Data are means ± SE.

symptoms and cardiovascular responses to hypoglycemia. Additionally, antecedent hypoglycemia can produce further widespread (i.e., neuroendocrine) reductions in the above physiological counterregulatory mechanisms in type 2 diabetic patients both before and after intensive therapy.

Three recent large multicentered trials have examined the effects of intensive glucose control with an average A1C <7.0% on macro- and microvascular complications in type 2 diabetes (9–11). All three studies identified an increased prevalence of hypoglycemia with lowering of A1C in type 2 diabetes (9–11). To date, there are no published prospective studies examining the effects of intensive glucose control (i.e., A1C <7.0%) on physiological responses to hypoglycemia in type 2 diabetes. Our study demonstrates that achieving an A1C of 6.7% with triple oral therapy (glipizide XL, metformin, and acarbose) for 6 months in the absence of exogenous insulin therapy can significantly reduce neuroendocrine, metabolic, and ANS responses to hypoglycemia. Furthermore, repeated episodes of relatively mild hypoglycemia (3.3 mmol/l) can further significantly reduce counterregulatory responses in type 2 diabetic patients, thus creating a syndrome of hypoglycemia-associated autonomic failure that occurs irrespective of moderate or tight glycemic control.

The patients in the present study were diagnosed with type 2 diabetes for a mean of 6 ± 2 years, which was similar to Spyer et al. (15) and Israelian et al. (17) but of a shorter duration than other recent studies investigating counterregulatory responses to hypoglycemia in type 2 diabetes (12–14,16). Thus, the present results provide data in a group of more recently diagnosed individuals whom may be predicted to benefit most from rigorous metabolic control. Additionally, it should be noted that the results in this present study are applicable to a group of patients whom underwent a period of significant glycemic control with a specific triple oral therapy and lifestyle change regimen. Thus, we cannot determine whether other therapeutic regimens (i.e., with insulin, thiazolidinediones, and/or agents that increase GLP-1 axis activity) would have produced similar results. Intensive therapy in this study had marked effects on blunting ANS responses to hypoglycemia. The key counterregulatory hormone epinephrine was reduced by ~50%. Similarly MSNA was reduced by ~66%, and hypoglycemic symptom scores were blunted by ~40%. Additionally, blood pressure and heart rate responses were also significantly blunted by intensive therapy. The above results demonstrate that central sensing of hypoglycemia combined with end-organ responses were both reduced by intensive therapy. The

reduced sympathetic nervous system activity also affected important metabolic counterregulatory mechanisms during hypoglycemia after intensive therapy. EGP was not measurable and lipolysis (NEFA, glycerol) together with glycogenolysis (lactate) were reduced by ~30% after intensive therapy. However, it should be noted that with the exception of epinephrine (which was lower during postintensive therapy compared with control), intensive therapy reduced the exaggerated counterregulatory responses observed in the preintensive therapy patients to the usual physiological responses observed in the control subjects. Additionally, we would like to point out that the above metabolic findings may have been caused by a combination of reduced ANS input and improvement in glucotoxicity/insulin sensitivity (32,33). We did not identify any effects of intensive therapy to significantly blunt other neuroendocrine responses (glucagon, cortisol, growth hormone, norepinephrine, and pancreatic polypeptide). With the exception of cortisol, levels of the above neuroendocrine hormones were not different from age- and BMI-matched nondiabetic individuals. Spyer et al. (15) also reported similar findings in a group of type 2 diabetes with an A1C of 7.4%. However, Israelian et al. (17) reported that both glucagon and growth hormone responses were blunted during similar hypoglycemic conditions to this study in type 2 diabetic subjects. The fact that the blunting effects of intensive therapy on counterregulatory responses in this study were confined almost exclusively to the sympathetic nervous system is different to the situation in type 1 diabetes where intensive therapy has been reported to result in a more widespread blunting of neuroendocrine responses during hypoglycemia (34). The reasons for the targeted effects on the sympathetic nervous system are not apparent from the present study. Previous work (13,14) has determined that the threshold for counterregulatory hormone release in type 2 diabetes remain elevated, even during relatively good glycemic control (A1C 7.4%). Thus, we believe that it is unlikely that the depth of hypoglycemia in our study (3.3 mmol/l) could have mitigated against finding a difference in neuroendocrine responses after intensive therapy. In addition, the magnitude of the neuroendocrine responses was sufficiently robust to have been able to determine a difference if one had been present. However, we cannot exclude the possibility that deeper hypoglycemia may have provoked a more widespread difference in maximal neuroendocrine responses between the preintensive therapy and postintensive therapy treatment groups (13,14).

The second part of our study addressed a possible mechanism for our findings of reduced counterregulatory mechanisms during hypoglycemia after intensive therapy. We tested the hypothesis that antecedent hypoglycemia was a mechanism responsible for acquired counterregulatory failure during hypoglycemia in type 2 diabetes. Self-reported blood glucose monitoring of four to six times per day had demonstrated an aggregate frequency of hypoglycemia of 36–48 episodes per month or up to 3.2 events per patient a month. More than 95% of these episodes were in the range of 2.8–3.9 mmol/l. Although this level of hypoglycemia is often considered "mild" in clinical practice, these present results clearly demonstrate the profound blunting effects of a plasma glucose of 3.3 mmol/l on subsequent physiological responses to hypoglycemia. Epinephrine and symptom responses were blunted by antecedent hypoglycemia in both preintensive therapy and postintensive therapy studies. Of note, despite equivalent insulinemia and glycemia, antecedent hypoglycemia blunted the fall of C-peptide during day 2 hypoglycemia in both preintensive therapy and postintensive therapy studies. This obviously causes some concern because suppression of endogenous insulin during hypoglycemia is a primary physiological counterregulatory defense. MSNA was substantially reduced during day 2 hypoglycemia in preintensive therapy. However, due to the inherent blunting effects of intensive therapy, MSNA was substantially suppressed during day 1 hypoglycemia in postintensive therapy and was not further reduced during day 2 hypoglycemia.

Cortisol and glucagon responses were significantly reduced by antecedent hypoglycemia in both preintensive therapy and postintensive therapy studies. In addition to the above, growth hormone and pancreatic polypeptide (a marker of parasympathetic activity) were both blunted by antecedent hypoglycemia in nondiabetic control studies. Our present findings extend the elegant studies of Segel et al. (16) whom also described blunting of ANS and neuroendocrine responses after antecedent hypoglycemia in longer duration, moderately controlled (A1C 8.6 ± 1.1%) type 2 diabetic patients. The widespread reduction of ANS and neuroendocrine responses after day 1 hypoglycemia also led to significant blunting of metabolic counterregulatory mechanisms (glucose kinetics, lipolysis, and glycogenolysis) in both preintensive therapy and postintensive therapy studies. As discussed, type 2 diabetic patients typically have higher thresholds (i.e., increased plasma glucose values) for counterregulatory defenses against hypoglycemia (7). This is an important protective mechanism that serves to reduce hypoglycemia in type 2 diabetes. The findings of increased MSNA, cortisol, and symptom scores coupled with elevated EGP, lipolysis, and glycogenolysis in preintensive therapy compared with the nondiabetic control subjects are consistent with higher plasma glucose thresholds and/or glucotoxicity providing added protection against hypoglycemia in these individuals. Thus, the finding that antecedent hypoglycemia and intensive glucose control reduced counterregulatory defenses (e.g., symptoms, EGP, and MSNA) back down to normal control values indicates that the risk for iatrogenic hypoglycemia had been increased as important physiological protective mechanisms against hypoglycemia had been removed in these type 2 diabetic patients.

A limitation of this study was that cognitive function was not formally assessed during our repeat hypoglycemia studies before and after intensive therapy. We did not identify any gross changes in cognitive function within our type 2 diabetic patients or healthy control subjects during any of our hypoglycemia studies. Whether this indicates that cognitive function is relatively preserved during repeated hypoglycemia and intensive therapy or that more sophisticated methodology is needed to detect differences in cognitive function will require further study.

In summary, this present study has demonstrated that 6-month intensive glycemic control with triple oral combination therapy to near-normal A1C levels can result in substantial reductions of epinephrine responses during hypoglycemia in individuals with type 2 diabetes. In addition, the exaggerated neuroendocrine, ANS, and metabolic counterregulatory responses that were present in the preintensive therapy group (and thus acting as increased defenses against hypoglycemia) were reduced to levels similar to the nondiabetic control group. Near normalization of A1C resulted in an increased frequency of ~3.0 hypoglycemic episodes per patient month by study end. Our results clearly demonstrate that antecedent hypoglycemia can also induce ANS, neuroendocrine, and metabolic counterregulatory failure in type 2 diabetic patients with either elevated or near-normal glycemic control. Furthermore, the combination of repeated hypoglycemia and intensive glycemic control produces additive effects to further reduce physiological defenses against subsequent hypoglycemia. Therefore, we would conclude that antecedent hypoglycemia appears to be the likely cause of the blunted sympathoadrenal counterregulatory responses occurring during hypoglycemia after intensive treatment in our type 2 diabetic patients. Additionally, even relatively mild hypoglycemia (3.3 ± 0.1 mmol/l) can produce significant blunting of subsequent counterregulatory mechanisms in type 2 diabetes and increase the risk for future hypoglycemia. This further reinforces the therapeutic goal of achieving good glycemic control while minimizing the occurrence of any hypoglycemia.

ACKNOWLEDGMENTS

This work was supported in part by National Institutes of Health Grants R01-DK-069803, M01-RR-000095, P01-HL-056693, and P60-DK-020593 and by an award from the Juvenile Foundation Research Foundation International/Veterans Affairs

No potential conflicts of interest relevant to this article were reported.

We are thankful for the expert technical assistance of Eric Allen, Pam Venson, and Wanda Snead. We also thank the nursing staff of the Vanderbilt GCRC, Caroll Moffat, Linda Balch, and Jerri Brown for superb dietary and diabetes management of our patients.

REFERENCES

1. Diabetes Control and Complication Trial Research Group: The effect of intensive treatment of diabetes on the development and progression of long-term complications in insulin-dependent diabetes mellitus. *N Engl J Med* 329:977–986, 1993
2. U.K. Prospective Study Group: Intensive blood-glucose control with sulfonylureas or insulin compared with conventional treatment and risk of complications in patients with type 2 diabetes (UKPDS). *Lancet* 352:837–853, 1998
3. American Diabetes Association: Standards of medical care in diabetes. *Diabetes Care* 31:S3–S78, 2008
4. Diabetes Control and Complications Trial Research Group: Epidemiology of severe hypoglycemia in the Diabetes Control and Complications Trial. *Am J Med* 90:450–459, 1991
5. Diabetes Control and Complications Trial (DCCT) Research Group: Hypoglycemia in the Diabetes Control and Complications Trial. *Diabetes* 46:271–286, 1997

6. Gabriely I, Shamoon H: Hypoglycemia in diabetes: common, often unrecognized. *Cleveland Clin J Med* 71:335–342, 2004

7. Briscoe VJ, Davis SN: Hypoglycemia in type 1 and type 2 diabetes: physiology, pathophysiology and management. *Clinical Diabetes* 24:115–121, 2006

8. Briscoe VJ, Davis SN: *Hypoglycemia in Type 1 Diabetes in Adults: Principles and Practice.* Jabbour S, Stephens E, Hirsch I, Goldstein B, Garg S, Riddle M, Eds. New York, Taylor 7 Francis Informa, 2008

9. Gerstein HC, Pogue J, Mann JF, Lonn E, Dagenais GR, McQueen M, Yusuf S, HOPE Investigators: The relationship between dysglycaemia and cardiovascular and renal risk in diabetic and non-diabetic participants in the HOPE study: a prospective epidemiological analysis. *Diabetologia* 48:1749–1755, 2005

10. Action to Control Cardiovascular Risk in Diabetes Study Group: Effects of intensive glucose lowering in type 2 diabetes. *N Engl J Med* 358:2545–2559, 2008

11. ADVANCE Collaborative Group: Intensive blood glucose control and vascular outcomes in patients with type 2 diabetes. *N Engl J Med* 358:2560–2572, 2008

12. Burge MR, Sobhy TA, Qualls CR, Schade DS: Effect of short-term glucose control on glycemic thresholds for epinephrine and hypoglycemic symptoms. *J Clin Endocrinol Metabol* 86:5471–5478, 2001

13. Levy CJ, Kinsley BT, Bajaj A, Simonson DC: Effect of glycemic control on glucose counterregulation during hypoglycemia in NIDDM. *Diabetes Care* 21:1330–1338, 1998

14. Korzon-Burakowska A, Hopkins D, Matyka K, Lomas J, Pernet A, Macdonald I, Amiel S: Effects of glycemic control on protective responses against hypoglycemia in type 2 diabetes. *Diabetes Care* 21:283–290, 1998

15. Spyer G, Hattersley AT, MacDonald IA, Amiel S, MacLeod KM: Hypoglycaemic counter-regulation at normal blood glucose concentrations in patients with well controlled type-2 diabetes. *Lancet* 365:1970–1974, 2000

16. Segel SA, Peramore DS, Cryer PE: Hypoglycemia-associated autonomic failure in advanced type 2 diabetes. *Diabetes* 51:724–733, 2002

17. Israelian Z, Szoke E, Woerle J, Bokhari S, Shorr M, Schwenke D, Cryer PE, Gerich J, Meyer C: Multiple defects in counterregulation of hypoglycemia in modestly advanced type 2 diabetes mellitus. *Metabolism* 55:593–598, 2006

18. Abumrad NN, Rabin D, Diamond MC, Lacy WW: Use of a heated superficial hand vein as an alternative site for measurement of amino acid concentration and for the study of glucose and alanine kinetics in man. *Metabolism* 30:936–940, 1981

19. DeFronzo R, Tobin K, Andres R: Glucose clamp technique: a method for quantifying insulin secretion and resistance. *Am J Physiol* 237:E216–E223, 1979

20. Amiel SA, Tambolane WV, Simonson DC, Sherwin R: Defective glucose counterregulation after strict control of insulin-dependent diabetes mellitus. *N Engl J Med* 316:1376–1383, 1987

21. Wallin BG, Sundlof G, Eriksson BM, Dominiak P, Grobecker H, Lindblad LE: Plasma noradrenaline correlates to sympathetic muscle nerve activity in normotensive man. *Acta Physiol Scand* 111:69–73, 1981

22. Sandoval DA, Ertl AC, Richardson MA, Tate DB, Davis SN: Estrogen blunts neuroendocrine and metabolic responses to hypoglycemia. *Diabetes* 52:1749–1755, 2003

23. Wall JS, Steele R, Debodo RD, Altszuler N: Effect of insulin on utilization and production of circulating glucose. *Am J Physiol* 189:43–50, 1957

24. Aguilar-Parada E, Eisentraut AM, Unger RH: Pancreatic glucagon secretion in normal and diabetic subjects. *Am J Med Sci* 257:415–419, 1969

25. Wide L, Porath J: Radioimmunoassay of proteins with the uses of sephadex-coupled antibodies. *Biochim Biophys Acta* 130:257–260, 1966

26. Causon R, Caruthers M, Rodnight R: Assay of plasma catecholamines by liquid chromatography with electrochemical detection. *Anal Biochem* 116:223–226, 1982

27. Hunter W, Greenwood F: Preparation of [^{131}I]-labeled human growth hormone of high specific activity. *Nature* 194:495–496, 1962

28. Hagopian W, Lever E, Cen D, Emmonoud D, Polonsky K, Pugh W, Moosa A, Jaspan J: Predominance of renal and absence of hepatic metabolism of pancreatic polypeptide in the dog. *Am J Physiol* 245:171–177, 1983

29. Lloyd B, Burrin J, Smythe P, Alberti KGMM: Enzymatic fluorometric continuous flow assays for blood glucose, lactate, pyruvate, alanine, glycerol and 2-hydroxybutyrate. *Clin Chem* 24:1724–1729, 1978

30. Ho RJ: Radiochemical assay of long chain fatty acids using ^{63}NI as tracer. *Anal Biochem* 26:105–113, 1970

31. Deary L, Hepburn D, Macleod K, Frier BM: Partitioning the symptoms of hypoglycemia using multi-sample confirmatory factor analysis. *Diabetologia* 36:771–770, 1993

32. Hawkins M, Gabriely L, Wozniak R, Reddy K, Rossetti L, Shamoon H: Glycemic control determines hepatic and peripheral glucose effectiveness in type 2 diabetic subjects. *Diabetes* 51:2179–2189, 2002

33. Donath MY, Schumann DM, Faulenback M, Ellingsgaard H, Perren A, Ehses JA: Islet inflammation in type 2 diabetes: from metabolic stress to therapy. *Diabetes Care* 31:S161–S164, 2008

34. Davis MR, Mellman M, Shamoon H: Further defects in counterregulatory response induced by recurrent hypoglycemia in IDDM. *Diabetes* 41:1335–1340, 1992

Type 1 Diabetic Drivers With and Without a History of Recurrent Hypoglycemia-Related Driving Mishaps

Physiological and performance differences during euglycemia and the induction of hypoglycemia

Daniel J. Cox, PhD[1]
Boris P. Kovatchev, PhD[1]
Stacey M. Anderson, MD[2]

William L. Clarke, MD[3]
Linda A. Gonder-Frederick, PhD[1]

OBJECTIVE — Collisions are more common among drivers with type 1 diabetes than among their nondiabetic spouses. This increased risk appears to be attributable to a subgroup of drivers with type 1 diabetes. The hypothesis tested is that this vulnerable subgroup is more at risk for hypoglycemia and its disruptive effects on driving.

RESEARCH DESIGN AND METHODS — Thirty-eight drivers with type 1 diabetes, 16 with (+history) and 22 without (−history) a recent history of recurrent hypoglycemia-related driving mishaps, drove a virtual reality driving simulator and watched a videotape of someone driving a simulator for 30-min periods. Driving and video testing occurred in a double-blind, randomized, crossover manner during euglycemia (5.5 mmol/l) and progressive hypoglycemia (3.9–2.5 mmol/l). Examiners were blind to which subjects were +/−history, whereas subjects were blind to their blood glucose levels and targets.

RESULTS — During euglycemia, +history participants reported more autonomic and neuroglycopenic symptoms ($P \leq 0.01$) and tended to require more dextrose infusion to maintain euglycemia with the same insulin infusion ($P < 0.09$). During progressive hypoglycemia, these subjects demonstrated less epinephrine release ($P = 0.02$) and greater driving impairments ($P = 0.03$).

CONCLUSIONS — Findings support the speculation that there is a subgroup of type 1 diabetic drivers more vulnerable to experiencing hypoglycemia-related driving mishaps. This increased vulnerability may be due to more symptom "noise" (more symptoms during euglycemia), making it harder to detect hypoglycemia while driving; possibly greater carbohydrate utilization, rendering them more vulnerable to experiencing hypoglycemia; less hormonal counterregulation, leading to more profound hypoglycemia; and more neuroglycopenia, rendering them more vulnerable to impaired driving.

Diabetes Care 33:2430–2435, 2010

W orldwide driving collisions account for 1.2 million fatalities and 50 million injuries annually (1). Drivers with type 1 diabetes have more driving mishaps (2). In both Europe and the U.S. type 1 diabetic drivers have been found to have more than twice as many collisions as their nondiabetic spouses (3) possibly because mild hypoglycemia significantly affects cognitive-motor functioning in general (4–6) and the cognitive-motor skills relevant to driving a car in particular (7,8). Severe hypoglycemia precludes safe driving and can contribute to vehicular fatalities (9). Further, mild hypoglycemia can impair judgment as to whether or not to drive (10,11).

Just as some individuals with type 1 diabetes are more vulnerable to experiencing severe hypoglycemia (12), some individuals may be more vulnerable to hypoglycemia-related driving mishaps. This speculation is supported by the U.S.-European survey (3) in which only 27% of the type 1 diabetic drivers reported vehicular collisions in the previous 2 years (3) and a prospective study in which only 22% of the sample reported a collision during the 12-month observation (13). In a previous study of hypoglycemia and driving, we conducted post hoc analyses comparing individuals with a recent history of no driving mishaps versus individuals with a history of multiple driving mishaps (14). Those with a +history were more likely to be female ($P = 0.02$), tended to demonstrate greater carbohydrate utilization ($P = 0.07$) and less epinephrine release ($P = 0.11$), and drove significantly worse during hypoglycemia ($P = 0.01$) (14). The present study was an a priori hypothesis-testing replication comparing subjects with or without a recent history of recurrent hypoglycemia-related driving mishaps, using a similar methodology, to test whether +history type 1 diabetic drivers were *1*) more vulnerable to experiencing hypoglycemia through greater carbohydrate utilization, *2*) more likely to be female, *3*) more vulnerable to progressive hypoglycemia because of a smaller counterregulatory epinephrine response, *4*) less aware of hypoglycemia due to fewer symptoms (autonomic and neuroglycopenic) during hypoglycemia, and *5*) more impaired while driving during hypoglycemia.

RESEARCH DESIGN AND METHODS — Forty-two adults with type 1 diabetes were recruited through regional advertisements. Inclusion criteria

From the [1]Department of Psychiatry and Neurobehavioral Sciences, University of Virginia Health Sciences Center, Charlottesville, Virginia; the [2]Department of Medicine, University of Virginia Health Sciences Center, Charlottesville, Virginia; and the [3]Department of Pediatrics, University of Virginia Health Sciences Center, Charlottesville, Virginia.
Corresponding author: Daniel J. Cox, djc4f@virginia.edu.
Received 19 November 2009 and accepted 3 August 2010. Published ahead of print at http://care.diabetesjournals.org on 19 August 2010. DOI: 10.2337/dc09-2130.

were that subjects *1*) had type 1 diabetes for at least 1 year, *2*) were between the ages of 21 and 70, *3*) drove a minimum of 6,000 miles a year, and *4*) either reported no driving mishaps (no collisions, citations, or automatic driving where they drove from point A to B with no recollection or someone else took over control of the vehicle due to hypoglycemia) in the past 12 months (−history group) or reported at least two such mishaps in the past 12 months (+history group). Further, because we were going to expose subjects to hypoglycemia (~2.2 mmol/l) through insulin infusion and take frequent blood samples, we excluded subjects with hematocrit <38% for men or <36% for women, the presence of an electronic pacemaker or >5% atrial or ventricular ectopy, and pregnant females. Four subjects prematurely discontinued testing: three had insufficient intravenous access for the hyperinsulinemic clamp procedure and one experienced lower extremity muscle twitching resulting from acute or chronic hypomagnesemia. The resulting sample of 38 participants had a mean age of 42.5 ± 12 years (median 42 years, range 21–66 years), disease duration of 21.6 ± 9.4 years (median 20 years, range 1–52 years), and A1C of 7.4 ± 0.8%. As illustrated in Table 1, the +/−history groups did not differ on any diabetes, hypoglycemia, or driving parameters other than +history subjects reported more episodes of severe hypoglycemia and driving mishaps in the previous 12 months.

Procedure

After signing an institutional review board–approved consent form, participants completed an outpatient screening evaluation including a medical history, physical examination, 12-lead electrocardiogram, and laboratory evaluation with A1C, complete blood count, and a comprehensive metabolic panel. They were also introduced to and rehearsed using the simulator.

For the 48 h before admission, subjects were instructed to avoid hypoglycemia by reducing total insulin by 10%, routinely testing blood glucose five times a day, and eating prophylactically 10 g of carbohydrates when blood glucose fell to <5.5 mmol/l. Intermediate and long-acting insulins were discontinued 24 and 36 h before hospitalization, respectively. During this preadmission period and hospital admission, only short- and rapid-acting insulins were used.

Table 1—*Subjects' descriptive characteristics*

Variables	−History	+History	*P* value
N	22	16	
Age (years)	42 ± 12.9	42 ± 12.8	NS
Sex (% female)	34% (7)	62% (10)	NS
Education/year	15 ± 2.6	16 ± 2.2	NS
A1C	7.1 ± 0.8	7.5 ± 0.9	NS
Diabetes duration (years)	21 ± 9.4	21 ± 10.8	NS
Insulin (units/day)	42 ± 15.5	42 ± 32.3	NS
BMI	27 ± 5.2	26 ± 4.2	Ns
Hypoglycemia awareness*	82% (18)	75% (12)	NS
Severe hypoglycemia† in past 12 months	0.5 ± 0.7	1.6 ± 2.2	<0.03
Subjective neuropathy	23% (5)	44% (7)	NS
Objective neuropathy	9% (2)	19% (3)	NS
Retinopathy	41% (9)	25% (4)	NS
Laser eye therapy	4% (1)	12% (2)	NS
Driving experience (years)	27	27	NS
Miles driven per year	18.5714 ± 12.040	17.7308 ± 16.133	NS
Self-monitored blood glucose before driving‡	1.3	1.7	NS
Fast-acting sugar in car‡	2.0	3.0	NS
No. mild hypoglycemia while driving in past 6 months	0.7	1.1	NS
No. driving mishaps in past 12 months	0	2.8	0.0001
Hypoglycemic nadir (mmol/l)	2.7 ± 0.9	2.6 ± 0.3	
Peak epinephrine during hypoglycemia	345 ± 178	217 ± 137	0.05
Self-treatment during hypoglycemic drive	59% (13)	44% (7)	NS

Data are means ± SD or % (*n*) unless otherwise indicated. *Hypoglycemia awareness was defined using the criteria reported by Clarke et al. (25). †Diabetes Control and Complications Trial criteria for severe hypoglycemia was used, i.e., episodes where individual was unable to treat himself or herself, either because he or she was stuporous, was unconscious, or had a seizure. ‡Mean rating on a scale where 1 is always, 2 is frequently, 3 is seldom, and 4 is never.

Subjects were admitted to the University of Virginia General Clinical Research Center at 4:00 P.M. on the evening before the hyperinsulinemic clamping procedure. Subjects were instructed on and given time to again practice driving the simulator and rating nine common symptoms of hypoglycemia on a 0–6 scale into a hand-held computer. Subjects were then provided with a standardized (50% carbohydrate, 20% protein, and 30% fat) eucaloric, caffeine-free meal at 6:00 P.M. and a bedtime snack at 9:00 P.M. Subjects were allowed glucose-free, caffeine-free drinks throughout the evening and retired at 11:00 P.M. Subjects were not allowed to eat any additional food during hospitalization other than that provided by the General Clinical Research Center or that required to treat blood glucose <5.5 mmol/l. Two intravenous lines were placed in the nondominant hand and arm for overnight infusion of insulin and hourly blood sampling to maintain glucose between 5.6 and 8.3 mmol/l.

On the first morning of testing, subjects were awakened at ~7:00 A.M. and given time to freshen up. They remained fasting until after the study procedures were completed. Immediately before testing, an additional retrograde hand intravenous line was inserted. Activated charcoal packets were affixed over this intravenous area for arterialized sampling of blood glucose every 5 min and epinephrine every 10 min (15). Euglycemia, with a plasma glucose goal of 6.1 mmol/l (110 mg/dl), was achieved and maintained using variable 20% dextrose infusion (16). After glucose and insulin stabilization, subjects performed 30 min of testing. Subsequently, dextrose infusion was slowed or discontinued to ensure a steady descent into hypoglycemia at a blood glucose rate of fall of 0.055 mmol/l/min. Progressive hypoglycemia testing began when blood glucose reached 3.9 mmol/l (70 mg/dl) and ended 30 min later at a blood glucose nadir of 2.5 mmol/l (45 mg/dl) (16). Progressive hypoglycemia,

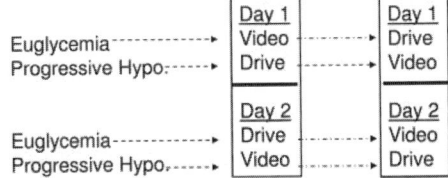

Figure 1—*Randomized, crossover design controlling for practice and antecedent hypoglycemia effects influencing condition effects. Hx, history; Hypo, hypoglycemia.*

rather than the traditional hypoglycemia clamp (4,5), was used because it was thought to be more similar to real-world conditions. Euglycemia testing always preceded hypoglycemia testing to avoid the affect of any lingering neuroglycopenia on performance during euglycemia. The same procedures were followed on the second day of testing. Testing was done on 2 consecutive days to avoid losing subjects due to rescheduling a second hospitalization. Figure 1 depicts the randomized crossover research design. Hypoglycemic driving was equally as likely to occur on day 1 or 2 among +/−hypoglycemia subjects, thus negating any antecedent hypoglycemia or practice effect having an impact on a group effect.

During the testing periods, subjects either drove the simulator or sat in the simulator and watched a videotape of someone else driving a simulator. At 0, 10, 20, and 30 min into testing, subjects rated four autonomic symptoms (sweatiness, pounding heart, jittery/tension, and trembling) and five neuroglycopenic symptoms (uncoordination, visual difficulty, lightheadedness, difficulty concentrating, and confusion) on a 0 (not at all) to 6 (extremely) scale. If subjects believed they were experiencing low blood glucose any time during testing they were instructed to self-treat with an orange drink (sugar-free placebo).

Subjects were told their blood glucose was going to be raised and lowered for testing throughout the study but were kept blind to their actual blood glucose and targeted blood glucose levels. Researchers conducting the testing were kept blind to whether subjects had or did not have a recent history of hypoglycemia-related driving mishaps.

The Atari Research Driving Simulator is an interactive, fixed-platform, virtual reality simulator that generates reliable, accurate, sensitive, and valid driving performance data (7,8,17–21). The simulator has three 25-inch computer screens that provide a 160° visual field, along with a programmed rearview mirror depicting rear traffic. The driving environment is realistic, incorporating a typical-sized steering wheel, gas and brake pedals, seat, and seat belt. Driving performance feedback is provided visually through the three screens that update at a rate of 60 times/s, audibly through quadraphonic speakers delivering engine, tire, and road noises, and kinesthetically through forced feedback from the steering wheel and pedal pressure. The simulator records three steering variables (SD of lane position, driving off road, and veering across the midline), three braking variables (inappropriate braking while on the open road, missed stopped signals, and collisions), and four speed control variables (exceeding speed limit, SD of speed, time at stop sign deciding when to turn left, and time to execute a left turn).

Outcome variables
With use of the algorithm of DeFronzo et al. (22), an individual's metabolic demand was determined and reported as glucose utilization rates in milligrams per kilogram per minute. Plasma epinephrine was measured using a single isotope derivative method (15).

As in previous studies that discriminated high-risk subjects and predicted future driving collisions (7,8,14,17–21), 32 we generated and analyzed a composite impaired driving score (IDS) to compare the various aspects of driving poorly. To compute the IDS, a subject's performance on each variable (e.g., SD of speed) was converted into a z score based on all subjects' performances on that variable during euglycemia and hypoglycemia. The z scores for all variables were then summed for each subject from each test drive, generating the IDS. Thus, an IDS of 0 represents average driving, an IDS <0 represents better than average driving (e.g., an IDS of −1 represents driving performance 1 SD per variable better than average), and an IDS >0 represents worse than average driving.

To evaluate whether +history subjects differed from −history subjects across euglycemia and hypoglycemia, two between (group) × two within (conditions) repeated-measures ANCOVAs were performed, with subject's average blood glucose for that condition used as the covariate.

RESULTS

Carbohydrate utilization
+History subjects demonstrated a trend toward greater carbohydrate utilization (F = 3.064, P = 0.089,). +History subjects demonstrated 16.1% greater carbohydrate utilization to maintain euglycemia than −History subjects.

Driving performance
Although +history subjects drove just as well as −history subjects during euglycemia, they demonstrated a marked impairment in performance during progressive hypoglycemia (group × condition F = 5.0, P = 0.03). As illustrated in Fig. 2, +history subjects' driving performance worsened almost 2.5 SDs from euglycemia to hypoglycemia, whereas −history subjects demonstrated no driving impairment, driving slightly (but not significantly) better during hypoglycemia.

Epinephrine response
Peak epinephrine released was greater during hypoglycemia than during the euglycemic condition (condition F = 57.35, P < 0.0001), and +history subjects released less epinephrine during hypoglycemia (group × condition F = 6.05, P = 0.02). However, post hoc analyses of peak epinephrine response during hypoglycemia (sex × group F = 2.938, P = 0.097) indicates that this reduced epinephrine response by +history subjects was primarily due to women, with mean peak epinephrine levels for male and female −history and male +history subjects of 382, 329, and 316 pg/ml, respectively, but 168 pg/ml for female +history subjects.

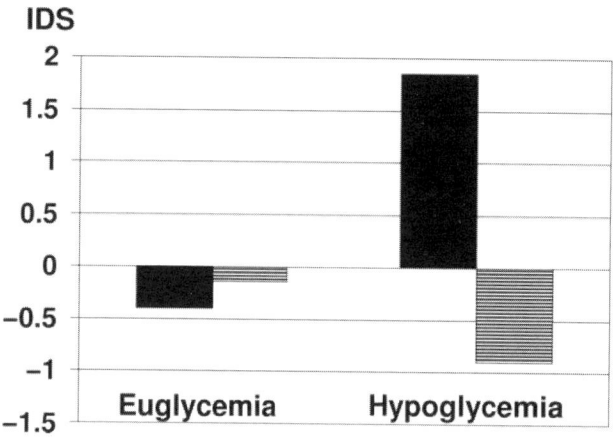

Figure 2—*IDS during euglycemic and hypoglycemic conditions for +/−history subjects.* ■, *+history;* ▤, *−history.*

Symptom perception

+History subjects reported more autonomic symptoms than −history subjects ($F = 7.79$, $P = 0.009$) with a near significant interaction ($F = 3.95$, $P = 0.055$). As seen in Fig. 3, +history subjects tended to report more symptoms during euglycemia than during hypoglycemia, whereas −history subjects demonstrated the anticipated increase in autonomic symptoms during hypoglycemia. Neuroglycopenic symptoms followed a similar pattern: +history subjects tended to report more neuroglycopenic symptoms than −history subjects (group $F = 2.9$, $P = 0.09$), with a significant interaction ($F = 4.00$, $P = 0.05$). Figure 3 illustrates that +history subjects reported more neuroglycopenic symptoms during euglycemia than during hypoglycemia, whereas −history subjects demonstrated the anticipated increase in perceived neuroglycopenic symptoms with hypoglycemia. Contrasts indicated that +history subjects reported more autonomic ($P <$ 0.001) and neuroglycopenic ($P = 0.018$) symptoms during euglycemia than −history subjects.

If we assume that hypoglycemic symptom perception in part contributes to self-treatment, self-treatment and symptom perception while driving during hypoglycemia were similar. Both +/−history groups were equally likely to self-treat with the soft drink (44%/59%, respectively, $P = 0.35$) while driving during hypoglycemia.

CONCLUSIONS — This study demonstrated that type 1 diabetic drivers with a history of recurrent hypoglycemia-related driving mishaps during the previous year differed on several basic levels from drivers with no such history. However, it is important to point out that these groups did not differ in terms of general demographic variables (e.g., age, education, and BMI), diabetes parameters (e.g., duration of disease, A1C, insulin regimens, hypoglycemia unawareness, and

long-term complications), or driving parameters (e.g., driving history or miles driven) (Table 1). The exception was that the +history subjects reported three times more episodes of severe hypoglycemia during the previous year.

Although the +history group demonstrated equivalent driving performance during euglycemia, relative to the −history group, their overall driving performance during the 30-min induction of hypoglycemia from 3.9 to 2.5 mmol/l was worse. Our design did not allow us to determine at what blood glucose level this impairment first manifested itself. In contrast, our −history group did not demonstrate a decay.

Drivers with a positive history of mishaps tended to require more infused dextrose to maintain euglycemia during similar insulin challenges, suggesting that these individuals may be more vulnerable to hypoglycemia due to increased glucose utilization. When exposed to progressive mild hypoglycemia, they released less epinephrine, possibly making them more likely to slip into deeper hypoglycemia. Further, when they were experiencing progressive mild hypoglycemia, they demonstrated greater neuroglycopenia as suggested by a significant worsening of driving performance by 2.5 SD.

Drivers with and without a history of hypoglycemia-related driving mishaps did differ significantly in symptom perception during euglycemia but were symptomatically equivalent during progressive hypoglycemia. Detection of autonomic and neuroglycopenic symptoms is a key way for individuals with type 1 diabetes to recognize hypoglycemia during routine functioning (23). Not only did +history drivers fail to detect an increase in symptoms during the induction of hy-

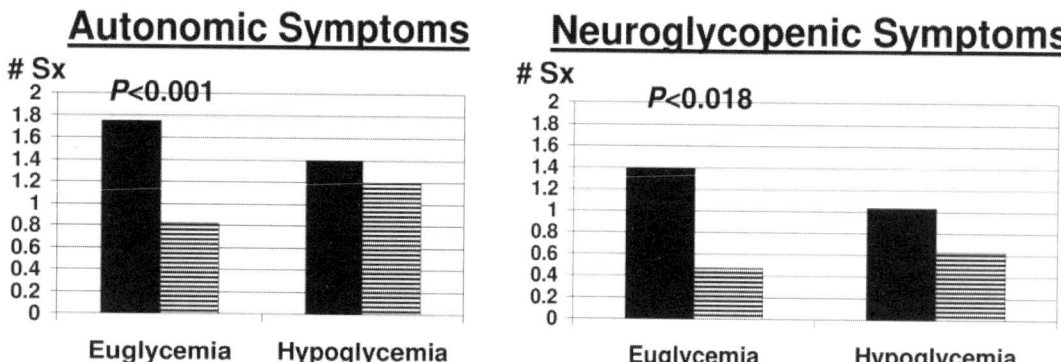

Figure 3—*Mean number of significant autonomic and neuroglycopenic symptoms endorsed while driving under euglycemic and hypoglycemic conditions for +/−history subjects, with P levels reflecting differences between groups at euglycemia.* ■, *+history;* ▤, *−history. Sx represents the mean number of symptoms.*

poglycemia, but they also actually reported more such symptoms during euglycemia than −History drivers. It is as if the former group has to deal with symptom "noise," i.e., a background of symptoms occurring during euglycemia that may make it difficult to detect the "signal" of hypoglycemia, in other words a poor symptom-to-noise ratio. It is not clear from the present study whether this is a general condition for these individuals or if there is something unique to driving that triggers this inversion of symptom perception. Despite these differences in epinephrine release and perceived symptoms, −history (59%) and +history (44%) subjects were similarly likely to self-treat. This may be because self-treatment of hypoglycemia seems to be related to detected difficulties driving and not classic symptoms of hypoglycemia (24). Further, this relatively low rate of self-treatment while hypoglycemic is consistent with the subjects' self-report that they seldom carried fast-acting glucose in their car, along with previously reported data indicating that drivers are willing to drive with low blood glucose (10).

Because a recent history of hypoglycemia-related driving mishaps heralds the likelihood of future driving mishaps (1,3,13), these findings have several clinical implications: Such high-risk drivers *1*) may require more robust carbohydrate dosing to prevent or to treat hypoglycemia, *2*) should be counseled in terms of an appropriate blood glucose threshold when not to begin driving, e.g., 5 mmol/l, which would vary depending on the length of the drive and whether their blood glucose will be rising or falling during the course of the drive, and *3*) should be encouraged to immediately stop driving if blood glucose falls to <4 mmol/l, treat themselves with sufficient fast-acting carbohydrates, and not resume driving until blood glucose is >5 mmol/l.

Limitations of this study should be considered. First, like most insulin clamp studies, these data represent a single observation in a laboratory setting. Therefore, the external validity of these findings cannot be confirmed. Second, this study was partially based on driving a simulator, not an actual car with real-life traffic and driving demands/risks. Third, this was a relatively small sample of only 38 adult drivers with type 1 diabetes. This small sample size may not have had sufficient power to identify small but potentially important differences between these two groups, such as differences in sex

(−history = 34% women as compared with 62% for +history group). Finally, although this crossover design controlled for effects of antecedent hypoglycemia, an alternative design would have been to separate testing days by 2 weeks while rigorously avoiding hypoglycemia for 2 weeks before each testing. However, these limitations are offset by the fact that these a priori findings replicate previous post hoc analyses with an independent sample and different research staff but using similar methodologies and technologies (14). In addition, the simulator used in this study has been found to predict on-road driving behaviors (21) and predict future collisions (20). Given the potential gravity of the consequences of hypoglycemia-related collisions (9), it would seem clinically prudent to use these findings as a guide when working with individuals who are at a higher risk for hypoglycemia while driving, despite these methodological limitations.

Acknowledgments— This work was supported by the National Institutes of Health (General Clinical Research Center grant RR-000847 and National Institute of Diabetes and Digestive and Kidney Diseases grants R01-DK-28288 and R01-DK-51562).

No potential conflicts of interest relevant to this article were reported.

D.J.C. oversaw the project and wrote the manuscript. B.K. conducted data analysis and revised/edited the manuscript. S.M.A. led the inpatient patient management. W.L.C. provided medical oversight for the project. L.A.G.-F. coordinated data collection.

References
1. 1.2 m killed on the road every year [article online], 2006. Available from http://archive.gulfnews.com/indepth/trafficwatch/Accidents/10028835.html. Accessed 19 February 2007
2. Songer TJ, Dorsey RR. High risk characteristics for motor vehicle crashes in persons with diabetes by age. Annu Proc Assoc Adv Automot Med 2006;50:335–351
3. Cox DJ, Penberthy JK, Zrebiec J, Weinger K, Aikens JE, Frier B, Stetson B, DeGroot M, Trief P, Schaechinger H, Hermanns N, Gonder-Frederick L, Clarke W. Diabetes and driving mishaps: frequency and correlations from a multinational survey. Diabetes Care 2003;26:2329–2334
4. Lobmann R, Smid HG, Pottag G, Wagner K, Heinze HJ, Lehnert H. Impairment and recovery of elementary cognitive function induced by hypoglycemia in type-1 diabetic patients and

healthy controls. J Clin Endocrinol Metab 2000;85:2758–2766
5. Gold AE, Deary IJ, MacLeod KM, Thomson KJ, Frier BM. Cognitive function during insulin-induced hypoglycemia in humans: short-term cerebral adaptation does not occur. Psychopharmacology 1995;119:325–333
6. Gonder-Frederick LA, Cox DJ, Driesen NR, Ryan CM, Clarke WL. Individual differences in neurobehavioral disruption during mild and moderate hypoglycemia in adults with IDDM. Diabetes 1994;43:1407–1412
7. Cox DJ, Gonder-Frederick L, Clarke W. Driving decrements in type I diabetes during moderate hypoglycemia. Diabetes 1993;42(2):239–243
8. Cox DJ, Gonder-Frederick LA, Kovatchev BP, Julian DM, Clarke WL. Progressive hypoglycemia's impact on driving simulation performance. Occurrence, awareness and correction. Diabetes Care 2000;23:163–170
9. Cox DJ, Kovatchev BK, Vandecar K, Gonder-Frederick L, Ritterband R, Clarke W. Hypoglycemia preceding fatal car collisions. Diabetes Care 2006;29:467–468
10. Clarke WL, Cox DJ, Gonder-Frederick LA, Kovatchev B. Hypoglycemia and the decision to drive a motor vehicle by persons with diabetes. JAMA 1999;282:750–754
11. Weinger K, Kinsley BT, Levy CJ, Bajaj M, Simonson DC, Cox DJ, Ryan CM, Jacobson AM. The perception of safe driving ability during hypoglycemia in patients with type 1 diabetes mellitus. Am J Med 1999;107:246–253
12. Cryer PE, Davis SN, Shamoon H. Hypoglycemia in diabetes. Diabetes Care 2003;26:1902–1912
13. Cox DJ, Ford D, Gonder-Frederick LA, Clark WL, Mazze R, Weinger K, Ritterband L. Driving mishaps among individuals with type 1 diabetes mellitus: a prospective study. Diabetes Care 2009;32:2177–2180
14. Cox DJ, Kovatchev BP, Gonder-Frederick LA, Clarke WL. Physiological and performance differences between drivers with type 1 diabetes mellitus (T1DM) with and without a recent history of driving mishaps: an exploratory study. Can J Diabetes 2003;27:23–29
15. Cryer PE, Santiago JV, Shah S. Measurement of norepinephrine and epinephrine in small volumes of human plasma by a single isotope derivative method: response to the upright posture. J Clin Endocrinol Metab 1974;39:1025–1029
16. Anderson SM, Clarke WL, Cox DJ, Gonder-Frederick LA, Kovatchev BP. Development of a novel glucose clamping technique for steady hypoglycemic descent. Diabetes 2004;53:A485
17. Cox DJ, Quillian WC, Thorndike FP, Ko-

vatchev BP, Hanna G. Evaluating driving performance of outpatients with Alzheimer's disease. J Am Board Fam Pract 1998;11:264–271

18. Quillian WC, Cox DJ, Kovatchev BP, Phillips C. The effects of age and alcohol intoxication on simulated driving performance, awareness and self-restraint. Age Ageing 1999;28:59–66

19. Cox DJ, Merkel RL, Moore M, Thorndike F, Muller C, Kovatchev B. Relative benefits of stimulant therapy with OROS methylphenidate versus mixed amphetamine salts extended release in improving the driving performance of adolescent drivers with at-tention-deficit/hyperactivity disorder. Pediatrics 2006;118:e704–e710

20. Cox DJ, Broshek DK, Kiernan BP, Kovatchev BP, Guerrier J, Giulano A, George C. Specific driving impairments with progressive age. Adv Med Psychother Psychodiagn 2002;11:107–122

21. Cox DJ, Taylor P, Kovatchev B. Driving simulation performance predicts future accidents among older drivers. J Am Geriatr Soc 1999;47:381–382

22. DeFronzo RA, Tobin JD, Andres R. Glucose clamp technique: a method for quantifying insulin secretion and resistance. Am J Physiol 1979;237:E214–E223

23. Gonder-Frederick LA, Cox DJ, Bobbitt SA, Pennebaker JW. Blood glucose symptom beliefs of diabetic patients: accuracy and implications. Health Psychol 1986;5: 327–341

24. Cox DJ, Gonder-Frederick LA, Kovatchev BP, Clarke WL. Self-treatment of hypoglycemia while driving. Diabetes Res Clin Pract 2001;54:17–26

25. Clarke WL, Cox DJ, Gonder-Frederick LA, Julian D, Schlundt D, Polonsky W. Reduced awareness of hypoglycemia in adults with IDDM. A prospective study of hypoglycemic frequency and associated symptoms. Diabetes Care 1995;18:517–522

The Impact of Frequent and Unrecognized Hypoglycemia on Mortality in the ACCORD Study

ELIZABETH R. SEAQUIST, MD[1]
MICHAEL E. MILLER, PHD[2]
DENISE E. BONDS, MD[3]
MARK FEINGLOS, MD, CM[4]

DAVID C. GOFF JR., MD, PHD[5]
KEVIN PETERSON, MD[6]
PETER SENIOR, MBBS, PHD[7]
FOR THE ACCORD INVESTIGATORS

OBJECTIVE—The aim of this study was to examine the relationship between frequent and unrecognized hypoglycemia and mortality in the Action to Control Cardiovascular Risk in Diabetes (ACCORD) study cohort.

RESEARCH DESIGN AND METHODS—A total of 10,096 ACCORD study participants with follow-up for both hypoglycemia and mortality were included. Hazard ratios (95% CIs) relating the risk of death to the updated annualized number of hypoglycemic episodes and the updated annualized number of intervals with unrecognized hypoglycemia were obtained using Cox proportional hazards regression models, allowing for these hypoglycemia variables as time-dependent covariates and controlling for the baseline covariates.

RESULTS—Participants in the intensive group reported a mean of 1.06 hypoglycemic episodes (self-monitored blood glucose <70 mg/dL or <3.9 mmol/L) in the 7 days preceding their regular 4-month visit, whereas participants in the standard group reported an average of 0.29 episodes. Unrecognized hypoglycemia was reported, on average, at 5.8% of the intensive group 4-month visits and 2.6% of the standard group visits. Hazard ratios for mortality in models including frequency of hypoglycemic episodes were 0.93 (95% CI 0.9–0.97; $P < 0.001$) for participants in the intensive group and 0.98 (0.91–1.06; $P = 0.615$) for participants in the standard group. The hazard ratios for mortality in models, including unrecognized hypoglycemia, were not statistically significant for either group.

CONCLUSIONS—Recognized and unrecognized hypoglycemia was more common in the intensive group than in the standard group. In the intensive group of the ACCORD study, a small but statistically significant inverse relationship of uncertain clinical importance was identified between the number of hypoglycemic episodes and the risk of death among participants.

Diabetes Care 35:409–414, 2012

H ypoglycemia has long been believed to cause serious consequences in patients with diabetes who receive insulin. Severe episodes of hypoglycemia requiring the assistance of another have been shown to be associated with an increased risk of mortality in both the Action to Control Cardiovascular Risk in Diabetes (ACCORD) (1) and the Action in Diabetes and Vascular Disease: Preterax and Diamicron Modified Release Controlled Evaluation (ADVANCE) (2) studies, where the impact of glycemic control on cardiovascular outcomes was examined in participants with type 2 diabetes. However, more recent evidence suggests that recurrent hypoglycemia that occurs over a few days to weeks actually may provide some protection during future episodes of hypoglycemia, at least in patients with type 1 diabetes (3,4). It is well known that recurrent episodes of hypoglycemia blunt the counterregulatory hormonal response during subsequent hypoglycemia (5), which reduces the symptoms associated with the event and may decrease its impact on the cardiovascular system. Whether recurrent hypoglycemia has such an impact on patients with type 2 diabetes is unknown.

The ACCORD study dataset offers a unique opportunity to examine the effect of recurrent hypoglycemia on mortality in individuals with type 2 diabetes. In the ACCORD study, participants were randomly assigned to an intensive group, in which the hemoglobin A_{1c} (HbA_{1c}) target was <6.0%, or to a standard group, in which the HbA_{1c} target was between 7.1 and 7.9%. During the 3.4 years of the intervention, the incidence of severe hypoglycemia was three times greater in the intensive than in the standard group (1). The ACCORD study was stopped earlier than planned because 20% more deaths were noted to occur in the intensive versus the standard group. Previous analysis has demonstrated that this increase in mortality was not related to the increase in severe hypoglycemia that also was noted in the intensive group (6), but the relationship between recurrent and milder hypoglycemic episodes and mortality is unknown.

In this article, we examine the relationship between participants who experienced frequent and unrecognized hypoglycemia as a surrogate for recurrent hypoglycemia over a short period of time and mortality risk in the ACCORD study cohort. To perform this analysis, we quantified hypoglycemia exposure and identified participants with unrecognized hypoglycemia (as a marker for recurrent hypoglycemia). We then determined whether mortality risk was different in those with or without intervals of unrecognized hypoglycemia.

From the [1]Department of Medicine, University of Minnesota, Minneapolis, Minnesota; the [2]Department of Biostatistical Sciences, Division of Public Health Sciences, Wake Forest School of Medicine, Winston-Salem, North Carolina; the [3]National Heart, Lung, and Blood Institute, Bethesda, Maryland; the [4]Division of Endocrinology, Metabolism, and Nutrition, Duke University Medical Center, Durham, North Carolina; the [5]Department of Internal Medicine, Wake Forest University School of Medicine, Winston-Salem, North Carolina; the [6]Department of Family Medicine, University of Minnesota, Minneapolis, Minnesota; and the [7]Department of Medicine, Division of Endocrinology, University of Alberta School of Medicine, Edmonton, Alberta, Canada.
Corresponding author: Elizabeth R. Seaquist, seaqu001@umn.edu.
Received 27 May 2011 and accepted 1 November 2011.
DOI: 10.2337/dc11-0996. Clinical trial reg. no. NCT00000620, clinicaltrials.gov.
This article contains Supplementary Data online at http://care.diabetesjournals.org/lookup/suppl/doi:10.2337/dc11-0996/-/DC1.

RESEARCH DESIGN AND
METHODS—The rationale, design, and entry criteria for the ACCORD trial have been described elsewhere (1). In brief, the ACCORD trial was conducted at 77 sites in the U.S. and Canada. Between January 2001 and October 2005, 10,251 participants with type 2 diabetes and who had a previous cardiovascular event (35%), anatomical evidence of atherosclerosis, left ventricular hypertrophy, albuminuria, at least two additional cardiovascular risk factors, and a current HbA_{1c} level at 7.5–11.0% were enrolled. Key exclusion criteria included frequent or serious hypoglycemic events or other serious illnesses. Participants were randomly assigned to either an intensive strategy, aiming to achieve an HbA_{1c} <6.0%, or a standard strategy, aiming to maintain an HbA_{1c} level between 7.0 and 7.9%. In addition, in a double two-by-two factorial design, all participants were enrolled in either a randomized blood pressure trial comparing an intensive with a standard blood pressure treatment strategy or a randomized lipid trial comparing treatment with fenofibrate versus placebo while maintaining good control of LDL cholesterol, mainly with simvastatin. The primary end point of all components of the ACCORD trial is a composite of cardiovascular mortality, nonfatal myocardial infarction, or nonfatal stroke. All-cause mortality is a predefined secondary end point. This report was limited to 10,096 ACCORD trial participants who had follow-up for both hypoglycemia and mortality. All follow-up data until the final closeout visit in 2009 were used in these analyses.

Definition and reporting of hypoglycemia
Participants were asked at every visit if they had experienced episodes of low blood glucose. A full description of the review of such events, including the adjustment of therapeutic goals in response to severe hypoglycemia, has been previously reported (7). That report focused on symptomatic, severe hypoglycemic events requiring medical assistance (hospitalization, visit to the emergency department, or treatment by medical personnel including emergency medical technicians either in a clinical setting or at home), which was defined in the ACCORD trial as either a blood glucose <50 mg/dL (2.8 mmol/L) or symptoms that promptly resolved with oral carbohydrate, intravenous glucose, or glucagon. In addition to this characterization of severe hypoglycemic episodes, at

each 4-month visit, participants were queried about the following four areas:

1. Since the last call or visit, how many times per week, on average, has the participant checked his/her blood sugar?
2. How many hypoglycemic episodes (SMBG [self-monitoring of blood glucose] <70 mg/dL or <3.9 mmol/L) did the participant have in the last 7 days?
3. Since the last visit or call, how many times per week, on average, did the participants report having minor, but uncomfortable symptoms suggesting hypoglycemia?
4. Did any of reported hypoglycemic episodes occur without warning symptoms?

This report made use of the information collected in response to the above questions to define variables representing hypoglycemic episodes characterized by low blood glucose but not requiring medical assistance and hypoglycemia unawareness. Question 3 was not introduced until June 2005. As such, follow-up for mortality before 1 June 2005 was censored for analyses involving that variable, excluding those who died before this date and starting follow-up at the time when use of the questionnaire was initiated.

To obtain time-dependent variables representing the hypoglycemic episodes characterized by low blood glucose, but not requiring medical assistance, we used all data for any visit where a blood glucose level had been checked at least once per week (question 1). Because those who live longer naturally will accumulate more episodes, variables were defined that represented the updated annualized number of episodes reported in response to question 2. We also created an additional variable to use in sensitivity analyses, in which we used only participants who reported checking ≥7 or more times per week on at least 90% of visits. We defined hypoglycemia unawareness in terms of *1*) a positive response to question 2 and *2*) a positive response to question 4 or a response of zero to question 3. For this variable, we also created a variable representing the updated annualized number of 4-month intervals in which the participant reported hypoglycemia unawareness.

Baseline covariates
Baseline characteristics used in these analyses were those identified by Riddle et al. (8) as being predictive of mortality in the

ACCORD study, including demographic and anthropometric characteristics (age, race, education level, and BMI), medical history (smoking history, history of cardiovascular disease, history of congestive heart failure, or previous amputation), and laboratory and clinical measures (urine albumin-to-creatinine ratio, HbA_{1c} level, and serum creatinine). This model also contained terms representing whether the clinic was part of an integrated health plan and group assignments within either the blood pressure or lipid trial.

Statistical analysis
All statistical analyses were conducted at the coordinating center with the use of SAS software (version 9.2; SAS Institute, Cary, NC). All analyses were conducted separately within the intensive and standard glycemia groups.

Across the full period of follow-up, we calculated the cumulative number of reports of low blood glucose by the subject in response to question 2 (listed above) and determined the percentage of participants who died for several ranges of cumulative episodes (0, 0–5, 6–10, 11–15, 16–20, and >20). Likewise, we tabulated the total number of assessment intervals during follow-up (each interval was 4 months long) where the participant experienced hypoglycemia unawareness. The percentage of participants who died was calculated for each cumulative number of intervals.

Within glycemia treatment groups, hazard ratios (95% CI) relating the risk of death to the updated annualized number of hypoglycemic episodes and the updated annualized number of intervals of hypoglycemia unawareness were obtained using Cox proportional hazards regression models, allowing for these hypoglycemia variables as time-dependent covariates and controlling for the baseline covariates identified by Riddle et al. (8). The series of models that were fitted included baseline covariates plus each of the following as additional factors entered into the model: *1*) updated annualized number of hypoglycemic episodes; *2*) updated annualized number of intervals of hypoglycemia unawareness; *3*) updated annualized number of hypoglycemic episodes, a time-varying covariate representing hypoglycemia requiring medical assistance, and the interaction between these two variables; and *4*) updated annualized number of intervals of hypoglycemia unawareness, a time-varying covariate representing hypoglycemia requiring medical assistance, and the interaction between these two variables.

RESULTS—For 10,096 participants with follow-up for hypoglycemia and mortality, there were 780 participants who experienced at least one event of hypoglycemia that required medical assistance (565 participants from the intensive group and 215 from the standard group) (9). Participants from the intensive group reported checking their blood glucose, on average, 17.6 times per week (Table 1), whereas participants from the standard group checked their blood glucose 12.7 times per week. Participants from the intensive group reported a mean of 1.06 hypoglycemic episodes (SMBG <70 mg/dL or <3.9 mmol/L) in the 7 days preceding their regular 4-month visit, whereas participants from the standard group reported an average of 0.29 episodes. Hypoglycemia unawareness was reported, on average, at 5.8% of the intensive group 4-month visits and 2.6% of the standard group visits.

Table 2 reports the number of participants who were alive or deceased relative to the number of reported hypoglycemic episodes at the end of the final follow-up interval. This information is followed by the same tabulation for the number of 4-month intervals where the participant was unaware of their hypoglycemic symptoms. Note that the number of participants used for this second variable is less than that for the first because question 3 was added late in follow-up, and some participants had already dropped out or were deceased by that time. These results suggest that there may be an inverse relationship between the cumulative number of hypoglycemic episodes and death, particularly in the intensive group, but this result could be attributed to the fact that those who live longer are able to accumulate more events. For this reason, the results from the proportional

hazards regression models using updated annualized variables may be of greater interest than these tabulations. When we controlled for the baseline covariates that predicted mortality in the ACCORD study cohort (8), we continued to see evidence of an inverse relationship between mortality, particularly in the intensive group, and both the updated annualized number of hypoglycemic events and the updated annualized number of 4-month intervals where participants were unaware of hypoglycemia (see Supplementary Tables 1 and 2 for the model involving only baseline covariates).

Table 3 reports the hazard ratios relating the risk of death to the updated annualized number of hypoglycemic episodes and the updated annualized number of intervals of hypoglycemia unawareness using Cox proportional hazards regression models. All models control for the baseline covariates contained in the Supplementary Tables. With model 1, participants in the intensive group were found to have a significantly lower risk of death as the annualized number of hypoglycemic episodes increased. Such a relationship was not seen in the standard group (model 5). In model 2, we included a time-dependent variable representing a previous history of severe hypoglycemia requiring medical attention and the interaction between the annualized number of hypoglycemic episodes and this variable. Because the interaction term is statistically significant ($P = 0.048$), we conclude that a previous event requiring medical assistance modified the relationship between the mortality risk and the annualized number of hypoglycemic episodes in the intensive group. In the intensive group, more frequent hypoglycemia reduced the risk of death more in participants with a history of a hypoglycemic event requiring medical assistance than in those without this previous event. In the

standard group, more frequent hypoglycemia increased the risk of death more in participants with a history of a hypoglycemic event requiring medical assistance, whereas it reduced the risk of death in those without this previous event. This apparent differential relationship with mortality is not significantly different between these two groups within participants in the standard group (interaction $P = 0.10$). A significant relationship was found between the annualized number of intervals of unrecognized hypoglycemia and the risk of death after controlling for baseline covariates in the intensive group, where there is a 31% (hazard ratio 0.69 [95% CI 0.48–1.00]) reduction in the risk of death associated with each additional report of unrecognized hypoglycemia; however, the CI for this estimate is quite wide.

All analyses were performed for the group as a whole and for a subgroup of those participants who reported checking seven or more times per week on at least 90% of visits (see Supplementary Fig. 1 for a flowchart of the number of participants used in each analysis). This sensitivity analysis did not change the direction of estimates reported in Table 3; however, the interaction term in model 6 was statistically significant under this restriction.

CONCLUSIONS—In this analysis, we found a lower risk of death in those ACCORD study subjects randomly assigned to the intensive treatment group who experienced more episodes of hypoglycemia. Such a relationship was not seen in the standard group. We also found that in participants of the intensive group, the reduction in mortality risk associated with an increased number of hypoglycemic events was more pronounced among those experiencing a previous hypoglycemic event requiring medical assistance than among those without this previous

Table 1—*Hypoglycemia characteristics by glycemia group*

Characteristics	Intensive glycemia (n = 5,045)		Standard glycemia (n = 5,051)	
	Mean (SD)	Median (minimum–maximum)	Mean (SD)	Median (minimum–maximum)
Frequency of checking blood glucose in the previous 7 days	17.6 (6.8)	16.6 (1.0–53.7)	12.7 (5.3)	12.5 (1.0–49.2)
Hypoglycemic episodes (SMBG <70 mg/dL or <3.9 mmol/L) in the previous 7 days	1.06 (0.98)	0.82 (0–7.8)	0.29 (0.49)	0.1 (0–8.0)
Proportion of visits in which hypoglycemia unawareness was reported (%)*	5.8		2.6	

*Restricted to visits after 1 June 2005.

Table 2—*Number of participants deceased by cumulative number of hypoglycemic episodes and levels of hypoglycemia unawareness*

	Intensive glycemia (n = 5,045)		Standard glycemia (n = 5,051)	
	Alive	Deceased [n (%)]	Alive	Deceased [n (%)]
Cumulative number of hypoglycemic episodes				
0	491	57 (10.40)	1,794	133 (6.9)
0–5	1,026	112 (9.84)	1,906	123 (6.06)
6–10	841	80 (8.69)	561	32 (5.40)
11–15	650	46 (6.61)	227	9 (3.81)
16–20	445	28 (5.92)	106	8 (7.02)
>20	1,222	47 (3.7)	149	4 (1.97)
Number of 4-month intervals where the participant was unaware				
0	3,082	223 (6.75)	3,856	215 (5.28)
1	985	50 (4.83)	626	24 (3.69)
2	351	17 (4.62)	188	10 (5.05)
3	132	6 (4.35)	45	0
4	62	1 (1.59)	7	0
5–10	50	0	10	0

event, but this differential relationship related to a previous event requiring medical assistance was not statistically significant in the standard group. This is in contrast to the positive relationship previously identified between mortality and episodes of severe hypoglycemia requiring medical assistance in both treatment groups (6). These observations suggest that the glycemic target may modify the relationship between mortality and severe hypoglycemia in patients with type 2 diabetes, particularly in patients who experience frequent hypoglycemia.

In this study, hypoglycemia was defined as blood glucose <70 mg/dL or <3.9 mmol/L on a home glucose meter. Assuming the meters used conformed to the International Organization for Standardization guidelines (9), the actual glucose level could have been anywhere between 55 and 85 mg/dL or 3.1 and 4.7 mmol/L. Because participants did not follow a single specific schedule for home glucose testing, we cannot be certain that all episodes in which blood glucose was <70 mg/dL or 3.9 mmol/L were captured on the glucose meters. Participants in the intensive group performed more tests than did participants in the standard group, so it is possible that more normal glucose values were erroneously classified as hypoglycemia in this group. However, an equal number of low blood glucose values would have been erroneously classified as normal. Therefore, it

is unlikely that more frequent testing in the intensive group led to an overestimation of the frequency of hypoglycemia. Of interest, the relationship between the number of hypoglycemic episodes experienced in the past 7 days (Table 1) in the intensive versus standard group is similar to the relationship previously defined for the annual incidence of severe hypoglycemia between these groups (6), providing evidence that any overestimation of hypoglycemia occurred equally in both groups.

What factors could be responsible for the observation that frequent hypoglycemia reduces the risk of mortality in participants randomly assigned to a more intensive glucose target? One possibility is that participants in the intensive group were seen more frequently than participants in the standard group and, consequently, may have had more opportunity to learn how to treat and prevent future episodes of hypoglycemia. Such education may have attenuated the severity of future episodes of hypoglycemia and any associated adverse outcomes. Frequency of hypoglycemia is known to increase with improved glycemic control, so it also is possible that participants in the intensive group who did not experience frequent hypoglycemia had comorbidities like cognitive impairment that both increase mortality risk (10) and impair adherence to the complex treatment regimens required to achieve a HbA_{1c} level <6.0%.

It also is possible that the counterregulatory response to hypoglycemia is blunted in participants of the intensive group because of their frequent exposure to hypoglycemia, and, as a result, any impact of this stress on cardiovascular function may be reduced.

The definition of hypoglycemia unawareness depended on participants remembering at a 4-month visit whether symptoms of hypoglycemia were present at a time the blood glucose was <70 mg/dL or <3.9 mmol/L on a home glucose meter at any time since the last visit. Such a recollection is subject to error, and this may explain why only a borderline relationship was found between mortality and the annualized number of intervals of unrecognized hypoglycemia. We did note a substantial reduction in the risk of death associated with each additional interval containing a report of unrecognized hypoglycemia in the intensive group, but the wide CI for this analysis probably reflects the imprecision in the measure.

The presence or absence of a previous episode of hypoglycemia requiring medical assistance in the intensive group had an impact on the reduction in mortality seen with increasing episodes of hypoglycemia. For participants in the intensive group with a previous event requiring medical assistance, every one-unit increase in the number of hypoglycemic episodes was associated with a 17.3% reduction in mortality. For participants in the intensive group without a previous event requiring medical assistance, every one-unit increase in the number of hypoglycemic episodes was associated with only a 6% reduction in mortality. The reason for this difference in mortality reduction is uncertain but could include changes in behavior in those who required the attention of a medical professional that made them more aware of impending hypoglycemia.

A history of severe hypoglycemia requiring medical assistance also had an impact on the relationship seen between mortality and increasing episodes of hypoglycemia in the standard group. For participants in the standard group with a history of severe hypoglycemia, the risk of death increased by 5.8% for every one-unit increase in the annualized number of hypoglycemic episodes. Participants in the standard group without a previous hypoglycemic event requiring medical assistance had an 8% reduction in the risk of death for each one-unit increase in the annualized number of hypoglycemic

Table 3—*Hazard ratios (95% CI) for mortality in models, including frequency of hypoglycemic episodes and levels of hypoglycemia unawareness**

	Intensive glycemia			
Variables	Model 1	Model 2†	Model 3	Model 4
Annualized number of hypoglycemic episodes	0.93 (0.90–0.97); $P < 0.001$	0.94 (0.91–0.98); $P = 0.003$		
Previous hypoglycemia requiring medical attention		1.78 (1.14–2.80); $P = 0.012$		1.13 (0.78–1.65); $P = 0.505$
Interaction term between previous hypoglycemia requiring medical attention and annualized number of hypoglycemic episodes		0.88 (0.78–1.00); $P = 0.048$		0.98 (0.68–1.42); $P = 0.912$
Annualized number of intervals of hypoglycemia unawareness			0.69 (0.48–1.00); $P = 0.047$	0.69 (0.47–1.03); $P = 0.068$

	Standard glycemia			
Variables	Model 5	Model 6‡	Model 7	Model 8
Annualized number of hypoglycemic episodes	0.98 (0.91–1.06); $P = 0.615$	0.92 (0.84–1.02); $P = 0.107$		
Previous hypoglycemia requiring medical attention		2.15 (1.31–3.53); $P = 0.003$		2.36 (1.45–3.83); $P = 0.001$
Interaction term between previous hypoglycemia requiring medical attention and annualized number of hypoglycemic episodes		1.15 (0.97–1.35); $P = 0.104$		1.11 (0.53–2.28); $P = 0.785$
Annualized number of intervals of hypoglycemia unawareness			0.81 (0.44–1.49); $P = 0.497$	0.77 (0.40–1.48); $P = 0.428$

*All results control for baseline covariates included in Supplementary Tables 1 and 2. Results are almost identical when sensitivity analyses are performed using only participants who checked their blood glucose at least seven times in a week. †If a participant in the intensive glycemia group experienced a previous hypoglycemic event requiring medical attention, then a one-unit increase in the annualized average number of episodes decreases their risk of death by 17.3% ($1 - 0.94 \times 0.88$). If the participant did not have a previous hypoglycemic event requiring medical assistance, then the effect is a 6% (1–0.94) reduction. ‡If a participant in the standard glycemia group experienced a previous hypoglycemic event requiring medical attention, then a one-unit increase in the annualized average number of episodes increases their risk of death by 5.8% (0.92×1.15). If the participant did not have a previous hypoglycemic event requiring medical assistance, then the effect is an 8% (1–0.92) reduction.

episodes. The reason for this difference is uncertain, but the data confirm, at least for subjects with a HbA$_{1c}$ target of 7.1–7.9%, the findings of the ADVANCE study, in which severe hypoglycemia was found to be a marker of increased vulnerability to adverse outcomes (2).

In the ADVANCE study, severe hypoglycemia was associated with increased mortality from any cause and specifically from cardiovascular disease (2). Similar to the ACCORD study, severe hypoglycemia was more common in the ADVANCE study participants randomly assigned to the intensive glycemic target, but the annual death rates were lower among participants in the intensive group who experienced severe hypoglycemia than among participants in the standard group who experienced severe hypoglycemia. In the ADVANCE study, minor hypoglycemia was associated with a significant reduction in the rate

of death and macrovascular events for the entire study population, although whether the relationship was the same in the standard and the intensive groups was not reported. Minor hypoglycemia occurred more than once in almost one-half of the ADVANCE study participants who experienced this event, and although an association between recurrent modest hypoglycemia and mortality in the ADVANCE study was not reported, it is possible that the benefits of minor hypoglycemia on mortality risk could be greatest in those who experienced recurrent episodes.

Our study has many strengths, including the large sample size, the diverse population, and the standardized methods used to collect information about outcomes. We were limited in our ability to accurately determine the number and duration of hypoglycemic episodes experienced by the ACCORD study participants.

We found no difference between the results calculated from the whole group and those calculated from participants who reported checking at least seven times per week on at least 90% of visits. Although this latter finding provides some assurance that our conclusions were not biased by the frequency of checking, it is likely that a more meaningful difference could be found between hypoglycemia and mortality if the dataset included multiple daily glucose records from all participants. In addition, our observations do not eliminate the possibility that specific subgroups of ACCORD study participants differ in how hypoglycemia frequency and unrecognized hypoglycemia affects mortality risk. Perhaps future collaboration between the ACCORD trial, ADVANCE trial, and Veterans Affairs Diabetes Trial (VADT) investigators will provide insights into this possibility.

In conclusion, we found a significant inverse relationship between the number of hypoglycemic episodes and the risk of death among participants in the intensive group of the ACCORD trial. However, because hypoglycemia can lead to confusion, coma, and death, this observation does not mean that clinical practice should change to purposefully include frequent episodes of hypoglycemia in patients with type 2 diabetes at high risk for cardiovascular events. Optimal diabetes care should strive to achieve individualized glycemic targets without episodes of hypoglycemia.

Acknowledgments—This work was supported by grants (N01-HC-95178, N01-HC-95179, N01-HC-95180, N01-HC-95181, N01-HC-95182, N01-HC-95183, N01-HC-95184, IAA-Y1-HC-9035, and IAA-Y1-HC-1010) from the National Heart, Lung, and Blood Institute and by other branches of the National Institutes of Health, including the National Institute of Diabetes and Digestive and Kidney Diseases, the National Institute on Aging, and the National Eye Institute; by the Centers for Disease Control and Prevention; and by general clinical research centers.

The following companies provided study medications, equipment, or supplies: Abbott Laboratories, Amylin Pharmaceutical, AstraZeneca, Bayer HealthCare, Closer Healthcare, GlaxoSmithKline, King Pharmaceuticals, Merck, Novartis, Novo Nordisk, Omron Healthcare, sanofi-aventis, and Schering-Plough.

M.E.M. has served as a consultant for Roche. No other potential conflicts of interest relevant to this article were reported.

E.R.S. collected data, contributed to the data analysis, drafted the manuscript, and is the guarantor of the article. M.E.M. performed data analysis and drafted the manuscript. D.E.B. and D.C.G. reviewed and edited the manuscript. M.F. and K.P. collected data and contributed to the manuscript. P.S. contributed to the data interpretation and revision of the manuscript.

References

1. Gerstein HC, Miller ME, Byington RP, et al.; Action to Control Cardiovascular Risk in Diabetes Study Group. Effects of intensive glucose lowering in type 2 diabetes. N Engl J Med 2008;358:2545–2559
2. Zoungas S, Patel A, Chalmers J, et al.; ADVANCE Collaborative Group. Severe hypoglycemia and risks of vascular events and death. N Engl J Med 2010;363:1410–1418
3. Jones TW, Borg WP, Borg MA, et al. Resistance to neuroglycopenia: an adaptive response during intensive insulin treatment of diabetes. J Clin Endocrinol Metab 1997;82:1713–1718
4. Fanelli CG, Paramore DS, Hershey T, et al. Impact of nocturnal hypoglycemia on hypoglycemic cognitive dysfunction in type 1 diabetes. Diabetes 1998;47:1920–1927
5. Cryer PE. Banting Lecture: Hypoglycemia: the limiting factor in the management of IDDM. Diabetes 1994;43:1378–1389
6. Bonds DE, Miller ME, Bergenstal RM, et al. The association between symptomatic, severe hypoglycaemia and mortality in type 2 diabetes: retrospective epidemiological analysis of the ACCORD study. BMJ 2010;340:b4909
7. Bonds DE, Kurashige EM, Bergenstal R, et al.; ACCORD Study Group. Severe hypoglycemia monitoring and risk management procedures in the Action to Control Cardiovascular Risk in Diabetes (ACCORD) trial. Am J Cardiol 2007;99:80i–89i
8. Riddle MC, Ambrosius WT, Brillon DJ, et al.; Action to Control Cardiovascular Risk in Diabetes Investigators. Epidemiologic relationships between A1C and all-cause mortality during a median 3.4-year follow-up of glycemic treatment in the ACCORD trial. Diabetes Care 2010;33:983–990
9. International Organization for Standardization. *In Vitro Diagnostic Test Systems: Requirements for Blood-Glucose Monitoring Systems for Self-Testing in Managing Diabetes Mellitus.* Geneva, World Health Org., 2003 (ISO rep. no. 15197)
10. Sachs GA, Carter R, Holtz LR, et al. Cognitive impairment: an independent predictor of excess mortality: a cohort study. Ann Intern Med 2011;155:300–308

Reducing Rates of Severe Hypoglycemia in a Population-Based Cohort of Children and Adolescents With Type 1 Diabetes Over the Decade 2000–2009

Susan M. O'Connell, mrcpi, md[1,2]
Matthew N. Cooper, bca, bsc[2]
Max K. Bulsara, phd, msc[3]

Elizabeth A. Davis, fracp, phd[1,2]
Timothy W. Jones, md, dch, fracp[1,2]

OBJECTIVE—To examine rates of severe hypoglycemia (SH) in a large population-based cohort of children with type 1 diabetes and relationships to HbA$_{1c}$.

RESEARCH DESIGN AND METHODS—Data from 1,683 children (mean [SD] age at diagnosis 10.5 [4.2]; range 1–18 years) from 2000 to 2009 were analyzed from the Western Australian Children's Diabetes Database. Rates of SH were related to HbA$_{1c}$ using negative binomial regression.

RESULTS—A total of 7,378 patient-years of data and 780 SH events were recorded. The rate of SH per 100 patient-years peaked at 17.3 in 2001 and then declined from 2004 to a nadir of 5.8 in 2006. HbA$_{1c}$ <7% was not associated with higher risk of SH (incidence rate ratio 1.2 [95% CI 0.9–1.6], $P = 0.29$) compared with HbA$_{1c}$ of 8–9%.

CONCLUSIONS—In a sample of youth with type 1 diabetes, there has been a decrease in rates of SH and a weaker relationship with glycemic control than previously observed.

Diabetes Care 34:2379–2380, 2011

The threat of hypoglycemia as a consequence of insulin treatment is a major barrier to optimizing glycemic control in type 1 diabetes (1). Previous studies have demonstrated a close relationship between glycemic control and increased rates of severe hypoglycemia (SH) (2). In the 1990s, increased emphasis on strict glycemic control was paralleled with an increase in the rate of SH, particularly in younger children (<6 years) (3,4). Therapies have changed, however, and the objectives in this study were to examine contemporary rates of SH in a large population-based cohort of pediatric type 1 diabetes and changes over the past decade and to investigate relationships with glycemic control.

RESEARCH DESIGN AND METHODS

All children with type 1 diabetes aged ≤18 years attending Princess Margaret Hospital for Children from 2000 to 2009 were prospectively included in the study. Princess Margaret Hospital for Children is the only pediatric referral center for diabetes in Western Australia, with a case ascertainment of 99.9% (5). Consent for data to be entered into the database was obtained from all parents, and the study was approved by the institution's ethics committee.

SH was strictly defined as a hypoglycemic event leading to loss of consciousness or seizure. For each patient, SH events were counted if they were reported during any clinical visit after the 1 January 2000. Subjects exited the study upon turning 18 years, permanently leaving the state, or if 12 months had elapsed since their last clinic visit. The number of patient-years contributed by each respective clinic visit was calculated as the number of days elapsed since the previous visit.

All children attending the center are managed by a multidisciplinary diabetes care team. The children and parents were advised to keep a logbook of blood glucose levels (BGL) and insulin doses and to record all atypical events such as episodes of hypoglycemia or illness. They were taught to obtain a BGL, if possible, to confirm hypoglycemia. They were seen in the clinic every 3 months, and data on all diabetes outcomes, including hypoglycemia events and treatment types, were recorded in the Western Australian Children's Diabetes Database.

HbA$_{1c}$ was determined at each clinic visit by agglutination inhibition immunoassay (nondiabetic reference <6.2%; Ames DCA 2000).

Statistical analysis

Annual SH incidence rates were calculated by obtaining the total number of SH events and dividing by the total length of follow-up represented by each clinic visit recorded in that year. Initial analyses involved revisiting previously identified risk factors by applying negative binomial regression methodology, as already described (3), to the new data. This was the basis of defining the final models for effect size estimates and age by treatment interaction analysis (6). Analyses were performed using R 2.11.1 and Stata 10 software (StataCorp 2007, Stata Statistical Software: Release 10; StataCorp LP, College Station, TX).

RESULTS—The study included 1,683 children (51% boys). In total, 7,378 patient-years of data were available for analysis, and 780 SH events occurred during the decade. Of all patients, 77.4% had no episodes, 11.8% had one event, 5.2% had two events, and 5.6% had three

From the [1]Department of Endocrinology and Diabetes, Princess Margaret Hospital for Children, Perth, Western Australia, Australia; the [2]Diabetes and Endocrinology Division, Telethon Institute for Child Health Research, Centre for Child Health Research, The University of Western Australia, Perth, Western Australia, Australia; and the [3]Department of Biostatistics, Institute of Health and Rehabilitation Research, University of Notre Dame, Fremantle, Western Australia, Australia.
Corresponding author: Timothy W. Jones, tim.jones@health.wa.gov.au.
Received 19 April 2011 and accepted 17 August 2011.
DOI: 10.2337/dc11-0748

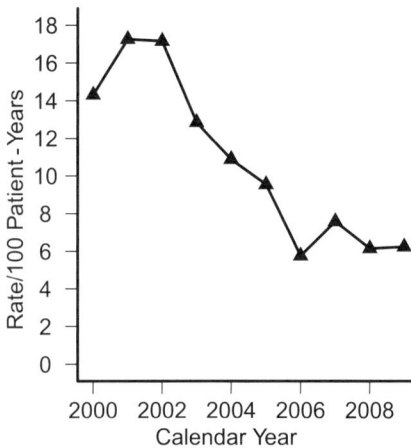

Figure 1—*Rates of severe hypoglycemia by calendar year.*

or more episodes. The incidence rate for SH (Fig. 1), adjusted for age and sex, decreased by an average of 14% per year compared with previous year for the first 7 years ($z = 5.33$, $P < 0.001$) and did not change after that time ($P = 0.446$).

Univariate analysis quantified the annual rate of decline in the SH incidence rate over the decade as 12.1% (95% CI 8.7–15.4, $P < 0.001$) per year.

The mean HbA_{1c} level for the decade was 8.3% (SD 1.5%), with only minor fluctuations. After adjusting for age and sex, the overall trend showed a decline in mean HbA_{1c} levels of 0.07% per year (95% CI 0.009–0.15; $P = 0.03$). Multivariate analysis, adjusting for age and treatment type, showed an HbA_{1c} <7% was not significantly associated with higher risk of SH (incidence rate ratio 1.2 [0.9–1.6]; $P = 0.29$) compared with the reference group of HbA_{1c} 8–9%, which was the average level in our cohort across the decade.

There was no relationship between age and risk of SH and no sex difference. Children with duration of diabetes >1 year had a significantly higher risk (incidence rate ratio 3.7 [95% CI 2.4–5.7]; $P < 0.001$ for 1–5 years, increasing thereafter), than those with duration of diabetes <1 year. In adolescents (>13 years), pump therapy was associated with a reduced incidence of SH (64% lower, $P = 0.048$).

CONCLUSIONS—The primary objective of this study was to determine incidence rates of SH in a population-based sample of pediatric type 1 diabetes during a period when there were changes to treatment regimens. This is one of the largest population-based cohorts for which clinical data have been collected prospectively, and this report follows on from rates previously reported for 1992–2002 (3) and 1992–1995 (4). The reduction in the hypoglycemia rate may have resulted from changes in clinical practice (e.g., new insulin regimens, more intensive glucose monitoring, improved management guidelines), but this remains speculative.

Despite the decrease in SH rates, glycemic control has remained relatively static since the middle of the decade. This is similar to a recent report from the Hvidoere group demonstrating no recent improvement in glycemic control (7,8). An important finding was that compared with past studies, the relationship between glycemic control and the risk of SH is now weaker, with no significant increased risk of SH associated with improved glycemic control range from 8–9% to <7%. Another change has been the reduced risk of SH in children aged <6 years (3). This is an important observation in view of concerns regarding the potential effect of hypoglycemia on the developing brain (9).

In summary, in a population-based sample of pediatric type 1 diabetes, rates of SH have decreased during the past decade, and the previously close relationship between tight glycemic control and risk of severe events is now weaker. Although the data are encouraging and suggest that the risk of SH is in part being reduced with modern therapy, the risk remains significant and fear of hypoglycemia continues to be a barrier to optimal glycemic control.

Acknowledgments—S.O'C. received a fellowship grant from Novo Nordisk Ltd. in 2010. No other potential conflicts of interest relevant to this article were reported.

S.O'C. collected and researched data and wrote the manuscript. M.N.C. performed statistical analysis, generated the figures, and reviewed and edited the manuscript. M.K.B. provided methodologic, data, and statistical support based on previous publications. E.A.D. contributed to study design, data collection, analysis, and discussion. T.W.J. contributed to study design, data collection and analysis, and reviewed and edited the manuscript.

The authors thank Nirubasini Paramalingam, Telethon Institute for Child Health Research, The University of Western Australia, for assistance with data extraction.

References
1. Cryer PE. Hypoglycaemia: the limiting factor in the glycaemic management of type I and type II diabetes. Diabetologia 2002;45: 937–948
2. Nathan DM, Zinman B, Cleary PA, et al.; Diabetes Control and Complications Trial/ Epidemiology of Diabetes Interventions and Complications (DCCT/EDIC) Research Group. Modern-day clinical course of type 1 diabetes mellitus after 30 years' duration: the Diabetes Control and Complications Trial/ Epidemiology of Diabetes Interventions and Complications and Pittsburgh Epidemiology of Diabetes Complications experience (1983–2005). Arch Intern Med 2009;169:1307–1316
3. Bulsara MK, Holman CD, Davis EA, Jones TW. The impact of a decade of changing treatment on rates of severe hypoglycemia in a population-based cohort of children with type 1 diabetes. Diabetes Care 2004; 27:2293–2298
4. Davis EA, Keating B, Byrne GC, Russell M, Jones TW. Hypoglycemia: incidence and clinical predictors in a large population-based sample of children and adolescents with IDDM. Diabetes Care 1997;20:22–25
5. Kelly HA, Byrne GC. Incidence of IDDM in Western Australia in children aged 0–14 yr from 1985 to 1989. Diabetes Care 1992;15: 515–517
6. Altman DG, Bland JM. Interaction revisited: the difference between two estimates. BMJ 2003;326:219
7. de Beaufort CE, Swift PG, Skinner CT, et al.; Hvidoere Study Group on Childhood Diabetes 2005. Continuing stability of center differences in pediatric diabetes care: do advances in diabetes treatment improve outcome? The Hvidoere Study Group on Childhood Diabetes. Diabetes Care 2007; 30:2245–2250
8. Mortensen HB, Hougaard P; The Hvidøre Study Group on Childhood Diabetes. Comparison of metabolic control in a cross-sectional study of 2,873 children and adolescents with IDDM from 18 countries. Diabetes Care 1997;20:714–720
9. Silverstein J, Klingensmith G, Copeland K, et al.; American Diabetes Association. Care of children and adolescents with type 1 diabetes: a statement of the American Diabetes Association. Diabetes Care 2005;28:186–212

Insulin-Induced Hypoglycemia and Its Effect on the Brain
Unraveling Metabolism by In Vivo Nuclear Magnetic Resonance

Raimund I. Herzog,[1] Robert S. Sherwin,[1] and Douglas L. Rothman[2]

Hypoglycemia, a frequent occurrence during modern intensive insulin therapy, remains the major limiting factor in achieving optimal glucose control in type 1 diabetic patients as well as in patients with long-standing type 2 diabetes. This has been a challenge for clinicians and investigators since several large population-based studies such as the Diabetes Control and Complications Trial and UK Prospective Diabetes Study established the long-term benefits of tight glycemic control many years ago (1,2). More recently, studies of intensive glucose control in patients with diabetes of several years duration have—to the surprise to many—been either terminated because of increased mortality in the intensive control arm or because worse outcomes were revealed in regard to the clinical end points (3,4). In a parallel development, we have gone, over the course of 10 years, from embracing stringent inpatient glucose control via insulin infusion protocols in the intensive care setting (5) to realizing that not everybody may benefit equally from such an intervention, since the increased incidence of profound hypoglycemia is the limiting factor (6). In fact, a recent systematic review of 21 trials of intensive insulin therapy by Kansagara et al. (7) found a sixfold higher risk of severe hypoglycemic events in patients undergoing such therapy. Faced with a clinical dilemma of such proportion, it appears that we may need to readdress our hypotheses, and we need to conduct mechanistic studies that allow us to identify therapies that are effective but minimize the exposure of patients to the heightened risk of hypoglycemia. Understanding the regulation of glucose metabolism in the brain and how it responds to hypoglycemia in this context is of particular relevance because of the brain's exquisite dependence on glucose as an energy substrate and its integrative function in whole body fuel homeostasis (8).

The brain poses particular challenges because, due to limited glucose transport activity in the blood brain barrier and high rates of cellular glucose metabolism, the concentrations of glucose in human brain interstitial fluid are only about a fifth of those in plasma, making the brain highly vulnerable to a drop in glucose supply (9). Magnetic resonance spectroscopy (MRS), which allows monitoring of glucose and other substrate metabolism in vivo offers the unique opportunity to study glucose metabolism behind the blood brain barrier in real time. Using the stable ^{13}C isotope as a tracer, labeled glucose or other substrates are infused and label appearance in the metabolite pools of glutamate and glutamine can be observed over time. Fitting of these data with a mathematical model of metabolism allows calculation of substrate-specific metabolism as well as compartmentation of metabolism between the two major brain cell types, neurons and glia (Fig. 1).

To test whether moderate hypoglycemia can reduce human brain energy production, van de Ven et al. (10) used ^{13}C MRS to study glucose metabolism in healthy control subjects during euglycemia and hypoglycemia using a hyperinsulinemic clamp to maintain stable glycemia. Eight subjects served as their own controls and were studied at a glucose level of 5 mM and at 3 mM, thereby reducing the confounding influence of interindividual variability. Interestingly, the authors were not able to detect a difference between tricarboxylic acid (TCA) cycle activity under euglycemic and hypoglycemic conditions. They suggest that oxidative brain metabolism was not impaired in a way that would have resulted in decreased production of ATP further downstream, in seeming contradiction with results showing impaired cortical function in control subjects at similar levels of hypoglycemia (11,12).

There are several potential explanations for the paradoxical results of van de Ven et al. (10), including the brain region observed and a switch of cerebral metabolism to alternate substrates. An important point to keep in mind is that most current MRS studies are focused on the brain tissue most adjacent to the nuclear magnetic resonance (NMR) coil, the occipital cortex. Because we know from animal studies and human positron emission tomography studies (13) that metabolic activity can vary substantially from region to region and change when local activity is stimulated (14), we must ask ourselves how the current observations can be applied from the occipital cortex to other areas of the brain. Several human studies using functional magnetic resonance imaging, which uses blood oxygen tension differences as a surrogate of regional activation, support the notion that changes in the activation patterns of the brain under acute hypoglycemia do occur (15,16). It is therefore likely that with the advent of more localized NMR spectroscopy we will be able to further delineate regional differences of metabolism.

We must also take into consideration that energy substrates other than glucose may increase their contribution

From the [1]Section of Endocrinology, Department of Internal Medicine, Yale University School of Medicine, New Haven, Connecticut; and the [2]Department of Diagnostic Radiology, Yale University School of Medicine, New Haven, Connecticut.
Corresponding author: Raimund I. Herzog, raimund.herzog@yale.edu.

DOI: 10.2337/db11-0498

See accompanying original article, published in Diabetes 2011;60:1467–1473.

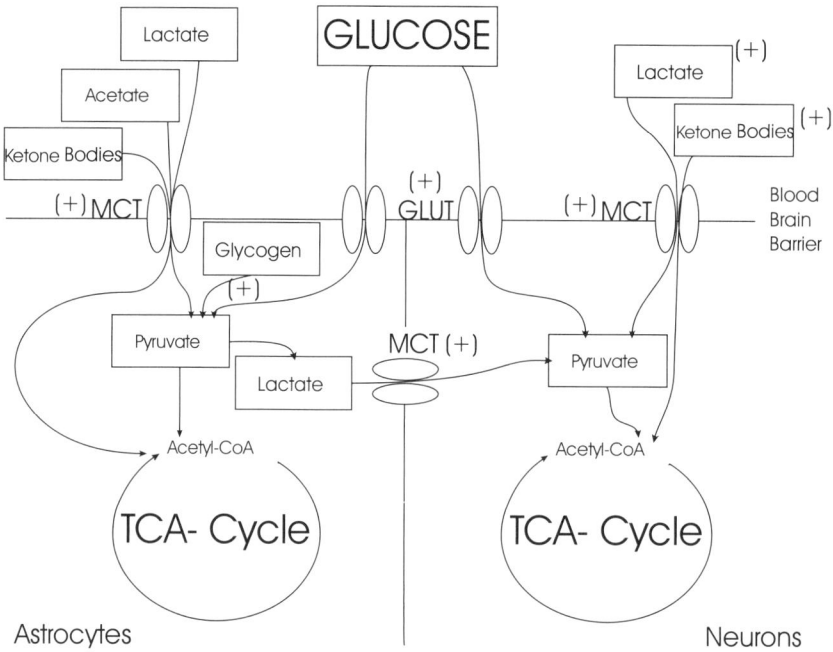

FIG. 1. Two-compartment model of brain metabolic fluxes along with pathways that have been proposed to be upregulated in intensively treated type 1 diabetes. Both astrocytes and neurons are dependent on glucose as a metabolic substrate, but neurons to a higher degree than astrocytes—particularly under hypoglycemia. Storage of glycogen allows astrocytes to provide neurons with an energy reserve that can be quickly mobilized and transferred during times of intense activity as well as during hypoglycemia; whether its levels are increased in type 1 diabetes still remains unclear (17). Monocarboxylic acid transporters (MCTs) along the blood brain barrier allow uptake of acetate, lactate, and ketone bodies and may be upregulated in type 1 diabetes (18,24) allowing increased alternate fuel consumption during hypoglycemia (indicated by +). Glucose transporters (GLUT) may be upregulated in a similar fashion in type 1 diabetes (20).

to TCA cycle activity, which in the brain is composed of separate and cooperative glial and neuronal compartments. For a schematic representation of these changes, see Fig. 1. Astrocytes (a form of glial cell predominant in the cerebral cortex) have emerged as playing a potentially important role by temporarily supplying neurons with fuel derived from stored glycogen, which could provide extra substrate during a hypoglycemic period (17). A reduction of astrocytic glucose metabolism to spare glucose for the neuron is also possible, and changes in the balance between neuronal and astrocyte glucose oxidation in animal models during hypoglycemia have been reported by our group (18). An alternative possibility is that there was an increase in the metabolism of lactate derived from the circulation, which increased by 50% under hypoglycemia. It has been reported that an infusion of lactate given to subjects during a comparable clamp study was able to alleviate cognitive dysfunction (19). We note that based on MRS measurements of glucose transport activity (20,21), the reduction in net glucose transport at 3 mmol/L plasma glucose levels would reduce glucose uptake on the order of 5–10%. Although van de Ven et al. indirectly calculate an up to 5% contribution of lactate, direct measurement of lactate metabolism by ^{13}C MRS (22) as well as arteriovenous difference methods (23) suggest that at the lactate levels achieved in the hypoglycemia portion of the study by van de Ven et al. the contribution of lactate oxidation is most likely greater and can support close to 10% of neuronal metabolic needs.

A more comprehensive understanding of the adaptations of brain fuel metabolism to acute and recurrent hypoglycemia will likely serve as the foundation for the development of more specific therapeutic interventions that avert the negative impact of neuroglycopenia in patients receiving insulin therapy.

ACKNOWLEDGMENTS

No potential conflicts of interest relevant to this article were reported.

REFERENCES

1. The Diabetes Control and Complications Trial Research Group. The effect of intensive treatment of diabetes on the development and progression of long-term complications in insulin-dependent diabetes mellitus. N Engl J Med 1993;329:977–986
2. UK Prospective Diabetes Study (UKPDS) Group. Intensive blood-glucose control with sulphonylureas or insulin compared with conventional treatment and risk of complications in patients with type 2 diabetes (UKPDS 33). Lancet 1998;352:837–853
3. Gerstein HC, Miller ME, Genuth S, et al.; ACCORD Study Group. Long-term effects of intensive glucose lowering on cardiovascular outcomes. N Engl J Med 2011;364:818–828
4. Yakubovich N, Gerstein HC. Serious cardiovascular outcomes in diabetes: the role of hypoglycemia. Circulation 2011;123:342–348
5. van den Berghe G, Wouters P, Weekers F, et al. Intensive insulin therapy in the critically ill patients. N Engl J Med 2001;345:1359–1367
6. Finfer S, Chittock DR, Su SY, et al.; NICE-SUGAR Study Investigators. Intensive versus conventional glucose control in critically ill patients. N Engl J Med 2009; 360:1283–1297
7. Kansagara D, Fu R, Freeman M, Wolf F, Helfand M. Intensive insulin therapy in hospitalized patients: a systematic review. Ann Intern Med 2011; 154:268–282
8. Cryer PE. Hypoglycemia in type 1 diabetes mellitus. Endocrinol Metab Clin North Am 2010;39:641–654
9. Abi-Saab WM, Maggs DG, Jones T, et al. Striking differences in glucose and lactate levels between brain extracellular fluid and plasma in conscious human subjects: effects of hyperglycemia and hypoglycemia. J Cereb Blood Flow Metab 2002;22:271–279

10. van de Ven KCC, de Galan BE, van der Graaf M, et al. Effect of acute hypoglycemia on human cerebral glucose metabolism measured by ^{13}C magnetic resonance spectroscopy. Diabetes 2011;60:1467–1473

11. Sommerfield AJ, Deary IJ, McAulay V, Frier BM. Moderate hypoglycemia impairs multiple memory functions in healthy adults. Neuropsychology 2003;17:125–132

12. Kodl CT, Seaquist ER. Cognitive dysfunction and diabetes mellitus. Endocr Rev 2008;29:494–511

13. Cranston I, Reed LJ, Marsden PK, Amiel SA. Changes in regional brain (18) F-fluorodeoxyglucose uptake at hypoglycemia in type 1 diabetic men associated with hypoglycemia unawareness and counter-regulatory failure. Diabetes 2001;50:2329–2336

14. Wang J, Jiang L, Jiang Y, Ma X, Chowdhury GM, Mason GF. Regional metabolite levels and turnover in the awake rat brain under the influence of nicotine. J Neurochem 2010;113:1447–1458

15. Anderson AW, Heptulla RA, Driesen N, et al. Effects of hypoglycemia on human brain activation measured with fMRI. Magn Reson Imaging 2006;24:693–697

16. Driesen NR, Goldberg PA, Anderson AW, et al. Hypoglycemia reduces the blood-oxygenation level dependent signal in primary auditory and visual cortex: a functional magnetic resonance imaging study. J Neurosci Res 2007;85:575–582

17. Herzog RI, Chan O, Yu S, Dziura J, McNay EC, Sherwin RS. Effect of acute and recurrent hypoglycemia on changes in brain glycogen concentration. Endocrinology 2008;149:1449–1504

18. Jiang L, Herzog RI, Mason GF, et al. Recurrent antecedent hypoglycemia alters neuronal oxidative metabolism in vivo. Diabetes 2009;58:1266–1274

19. Maran A, Cranston I, Lomas J, Macdonald I, Amiel SA. Protection by lactate of cerebral function during hypoglycaemia. Lancet 1994;343:16–20

20. Gruetter R, Novotny EJ, Boulware SD, et al. Direct measurement of brain glucose concentrations in humans by ^{13}C NMR spectroscopy. Proc Natl Acad Sci USA 1992;89:1109–1112

21. de Graaf RA, Mason GF, Patel AB, Rothman DL, Behar KL. Regional glucose metabolism and glutamatergic neurotransmission in rat brain in vivo. Proc Natl Acad Sci USA 2004;101:12700–12705

22. Boumezbeur F, Petersen KF, Cline GW, et al. The contribution of blood lactate to brain energy metabolism in humans measured by dynamic ^{13}C nuclear magnetic resonance spectroscopy. J Neurosci 2010;30:13983–13991

23. van Hall G, Strømstad M, Rasmussen P, et al. Blood lactate is an important energy source for the human brain. J Cereb Blood Flow Metab 2009;29:1121–1129

24. Mason GF, Petersen KF, Lebon V, Rothman DL, Shulman GI. Increased brain monocarboxylic acid transport and utilization in type 1 diabetes. Diabetes 2006;55:929–934

Hypoglycemia in Type 1 Diabetes

Rory J. McCrimmon[1] and Robert S. Sherwin[2]

In subjects with type 1 diabetes, autoimmune destruction of pancreatic β-cells leads eventually to an absolute requirement for insulin replacement therapy. Insulin delivered exogenously is not subject to normal physiological feedback regulation, so it may induce hypoglycemia even in the presence of an intact counterregulatory response. The average individual with type 1 diabetes experiences about two episodes of symptomatic hypoglycemia per week, a figure that has not changed substantially in the last 20 years (1). Severe hypoglycemia (requiring help for recovery) has an annual prevalence of 30–40% and an annual incidence of 1.0–1.7 episodes per patient per year (1). This risk is increased markedly with the increasing duration of the disease and strict glycemic control. In subjects with type 2 diabetes, the increasing duration of the disease and the more widespread use of insulin therapy also increase the risk of severe hypoglycemia. This is reflected in a recent survey in Tayside, Scotland, which found the proportion of severe hypoglycemic episodes needing emergency medical assistance was similar between type 1 and insulin-treated type 2 diabetic patients (2).

The experience of hypoglycemia is not limited to a transient impairment of cognition. We now recognize that hypoglycemia carries with it a recognized morbidity and mortality (3) and creates a negative mood-state characterized by reduced energy and increased tension (4). This may explain why hypoglycemia is greatly feared by individuals with diabetes; so much so that the fear of hypoglycemia is rated with the same degree of concern as the development of sight-threatening retinopathy or end-stage renal disease. This fear of hypoglycemia influences an individual's ability to adhere to optimal insulin replacement regimens and to put in place those measures required to achieve near-normal glucose control. In this way, hypoglycemia has emerged as a major obstacle to achieving the goals of intensive insulin therapy in everyday clinical practice.

In this review, we briefly describe the primary defects in hypoglycemia counterregulation, which are almost universally present in individuals with type 1 diabetes and, within this context, subsequently provide a general overview of the current state of research into the more basic mechanisms underlying the detection of hypoglycemia. Our focus tends to be on research into animal models, reflecting the focus of recent activity in this area. Animal models are a valuable tool for dissecting the molecular mechanisms involved in glucose sensing. To date, most animal models seem to show a similar hierarchy of responses to acute hypoglycemia—as well as developing similar defects to repeated hypoglycemia—as their human counterparts (5). However, species differences, particularly in brain metabolism given the unique size and metabolic demands of the human brain or in islet substructure, mean that data gleaned from animal studies still require further validation in human subjects before they can be confidently translated into clinical practice. A recent clinical review of hypoglycemia research (6) provides a detailed discussion on the clinical trials in human subjects.

Abnormal glucose counterregulation in diabetes. In nondiabetic individuals, hypoglycemia initiates a classic negative feedback counterregulatory response in which the fall in glucose leads to a series of neurohumoral and behavioral responses designed to restore normal glucose levels. Key steps in this homeostatic response are the suppression of endogenous insulin secretion and a stimulus to the secretion of the counterregulatory hormones, glucagon and epinephrine, which act rapidly to stimulate endogenous glucose production and to limit peripheral glucose utilization, thus increasing glucose delivery to the brain.

Three major defects in this homeostatic response contribute to the high frequency of hypoglycemia in type 1 diabetes. Firstly, the loss of β-cell insulin secretion and the need for exogenous insulin therapy mean that hypoglycemia is more likely to develop because of unregulated and sustained hyperinsulinemia. Secondly, within 5 years of disease diagnosis, almost all individuals with type 1 diabetes fail to generate an adequate glucagon response to hypoglycemia (7). Glucagon is the principal rapid-acting counterregulatory hormone, and the portal insulin-to-glucagon ratio is the major determinant of hepatic glucose production. Reduced or absent glucagon release results in a marked impairment of glucose recovery from hypoglycemia (8). A number of intra- and extra-pancreatic factors are thought to contribute to this defect. Briefly, a failure in local regulation of β- to α-cell signaling by insulin, zinc, and possibly the neurotransmitter γ-aminobutyric acid (GABA) during hypoglycemia probably play the dominant role in the genesis of this defect, particularly as it seems to track with the progressive loss of β-cell function (9). However, recent data suggest that the inhibitory effect of exogenous insulin on α-cell glucagon release is in part mediated at the level of the ventromedial hypothalamus (VMH) (10). Thus, the loss of glucagon response to insulin-induced hypoglycemia in C-peptide–deficient type 1 diabetic patients may to be due to the simultaneous increase in insulin levels both within the islet and the VMH. In addition, evidence exists of a local intra-islet sympathetic neuropathy (11), which may contribute in part to impaired glucagon release during hypoglycemia. Again, species differences in islet substructure in rodents limit our transla-

From the [1]Biomedical Research Institute, University of Dundee, Dundee, Scotland; and the [2]Department of Internal Medicine, Yale University, New Haven, Connecticut.

Corresponding author: Rory J. McCrimmon, r.mccrimmon@cpse.dundee.ac.uk.

Received 21 January 2010 and accepted 3 July 2010.

DOI: 10.2337/db10-0103

tion of these findings to human physiology, but the recognition that a number of defects may contribute to the loss of α-cell glucagon secretion during hypoglycemia opens up the possibility of novel therapeutic approaches, such as stimulation of central nervous system (CNS) sensing mechanisms. The selective inability of the α-cell to respond appropriately to a hypoglycemic challenge is a hallmark of type 1 (8) and long-duration type 2 diabetes (12), which remains poorly understood. Thirdly, the major defect in the counterregulatory response to hypoglycemia in diabetes is a reduced autonomic response. This affects the majority of individuals with type 1 diabetes by 10 years disease duration (7). Hypoglycemia normally leads to activation of the autonomic nervous system resulting in increased hepatic glucose production and reduced glucose uptake in peripheral tissues. In liver stimulation, sympathetic nervous system activation increases both glycogenolysis and gluconeogenesis; the latter via a simultaneous increase in the delivery of gluconeogenic substrates and free fatty acids (13). The autonomic response is closely associated with the generation of a symptomatic response to hypoglycemia and, as such, when this response becomes impaired there is usually reduced awareness of hypoglycemia as well as a reduction in catecholamine release. This association means the autonomic response to hypoglycemia is critically important in individuals with type 1 diabetes. As will be discussed later in this review, a defective autonomic counterregulatory response results primarily from prior exposure to hypoglycemia per se (14), a situation that occurs most frequently during intensive insulin therapy. This sets up a vicious cycle whereby hypoglycemia increases the likelihood of subsequent hypoglycemia.

Thus, the glucose counterregulatory defense against hypoglycemia in individuals with diabetes becomes impaired at almost every level and rendered even more defective through intensive insulin therapy. In the following sections, we will examine some of the basic mechanisms underlying the detection of hypoglycemia. In vivo and ex vivo animal models have been used to ask the questions, where does the body sense fluctuations in glucose levels, how is glucose sensed, and why does this mechanism become impaired following recurrent hypoglycemia?

The molecular biology of hypoglycemia detection
Hypoglycemia sensors. It is currently believed that hypoglycemia is detected by specialized cells/neurons located within discrete regions of the CNS and periphery, and it seems likely that these cells are linked together in some way providing an integrated mechanism for monitoring whole-body glucose and/or fuel homeostasis (Fig. 1). In an excellent recent review of this integrative glucose-sensing network, Watts and Donovan (15) describe how peripheral, hindbrain, and hypothalamic glucose sensors form a classical sensory-motor integrative pathway. They illustrate how forebrain integrative networks might modify hindbrain glucose-sensing autonomic reflex loops. This model could explain how different stressors (e.g., hypoglycemia and exercise) might interact, and why defective hypoglycemia counterregulation could arise through defects in these forebrain integrative networks.

To date, glucose sensors in the periphery, apart from the pancreatic β-cell, have been found in the intestine, hepatoportal vein, and carotid body (7). Within the CNS, ex-vivo electrophysiological studies have identified a num-

ber of areas in the brain that contain neurons sensitive to local changes in glucose (7). One brain region in particular, the VMH, appears to plays a crucial role during hypoglycemia and was the subject of a recent review (16). The specialized glucose-sensing neurons in the CNS have been broadly defined as either glucose-excited (GE), which increases their action potential frequency when glucose rises, or glucose-inhibited (GI), which increases their action potential frequency when glucose levels fall (17). These neurons are liable to react in a coordinated manner to alterations in the glucose level to which they are exposed. The neurons also respond to other metabolites such as lactate and β-hydroxybutyrate, as well as hormones such as insulin, leptin, and possibly glucagon-like peptide 1, reflecting the central role they play in responding to alterations in fuel supply and in maintaining glucose homeostasis. From an evolutionary perspective, it seems very likely that these neurons have developed to ensure an adequate supply of fuel to the brain during periods of prolonged starvation because of the limited capacity of the brain to store fuel in depots such as glycogen or fat. In this context, the ability to integrate many different aspects of human metabolism is essential to ensure a continuous supply of glucose to the brain.

Hypoglycemia sensing
The hypothalamic β-cell. A number of mechanisms may underlie glucose sensing by GE/GI neurons in the CNS. These are not necessarily distinct or redundant mechanisms and, at least in the authors' opinion, probably all play some role in the detection of hypoglycemia. Most studies indicate that the principal glucose-sensing mechanism within these specialized neurons parallels that used by the pancreatic β-cell, namely in the critical roles for glucokinase (GK) (18), the ATP-sensitive potassium channel (K_{ATP}) (19), and AMP-activated protein kinase (AMPK) (20) (Fig. 2). The pancreatic isoform of GK (the critical regulator of glycolytic production of ATP and K_{ATP} channel activity in the pancreatic β-cell) is expressed in the majority of glucose-sensing neurons as is mRNA for sulfonurea receptor (SUR)-1 and Kir6.2 subunits of the K_{ATP} channel (21). Pharmacological or adenoviral manipulation of GK modulates hypothalamic glucose-sensing neurons ex-vivo, and selective down-regulation of GK using RNA interference in the VMH of rats suppresses the counterregulatory response to acute hypoglycemia (22). In addition, down-regulating GK in primary VMH neuronal cultures using RNA interference leads to the loss of all demonstrable glucose-sensing (GE and GI) activity (18). Similarly, electrophysiological studies of rat (23) and mouse hypothalamic slice preparations (24) demonstrate that sulfonylureas modulate the firing rate of glucose-sensing neurons, and local in vivo application of a K_{ATP} channel blocker to the VMH suppresses, while the opening of the K_{ATP} channel amplifies the glucose counterregulatory response to acute hypoglycemia (7). GLUT-2, the high-capacity, low-affinity GLUT of the pancreatic β-cell, may also play a role in central glucose sensing (25), although limitations in the transgenic model employed in this study and the difficulty in detecting GLUT-2 in the brain mean this data needs replicating.

Evidence is also emerging for an important role for AMPK in glucose sensing, particularly during hypoglycemia. AMPK is an ancient, highly conserved serine/threonine kinase that is activated during cellular energy depletion and acts to suppress ATP-consuming pathways and to activate ATP-generating pathways. Hypothalamic

Hypoglycemia
Development

Hypoglycemia
Sensing

Glucose Counter-
regulation

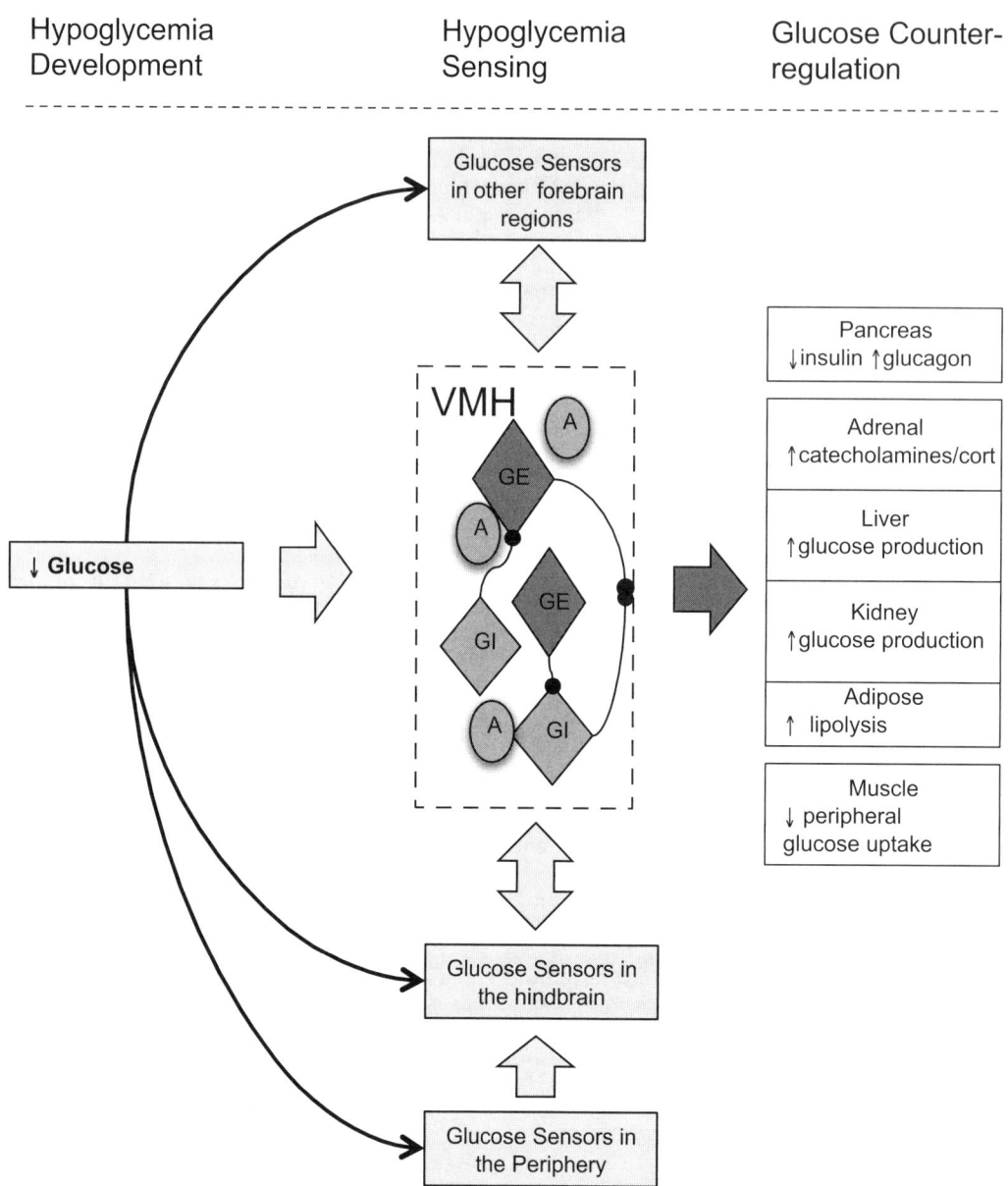

FIG. 1. Integrative model of hypoglycemia detection. A falling glucose is detected by peripheral and central glucose-sensing cells/neurons. Peripheral glucose sensors signal back to glucose-sensing regions of the hindbrain in turn activating efferent pathways that initiate a counterregulatory response. At the same time, glucose sensors in the hypothalamus, such as those in the VMH and other forebrain regions, detect falling glucose, also activating efferent pathways that initiate a counterregulatory response. Integrative pathways between hindbrain, hypothalamic, and other forebrain regions are reciprocally connected and can modulate responses to the hypoglycemic signal. Glucose-sensing regions in the brain, such as the VMH, contain GE and GI neurons and an astrocytic support structure. A, astrocytic.

AMPK is activated in response to fasting or central glucoprivation. During hypoglycemia, local in vivo pharmacological activation of AMPK in the VMH amplifies counterregulatory responses while selective AMPK downregulation in the VMH suppresses the responses (7). It has been suggested that AMPK acts as the dominant glucose sensor in GI neurons (26), however loss of glucose-sensing ability in transgenic mouse models with selective loss of AMPK in classical hypothalamic GE neurons (27) and pancreatic β-cells (28) would seem to suggest that AMPK acts as a functional glucose sensor within both GI and GE neurons (7).

The "glucose" signal. In addition to the classical pathway of glucose sensing, Burdakov et al. (29) have proposed the novel and intriguing hypothesis that glucose,

independent of its oxidation, may modulate the action potential in glucose-sensing neurons. Glucose transport into the neuron is thought to be coupled directly with the transmembrane movement of ions, such as those used by sodium glucose cotransporters (SGLTs). Given intracerebroventricular, phloridizin, a nonselective inhibitor of SGLTs, increased food intake in rats and inhibited VMH GE neurons (29), while α-methylglucopyranoside, a nonmetabolizable substrate of SGLTs, excited GE neurons in primary rat hypothalamic cultures (30). Alternatively, glucose might bind to an extra-cellular receptor that could alter electrical activity without transporting the glucose into the neuron (29). Whether glucose sensing in the brain occurs primarily through this mechanism, or whether glucose per se might act to potentiate the signal induced

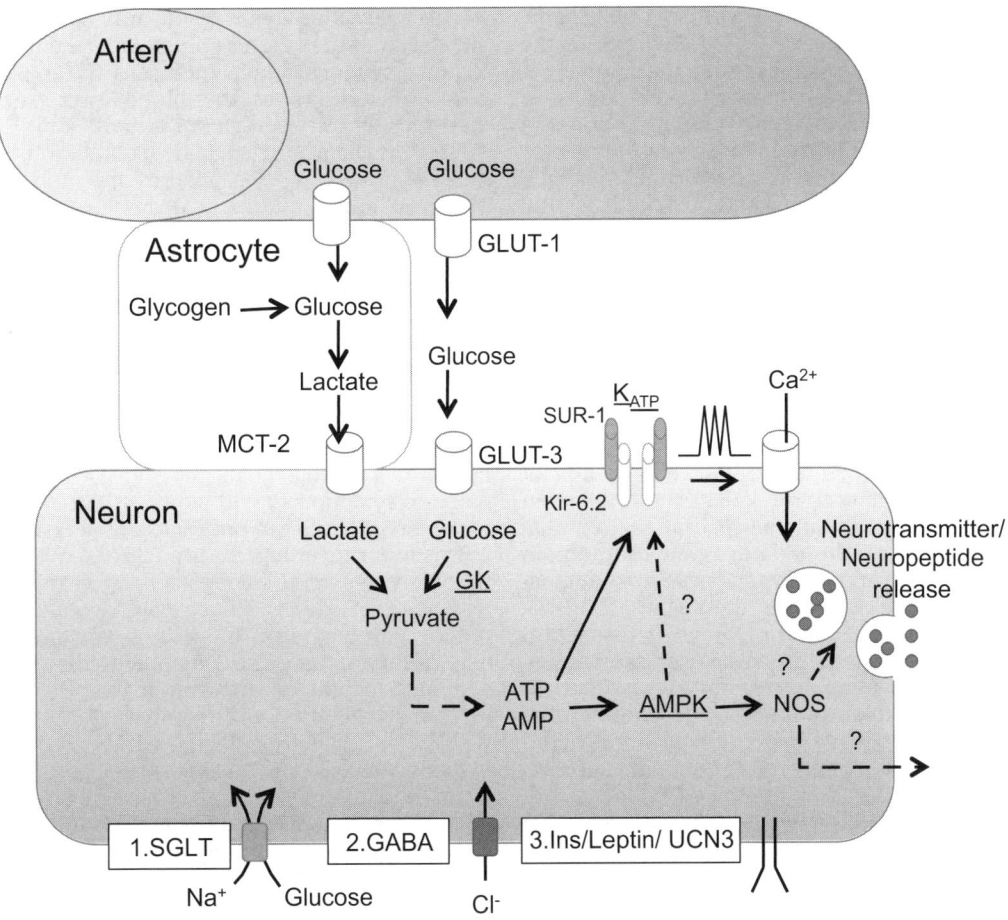

FIG. 2. A simplified model of glucose-sensing mechanisms present in the brain. Glucose from the arterial supply is transported either directly into neurons via GLUT-3 (possibly GLUT-2) or indirectly as lactate generated through glycolysis in astrocytes. Glucose is phosphorylated by GK, a key regulatory step in glucose sensing, before undergoing oxidative-phosphorylation to generate ATP. ATP closes the SUR-1–selective K_{ATP}, leading to membrane depolarization, calcium influx, and release of neurotransmitters and/or neuropeptides. In addition, AMP-to-ATP ratios are monitored by AMPK, activation that during hypoglycemia stimulates the production of nitric oxide and may act via the K_{ATP} channel or directly to stimulate neurotransmitter release. Additional mechanisms that may modulate this basic glucose-sensing mechanism include: *1*) SGLTs, *2*) GABAergic inhibition (or modulation by other neurotransmitters such as norepinephrine), and *3*) the actions of hormones such as insulin and leptin and neuropeptides such as urocortin 3. CI⁻, chloride; Ins, insulin; MCT, monocarboxylate transporters; NOS, nitric oxide synthase; UCN3, urocortin 3.

by the oxidation of glucose in sensing neurons, remains to be determined.

Astrocytic glucose sensing. Finally, it is well established that within the CNS, astrocytes and neurons (and blood vessels) work together as functional units. Importantly, the cerebral blood vessels delivering glucose to the brain are almost completely surrounded by a network of astrocytic foot processes. This raises the possibility that glucose may regulate sensing neurons at least in part indirectly via astrocytes. Tanycytes, for instance, are specialized astrocytic cells that line much of the floor of the third ventricle and express GLUT-2, GK, and the K_{ATP} channel and send long processes that terminate in the VMH. Tanycytes show reversible inhibition by third ventricular delivery of alloxan (taken up through GLUT-2) in a temporal pattern that parallels changes in the hormonal counterregulatory response to systemic 2-deoxyglucose (31). On the basis of these findings, Sanders et al. (31) have suggested that tanycytes may play a critical role in glucose sensing during hypoglycemia, transmitting the glucoprivic signal to neurons in the VMH, which then stimulate a counterregulatory response.

The current literature, taken together, would appear to suggest that the characteristic feature of glucose-sensing cells is the presence of GK and AMPK. Intriguingly, this would suggest that the glucose-sensing mechanism may be a universal mechanism even if the cell is activated or inhibited by glucose. Downstream signaling and the specific neurotransmitters/neuropeptides released would then determine the output of that glucose signal. It is important to note that this would also imply that a glucose-sensing neuronal population did not need to be directly involved in glucose homeostasis. Neuropeptide Y neurons are GI neurons that play a major role in stimulating food intake in response to glucoprivation, but there is no evidence to date indicating a direct role in the stimulus to hormonal counterregulation.

Hypoglycemia activation. Once a change in glucose is sensed, the neuron needs to communicate that signal to a downstream neuron in the pathway that eventually leads to glucose counterregulation. In general, neural communication relies on the release of classical neurotransmitters, such as GABA, glutamate, neuropeptides, or unconventional transmitters such as nitric oxide. GAD, the rate limiting enzyme in GABA synthesis, is expressed in 56% of GE and 36% of GI neurons (21). GABA levels in VMH interstitial fluid are decreased during acute hypoglycemia, and in vivo antagonism of the VMH GABA amplifies the counterregulatory hormone response to acute hypoglycemia (32). It is important here to note that the source of GABA input to the VMH during hypoglycemia is not as yet known and may arise from surrounding hypothalamic or other forebrain regions. Interestingly, recurrent hypoglycemia leads to a significant increase in GAD65 mRNA and protein (33 and 580%, respectively) in the VMH, while VMH GABA concentrations measured by microdialysis were more than threefold higher, suggesting that recurrent hypoglycemia results in increased VMH GABA inhibitory tone. Increased GABA tone could contribute to reduced action potential frequency in VMH glucose-sensing neurons with the net result of this being to suppress the counterregulatory response during subsequent hypoglycemia.

A single report (33) suggests that the excitatory output from glucose sensors such as the VMH may be glutamatergic, while excitatory input to the VMH from brain stem noradrenergic neurons may link peripheral to hypothalamic glucose sensors (34). In addition, caudal hindbrain serotonergic neurons express GK and project to sympathetic interomediolateral neurons in the spinal cord (35). Recently, it was reported that 6- or 20-days delivery of a selective serotonin reuptake inhibitor to normal Sprague-Dawley rats amplified the counterregulatory response to acute hypoglycemia and prevented the development of defective counterregulation in rats exposed to repeated hypoglycemic stress (35). Interestingly, human subjects with type 1 diabetes also show enhanced counterregulation to hypoglycemia following 6 weeks of selective serotonin reuptake inhibitor therapy (36). Finally, the unconventional transmitter nitric oxide may also provide a signal to downstream neurons (37).

Hypothalamic glucose-sensing neurons can also be regulated by local or peripheral release of neuropeptides. Davis et al. (38) was the first to demonstrate this in the context of the hypoglycemic stress response by showing the important regulatory role of systemic glucocorticoids, while Flannagan et al. (39) noted a potential role for systemic corticotrophin-releasing hormone (CRH). More recently it has been shown that VMH urocortin 3, also a member of the CRH family of neuropeptides, has a marked suppressive action on counterregulatory responses to acute hypoglycemia (40). Conversely, VMH microinjection of CRH, which acts primarily through CRH-receptor type 1, amplifies the counterregulatory response (41). Thus, there appears to be feedback inhibition to the hypothalamus of the hypoglycemic stimulus to counterregulation through the release of systemic and central peptides. It is likely that these mechanisms coexist because the stress response is at once essential to the survival of the species, and on the other hand, potentially highly toxic if sustained. It is therefore highly regulated at both the whole-body and cellular level.

Recurrent hypoglycemia and hypothalamic glucose sensing. Repeated hypoglycemia produces a downregulation of the hormonal counterregulatory response to subsequent hypoglycemia (14), while its strict avoidance can restore the response (42). Rodent studies indicate that changes in key brain glucose-sensing regions play a major role in mediating this phenomenon. Recurrent hypoglycemia markedly suppressed the counterregulatory response induced by local VMH perfusion with 2-deoxyglucose (43) and lowered the glucose level activating individual VMH glucose-sensing neurons (44).

This adaptation might result from increased transport of glucose and/or alternate fuel into the sensing neuron. Repeated hypoglycemia increases the expression of glucose transporters at the blood-brain barrier (45) and increases whole-brain glucose uptake (46) and the uptake of the monocarboxylic acid acetate (47). The effect on overall brain glucose transport has not, however, been observed in all studies (48), raising the possibility that there is regional variation in the brain of this response. Alternatively, the central glucose-sensing neurons might obtain additional metabolic substrates from more local sources such as brain glycogen. Brain glycogen levels were reported to increase following the restoration of normoglycemia (49), and this "super-compensation" could provide an additional fuel reserve. However, brain glycogen levels are very low (by necessity of the skull vault). In rodents, these levels also return to baseline within several hours of a hypoglycemic episode, a time when glucose counterregulation is still suppressed (50). This does not, however, exclude the possibility of accelerated astrocytic glycogen turnover and in turn increased delivery of lactate following repeated hypoglycemia. In addition, repeated activation of the AMPK cascade would be expected to induce mitochondrial biogenesis and increased metabolism of fatty acids (51). This potentially reduces neuronal demands for glucose, sparing it for other tasks. Interestingly, a recent study (52) comparing nondiabetic subjects with type 1 diabetic subjects who were unaware of their hypoglycemia found no difference in the overall rate of brain oxidative phosphorylation measured by ^{13}C nuclear magnetic resonance, although the study was undertaken under euglycemic conditions.

As described earlier, acute hypoglycemia also activates a number of pathways involved in the regulation of the neuroendocrine stress response. Glucocorticoids (38), CRH (39), and urocortin 3 (40) given under controlled euglycemic conditions (i.e., excluding hypoglycemia as a factor) can all induce defective counterregulation to next-day hypoglycemia. Activation of this family of neuropeptides plays an integral role in a number of different forms of stress, and they are tightly regulated. Studies in transgenic mice show that activation of CRH-R2 suppresses—whereas activation of CRH-R1 amplifies—the responses to a number of physiological stressors (53). Therefore, an alteration in the balance between CRH-R2– and CRH-R1–mediated actions, induced by glucocorticoids or the CRH neuropeptides, could lead to suppression of the glucose counterregulatory response during a subsequent exposure to hypoglycemia. This mechanism would explain why the depth and duration of hypoglycemia both contribute directly to the magnitude of the subsequent counterregulatory defect (increased antecedent stress response) (54), and why alternate stressors, such as exercise (55), induce similar changes.

These adaptations are not necessarily mutually exclusive and, given the complexity of the neuroendocrine response to hypoglycemia, it is likely that a number of adaptations at the cellular and whole systems levels all contribute to some degree in the development of defective counterregulation. In the authors' opinion, hypoglycemia initiates two primary adaptive responses, both of which are interlinked at many levels. The first results from hypoglycemia acting as an acute "starvation" signal leading to local cellular adaptations in the brain, such as an increased ability to use alternate fuels and changes to peripheral metabolism that would permit increased delivery of fuel substrates to the liver for the generation of glucose and ketone bodies. The second adaptation is a down-regulation of the stress response, which again takes place at both the cellular and whole systems levels and is designed to limit the potential of hypoglycemia to induce cell death. This later response is a very well-established response to repeated cellular stress and can be seen as a form of preconditioning or tolerance. These two principal adaptive responses also explain why there is likely to be regional variation in the effects of recurrent hypoglycemia. Neurons most affected by acute hypoglycemia (e.g., glucose-sensing neurons that are activated by hypoglycemia and drive the stress response) may show an enhanced dual effect of metabolic adaptation and feedback inhibition of the stress response caused by repeated hypoglycemia.

It is our belief that these changes are adaptive and not maladaptive and, to that extent, this would not be consistent with the current description of this phenomenon as hypoglycemia-associated autonomic failure. At a more basic level, repeated hypoglycemia is inducing hypoglycemia tolerance through preconditioning. This does not mean the individual is fully protected from the consequences of hypoglycemia. The problem is, of course, that the appearance of hypoglycemia in diabetes occurs when there is a marked hyper- rather than hypoinsulinemia. Hyperinsulinemia blocks peripheral generation of alternate fuels and, in the presence of impaired counterregulation, is more likely to induce severe and prolonged hypoglycemia. Under these conditions, brain extracellular fluid glucose levels are extremely low and, thus, there is the potential for cellular damage or even death. This is why the inability to exert feedback inhibition of insulin release and action during hypoglycemia is one of the key counterregulatory defects of type 1 diabetes.

Summary. Hypoglycemia remains a major obstacle to improved glycemic control in diabetes and, despite the development of novel short- and long-acting and insulin analogues and the more widespread use of pump therapy, the frequency of hypoglycemia in type 1 diabetes has not changed dramatically over the last 20 years. The challenge is to try and understand the mechanisms through which the body detects falling glucose and initiates a glucose counterregulatory response. Despite a few decades of research, these mechanisms are still poorly understood, as are the pathways through which different glucose-sensing regions communicate in order to integrate the whole-body response to hypoglycemia at a behavioral and a physiological level. A further challenge, but one that is crucial to the translation of this basic research into clinical practice, will be to examine candidate mechanisms in model systems that are more directly relevant to type 1 diabetes. There are currently no widely available therapies for the individual with type 1 diabetes who experiences recurrent severe hypoglycemia, so the need to develop such interventions is great.

ACKNOWLEDGMENTS

The research work of the authors is supported by research grants from the National Institute of Diabetes and Digestive and Kidney Diseases (69831, 20495, and 45735), the Juvenile Diabetes Research Foundation, and the American Diabetes Association.

No potential conflicts of interest relevant to this article were reported.

R.J.M. and R.S.S. wrote and edited the manuscript.

The authors thank the postdoctoral fellows and technical staff who contributed greatly to the research that underpins this review.

REFERENCES

1. Frier BM. The incidence and impact of hypoglycemia in type 1 and type 2 diabetes. International Diabetes Monitor 2009;21:210–218
2. Leese GP, Wang J, Broomhall J, Kelly P, Marsden A, Morrison W, Frier BM, Morris AD, DARTS/MEMO Collaboration. Frequency of severe hypoglycemia requiring emergency treatment in type 1 and type 2 diabetes: a population-based study of health service resource use. Diabetes Care 2003;26:1176–1180
3. McCrimmon RJ, Frier BM. Hypoglycaemia: the most feared complication of insulin therapy. Diabete Metab 1994;20:503–512
4. McCrimmon RJ, Frier BM, Deary IJ. Appraisal of mood and personality during hypoglycaemia in human subjects. Physiol Behav 1999;67:27–33
5. Powell AM, Sherwin RS, Shulman GI. Impaired hormonal responses to hypoglycemia in spontaneously diabetic and recurrently hypoglycemic rats: reversibility and stimulus specificity of the deficits. J Clin Invest 1993;92:2667–2674
6. Amiel SA. Hypoglycemia: from the laboratory to the clinic. Diabetes Care 2009;32:1364–1371
7. McCrimmon R. The mechanisms that underlie glucose sensing during hypoglycaemia in diabetes. Diabet Med 2008;25:513–522
8. Gerich JE, Langlois M, Noacco C, Karam JH, Forsham PH. Lack of glucagon response to hypoglycemia in diabetes: evidence for an intrinsic pancreatic alpha cell defect. Science 1973;182:171–173
9. Fukuda M, Tanaka A, Tahara Y, Ikegami H, Yamamoto Y, Kumahara Y, Shima K. Correlation between minimal secretory capacity of pancreatic beta-cells and stability of diabetic control. Diabetes 1988;37:81–88
10. Paranjape SA, Chan O, Zhu W, Horblitt AM, McNay EC, Cresswell JA, Bogan JS, McCrimmon RJ, Sherwin RS. Influence of insulin in the ventromedial hypothalamus on pancreatic glucagon secretion in vivo. Diabetes 2010;59:1521–1527
11. Mundinger TO, Mei Q, Figlewicz DP, Lernmark A, Taborsky GJ Jr. Impaired glucagon response to sympathetic nerve stimulation in the BB diabetic rat: effect of early sympathetic islet neuropathy. Am J Physiol Endocrinol Metab 2003;285:E1047–E1054
12. Segel SA, Paramore DS, Cryer PE. Hypoglycemia-associated autonomic failure in advanced type 2 diabetes. Diabetes 2002;51:724–733
13. Fanelli CG, De Feo P, Porcellati F, Perriello G, Torlone E, Santeusanio F, Brunetti P, Bolli GB. Adrenergic mechanisms contribute to the late phase of hypoglycemic glucose counterregulation in humans by stimulating lipolysis. J Clin Invest 1992;89:2005–2013
14. Heller SR, Cryer PE. Reduced neuroendocrine and symptomatic responses to subsequent hypoglycemia after 1 episode of hypoglycemia in nondiabetic humans. Diabetes 1991;40:223–226
15. Watts AG, Donovan CM. Sweet talk in the brain: glucosensing, neural networks, and hypoglycemic counterregulation. Front Neuroendocrinol 2010;31:32–43
16. Sherwin RS. Bringing light to the dark side of insulin: a journey across the blood-brain barrier. Diabetes 2008;57:2259–2268
17. Routh VH. Glucose-sensing neurons: are they physiologically relevant? Physiol Behav 2002;76:403–413
18. Kang L, Dunn-Meynell AA, Routh VH, Gaspers LD, Nagata Y, Nishimura T, Eiki J, Zhang BB, Levin BE. Glucokinase is a critical regulator of ventromedial hypothalamic neuronal glucosensing. Diabetes 2006;55:412–420
19. Ashford ML, Boden PR, Treherne JM. Tolbutamide excites rat glucoreceptive ventromedial hypothalamic neurones by indirect inhibition of ATP-K+ channels. Br J Pharmacol 1990;101:531–540
20. McCrimmon RJ, Shaw M, Fan X, Cheng H, Ding Y, Vella MC, Zhou L, McNay EC, Sherwin RS. Key role for AMP-activated protein kinase in the ventromedial hypothalamus in regulating counterregulatory hormone responses to acute hypoglycemia. Diabetes 2008;57:444–450
21. Kang L, Routh VH, Kuzhikandathil EV, Gaspers LD, Levin BE. Physiological and molecular characteristics of rat hypothalamic ventromedial nucleus glucosensing neurons. Diabetes 2004;53:549–559
22. Levin BE, Becker TC, Eiki J, Zhang BB, Dunn-Meynell AA. Ventromedial hypothalamic glucokinase is an important mediator of the counterregulatory response to insulin-induced hypoglycemia. Diabetes 2008;57:1371–1379
23. Song Z, Levin BE, McArdle JJ, Bakhos N, Routh VH. Convergence of pre- and postsynaptic influences on glucosensing neurons in the ventromedial hypothalamic nucleus. Diabetes 2001;50:2673–2681

24. Miki T, Liss B, Minami K, Shiuchi T, Saraya A, Kashima Y, Horiuchi M, Ashcroft F, Minokoshi Y, Roeper J, Seino S. ATP-sensitive K+ channels in the hypothalamus are essential for the maintenance of glucose homeostasis. Nat Neurosci 2001;4:507–512

25. Burcelin R, Thorens B. Evidence that extrapancreatic GLUT2-dependent glucose sensors control glucagon secretion. Diabetes 2001;50:1282–1289

26. Mountjoy PD, Bailey SJ, Rutter GA. Inhibition by glucose or leptin of hypothalamic neurons expressing neuropeptide Y requires changes in AMP-activated protein kinase activity. Diabetologia 2007;50:168–177

27. Claret M, Smith MA, Batterham RL, Selman C, Choudhury AI, Fryer LG, Clements M, Al-Qassab H, Heffron H, Xu AW, Speakman JR, Barsh GS, Viollet B, Vaulont S, Ashford ML, Carling D, Withers DJ. AMPK is essential for energy homeostasis regulation and glucose sensing by POMC and AgRP neurons. J Clin Invest 2007;117:2325–2336

28. Sun G, Tarasov AI, McGinty J, McDonald A, da Silva Xavier G, Gorman T, Marley A, French PM, Parker H, Gribble F, Reimann F, Prendiville O, Carzaniga R, Viollet B, Leclerc I, Rutter GA. Ablation of AMP-activated protein kinase alpha1 and alpha2 from mouse pancreatic beta cells and RIP2: Cre neurons suppresses insulin release in vivo. Diabetologia 2010; 53:924–936

29. Burdakov D, Luckman SM, Verkhratsky A. Glucose-sensing neurons of the hypothalamus. Philos Trans R Soc Lond B Biol Sci 2005;360:2227–2235

30. O'Malley D, Reimann F, Simpson AK, Gribble FM. Sodium-coupled glucose cotransporters contribute to hypothalamic glucose sensing. Diabetes 2006; 55:3381–3386

31. Sanders NM, Dunn-Meynell AA, Levin BE. Third ventricular alloxan reversibly impairs glucose counterregulatory responses. Diabetes 2004;53: 1230–1236

32. Chan O, Cheng H, Herzog R, Czyzyk D, Zhu W, Wang A, McCrimmon RJ, Seashore MR, Sherwin RS. Increased GABAergic tone in the ventromedial hypothalamus contributes to suppression of counterregulatory responses after antecedent hypoglycemia. Diabetes 2008;57:1363–1370

33. Tong Q, Ye C, McCrimmon RJ, Dhillon H, Choi B, Kramer MD, Yu J, Yang Z, Christiansen LM, Lee CE, Choi CS, Zigman JM, Shulman GI, Sherwin RS, Elmquist JK, Lowell BB. Synaptic glutamate release by ventromedial hypothalamic neurons is part of the neurocircuitry that prevents hypoglycemia. Cell Metab 2007;5:383–393

34. de Vries MG, Lawson MA, Beverly JL. Hypoglycemia-induced noradrenergic activation in the VMH is a result of decreased ambient glucose. Am J Physiol Regul Integr Comp Physiol 2005;289:R977–R981

35. Sanders NM, Wilkinson CW, Taborsky GJ Jr, Al-Noori S, Daumen W, Zavosh A, Figlewicz DP. The selective serotonin reuptake inhibitor sertraline enhances counterregulatory responses to hypoglycemia. Am J Physiol Endocrinol Metab 2008;294:E853–E860

36. Briscoe VJ, Ertl AC, Tate DB, Davis SN. Effects of the selective serotonin reuptake inhibitor fluoxetine on counterregulatory responses to hypoglycemia in individuals with type 1 diabetes. Diabetes 2008;57:3315–3322

37. Fioramonti X, Marsollier N, Song Z, Fakira KA, Patel RM, Brown S, Duparc T, Pica-Mendez A, Sanders NM, Knauf C, Valet P, McCrimmon RJ, Beuve A, Magnan C, Routh VH. Ventromedial hypothalamic nitric oxide production is necessary for hypoglycemia detection and counterregulation. Diabetes 2010;59:519–528

38. Davis SN, Shavers C, Costa F, Mosqueda-Garcia R. Role of cortisol in the pathogenesis of deficient counterregulation after antecedent hypoglycemia in normal humans. J Clin Invest 1996;98:680–691

39. Flanagan DE, Keshavarz T, Evans ML, Flanagan S, Fan X, Jacob RJ, Sherwin RS. Role of corticotrophin-releasing hormone in the impairment of counterregulatory responses to hypoglycemia. Diabetes 2003;52:605–613

40. McCrimmon RJ, Song Z, Cheng H, McNay EC, Weikart-Yeckel C, Fan X, Routh VH, Sherwin RS. Corticotrophin-releasing factor receptors within the ventromedial hypothalamus regulate hypoglycemia-induced hormonal counterregulation. J Clin Invest 2006;116:1723–1730

41. Cheng H, Zhou L, Zhu W, Wang A, Tang C, Chan O, Sherwin RS, McCrimmon RJ. Type 1 corticotropin-releasing factor receptors in the ventromedial hypothalamus promote hypoglycemia-induced hormonal counterregulation. Am J Physiol Endocrinol Metab 2007;293:E705–E712

42. Cranston I, Lomas J, Maran A, Macdonald I, Amiel SA. Restoration of hypoglycaemia awareness in patients with long-duration insulin-dependent diabetes. Lancet 1994;344:283–287

43. Borg MA, Borg WP, Tamborlane WV, Brines ML, Shulman GI, Sherwin RS. Chronic hypoglycemia and diabetes impair counterregulation induced by localized 2-deoxy-glucose perfusion of the ventromedial hypothalamus in rats. Diabetes 1999;48:584–587

44. Song Z, Routh VH. Recurrent hypoglycemia reduces the glucose sensitivity of glucose-inhibited neurons in the ventromedial hypothalamus nucleus. Am J Physiol Regul Integr Comp Physiol 2006;291:R1283–R1287

45. Kumagai AK, Kang YS, Boado RJ, Pardridge WM. Upregulation of blood-brain barrier GLUT1 glucose transporter protein and mRNA in experimental chronic hypoglycemia. Diabetes 1995;44:1399–1404

46. Boyle PJ, Kempers SF, O'Connor AM, Nagy RJ. Brain glucose uptake and unawareness of hypoglycemia in patients with insulin-dependent diabetes mellitus. N Engl J Med 1995;333:1726–1731

47. Mason GF, Petersen KF, Lebon V, Rothman DL, Shulman GI. Increased brain monocarboxylic acid transport and utilization in type 1 diabetes. Diabetes 2006;55:929–934

48. Segel SA, Fanelli CG, Dence CS, Markham J, Videen TO, Paramore DS, Powers WJ, Cryer PE. Blood-to-brain glucose transport, cerebral glucose metabolism, and cerebral blood flow are not increased after hypoglycemia. Diabetes 2001;50:1911–1917

49. Choi IY, Seaquist ER, Gruetter R. Effect of hypoglycemia on brain glycogen metabolism in vivo. J Neurosci Res 2003;72:25–32

50. Herzog RI, Chan O, Yu S, Dziura J, McNay EC, Sherwin RS. Effect of acute and recurrent hypoglycemia on changes in brain glycogen concentration. Endocrinology 2008;149:1499–1504

51. Zong H, Ren JM, Young LH, Pypaert M, Mu J, Birnbaum MJ, Shulman GI. AMP kinase is required for mitochondrial biogenesis in skeletal muscle in response to chronic energy deprivation. Proc Natl Acad Sci U S A 2002;99:15983–15987

52. Henry PG, Criego AB, Kumar A, Seaquist ER. Measurement of cerebral oxidative glucose consumption in patients with type 1 diabetes mellitus and hypoglycemia unawareness using (13)C nuclear magnetic resonance spectroscopy. Metabolism 2010;59:100–106

53. Bale TL, Vale WW. CRF and CRF receptors: role in stress responsivity and other behaviors. Annu Rev Pharmacol Toxicol 2004;44:525–557

54. Davis SN, Mann S, Galassetti P, Neill RA, Tate D, Ertl AC, Costa F. Effects of differing durations of antecedent hypoglycemia on counterregulatory responses to subsequent hypoglycemia in normal humans. Diabetes 2000; 49:1897–1903

55. Galassetti P, Mann S, Tate D, Neill RA, Costa F, Wasserman DH, Davis SN. Effects of antecedent prolonged exercise on subsequent counterregulatory responses to hypoglycemia. Am J Physiol Endocrinol Metab 2001;280: E908–E917

Hypoglycemia, Diabetes, and Cardiovascular Events

Cyrus V. Desouza, md[1]
Geremia B. Bolli, md[2]
Vivian Fonseca, md[3]

Diabetes is at epidemic proportions in the U.S. Patients with diabetes are at increased risk for micro- and macrovascular complications. The benefit of glycemic control in decreasing the risk for microvascular disease is well established. However, the role of glycemic control in decreasing macrovascular complications has been controversial. Several large clinical trials looking at this issue have either shown no benefit or even potential harm. The possibility of hypoglycemia as a risk factor for cardiovascular events is a topic of much debate. In this review article, we discuss the evidence for and against this hypothesis and the possible mechanisms that might be involved.

Patients with diabetes have an increased risk of cardiovascular disease. The link between glycemic control and microvascular complications has been firmly established (1,2). However, the association between glycemic control and macrovascular disease is mainly obtained from epidemiological studies, and intensive glucose control has often failed to reduce macrovascular events. Intensive glucose control invariably increases the risk of hypoglycemia and sometimes the severity of hypoglycemia (2) Several epidemiological studies and smaller prospective studies have linked hypoglycemia to increased cardiovascular risk (3–5). Recent large randomized trials looking at intensive glycemic control have either shown no benefit (Action in Diabetes and Vascular Disease: Preterax and Diamicron Modified Release Controlled Evaluation [ADVANCE] and Veterans Affairs Diabetes Trial [VADT]) or increased all cause mortality (Action to Control Cardiovascular Risk in Diabetes [ACCORD]) (6).

While the reason for the increased mortality is unclear and hypoglycemia has not been implicated as a cause of death, these studies have increased the debate about the degree of glycemic control required to decrease diabetes complications and the role of hypoglycemia in cardiovascular morbidity and mortality.

DEFINITION, INCIDENCE OF, AND RISK FACTORS ASSOCIATED WITH HYPOGLYCEMIA

The modern definition of hypoglycemia is plasma glucose <70 mg/dl (7–9). At plasma glucose below this threshold (60–65 mg/dl), the brain becomes neuroglycopenic and promotes secretion of counterregulatory hormones, primarily the adrenomedullary adrenaline and the neurotransmitter norepinephrine (along with glucagons, the "rapid" responses), which have relevant cardiovascular effects (9–11). This occurs in the absence of the warning symptoms of hypoglycemia, which normally occur at lower plasma glucose (<60 mg/dl) (9). If (even mild) hypoglycemia episodes recur often over time (e.g., once a day), the brain adapts to hypoglycemia with symptom responses at a lower-than-usual plasma glucose concentration (9). This shifting of brain glucose thresholds to higher levels (i.e., it takes a lower plasma glucose to activate symptom responses) is dangerous because it masks most of the mild hypoglycemia episodes until blood glucose decreases to ≤50 mg/dl. In turn, failure to sense symptoms of hypoglycemia in an early phase (hypoglycemia unawareness) increases the risk of prolonging duration and increasing frequency of hypoglycemia. These events

perpetrate a deleterious vicious circle leading to an increase in severe hypoglycemia with brain dysfunction (9,11). The response of adrenaline (and norepinephrine) in individuals with hypoglycemia unawareness is lower than in aware subjects (9), a finding that might be of cardiovascular protection.

The incidence of hypoglycemia is quite varied in the literature (supplementary Table 1, available in an online appendix at http://care.diabetesjournals.org/cgi/content/full/dc09-2082/DC1) (12), with lack of standardization of definition of hypoglycemia and its classification. The incidence of hypoglycemia in various trials reviewed in this article depends on the definitions of mild, moderate, and severe hypoglycemia. Most recent large trials have defined severe hypoglycemia as severe, whenever help from a third party is required, whereas mild episodes are those that are self-treated (supplementary Table 1 reports severe episodes).

Hypoglycemia has long been recognized as a major barrier to achieving normoglycemia with intensive therapy and has therefore been investigated in terms of its impact (particularly on cognitive function) and physiological counterregulation (7,11). In the Diabetes Control and Complications Trial (DCCT), patients in the intensive arm had a 65% incidence of severe hypoglycemia, compared with 35% in the conventional group (2,13). In the UK Diabetes Prospective Study, the rates of major hypoglycemic episodes were 0.7% in the conventional group, 1.4% in the glibenclamide group, and 1.8% in the group treated with insulin (1). In the 4-T study, median rates of hypoglycemia per patient per year were lowest in the basal insulin group (1.7), higher in the biphasic aspart insulin group (3.0), and highest in the prandial aspart insulin group (5.7) (14). An observational study of 383 patients reported that the duration of diabetes and the duration of insulin treatment were both positively correlated to hypoglycemic episodes (15). Thus, although in general in type 2 diabetes there is less hypoglycemia risk versus type 1 diabetes, the frequency of hypoglycemia increases with increased diabetes and insulin treatment duration in type 2 diabetes, approaching the figures of type 1 diabetes

From the [1]University of Nebraska Medical Center, Omaha, Nebraska; the [2]Section of Internal Medicine and Oncology, University of Perugia, Italy; and the [3]Tulane University Health Sciences Center, New Orleans, Louisiana.
Corresponding author: Cyrus Desouza, cdesouza@unmc.edu.
Received 11 November 2009 and accepted 9 March 2010.
DOI: 10.2337/dc09-2082

(8), primarily because of loss of glucagon responses to hypoglycemia. A retrospective cohort study of Medicaid enrollees, aged ≥65 years, who used insulin or sulfonylureas, identified 586 individuals with an episode of serious hypoglycemia (16). In this cohort, recent hospital discharge was the strongest predictor of subsequent hypoglycemia.

Mild hypoglycemic events are more common but less reported. One prospective study of 267 patients with both type 1 and type 2 diabetes reported 572 hypoglycemic events in 155 patients (17). Patients with type 1 diabetes had a mild hypoglycemic event rate of 42.89 events/patient/year and 1.15 severe hypoglycemic events/patient/year compared with 16.37 mild events/patient/year and 0.35 severe events/patient/year in subjects with type 2 diabetes. Predictors of diabetes in this group included previous hypoglycemia and duration of insulin therapy. A retrospective cross-sectional analysis in 1,055 patients with type 2 diabetes revealed a prevalence of hypoglycemic symptoms in 12% of diet-treated patients, 16% of patients using oral agents, and 30% of patients on insulin (18). Risk factors for hypoglycemia included insulin therapy, lower A1C at follow-up, younger age, and report of hypoglycemia at baseline visit (18).

The estimation of the incidence is complicated by the occurrence of hypoglycemia unawareness, which by its very nature makes it impossible to determine true incidence. Furthermore, many patients in trials may take corrective action to treat hypoglycemia in its early stages, without blood glucose testing, and may not record the occurrence of hypoglycemia. Therefore, all the above rates of hypoglycemia are likely to be underestimates.

Well-known risk factors for the development of hypoglycemia include exercise, alcohol, older age, renal dysfunction, infection, decreased intake of energy, and mental health issues, including dementia, depression, and psychiatric illnesses. In the ADVANCE trial, cognitive dysfunction increased the risk of hypoglycemia (hazard ratio 2.1).

EPIDEMIOLOGICAL EVIDENCE FOR THE ASSOCIATION BETWEEN HYPOGLYCEMIA AND CARDIOVASCULAR MORBIDITY — Recent studies such as VADT and ACCORD have brought to

the forefront the question of the role of hypoglycemia, if any, in increasing the risk for cardiovascular events. There are few studies looking at this question. Broadly, they can be divided into studies that look at the effect of hypoglycemia on cardiac ischemia, arrhythmias, and cerebral ischemia.

MYOCARDIAL ISCHEMIA, INFARCTION, AND ARRHYTHMIAS — The earliest study in 1932 reported chest pain consistent with myocardial ischemia in two of seven type 1 diabetic patients with known cardiovascular disease (19). However, other similar studies failed to confirm these findings (3,5). More recently, in a retrospective review of 14,670 patients with coronary artery disease, recruited for the Bezafibrate Infarction Prevention study (a secondary prevention prospective multicenter randomized placebo-controlled double-blind trial conducted to assess the efficacy of bezafibrate in reduction of coronary events conducted in Israel) over an 8-year mean follow-up, hypoglycemia (<70 mg/dl) was a predictor of increased all-cause mortality with a hazard ratio of 1.84, but not of increased coronary artery disease mortality (4). The Veterans Affairs Cooperative Study on Glycemic Control and Complications in Type II Diabetes showed that more cardiac events were documented in patients after institution of intensive glycemic control versus standard control (32 vs. 20%) (20). However, this was not significantly different, since the study was inadequately powered to study this question (20). In contrast, in the Bypass Angioplasty Revascularization Investigation 2 Diabetes (BARI 2D) trial, although severe hypoglycemia was more frequent in the insulin-provision group (9.2%) than in the insulin-sensitization group (5.9%), major cardiovascular events were not significantly different (21).

A few studies using continuous electrocardiogram monitoring and glucose monitoring have been performed recently. Desouza et al. (22) demonstrated that of 54 episodes of hypoglycemia, 10 were associated with symptoms or electrocardiogram evidence of ischemia, whereas only one episode of chest pain occurred during 59 episodes of hyperglycemia. Less studied is the "dead-in-bed" syndrome, which is defined as sudden nocturnal death in type 1 diabetes. In one study, 24 deaths of patients with type 1 diabetes under the age of 50 years were

studied (23). Two patients had irreversible hypoglycemic brain damage and died after artificial ventilation. Nineteen others were sleeping alone at the time of death, and 20 were found lying undisturbed (23). Gill et al. (24) demonstrated that, in patients with type 1 diabetes, severe hypoglycemia was associated with a prolonged corrected QT interval. Eight of those episodes also showed cardiac rate and rhythm abnormalities.

CEREBRAL ISCHEMIA, STROKE, AND DEMENTIA — Severe hypoglycemia has been known to induce focal neurological deficits and transient ischemic attacks, which are reversible with the correction of blood glucose. However, the question whether hypoglycemia increases the risk for stroke or dementia remains controversial. Recent evidence suggests that recurrent or severe hypoglycemia may predispose to long-term cognitive dysfunction and dementia. Whitmer et al. (25) conducted a longitudinal cohort study of 16,667 patients with type 2 diabetes looking at the relationship between hypoglycemia and dementia. The study found that the attributable risk of dementia between individuals with and without a history of hypoglycemia was 2.4% per year. Patients with multiple episodes of hypoglycemia had a graded increase in dementia risk (25). Conversely, severe cognitive dysfunction has been associated with increased risk of hypoglycemia. In the ADVANCE trial (type 2 diabetes), severe cognitive dysfunction increased the risk of severe hypoglycemia (hazard ratio 2.1) in patients with type 2 diabetes (26). The Fremantle diabetes study (type 2 diabetes) found that dementia was a risk factor for hypoglycemia. However, hypoglycemia itself was not found to increase the risk of getting dementia (27). In type 1 diabetes, some small studies show alterations in regional cerebral blood flow in patients with severe hypoglycemia; however, these are temporary and reversible (28).

In the DCCT, despite frequent hypoglycemia, intensively treated patients with type 1 diabetes did not experience cognitive decline. Some small studies show alterations in regional cerebral blood flow in patients with type 1 diabetes with severe hypoglycemia; however, these are temporary and reversible (28). It is unclear whether this finding can be extrapolated to type 2 diabetes. Thus, the role of hypoglycemia in increasing the risk for dementia is still controversial.

ROLE OF HYPOGLYCEMIA IN THE RESULTS OF RECENT CLINICAL TRIALS — Recently, several large randomized trials evaluating the effects of glycemic control on cardiovascular events have published their results (29–31).

The ACCORD trial randomized 10,251 participants with a history of cardiovascular events or significant cardiovascular risk to a strategy of intensive glycemic control or standard glycemic control (29). The ACCORD trial was halted because of a significant increase in all-cause mortality (22%) and cardiovascular mortality (35%) in the intensive treatment group. In both the intensive and standard treatment arms, participants with severe hypoglycemia had a higher mortality rate than those without severe hypoglycemia (29). However, the association between hypoglycemia and mortality is much more complex in this study. The relative risk of death associated with severe hypoglycemia was 1.28 for the intensive arm versus 2.87 for the standard arm in spite of larger number of severe hypoglycemic episodes in the intensive arm. This suggests that severe hypoglycemia in a certain subset of patients may be associated with mortality rather than the strategy of treatment used (intensive versus standard). However, these data are based on post hoc analysis, and the true cause of the increased mortality in these patients may never become obvious. The subset of patients most prone to the detrimental effects of hypoglycemia had several of the following characteristics: they were likely to be women, African American, older patients, or patients with a longer duration of diabetes and have higher A1C and high albumin-to-creatinine ratio.

VADT randomized 1,791 patients with type 2 diabetes to an intensive treatment group and a conventional treatment group (31). At the end of the study, there was no significant difference in cardiovascular events between the two treatment arms. As expected, there was an increased incidence of severe hypoglycemia in the intensive treatment group. Predictors for hypoglycemia included increased duration of diabetes, insulin treatment at baseline, low BMI, previous cardiovascular events, and high albumin-to-creatinine ratio.

The ADVANCE study randomized 11,140 participants to an intensive glycemic control arm and a standard glycemic control arm (30). Although there was an increased risk of hypoglycemia in the intensive treatment arm, there was no association between hypoglycemia and cardiovascular mortality (30). One explanation for the discrepancy between this finding and that in the ACCORD study is the extremely low number of patients (<3%) who had severe hypoglycemia in the intensive treatment arm, during the course of the entire trial.

It is therefore important to seek out the similarities and differences in the study design and patient population of these studies. Patients in the ADVANCE trial had a 2- to 3-year shorter duration of diabetes as well as a lower baseline A1C than patients in the ACCORD trial. The number of patients on insulin in the intensive arm versus the standard arm was 77 versus 55% in the ACCORD trail, 90 versus 74% in the VADT, and 41 versus 24% in the ADVANCE trial. Thus, the ADVANCE trial had a much smaller proportion of patients on insulin than ACCORD or VADT. This could in part account for the low level of hypoglycemia seen in the intensive arm of the ADVANCE trial (<3%) versus the ACCORD trail (16%) and VADT (21%). The DCCT enrolled type 1 diabetic patients on insulin treatment. In contrast to the UK Diabetes Prospective Study, VADT, and ACCORD, the DCCT had a relatively high risk for severe hypoglycemia in the "conventional" treatment group (0.19 episodes/patient-year) and a threefold increased risk in the "intensive" group (0.62 episodes/patient-year). Interestingly, the more frequent severe hypoglycemia in the intensive group was not associated with increased cardiovascular mortality (13) at later follow-up (1). This indirectly highlights the different cardiovascular risk of hypoglycemia in type 2 versus type 1 diabetes. Thus, it is clear that these trials had different treatment strategies to achieve risk factor modification. Perhaps we can now appreciate that the strategy used to achieve risk factor modification is important in how it affects patient outcomes. Moreover, the particular strategy's effect on a risk factor may not predict its effect on patient outcomes (32).

HYPOGLYCEMIA AND INPATIENT GLUCOSE CONTROL — Hyperglycemia is common in acutely ill patients and is associated with an increased morbidity and mortality (33). This has subsequently led to a large number of trials using various intensive insulin protocols to control inpatient blood glucose. However, results from these trials have increased the controversy over the risks versus benefit of tight inpatient glycemic control. Van den Berghe et al. (34) demonstrated that intensive insulin therapy in critically ill patients reduced morbidity and mortality. The DIGAMI (Diabetes Mellitus, Insulin Glucose Infusion in Acute Myocardial Infarction) study found that insulin-glucose infusion followed by intensive subcutaneous insulin in diabetic patients with acute myocardial infarction improved long-term survival (35). Conversely, the DIGAMI 2 study did not confirm superiority of insulin versus conventional treatment, but reaffirmed the importance of good glycemic control in prevention of cardiovascular events (36). The recently published NICE-SUGAR (Normoglycemia in Intensive Care Evaluation–Survival Using Glucose Algorithm Regulation) study found that intensive glucose control increased mortality among adults in the ICU (37). The Glucose Insulin in Stroke Trial (GIST)-U.K. looked at tight control of glucose in patients with acute stroke using an intensive insulin infusion protocol and found no benefit (38). The GIST-UK trial was underpowered to draw any firm conclusions. However, the sub-analysis of the mean change in glucose at 24 h showed that patients who had a decrease in plasma glucose of ≥2 mmol/l had a mortality rate of 34 versus 22% for those who had a <2 mmol/l decrease (38). This raises the question of hypoglycemia having a role in increased mortality in the inpatient setting.

Some recent studies looking at using intensive insulin infusions such as the volume and insulin therapy in severe sepsis and septic shock (VISEP) showed that the incidence of hypoglycemia was higher in the intensively treated group (39). A study by Kosiborod et al. (40), looking at 16,871 patients admitted with myocardial infarction, found that a J-shaped relationship existed between glucose and mortality. Incremental increases above 120 mg/dl and incremental declines below 70 mg/dl were found to be strongly associated with increased mortality. The slopes of these relationships were even steeper in patients with diabetes, suggesting hypoglycemia could contribute to increased mortality, especially in diabetic patients. In another study, a pooled analysis of over 4,200 patients from various myocardial infarction intervention studies, death occurred in 4.6% of the patients with hypoglycemia versus 1% of those who were considered euglycemic (81–199 mg/dl) (41). In contrast, a sub-analysis of the DIGAMI 2 data did not show hypoglycemia to be an independent risk factor for future morbidity or mortality in patients with type 2 diabetes and myocardial infarction (42).

Thus, the role of hypoglycemia in cardiovascular mortality in the inpatient setting is still controversial. Much of the variability in results is due to the different protocols used, differences in definition of hypoglycemia, as well as methodology of its detection and report, presence or absence of safeguards against hypoglycemia in the protocols, local training level of the personnel administering the protocols, and selected patient population. Hence, carefully constructed clinical trials to research this question are required. However, it is prudent to conclude from the available data that severe hypoglycemia should be avoided as much as possible in the inpatient setting.

MECHANISMS BY WHICH HYPOGLYCEMIA MAY AFFECT CARDIOVASCULAR EVENTS

— Hypoglycemia induces several counterregulatory responses. They include a decrease in pancreatic β-cell insulin secretion, an increase in pancreatic α-cell glucagon secretion, an increased sympathoadrenal response with acute plasma increase in adrenaline and norepinephrine (in addition to its elevated tissue turnover), as well as an increased secretion of ACTH/glucocorticoids. Besides these classical responses, there are several indirect changes induced by hypoglycemia that affect inflammatory cytokine secretion, endothelial function, coagulation, and fibrinolysis. All of these responses have potential adverse effects on cardiovascular morbidity and mortality and will be discussed in this section (Fig. 1).

THE SYMPATHOADRENAL RESPONSE

— Hypoglycemia stimulates the release of catecholamines, which have profound effects on the myocardium and blood vessels. Catecholamines increase myocardial contractility, myocardial workload, and cardiac output (Fig. 1). These effects can induce ischemia in the myocardium in patients with coronary vessel disease (3). The greater oxygen demand is not met because of the rigid vessels, but also

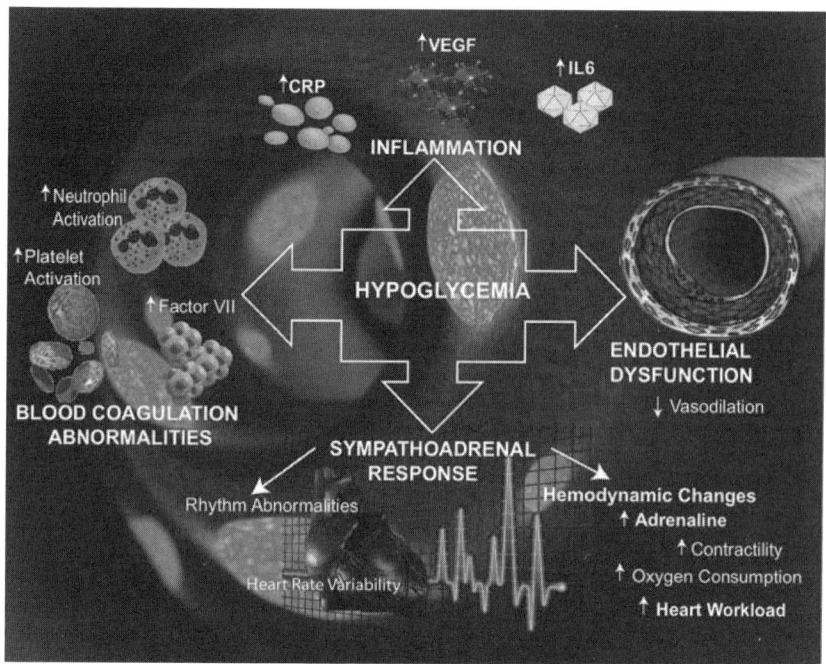

Figure 1—*Mechanisms by which hypoglycemia may affect cardiovascular events. Hypoglycemic events may trigger inflammation by inducing the release of C-reactive protein (CRP), IL-6, and vascular endothelial growth factor (VEGF). Hypoglycemia also induces increased platelet and neutrophil activation. The sympathoadrenal response during hypoglycemia increases adrenaline secretion and may induce arrhythmias and increase cardiac workload. Underlying endothelial dysfunction leading to decreased vasodilation may also contribute to cardiovascular risk.*

because of endothelial dysfunction with failure to vasodilate (Fig. 1).

Several studies have shown that hypoglycemia is associated with a significant lengthening of the corrected QT interval (QT_C) in subjects with and without diabetes (10,24). Other electrocardiographic abnormalities observed during hypoglycemia include a decrease in PR interval and moderate ST segment depressions (10). These changes are likely seen because of increased catecholamine release during hypoglycemia, and QT_C prolongation in particular could lead to a high risk of ventricular tachycardia and sudden death (43). These changes can be prevented or reversed by β blockade (43).

A few studies suggest that hyperinsulinemia and increased secretion of catecholamines may lead to hypokalemia during hypoglycemia, thus potentiating cardiac repolarization abnormalities. These effects can be reversed by β blockade and potassium replacement (43).

Cardiovascular autonomic neuropathy or impairment is associated with increased mortality. Effects of antecedent hypoglycemia on cardiac autonomic regulation may contribute to the occurrence of adverse cardiac events (44). Abnormalities in high-frequency and low-frequency heart

rate variability have been associated with hypoglycemia and increases catecholamine release (45). However, other studies did not find any associations between heart rate variability, hypoglycemia, and increased catecholamine release (10,46).

INFLAMMATION, COAGULATION, AND ENDOTHELIAL DYSFUNCTION DURING HYPOGLYCEMIA

— Inflammation has been associated with cardiovascular disease and diabetes. Several inflammatory markers including C-reactive protein, interleukin (IL)-6, IL-8, tumor necrosis factor (TNF)-α, and endothelin-1 have been shown to be increased during hypoglycemia (47,48). This increase in inflammatory cytokines could result in endothelial injury and abnormalities in coagulation, resulting in increased risk for cardiovascular events (Fig. 1). Certain growth factor levels such as vascular endothelial growth factor are also increased locally and in circulation after an episode of hypoglycemia (49). Furthermore, some cytokines such as IL-1 have been shown to increase the severity of hypoglycemia, thus perpetuating a positive feedback cycle (50).

Hypoglycemia induces abnormalities in platelet function and activation of the fibrinolytic system (51,52). Increased epinephrine levels lead to an increase in platelet activation, leukocyte mobilization, and blood coagulability (52). Many of these changes can be reversed by α or β blockade (52).

Recent studies suggest that endothelial function may be compromised during acute hypoglycemia. Vessel wall stiffness was found to be increased during hypoglycemia in patients with type 1 diabetes of longer duration than those with a shorter duration of diabetes (53). Thus, hypoglycemia may increase the risk of cardiovascular events, especially in a subset of patients with longer duration of diabetes. As discussed before, this has been suggested as a possible explanation for the results of ACCORD and VADT.

Inflammation, blood component, and functional abnormalities and endothelial dysfunction are closely interdependent. These abnormalities could potentially be aggravating factors that contribute to increased cardiovascular risk with severe hypoglycemia, especially when applied to the subset of patients with preexisting cardiovascular disease, longer duration of diabetes, and severe autonomic neuropathy (Fig. 1). However, most of these studies are short-duration acute observations and the long-term effects of hypoglycemia on inflammation, coagulation, and endothelial dysfunction are largely unknown and need to be studied.

CONCLUSIONS — The review of the literature and results from large randomized trials suggest that severe hypoglycemia is common during intensive therapy in type 1 and type 2 diabetes. This is true in the outpatient setting as well as the inpatient setting. Although smaller observational and epidemiological studies suggest an association between hypoglycemia and cardiovascular events, there is currently no evidence for causality. Larger clinical trials looking specifically at this question are required. The mechanisms that might be involved also need to be determined further. Our challenge in these patients is to lower blood glucose to near-normal values to lower the risk for long-term complications, but at the same time minimize hypoglycemia- and hypoglycemia-associated morbidity and mortality.

Acknowledgments— V.F. has received research support from GlaxoSmithKline, Novartis, Novo Nordisk, Takeda, Pfizer, sanofi-aventis, Eli Lilly, and the American Diabetes Association. He has also received honoraria for consulting and lectures from GlaxoSmithKline, Novartis, Novo Nordisk, Takeda, Pfizer, sanofi-aventis, Eli Lilly, and Daiichi Sankyo. C.V.D. has received honoraria from Novo Nordisk and Takeda for consulting. No other potential conflicts of interest relevant to this article were reported.

References

1. Gore MO, McGuire DK. The 10-year post-trial follow-up of the United Kingdom Prospective Diabetes Study (UKPDS): cardiovascular observations in context. Diab Vasc Dis Res 2009;6:53–55
2. Keen H. The Diabetes Control and Complications Trial (DCCT). Health Trends 1994;26:41–43
3. Egeli ES, Berkmen R. Action of hypoglycemia on coronary insufficiency and mechanism of ECG alterations. Am Heart J 1960;59:527–540
4. Fisman EZ, Motro M, Tenenbaum A, Leor J, Boyko V, Mandelzweig L, Sherer Y, Adler Y, Behar S. Is hypoglycaemia a marker for increased long-term mortality risk in patients with coronary artery disease? An 8-year follow-up. Eur J Cardiovasc Prev Rehabil 2004;11:135–143
5. Judson WE, Hollander W. The effects of insulin-induced hypoglycemia in patients with angina pectoris: before and after intravenous hexamethonium. Am Heart J 1956;52:198–209
6. Skyler JS, Bergenstal R, Bonow RO, Buse J, Deedwania P, Gale EA, Howard BV, Kirkman MS, Kosiborod M, Reaven P, Sherwin RS, American Diabetes Association, American College of Cardiology Foundation, American Heart Association. Intensive glycemic control and the prevention of cardiovascular events: implications of the ACCORD, ADVANCE, and VA Diabetes Trials: a position statement of the American Diabetes Association and a Scientific Statement of the American College of Cardiology Foundation and the American Heart Association. J Am Coll Cardiol 2009;53:298–304
7. American Diabetes Association. Standards of medical care in diabetes—2010. Diabetes Care 2010;33(Suppl. 1):11–61
8. Cryer PE. Hypoglycemia: still the limiting factor in the glycemic management of diabetes. Endocr Pract 2008;14:750–756
9. Rossetti P, Porcellati F, Bolli GB, Fanelli CG. Prevention of hypoglycemia while achieving good glycemic control in type 1 diabetes: the role of insulin analogs. Diabetes Care 2008;31(Suppl. 2):113–120
10. Laitinen T, Lyyra-Laitinen T, Huopio H, Vauhkonen I, Halonen T, Hartikainen J, Niskanen L, Laakso M. Electrocardiographic alterations during hyperinsulinemic hypo-glycemia in healthy subjects. Ann Noninvasive Electrocardiol 2008;13:97–105
11. Sherwin RS. Bringing light to the dark side of insulin: a journey across the blood-brain barrier. Diabetes 2008;57:2259–2268
12. Cryer PE. *Hypoglycemia in Diabetes: Pathophysiology, Prevalence and Prevention.* Alexandria, VA, American Diabetes Association, 2009
13. Hypoglycemia in the Diabetes Control and Complications Trial. The Diabetes Control and Complications Trial Research Group. Diabetes 1997;46:271–286
14. Holman RR, Farmer AJ, Davies MJ, Levy JC, Darbyshire JL, Keenan JF, Paul SK, 4-T Study Group. Three-year efficacy of complex insulin regimens in type 2 diabetes. N Engl J Med 2009;361:1736–1747
15. UK Hypoglycaemia Study Group. Risk of hypoglycaemia in types 1 and 2 diabetes: effects of treatment modalities and their duration. Diabetologia 2007;50:1140–1147
16. Shorr RI, Ray WA, Daugherty JR, Griffin MR. Incidence and risk factors for serious hypoglycemia in older persons using insulin or sulfonylureas. Arch Intern Med 1997;157:1681–1686
17. Donnelly LA, Morris AD, Frier BM, Ellis JD, Donnan PT, Durrant R, Band MM, Reekie G, Leese GP, DARTS/MEMO Collaboration. Frequency and predictors of hypoglycaemia in type 1 and insulin-treated Type 2 diabetes: a population-based study. Diabet Med 2005;22:749–755
18. Miller CD, Phillips LS, Ziemer DC, Gallina DL, Cook CB, El-Kebbi IM. Hypoglycemia in patients with type 2 diabetes mellitus. Arch Intern Med 2001;161:1653–1659
19. Strouse SSS, Katz LN, Rubinfield SH. Treatment of older diabetic patients with cardiovascular disease. JAMA 1932;98:1703–1706
20. Abraira C, Colwell J, Nuttall F, Sawin CT, Henderson W, Comstock JP, Emanuele NV, Levin SR, Pacold I, Lee HS. Cardiovascular events and correlates in the Veterans Affairs Diabetes Feasibility Trial. Veterans Affairs Cooperative Study on Glycemic Control and Complications in Type II Diabetes. Arch Intern Med 1997;157:181–188
21. BARI 2D Study Group, Frye RL, August P, Brooks MM, Hardison RM, Kelsey SF, MacGregor JM, Orchard TJ, Chaitman BR, Genuth SM, Goldberg SH, Hlatky MA, Jones TL, Molitch ME, Nesto RW, Sako EY, Sobel BE. A randomized trial of therapies for type 2 diabetes and coronary artery disease. N Engl J Med 2009;360:2503–2515
22. Desouza C, Salazar H, Cheong B, Murgo J, Fonseca V. Association of hypoglycemia and cardiac ischemia: a study based on continuous monitoring. Diabetes Care 2003;26:1485–1489
23. Tattersall RB, Gill GV. Unexplained deaths of type 1 diabetic patients. Diabet Med 1991;8:49–58
24. Gill GV, Woodward A, Casson IF, Weston PJ. Cardiac arrhythmia and nocturnal hy-

poglycaemia in type 1 diabetes: the 'dead in bed' syndrome revisited. Diabetologia 2009;52:42–45

25. Whitmer RA, Karter AJ, Yaffe K, Quesenberry CP Jr, Selby JV. Hypoglycemic episodes and risk of dementia in older patients with type 2 diabetes mellitus. JAMA 2009;301:1565–1572

26. de Galan BE, Zoungas S, Chalmers J, Anderson C, Dufouil C, Pillai A, Cooper M, Grobbee DE, Hackett M, Hamet P, Heller SR, Lisheng L, Macmahon S, Mancia G, Neal B, Pan CY, Patel A, Poulter N, Travert F, Woodward M. Cognitive function and risks of cardiovascular disease and hypoglycaemia in patients with type 2 diabetes: the Action in Diabetes and Vascular Disease: Preterax and Diamicron Modified Release Controlled Evaluation (ADVANCE) trial. Diabetologia 2009;52: 2328–2336

27. Bruce DG, Davis WA, Casey GP, Clarnette RM, Brown SG, Jacobs IG, Almeida OP, Davis TM. Severe hypoglycaemia and cognitive impairment in older patients with diabetes: the Fremantle Diabetes Study. Diabetologia 2009;52:1808–1815

28. MacLeod KM, Hepburn DA, Deary IJ, Goodwin GM, Dougall N, Ebmeier KP, Frier BM. Regional cerebral blood flow in IDDM patients: effects of diabetes and of recurrent severe hypoglycaemia. Diabetologia 1994;37:257–263

29. Action to Control Cardiovascular Risk in Diabetes Study Group, Gerstein HC, Miller ME, Byington RP, Goff DC Jr, Bigger JT, Buse JB, Cushman WC, Genuth S, Ismail-Beigi F, Grimm RH Jr, Probstfield JL, Simons-Morton DG, Friedewald WT. Effects of intensive glucose lowering in type 2 diabetes. N Engl J Med 2008;358: 2545–2559

30. ADVANCE Collaborative Group, Patel A, MacMahon S, Chalmers J, Neal B, Billot L, Woodward M, Marre M, Cooper M, Glasziou P, Grobbee D, Hamet P, Harrap S, Heller S, Liu L, Mancia G, Mogensen CE, Pan C, Poulter N, Rodgers A, Williams B, Bompoint S, de Galan BE, Joshi R, Travert F. Intensive blood glucose control and vascular outcomes in patients with type 2 diabetes. N Engl J Med 2008;358:2560–2572

31. Duckworth W, Abraira C, Moritz T, Reda D, Emanuele N, Reaven PD, Zieve FJ, Marks J, Davis SN, Hayward R, Warren SR, Goldman S, McCarren M, Vitek ME, Henderson WG, Huang GD, VADT Investigators. Glucose control and vascular complications in veterans with type 2 diabetes. N Engl J Med 2009;360:129–139

32. Krumholz HM, Lee TH. Redefining quality: implications of recent clinical trials. N Engl J Med 2008;358:2537–2539

33. Capes SE, Hunt D, Malmberg K, Gerstein HC. Stress hyperglycaemia and increased risk of death after myocardial infarction in patients with and without diabetes: a sys-

tematic overview. Lancet 2000;355:773–778

34. Van den Berghe G, Wilmer A, Hermans G, Meersseman W, Wouters PJ, Milants 1, Van Wijngaerden E, Bobbaers H, Bouillon R. Intensive insulin therapy in the medical ICU. N Engl J Med 2006;354:449–461

35. Malmberg K. Prospective randomised study of intensive insulin treatment on long term survival after acute myocardial infarction in patients with diabetes mellitus. DIGAMI (Diabetes Mellitus, Insulin Glucose Infusion in Acute Myocardial Infarction) Study Group. BMJ 1997;314:1512–1515

36. Malmberg K, Rydén L, Wedel H, Birkeland K, Bootsma A, Dickstein K, Efendic S, Fisher M, Hamsten A, Herlitz J, Hildebrandt P, MacLeod K, Laakso M, Torp-Pedersen C, Waldenström A, DIGAMI 2 Investigators. Intense metabolic control by means of insulin in patients with diabetes mellitus and acute myocardial infarction (DIGAMI 2): effects on mortality and morbidity. Eur Heart J 2005;26:650–661

37. NICE-SUGAR Study Investigators, Finfer S, Chittock DR, Su SY, Blair D, Foster D, Dhingra V, Bellomo R, Cook D, Dodek P, Henderson WR, Hébert PC, Heritier S, Heyland DK, McArthur C, McDonald E, Mitchell I, Myburgh JA, Norton R, Potter J, Robinson BG, Ronco JJ. Intensive versus conventional glucose control in critically ill patients. N Engl J Med 2009;360:1283–1297

38. Gray CS, Hildreth AJ, Sandercock PA, O'Connell JE, Johnston DE, Cartlidge NE, Bamford JM, James OF, Alberti KG, GIST Trialists Collaboration. Glucose-potassium-insulin infusions in the management of post-stroke hyperglycaemia: the UK Glucose Insulin in Stroke Trial (GIST-UK). Lancet Neurol 2007;6:397–406

39. Brunkhorst FM, Engel C, Bloos F, Meier-Hellmann A, Ragaller M, Weiler N, Moerer O, Gruendling M, Oppert M, Grond S, Olthoff D, Jaschinski U, John S, Rossaint R, Welte T, Schaefer M, Kern P, Kuhnt E, Kiehntopf M, Hartog C, Natanson C, Loeffler M, Reinhart K, German Competence Network Sepsis (SepNet). Intensive insulin therapy and pentastarch resuscitation in severe sepsis. N Engl J Med 2008;358:125–139

40. Kosiborod M, Inzucchi SE, Krumholz HM, Xiao L, Jones PG, Fiske S, Masoudi FA, Marso SP, Spertus JA. Glucometrics in patients hospitalized with acute myocardial infarction: defining the optimal outcomes-based measure of risk. Circulation 2008;117:1018–1027

41. Pinto DS, Skolnick AH, Kirtane AJ, Murphy SA, Barron HV, Giugliano RP, Cannon CP, Braunwald E, Gibson CM, TIMI Study Group. U-shaped relationship of blood glucose with adverse outcomes among patients with ST-segment elevation myocardial infarction. J Am Coll Cardiol 2005;46:178–180

42. Mellbin LG, Malmberg K, Waldenström A, Wedel H, Rydén L, DIGAMI 2 Investigators. Prognostic implications of hypoglycaemic episodes during hospitalisation for myocardial infarction in patients with type 2 diabetes: a report from the DIGAMI 2 trial. Heart 2009;95:721–727

43. Robinson RT, Harris ND, Ireland RH, Lee S, Newman C, Heller SR. Mechanisms of abnormal cardiac repolarization during insulin-induced hypoglycemia. Diabetes 2003;52:1469–1474

44. Adler GK, Bonyhay I, Failing H, Waring E, Dotson S, Freeman R. Antecedent hypoglycemia impairs autonomic cardiovascular function: implications for rigorous glycemic control. Diabetes 2009;58:360–366

45. Vlcek M, Radikova Z, Penesova A, Kvetnansky R, Imrich R. Heart rate variability and catecholamines during hypoglycemia and orthostasis. Auton Neurosci 2008; 143:53–57

46. Koivikko ML, Karsikas M, Salmela PI, Tapanainen JS, Ruokonen A, Seppänen T, Huikuri HV, Perkiömäki JS. Effects of controlled hypoglycemia on cardiac repolarisation in patients with type 1 diabetes. Diabetologia 2008;51:426–435

47. Galloway PJ, Thomson GA, Fisher BM, Semple CG. Insulin-induced hypoglycemia induces a rise in C-reactive protein. Diabetes Care 2000;23:861–862

48. Razavi Nematollahi L, Kitabchi AE, Kitabchi AE, Stentz FB, Wan JY, Larijani BA, Tehrani MM, Gozashti MH, Omidfar K, Taheri E. Proinflammatory cytokines in response to insulin-induced hypoglycemic stress in healthy subjects. Metabolism 2009;58:443–448

49. Dantz D, Bewersdorf J, Fruehwald-Schultes B, Kern W, Jelkmann W, Born J, Fehm HL, Peters A. Vascular endothelial growth factor: a novel endocrine defensive response to hypoglycemia. J Clin Endocrinol Metab 2002;87:835–840

50. Del Rey A, Roggero E, Randolf A, Mahuad C, McCann S, Rettori V, Besedovsky HO. IL-1 resets glucose homeostasis at central levels. Proc Natl Acad Sci U S A 2006;103: 16039–16044

51. Dalsgaard-Nielsen J, Madsbad S, Hilsted J. Changes in platelet function, blood coagulation and fibrinolysis during insulin-induced hypoglycaemia in juvenile diabetics and normal subjects. Thromb Haemost 1982;47:254–258

52. Fisher BM, Hepburn DA, Smith JG, Frier BM. Responses of peripheral blood cells to acute insulin-induced hypoglycaemia in humans: effect of alpha-adrenergic blockade. Horm Metab Res Suppl 1992; 26:109–110

53. Sommerfield AJ, Wilkinson IB, Webb DJ, Frier BM. Vessel wall stiffness in type 1 diabetes and the central hemodynamic effects of acute hypoglycemia. Am J Physiol Endocrinol Metab 2007;293:E1274–E1279

Hypoglycemia Aggravates Critical Illness-Induced Neurocognitive Dysfunction

Thomas Duning, md[1]
Ingeborg van den Heuvel, md[2]
Annabelle Dickmann[2]
Thomas Volkert, md[2]
Carola Wempe, md[2]

Julia Reinholz, md[1]
Hubertus Lohmann, md[1]
Hendrik Freise, md[2]
Björn Ellger, md, phd[2]

OBJECTIVE — Tight glycemic control (TGC) in critically ill patients is associated with an increased risk of hypoglycemia. Whether those short episodes of hypoglycemia are associated with adverse morbidity and mortality is a matter of discussion. Using a case-control study design, we investigated whether hypoglycemia under TGC causes permanent neurocognitive dysfunction in patients surviving critical illness.

RESEARCH DESIGN AND METHODS — From our patient data management system, we identified adult survivors treated for >72 h in our surgical intensive care unit (ICU) between 2004 and 2007 (n = 4,635) without a history of neurocognitive dysfunction or structural brain abnormalities who experienced at least one episode of hypoglycemia during treatment (hypo group) (n = 37). For each hypo group patient, one patient stringently matched for demographic- and disease-related data were identified as a control subject. We performed a battery of neuropsychological tests investigating five areas of cognitive functioning in both groups at least 1 year after ICU discharge. Test results were compared with data from healthy control subjects and between groups.

RESULTS — Critical illness caused neurocognitive dysfunction in all tested domains in both groups. The dysfunction was aggravated in hypo group patients in one domain, namely that of visuospatial skills ($P < 0.01$). Besides hypoglycemia, both hyperglycemia ($r = -0.322$; $P = 0.005$) and fluctuations of blood glucose ($r = -0.309$; $P = 0.008$) were associated with worse test results in this domain.

CONCLUSIONS — Hypoglycemia was found to aggravate critical illness–induced neurocognitive dysfunction to a limited, but significant, extent; however, an impact of hyperglycemia and fluctuations of blood glucose on neurocognitive function cannot be excluded.

Diabetes Care 33:639–644, 2010

Since the concept of tight glycemic control (TGC) was introduced in critical care medicine in 2001 (1), its implementation in daily clinical practice has been the subject of a vivid discussion. Several single-center trials in different patient populations largely confirmed the clinical benefits, at least when patients were treated for a few days or longer in an intensive care unit (ICU) (2). Numerous studies have suggested plausible mechanisms behind the clinical benefits (3). However, a recent multicenter trial failed to confirm the strict blood glucose targets (4), and two multicenter trials have been preliminarily stopped because of a high incidence of hypoglycemic episodes (5).

Indeed, hypoglycemia appears as the major side effect of any effort to regulate blood glucose levels with insulin, whatever the blood glucose levels aimed for (2). Although numerous algorithms are available to minimize this risk (6), the fear of hypoglycemia-induced mortality and permanent disability largely impedes the implementation of TGC in daily routine. Scientific evidence supporting the common notion that hypoglycemia is responsible for an increased mortality and profound permanent neurocognitive dysfunction rather than it being just a marker of severity of illness is poor and controversial, however. Efforts to substantiate any evidence are based on post hoc analyses, since confirmation from prospective randomized, controlled trials is precluded for obvious ethical reasons. Some studies imply that any mortality benefits of TGC might be outweighed when the incidence of hypoglycemia is very high (7); however, other analyses revealed conflicting results in this respect (8). Besides direct effects on mortality, neuroglycopenia might cause neuronal damage and at least subtle permanent neurocognitive impairment that potentially affects life quality after discharge. From diabetes, it is known that neuroglycopenia might have a permanent effect on neurocognitive function, at least when it occurs repetitively. Since diabetes and critical illness–induced dysregulations of glucose homeostasis represent substantially different entities, it is inappropriate to extrapolate these data to the ICU population. Cognitive impairment is a relevant problem of patients surviving critical illness in general (9). Currently, there are no data available on the specific impact of hypoglycemic events during treatment in ICU on long-term neurocognitive function. Using a case-control design, we investigated whether hypoglycemic episodes under TGC induce or aggravate permanent neurocognitive deficits in patients surviving critical illness.

RESEARCH DESIGN AND METHODS

— The work was approved by the local ethics committee, and written informed consent was obtained from all patients prior to neurocognitive testing.

All patients in the surgical ICU of our university hospital are treated according to our institutional TGC protocol (analog to [1]), aiming for blood glucose between 80 and 110 mg/dl using insulin infusions as necessary. Blood glucose was measured

From the [1]Department of Neurology, University Hospital of Muenster, Muenster, Germany; and the [2]Department of Anesthesiology and Intensive Care Medicine, University Hospital of Muenster, Muenster, Germany.
Corresponding author: Björn Ellger, ellger@anit.uni-muenster.de.
Received 18 September 2009 and accepted 10 December 2009. Published ahead of print at http://care.diabetesjournals.org on 23 December 2009. DOI: 10.2337/dc09-1740. Clinical trial reg. no. NCT00662922, clinicaltrials.gov.
T.D. and I.v.d.H. contributed equally to this article.

Table 1—*Cognitive domains and tests: results of neurocognitive testing*

	Hypo group			Control group			
	Score (percentile)	Evaluation	Z scores	Score (percentile)	Evaluation	Z scores	P
Dementia screening			0.006			−0.003	0.969
Mini-mental state examination	28.4	Close below average		28.8	Close below average		0.909
Boston Naming Test	13.8	Normal		13.9	Normal		0.871
Attention and working memory			−0.039			−0.045	0.774
Nuernberg Gerontopsychological Inventory							
Digit symbol substitution	30.0 (56.7)	Normal		31.1 (60.7)	Normal		0.770
Color word interference task (reading)	39.8 (10.2)	Far below average		40.0 (12.5)	Far below average		0.861
Color word interference task (color naming)	53.3 (28.4)	Close below average		52.8 (26.6)	Close below average		0.608
Wechsler Memory Scale (revised)							
Digit span forward	11.6 (51.7)	Normal		12.6 (54.4)	Normal		0.156
Digit span backward	10.7 (40.6)	Close below average		11.6 (42.0)	Close below average		0.892
Trail-making test (A)	60.1 (13.9)	Far below average		59.6 (13.0)	Far below average		0.270
Executive function			−0.001			−0.007	0.991
Color word interference task (interference condition)	17.5 (47.9)	Normal		19.5 (51.3)	Normal		0.421
Regensburg Word Fluency Test (letter fluency) (S)	14.2 (28.4)	Close below average		14.2 (28.4)	Close below average		1.000
Trail-making test (B)	117.0 (27.8)	Close below average		110.8 (25.6)	Close below average		0.792
Visuospatial skills			−2.084			−0.145	0.001
Rey Osterrieth Complex Figure Test							
Copy	20.4			24.7			0.007
Delayed recall	9.4 (22.8)	Close below average		14.5 (29.9)	Close below average		0.002
Difference copy (delayed)	−54.3%			−41.9% (4.2)			0.043
Verbal learning and memory			−0.027			−0.064	0.807
Auditory verbal learning test (German)							
Recall trial 1	4.9 (30.2)	Close below average		5.5 (38.4)	Close below average		0.503
Recall trial 5	10.7 (31.1)	Close below average		10.5 (28.8)	Close below average		0.543
Total trials 1–5	38.0 (30.4)	Close below average		38.7 (32.1)	Close below average		0.527
Delayed recall	8.5 (13.8)	Far below average		9.0 (15.0)	Far below average		0.240
Recognition (true positives, false positives)	10.9 (30.5)	Close below average		10.9 (30.5)	Close below average		1.000

in full blood drawn from an arterial line with an ABL blood gas analyzer (glucose oxidase method with amperometric reading, range 7–540 mg/dl, coefficient of variance <10% for lower detection limit; Radiometer, Copenhagen, Denmark). Quality checks of the device were performed according to the instruction manual.

We identified all patients who suffered from at least one episode of hypoglycemia (blood glucose ≤40 mg/dl) (labeled the hypo group) between 1 January 2004 and 31 December 2007 from our patient data management system. Patients were selected to undergo a battery of validated neuropsychological tests that were designed to assess a full range of cog-

nitive functions (Table 1) at least 1 year after discharge from the unit. To diagnose patients with manifest neurological deficits, a short neurological examination was performed (sensory and motor responses, reflexes including Babinski's sign, and examination of posture and movements). We included all patients, aged between 18 and 80 years, upon admission who were treated for at least 72 h in the ICU. We excluded patients who did not survive until the scheduled time point of testing or had a medical history or medical condition potentially biasing neurocognitive testing, such as neurocognitive, neurodegenerative (Alzheimer's or Parkinson's disease), psychiatric disorders (drug abuse, depression, and schizophre-

nia and the use of respective medication), severe liver disease (ammonia three times the upper limit of normal or Child C liver insufficiency), or end-stage kidney failure. Patients after neurotrauma, intracranial hemorrhage, stroke, intracranial surgery, and other structural brain lesions were also excluded.

For each hypo group patient, a matching partner (control group) without any hypoglycemic event meeting the same inclusion and exclusion criteria was identified from the database according to strict demographic- and illness-related matching criteria (Table 2).

We recorded and calculated duration (time from last blood glucose above hypoglycemia threshold before, to first

Table 2—*Matching criteria*

Demography	
Sex	Male/female
Age (classified in groups)	<40; 41–60; 61–75; >75 years
Simplified acute physiology score (maximum simplified acute physiology score, classified in groups)	<7; 8–14; >14
Year of ICU treatment	
Disease-related criteria	
Type of surgery	Elective surgery/emergency surgery
Cardiopulmonary resuscitation	Yes/no
Type 1 or type 2 diabetes	Yes/no
Length of stay in ICU*	
Mean morning blood glucose*	
Duration of sedation (classified in groups)	<3 days; 3–7 days; 1–2 weeks; >2 weeks
Respiratory failure (classified by Horrowitz Index in groups)†	>300; 200–300; <200
Cardiovascular failure†	Catecholamine therapy: yes/no; mechanical assist device: yes/no
Renal failure†	Hemodialysis of any kind: yes/no; classified by RIFLE criteria
Hepatic failure (classified by laboratory liver testing, classified in four groups)	All values <2.5 ULN, one value 2.5–5 ULN, one value >5 ULN, all values >5 ULN
Medication	Steroids: yes/no; immunosuppressants: yes/no

*Smallest possible difference. †At time of hypoglycemia ±3 days. ULN, upper limit of normal. RIFLE, Risk, Injury, Failure, Loss, and End-stage classification for acute renal dysfunction.

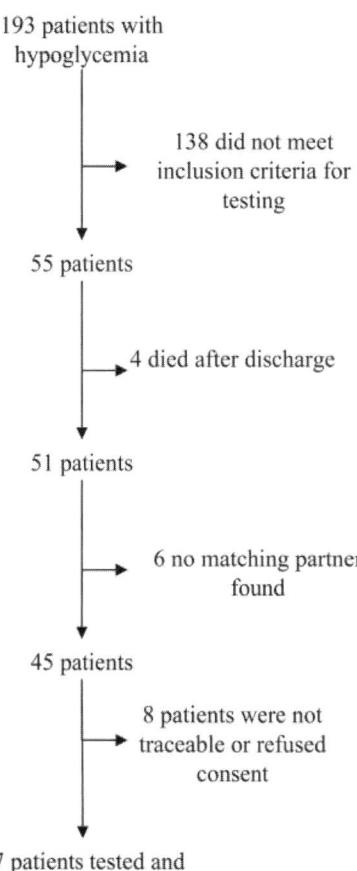

Figure 1—*Flow chart of patient inclusion in the hypo group.*

blood glucose >40 mg/dl after a hypoglycemic reading), number and severity of hypoglycemia (minimum blood glucose during treatment), mean blood glucose over the whole ICU stay, mean morning blood glucose, maximum blood glucose, Δblood glucose (difference between the minimum blood glucose and maximum blood glucose within 6 h following hypoglycemia), and the difference between minimum and maximum blood glucose during ICU treatment.

Neuropsychological assessment
One investigator, who was unaware of the allocation of the patients, conducted the neuropsychological tests. Test results were primarily analyzed by the same investigator and supervised by an experienced clinical neuropsychologist. Performances in five major areas of cognitive functioning were evaluated. Cognitive domains and their particular tests are listed in Table 1. Concerning the Rey Osterrieth Complex Figure Test, we also calculated the relative difference between both test results since results of delayed recall performance can be influenced by an impairment of initial copying. Additionally, test results from patients were compared with published normative data for age, sex, and educational level. A de-

tailed description of each test can be found in the book by Lezak (10).

Statistical analyses
Data were tested for normal distribution with the Shapiro-Wilk Test. To determine meaningful composite scores of cognitive domains, we performed a principal component analysis using the single test results, followed by an oblique (Oblimin with Kaiser normalization) rotation. The same test was not included in more than one composite score. The resulting five factors of the principal component analysis were Z transformed (mean score of 0 and an SD of 1). For timed tests, the sign of the Z score was reversed so that improved performance resulted in a higher score in all tests.

Primary analysis assessed differences in neurocognitive test results between groups with either paired t test or Mann-Whitney U test as appropriate. Secondary analyses were carried out to test the relation of hypoglycemia severity, length of hypoglycemic episode, and the number of hypoglycemic events to neurocognitive scores and whether maximum glucose values, Δblood glucose, or the difference between minimum and maximum blood glucose were associated with worse test results by means of Pearson's correlation.

Test results of the ICU patients were compared with published normative data for age, sex, and educational level. Differences were expressed semi-quantitatively as normal, close below average, or far below average, respectively. Test results are given as means ± SD. A two-tailed P value <0.05 was considered significant. All data were analyzed using SPSS Statistics version 15.0.

RESULTS — A total of 4,635 patients were treated in our ICU in the study period for >72 h, 193 of whom experienced at least one episode of hypoglycemia (4.2%). Thirty-seven hypo group patients met inclusion criteria, fulfilled no exclusion criteria, and one matching control partner could be identified for each (Fig. 1). Demographic data were as follows (means ± SE): 44 male and 30 female subjects, age 66.3 ± 1.3 years, simplified acute physiology score 39 ± 2.3, length of stay on ICU 15.2 ± 1.6 days, and 32% had diabetes. Admission blood glucose (167.8 ± 7.8 vs. 167.0 ± 8.3 mg/dl; P =

0.941), mean morning blood glucose (131.7 ± 3.0 vs. 126.5 ± 2.6 mg/dl; P = 0.196), and mean blood glucose (139.0 ± 3.0 vs. 137.1 ± 2.5; P = 0.644) did not differ between groups. Mean maximum blood glucose was significantly higher in the hypo group than in the control group (297.8 ± 14.9 vs. 249.8 ± 10.7 mg/dl; P = 0.017). Demographic data did not differ between groups, as patients were matched accordingly.

None of the patients revealed manifest neurological deficits in the neurological examination. Neurocognitive tests in both patient groups showed impaired neurocognitive function in several domains compared with age-matched healthy control subjects (Table 1). Analyses of differences between both patient groups in the five neurocognitive domains revealed solely a significant impairment of visuospatial skills in the hypo compared with the control group (P = 0.001). Within the single subtests, results of both copy (P = 0.007) and delayed (P = 0.002) recall of the Rey Osterrieth Complex Figure Test were lower in the hypo than in the control group. The relative difference between copy and delayed recall also significantly differed between both groups (hypo group < control group; P = 0.043). Results of all other tests did not differ between groups (Table 1).

Solely within the hypoglycemic group, the maximum blood glucose and the difference between minimum and maximum blood glucose serving as rough surrogates for the quality of glycemic control during ICU treatment were negatively correlated with visual-spatial processing parameters. Neither the number nor the duration of hypoglycemic episodes showed a significant correlation. Severity of hypoglycemia was also not significantly associated with visuospatial performance but did show a negative trend (Table 3). In the control group, no correlations between parameters of glycemic control and the performance in the neurocognitive tests were found.

CONCLUSIONS — In the current case-control study, we found that patients who experienced one or more hypoglycemic events during ICU treatment showed an aggravation of critical illness–induced neurocognitive dysfunction compared with patients who did not experience hypoglycemia. Both groups showed significant neurocognitive dysfunctions in all

Table 3—*Correlation of the parameters of glycemic control with Rey Osterrieth Complex Figure Test results in the hypo group*

	r	P
Mean morning blood glucose	−0.055	0.747
Mean blood glucose	0.116	0.494
Number of hypoglycemic episodes	−0.097	0.414
Duration of hypoglycemic episode	−0.293	0.154
Maximum blood glucose during treatment	−0.322	0.005
Minimum blood glucose during treatment	−0.299	0.072
Difference maximum/ minimum blood glucose	−0.309	0.001
ΔBlood glucose	0.052	0.765

domains compared with healthy control subjects, but hypo group patients had an additional deficit in visuospatial skills. Since tests were done at least 1 year after ICU discharge, these impairments must be considered long term if not permanent.

Former studies investigating the consequences of hypoglycemia under TGC in the critically ill have revealed conflicting results (7,8); however, they have been primarily focused on mortality and gross somatic morbidity. Data on the positive effects of TGC on mortality from prior trials could not be confirmed by the recent multicenter trial Normoglycaemia in Intensive Care Evaluation–Survival Using Glucose Algorithm Regulation (NICE-SUGAR) (4), which investigated the impact of a strict versus a more liberal TGC protocol. NICE-SUGAR revealed a higher mortality in the strict TGC group. The high incidence of hypoglycemia in the strict TGC group might be considered one possible explanation for this controversy. Similarly, from mathematical modeling, Krinsley concluded that negative effects of hypoglycemia might outweigh any benefits on mortality and gross morbidity when they occur in a critical incidence (7). Our study focuses on ICU survivors and is thus the first to explore the long-term effects of hypoglycemia under TGC during ICU treatment on subtle neuropsychological function. With the utilized test battery, we largely confirm and complement prior studies (9) demonstrating neurocognitive impairment in the tested domains in both critically ill patient groups compared with age-, sex-, and ed-

ucational level–matched healthy control subjects. Furthermore, we could show that in patients surviving the ICU without primary brain damage and preexisting neurocognitive deficits, critical illness–induced deficits of complex neurocognitive functions, in particular visuoconstructive performance as well as figural and spatial aspects of nonverbal memory, might be aggravated by even a single episode of hypoglycemia. Although the aggravation appears minor at first view and is restricted to one single domain, the impairment of visual-spatial processing might have a relevant impact on overall daily functioning (11). It could be associated with the evolution of further cognitive decline over time (12) and, thus, have a significant impact on patients' quality of life.

Recent studies have indicated that an impairment of visuoconstructive skills and both figural and spatial aspects of nonverbal memory are associated with temporal and hippocampal dysfunction (13). Neuroimaging has demonstrated that not all neurons and brain regions are equally sensitive to hypoglycemic injury but that there appears to be a selective vulnerability of especially those hippocampal and/or temporal neurons, followed by neurons in the basal ganglia (14,15). Although the reported abnormalities could be transient and reversible by glucose infusion, several studies in both animals and humans have consistently demonstrated hypoglycemia-induced permanent neuronal damage in regions of the hippocampus, especially in the dentate gyrus (16,17). Although most biochemical studies have focused on cell death, more recent studies indicate that mild, recurrent hypoglycemia can cause synaptic dysfunction even in the absence of neuronal death, particularly in hippocampal neurons (18). Repeated episodes of even moderate hypoglycemia in diabetic patients have been reported as being associated with a decline of intelligence quotient, persistent cognitive impairment, and other long-term effects such as mood changes and affected general well-being (19,20); however, since conflicting results have been published, assigning hypoglycemia as the sole cause of these findings is debatable. Some of the divergent results may be due to methodical issues with regards to the determination of cognitive function; other negative studies may not have been sufficiently long to detect a significant effect. On the other hand, the associations between intellectual disadvantage and episodes of hypoglycemia might exist simply because patients manage their insulin treatment less accurately. It is thus difficult to differentiate between effects of hypoglycemia and modest glycemic control comprising hyperglycemia, hypoglycemia, and blood glucose fluctuations. To conclude from clinical trials that persistent neurocognitive impairment in diabetic subjects is exclusively a consequence of (repeated) episodes of hypoglycemia is plausible but not imperative. Moreover, the underlying pathogenetic mechanisms of the long-term cognitive deficits remain largely unclear; some findings indicate that dopaminergic functional disturbance in the hippocampus (21) and changes in brain glucose transporters or astrocyte-neuron interactions may play a major role (14). The agreement between neurocognitive test results, their probable functional and structural neuroanatomic correlates, and the specific vulnerability of (para-) hippocampal neuron populations to hypoglycemic damage is striking, however.

Current data suggest that a great portion of ICU survivors in general develop persistent cognitive impairment (9,22); we also found neurocognitive impairment in various domains in both our patient groups compared with published normative data. Since critically ill patients, per se, seem to be at risk for neural damage, one might speculate that critical illness can induce a specific vulnerability of neurons to glucose deprivation. Our data show that hypoglycemic events under TGC aggravate these critical illness–induced neurocognitive deficits but that this is limited to one neurocognitive domain. Notwithstanding stringent matching criteria for demographic and severity of illness data including mean blood glucose, we cannot completely exclude confounders. Our groups differ in mean maximum and minimum glucose, suggesting that the hypo group experienced a worse quality of blood glucose control with more variability. Solely within the hypo group, we found a significant association of hyperglycemia and the difference between lowest and highest blood glucose with declined visuospatial skills, whereas for quantity and duration of hypoglycemic episodes, no such correlation was found. No correlations at all were found in our control group. Indeed, previous work showed that hyperglycemia in diabetes, too, is associated with adverse effects on the brain (23), neurocognitive impairment, and affected general well-being (19). Not only hypoglycemia but

also hyperglycemia, glucose fluctuations, and their treatments thus might have an impact on cognitive function of ICU survivors. Moreover, neural death is aggravated when glucose concentrations rise rapidly and hyperglycemia occurs after hypoglycemia ("glucose reperfusion injury" [24]). Notably, critically ill patients reveal increased insulin levels, and insulin has also been reported to accelerate neural cell death in the hippocampus during low glucose levels, suggesting that insulin might have a double-edged effect on neuron death dependent on glucose concentration (25). Our findings are in accordance with these data. Since exclusively in the hypo group a correlation of hyperglycemia and a surrogate parameter of the quality of glycemic control with neurocognitive dysfunction was found, we cannot rule out those parameters as relevant confounders of our findings. However, our hypothesis and design only allow to draw a causal link between hypoglycemia and neurocognitive impairment. It is undue to conclude causality between maximum blood glucose or glucose fluctuations from our data; we solely can allude to an association.

To unequivocally prove a causal relation between hypoglycemia and neurocognitive dysfunction, a prospective, randomized controlled trial would be required, but self-evident, ethical considerations preclude this approach. We thus have to rely on the available data from post hoc analysis with its limitations. Another limitation is the absence of brain imaging in all patients. Significant structural brain lesions are unlikely, however, since none of the patients revealed manifest neurological deficits during the study period. However, subtle structural cerebral lesions cannot completely be excluded.

In conclusion, neurocognitive dysfunction is common in patients surviving critical illness. Patients who experienced a hypoglycemic event during ICU treatment show a significant additional impairment in the visuospatial domain compared with patients who did not. In those patients, hyperglycemia and fluctuations of blood glucose levels were also associated with long-term visuospatial dysfunction and might thus confound this conclusion. Every effort should be put in implementing effective blood glucose control algorithms, largely avoiding hypoglycemia and hyperglycemia as well as large fluctuations of blood glucose.

Acknowledgments— The work was supported by a grant from the program "Innovative Medizinische Forschung," Faculty of Medicine, University of Muenster, Muenster, Germany.

No potential conflicts of interest relevant to this article were reported.

Part of the results of this study was presented at the yearly congress of the European Society of Anaesthesiology, Euroanesthesia ESA, Milan, Italy, 6–8 June 2009, and the Annual Congress of the German Society of Anesthesia and Intensive Care Medicine DGAI, DAC Nürnberg, Germany, 9–12 May 2009.

References
1. Van den Berghe G, Wouters P, Weekers F, Verwaest C, Bruyninckx F, Schetz M, Vlasselaers D, Ferdinande P, Lauwers P, Bouillon R. Intensive insulin therapy in the critically ill patients. N Engl J Med 2001;345:1359–1367
2. Griesdale DE, de Souza RJ, van Dam RM, Heyland DK, Cook DJ, Malhotra A, Dhaliwal R, Henderson WR, Chittock DR, Finfer S, Talmor D. Intensive insulin therapy and mortality among critically ill patients: a meta-analysis including NICE-SUGAR study data. CMAJ 2009;180:821–827
3. Vanhorebeek I, Langouche L, Van den Berghe G. Tight blood glucose control with insulin in the ICU: facts and controversies. Chest 2007;132:268–278
4. NICE-SUGAR Study Investigators, Finfer S, Chittock DR, Su SY, Blair D, Foster D, Dhingra V, Bellomo R, Cook D, Dodek P, Henderson WR, Hebert PC, Heritier S, Heyland DK, McArthur C, McDonald E, Mitchell I, Myburgh JA, Norton R, Potter J, Robinson BG, Ronco JJ. Intensive versus conventional glucose control in critically ill patients. N Engl J Med 2009; 360:1283–1297
5. Brunkhorst FM, Engel C, Bloos F, Meier-Hellmann A, Ragaller M, Weiler N, Moerer O, Gruendling M, Oppert M, Grond S, Olthoff D, Jaschinski U, John S, Rossaint R, Welte T, Schaefer M, Kern P, Kuhnt E, Kiehntopf M, Hartog C, Natanson C, Loeffler M, Reinhart K, the German Competence Network Sepsis (SepNet). Intensive insulin therapy and pentastarch resuscitation in severe sepsis. N Engl J Med 2008;358:125–139
6. Vogelzang M, Loef BG, Regtien JG, van der Horst IC, van Assen H, Zijlstra F, Nijsten MW. Computer-assisted glucose control in critically ill patients. Intensive Care Med 2008;34:1421–1427
7. Krinsley JS, Grover A. Severe hypoglycemia in critically ill patients: risk factors and outcomes. Crit Care Med 2007;35: 2262–2267
8. Vriesendorp TM, DeVries JH, van Santen S, Moeniralam HS, de Jonge E, Roos YB, Schultz MJ, Rosendaal FR, Hoekstra JB.

Evaluation of short-term consequences of hypoglycemia in an intensive care unit. Crit Care Med 2006;34:2714–2718

9. Hopkins RO, Ely EW, Jackson JC. The role of future longitudinal studies in ICU survivors: understanding determinants and pathophysiology of brain dysfunction. Curr Opin Crit Care 2007;13:497–502

10. Lezak MD. *Neuropsychological Assessment.* 4th ed. Oxford, U.K., Oxford University Press, 2004

11. Fukui T, Lee E. Visuospatial function is a significant contributor to functional status in patients with Alzheimer's disease. Am J Alzheimers Dis Other Demen 2009; 24:313–321

12. Hamilton JM, Salmon DP, Galasko D, Raman R, Emond J, Hansen LA, Masliah E, Thal LJ. Visuospatial deficits predict rate of cognitive decline in autopsy-verified dementia with Lewy bodies. Neuropsychology 2008;22:729–737

13. Boxer AL, Kramer JH, Du AT, Schuff N, Weiner MW, Miller BL, Rosen HJ. Focal right inferotemporal atrophy in AD with disproportionate visual constructive impairment. Neurology 2003;61:1485–1491

14. Suh SW, Hamby AM, Swanson RA. Hypoglycemia, brain energetics, and hypoglycemic neuronal death. Glia 2007;55: 1280–1286

15. Fujioka M, Okuchi K, Hiramatsu KI, Sakaki T, Sakaguchi S, Ishii Y. Specific changes in human brain after hypoglycemic injury. Stroke 1997;28:584–587

16. Bree AJ, Puente EC, Daphna-Iken D, Fisher SJ. Diabetes increases brain damage caused by severe hypoglycemia. Am J Physiol Endocrinol Metab 2009;297: E194–E201

17. Auer RN. Hypoglycemic brain damage. Metab Brain Dis 2004;19:169–175

18. McNay EC, Williamson A, McCrimmon RJ, Sherwin RS. Cognitive and neural hippocampal effects of long-term moderate recurrent hypoglycemia. Diabetes 2006; 55:1088–1095

19. Warren RE, Frier BM. Hypoglycaemia and cognitive function. Diabetes Obes Metab 2005;7:493–503

20. Lincoln NB, Faleiro RM, Kelly C, Kirk BA, Jeffcoate WJ. Effect of long-term glycemic control on cognitive function. Diabetes Care 1996;19:656–658

21. Robinson R, Krishnakumar A, Paulose CS. Enhanced dopamine D1 and D2 receptor gene expression in the hippocampus of hypoglycaemic and diabetic rats. Cell Mol Neurobiol 2009;29:365–372

22. Gunther ML, Jackson JC, Ely EW. The cognitive consequences of critical illness: practical recommendations for screening and assessment. Crit Care Clin 2007;23: 491–506

23. Malone JI, Hanna S, Saporta S, Mervis RF, Park CR, Chong L, Diamond DM. Hyperglycemia not hypoglycemia alters neuronal dendrites and impairs spatial memory. Pediatr Diabetes 2008;9:531–539

24. Suh SW, Gum ET, Hamby AM, Chan PH, Swanson RA. Hypoglycemic neuronal death is triggered by glucose reperfusion and activation of neuronal NADPH oxidase. J Clin Invest 2007;117:910–918

25. Tanaka Y, Takata T, Satomi T, Sakurai T, Yokono K. The double-edged effect of insulin on the neuronal cell death associated with hypoglycemia on the hippocampal slice culture. Kobe J Med Sci 2008;54:E97–E107

Hypoglycemia in Type 1 Diabetic Pregnancy

Role of preconception insulin aspart treatment in a randomized study

Simon Heller, md, frcp[1]
Peter Damm, md, dmsc[2]
Henriette Mersebach, md, phd[3]
Trine Vang Skjøth, md[3]
Risto Kaaja, md, phd[4]

Moshe Hod, md[5]
Santiago Durán-García, md, phd[6]
David McCance, md[7]
Elisabeth R. Mathiesen, md, dmsc[2]

OBJECTIVE — A recent randomized trial compared prandial insulin aspart (IAsp) with human insulin in type 1 diabetic pregnancy. The aim of this exploratory analysis was to investigate the incidence of severe hypoglycemia during pregnancy and compare women enrolled preconception with women enrolled during early pregnancy.

RESEARCH DESIGN AND METHODS — IAsp administered immediately before each meal was compared with human insulin administered 30 min before each meal in 99 subjects (44 to IAsp and 55 to human insulin) randomly assigned preconception and in 223 subjects (113 for IAsp and 110 for human insulin) randomly assigned in early pregnancy (<10 weeks). NPH insulin was the basal insulin. Severe hypoglycemia (requiring third-party assistance) was recorded prospectively preconception (where possible), during pregnancy, and postpartum. Relative risk (RR) of severe hypoglycemia was evaluated with a gamma frailty model.

RESULTS — Of the patients, 23% experienced severe hypoglycemia during pregnancy with the peak incidence in early pregnancy. In the first half of pregnancy, the RR of severe hypoglycemia in women randomly assigned in early pregnancy/preconception was 1.70 (95% CI 0.91–3.18, $P = 0.097$); the RR in the second half of pregnancy was 1.35 (0.38–4.77, $P = 0.640$). In women randomly assigned preconception, severe hypoglycemia rates occurring before and during the first and second halves of pregnancy and postpartum for IAsp versus human insulin were 0.9 versus 2.4, 0.9 versus 2.4, 0.3 versus 1.2, and 0.2 versus 2.2 episodes per patient per year, respectively (NS).

CONCLUSIONS — These data suggest that initiation of insulin analog treatment preconception rather than during early pregnancy may result in a lower risk of severe hypoglycemia in women with type 1 diabetes.

Diabetes Care 33:473–477, 2010

S evere hypoglycemia is common in pregnant women with type 1 diabetes, with observed rates up to 15 times those reported by the Diabetes Control and Complications Trial (1), and severe hypoglycemia occurs in 19–44% of patients treated with intensive insulin therapy during pregnancy (2). The risk of experiencing a severe event is usually highest in early pregnancy, particularly during the first trimester (3–5).

The risk factors that predict severe hypoglycemic episodes during pregnancy include duration of diabetes, a history of previous severe episodes (recurrent events), hypoglycemic unawareness, a change in insulin treatment (such as regimen or dosing) or a high insulin dose, and A1C <6.5% (4,6,7). However, because normoglycemia is universally recommended in diabetic pregnancy (8,9), with A1C levels between 4.0 and 6.0% advocated to optimize pregnancy outcome (10,11), minimizing the risk of severe hypoglycemia is a major challenge to those caring for pregnant women with type 1 diabetes.

Preconception care programs are associated with both reduced malformations and fewer early fetal losses in pregnant women with type 1 diabetes (12–14), perhaps due to improved glycemic control in the first stages of pregnancy. It is possible that working with women to improve metabolic control and optimize their insulin regimen before pregnancy might also help to reduce the high rate of severe episodes of hypoglycemia postconception, but this has yet to be demonstrated.

We recently completed a randomized, open-label, parallel-group, multinational, multicenter study investigating maternal and fetal outcomes in 322 women with type 1 diabetes treated with either prandial insulin aspart (IAsp) or human insulin (15–17). IAsp injected immediately before eating was as effective and well tolerated as human insulin administered 30 min before eating. Although the study was somewhat underpowered, there were strong trends toward improved postprandial glucose control and prevention of severe hypoglycemia in the IAsp group (15,16). This study supports the conclusions of trials in nonpregnant individuals with type 1 diabetes, which suggest that the advantages of rapid-acting insulin analogs are most likely to be seen in those with tight control (18–20).

The aim of this exploratory analysis was to compare the incidence of severe hypoglycemia during pregnancy between women enrolled into the trial either preconception or early in the first trimester. Finally, we also compared the effects of the different insulins on rates of severe hypoglycemia according to the time of enrollment of (pregnant) women into the study.

• •

From the [1]Northern General Hospital, Sheffield, U.K.; the [2]Rigshospitalet, University of Copenhagen, Copenhagen, Denmark; the [3]Novo Nordisk, Soeborg, Denmark; the [4]Helsinki University Central Hospital, Helsinki, Finland; the [5]Rabin Medical Center, Tel-Aviv University, Petah-Tiqva, Israel; the [6]University of Seville, Seville, Spain; and the [7]Royal Victoria Hospital, Belfast, U.K.

Corresponding author: Simon Heller, s.heller@sheffield.ac.uk.

Received 27 August 2009 and accepted 17 November 2009. Published ahead of print at http://care.diabetesjournals.org on 10 December 2009. DOI: 10.2337/dc09-1605.

RESEARCH DESIGN AND METHODS

— A total of 322 women with type 1 diabetes participated in this open-label, randomized, parallel-group, multinational, multicenter study conducted at 63 sites in 18 countries (15–17). The study was performed in accordance with the Declaration of Helsinki and was approved by the respective ethics committees and health authorities according to local regulations. Written informed consent was obtained from subjects before commencement of the study. Eligible subjects were aged ≥18 years, had insulin-treated type 1 diabetes for ≥12 months, and were either planning to become pregnant or were already pregnant with a singleton pregnancy (gestational age ≤10 weeks). A1C was ≤8% at confirmation of pregnancy. Subjects were randomly assigned (1:1) to mealtime IAsp (NovoRapid 100 IU/ml Penfill; Novo Nordisk) injected immediately before each meal or human insulin (human soluble insulin, Actrapid 100 IU/ml, 3 ml Penfill; Novo Nordisk) injected 30 min before each meal, in combination with NPH insulin (human isophane insulin, 100 IU/ml, 3 ml Penfill; Novo Nordisk) one to four times per day.

In this exploratory analysis, the intent-to-treat pregnant population included all randomly assigned subjects who were exposed to the trial drug and in whom pregnancy was confirmed at some point during the trial. This population consisted of 99 subjects randomly assigned before known pregnancy (44 to IAsp and 55 to human insulin) and 223 subjects randomly assigned in early pregnancy (113 to IAsp and 110 to human insulin).

Severe hypoglycemia was defined as an event requiring third-party assistance associated with plasma glucose <3.1 mmol/l and/or reversal of symptoms after food, glucagon, or intravenous glucose. Nocturnal hypoglycemia was defined as episodes occurring between midnight and 0600 h. Hypoglycemia was recorded prospectively preconception (where possible), during the first half of pregnancy (<20 weeks' gestation), during the second half of pregnancy (≥20 weeks' gestation), and postpartum. Subjects were followed throughout pregnancy with one visit per trimester and at 6 weeks postpartum. Hypoglycemic coma, glycemic control, duration of diabetes, and pretrial insulin regimen (use of analogs) were also recorded. Between study visits, the

women received routine diabetes and obstetric care according to local practice.

Statistical analyses

The primary end point in this study was severe hypoglycemia. Assuming an incidence of one severe hypoglycemic episode during pregnancy with 7 months of insulin treatment (21), 305 subjects were required to complete the trial to detect a treatment difference of 40% with a power of 80% (5% significance level). Assuming a dropout rate of ~20%, 380 subjects were to be randomly assigned.

In this analysis, rates of severe hypoglycemia were compared between those women randomly assigned preconception with those randomly assigned in early pregnancy and between treatment groups. Relative risk (RR) of severe hypoglycemia was estimated using a gamma frailty model with treatment as a factor. For women already pregnant at screening, delayed entry was used to account for the different observation periods. A Cox regression model accounted for recurrent aspects of episodes. Incidence of nocturnal severe hypoglycemia is presented here using descriptive statistics, as there were too few events for formal analysis. The observed rate is defined as number of episodes per patient per year. The relationship between history of severe hypoglycemia and episodes during pregnancy is based on subjects who had at least 30 days' preconception exposure to the trial drug, i.e., only those enrolled before pregnancy.

RESULTS

Baseline patient demographics

The study includes the 99 of the 189 subjects making up the preconception group who became pregnant during the 12 months specified in the original protocol (15). Age, A1C, BMI, and duration of diabetes were similar in subjects randomly assigned preconception or in early pregnancy and between treatment groups (Table 1).

Hypoglycemia in those randomly assigned preconception versus those randomly assigned in early pregnancy

Overall, 23% of subjects ($n = 73$) experienced at least one episode of severe hypoglycemia during the study, and many subjects experienced several episodes, including six subjects who experienced ≥10 episodes. Rates of severe hypoglycemia calculated for each week of pregnancy and postpartum are shown in Fig. 1A and B and are combined into rates in early pregnancy, late pregnancy, and postpartum in Fig. 1C. These rates appear to peak in early pregnancy, with low values in the second half of pregnancy except for a rise immediately before birth. Rates of severe hypoglycemia in the first and second halves of pregnancy are presented separately here. Rates of severe hypoglycemia in subjects randomly assigned preconception or early in pregnancy, respectively, were 1.7 versus 3.4 events per patient per year in the first half of pregnancy, 0.8 versus 0.9 events per pa-

Table 1—*Patient baseline demographics*

	IAsp + NPH		Human insulin + NPH	
	Randomly assigned preconception	Randomly assigned in early pregnancy	Randomly assigned preconception	Randomly assigned in early pregnancy
n	44	113	55	110
Age (years)	28.6 ± 3.7	29.2 ± 5.1	28.8 ± 4.3	29.2 ± 4.7
A1C (%)*	7.3 ± 1.0	6.8 ± 0.7	7.1 ± 1.2	6.8 ± 0.8
BMI (kg/m^2)	24.1 ± 3.6	25.2 ± 4.2	25.0 ± 4.0	24.4 ± 3.6
Duration of diabetes (years)	11.8 ± 6.4	12.4 ± 7.4	11.3 ± 6.7	12.0 ± 7.8
Pretrial insulin including insulin analogs	24 (54.5)	49 (43.3)	30 (54.5)	50 (45.5)
Dose (IU · kg^{-1} · 24 h^{-1})	0.79 ± 0.25	0.77 ± 0.27	0.75 ± 0.21	0.77 ± 0.27
Preconception exposure to trial drug (days)	153.8 ± 108.2	NA	110.3 ± 92.0	NA

Data are means ± SD or n (%). *A1C is from early pregnancy: at randomization in those randomly assigned in early pregnancy and at pregnancy confirmation in those randomly assigned preconception. NA, not applicable.

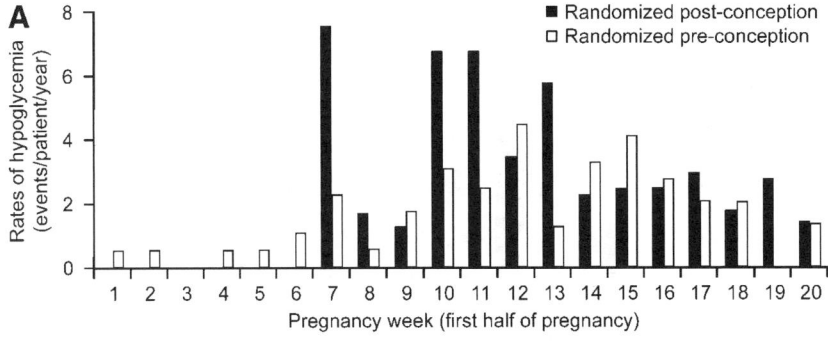

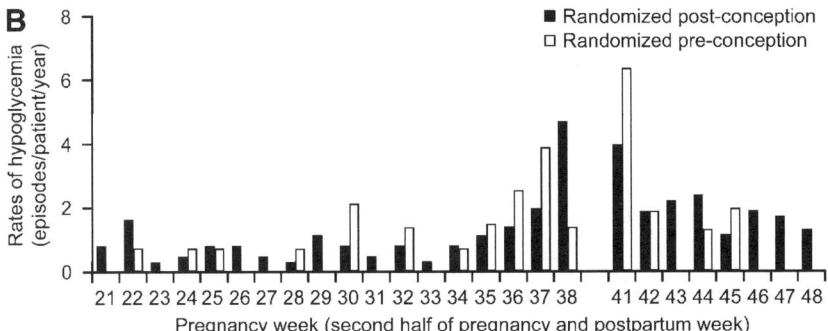

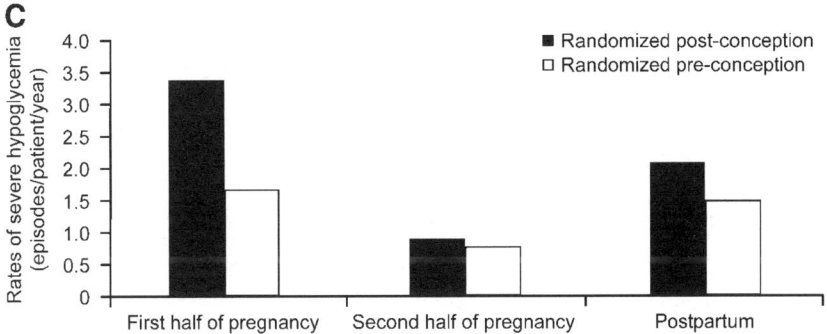

Figure 1—*Rate of severe hypoglycemia in pregnancy, grouped according to timing of randomization in the first half of pregnancy (A), in the second half of pregnancy and postpartum (B), and in the first and second half of pregnancy and postpartum (C).*

tient per year in the second half of pregnancy, and 1.5 versus 2.1 events per patient per year in the postpartum period (Fig. 1C).

In the first half of pregnancy, the estimated risk of severe hypoglycemia was 70% higher in subjects randomly assigned in early pregnancy versus those randomly assigned preconception (RR 1.70 [95% CI 0.91–3.18], $P = 0.097$); in the second half of pregnancy the RR was 1.35 (0.38–4.77) ($P = 0.640$). Observed rates for severe nocturnal hypoglycemia in subjects randomly assigned preconception versus postconception were 0.7 versus 0.9 events per patient per year, respectively, in the first half of pregnancy; 0.4 versus 0.2 events per patient per year in the second half of pregnancy; and 0.5

events per patient per year versus 0.6 postpartum.

Hypoglycemia in subjects treated with IAsp and those treated with human insulin

Subjects randomly assigned preconception had consistently lower observed rates of severe hypoglycemia with IAsp versus human insulin, respectively, preconception (0.9 vs. 2.4 events per patient per year), in the first half of pregnancy (0.9 vs. 2.4 events per patient per year), in the second half of pregnancy (0.3 vs. 1.2 events per patient per year), and postpartum (0.2 vs. 2.2 events per patient per year, NS for all) (Fig. 2). In subjects randomly assigned preconception, the estimated risk for severe hypoglycemia

during the first and second halves of pregnancy tended to be lower with IAsp than with human insulin (RR 0.37 [95% CI 0.10–1.32], $P = 0.13$ vs. 0.20 [0.02–1.85], $P = 0.16$, respectively). Estimated risk with IAsp was 66% lower for the preconception period (0.34 [0.07–1.71], $P = 0.19$ [NS]) and 92% lower postpartum (0.08 [0.01–0.84], $P = 0.04$) (Fig. 2).

Observed rates of severe nocturnal hypoglycemia in subjects treated with IAsp preconception were likewise consistently lower than those for human insulin–treated subjects preconception (0.3 vs. 1.5 events per patient per year), during the first half of pregnancy (0.1 vs. 1.2 events per patient per year), during the second half of pregnancy (0.1 vs. 0.7 events per patient per year), and postpartum (0.2 vs. 0.7 events per patient per year), respectively. The numbers in this group were too small for a meaningful analysis of statistical significance. In subjects randomly assigned in early pregnancy, rates of severe nocturnal hypoglycemia were similar for the IAsp and human insulin treatment groups during the first half of pregnancy (0.7 vs. 1.0 events per patient per year), the second half of pregnancy (0.2 vs. 0.2 events per patient per year), and postpartum (0.6 vs. 0.6 events per patient per year), respectively.

Rates of hypoglycemia were higher in subjects randomly assigned in early pregnancy to an insulin regimen differing from their previous treatment. In subjects who changed insulin regimens and were randomly assigned to IAsp, the hypoglycemia rate was 3.0 versus 2.1 events per patient per year for subjects who did not change regimens. The same values for those randomly assigned to human insulin in early pregnancy were 4.5 events per patient per year for subjects who changed regimens versus 3.3 events per patient per year for those already treated with human insulin.

History of severe hypoglycemia
Of subjects reporting episodes of severe hypoglycemia preconception (during the trial), 67% (10 of 15) had severe hypoglycemia during pregnancy versus only 9% (6 of 67) of subjects with no preconception episodes.

Hypoglycemic coma
Eight episodes of hypoglycemic coma were observed during pregnancy in this study (three episodes with IAsp and five episodes with human insulin), all in

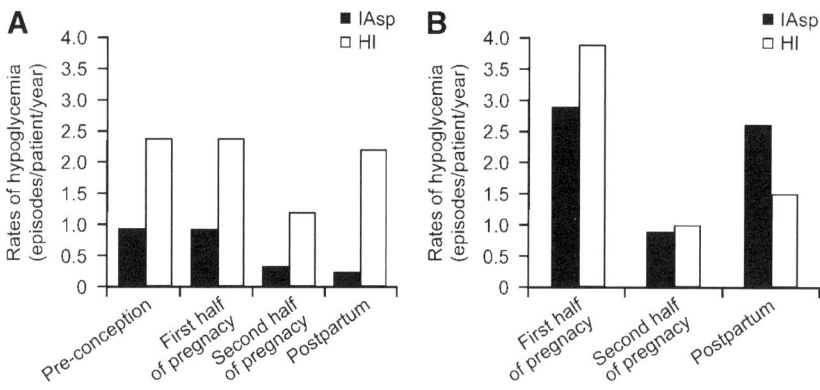

Figure 2—*Observed rates of severe hypoglycemia in subjects randomly assigned preconception (A) or early in pregnancy (B) treated with either IAsp or human insulin (HI).*

subjects randomly assigned in early pregnancy.

Glycemic control

During pregnancy, mean A1C and average plasma glucose levels were comparable between treatment groups throughout the study (Table 2). Plasma glucose was derived as the average of the 8-point profile for each subject. Profiles were taken on a normal weekday within the week before the visit and included values premeal, 90-min postmeal, at bedtime, and at 0200 h.

CONCLUSIONS — This exploratory analysis was based on data obtained from the largest randomized controlled trial to date involving an insulin analog in the treatment of pregnant women with type 1 diabetes. Despite the limitations imposed by the observational design, we believe that exploring the influence of the timing of entry into the trial on risk of hypoglycemia is clinically relevant. The data suggest that women enrolled in a clinical trial preconception experience fewer hypoglycemic episodes than those enrolled postconception. Although the RRs in women randomly assigned preconception are not statistically significant because of a lack of power, the marked trend to lower rates in this group is of interest.

It is well known that severe hypoglycemia is common during pregnancy and is most likely to occur during the first trimester (3,4). One observation from our data is that the incidence of severe hypo-

glycemia does not peak in early pregnancy in women who were enrolled preconception. This group had a low rate of severe hypoglycemic episodes comparable to the 1.3 events per patient per year seen in the nonpregnant background population (22).

It is possible that patients who entered the trial preconception were more motivated and experienced in diabetes self-management than those enrolling postconception, as represented by tighter control and less hypoglycemia. However, glycemic control (A1C and plasma glucose) was similar between those randomly assigned in early pregnancy and those randomly assigned preconception. An alternative explanation is that the extra professional input in the preconception period led to optimized insulin therapy and a lower risk of hypoglycemia. Although preconception counseling is associated with a reduced malformation rate in the offspring of women with type 1 diabetes (12–14), we are unaware of previous studies exploring the impact of preconception input on severe hypoglycemia during the ensuing pregnancy.

It is conceivable that subjects who changed their insulin regimen may have had higher rates of hypoglycemia than those who did not change their insulin regimen; however, the numbers of those taking the same insulin in the trial were too small to undertake formal comparisons. Nevertheless, switching to IAsp after human insulin treatment during pregnancy did not seem to worsen the risk of hypoglycemia, confirming the results of a smaller earlier study (23).

Our data show an apparent rise in hypoglycemia in the weeks immediately before birth. This finding might relate to a fall in insulin requirements in the immediate predelivery period. A further intriguing finding was that the benefit of a rapid-acting insulin analog (IAsp) associated with a lower risk of severe hypoglycemia than that with human insulin (20) tended to be most pronounced in women who were randomly assigned preconception. This result may be related to their experience with the use of insulin IAsp before the influence of the metabolic changes of pregnancy. The rate of severe hypoglycemia immediately postpartum was considerably higher than that in the last half of pregnancy and was also higher than that seen in observational data in nonpregnant diabetic populations (22), suggesting that women should focus on reducing their postpar-

Table 2—A1C and plasma glucose values

	IAsp + NPH		Human insulin + NPH	
	Randomly assigned preconception	Randomly assigned in early pregnancy	Randomly assigned preconception	Randomly assigned in early pregnancy
n	44	113	55	110
A1C (%)				
First visit	7.3 ± 1.0	6.8 ± 0.7	7.1 ± 1.2	6.8 ± 0.8
First trimester visit	6.3 ± 0.7	6.3 ± 0.6	6.2 ± 0.7	6.4 ± 0.7
Second trimester visit	6.0 ± 0.7	5.9 ± 0.7	6.0 ± 0.6	5.9 ± 0.7
Third trimester visit	6.2 ± 0.5	6.0 ± 0.7	6.2 ± 0.5	6.1 ± 0.7
Follow-up (6 weeks postpartum)	6.6 ± 0.7	6.5 ± 0.9	6.6 ± 0.8	6.4 ± 0.8
Average plasma glucose (mmol/l)				
First visit	7.9 ± 1.8	6.8 ± 1.7	7.9 ± 1.9	7.1 ± 1.4
First trimester visit	7.1 ± 1.6	6.6 ± 1.4	6.7 ± 1.7	6.6 ± 1.3
Second trimester visit	7.1 ± 1.2	6.7 ± 1.4	7.1 ± 1.5	6.8 ± 1.4
Third trimester visit	6.2 ± 1.0	6.2 ± 1.2	6.4 ± 1.3	6.4 ± 1.3

Data are means ± SD.

tum insulin dose and returning to preconception glycemic control goals.

This analysis suggests that the initiation of insulin analog treatment preconception as opposed to during early pregnancy results in a lower risk of severe hypoglycemia in women with type 1 diabetes. The reasons for this finding remain unclear but might include the influence of preconception planning. Although the limitations of exploratory analyses prevent any firm conclusions, these data suggest another potential advantage of prenatal care that is worthy of further investigation. The observation should also be taken into account in future clinical trials during pregnancy in women with type 1 diabetes.

Acknowledgments— S.H. has served on advisory boards for, received research funds from, and given lectures sponsored by Novo Nordisk. P.D. and E.R.M. are associated with Novo Nordisk as part of an advisory board. H.M. and T.V.S. are employees and shareholders of Novo Nordisk. No other potential conflicts of interest relevant to this article were reported.

References

1. ter Braak EW, Evers IM, Willem Erkelens D, Visser GH. Maternal hypoglycemia during pregnancy in type 1 diabetes: maternal and fetal consequences. Diabetes Metab Res Rev 2002;18:96–105
2. Persson B, Hansson U. Hypoglycaemia in pregnancy. Baillieres Clin Endocrinol Metab 1993;7:731–739
3. Kimmerle R, Heinemann L, Delecki A, Berger M. Severe hypoglycemia, incidence and predisposing factors in 85 pregnancies of type I diabetic women. Diabetes Care 1992;15:1034–1037
4. Evers IM, ter Braak EW, de Valk HW, van Der Schoot B, Janssen N, Visser GH. Risk indicators predictive for severe hypoglycemia during the first trimester of type 1 diabetic pregnancy. Diabetes Care 2002;25:554–559
5. Rosenn BM, Miodovnik M, Holcberg G, Khoury JC, Siddiqi TA. Hypoglycemia: the price of intensive insulin therapy for pregnant women with insulin-dependent diabetes mellitus. Obstet Gynecol 1995;85:417–422
6. Rayburn W, Piehl E, Jacober S, Schork A, Ploughman L. Severe hypoglycemia during pregnancy: its frequency and predisposing factors in diabetic women. Int J Gynaecol Obstet 1986;24:263–268
7. Nielsen LR, Pedersen-Bjergaard U, Thorsteinsson B, Johansen M, Damm P, Mathiesen ER. Hypoglycemia in pregnant women with type 1 diabetes: predictors and role of metabolic control. Diabetes Care 2008;31:9–14
8. American Diabetes Association. Standards of medical care in diabetes—2007 (Position Statement). Diabetes Care 2007;30 (Suppl. 1):S4–S41
9. National Institute for Health and Clinical Excellence (NICE). *Clinical Guidelines (2008): CG63 Diabetes in Pregnancy: Full Guideline* [article online], 2008. Available from http://guidance.nice.org.uk/CG63/NiceGuidance/pdf/English. Accessed 31 July 2009
10. Temple R, Aldridge V, Greenwood R, Heyburn P, Sampson M, Stanley K. Association between outcome of pregnancy and glycaemic control in early pregnancy in type 1 diabetes: population based study. BMJ 2002;325:1275–1276
11. Nielsen GL, Møller M, Sørensen HT. HbA1c in early diabetic pregnancy and pregnancy outcomes: a Danish population-based cohort study of 573 pregnancies in women with type 1 diabetes. Diabetes Care 2006;29:2612–2616
12. McElvy SS, Miodovnik M, Rosenn B, Khoury JC, Siddiqi T, Dignan PS, Tsang RC. A focused preconceptional and early pregnancy program in women with type 1 diabetes reduces perinatal mortality and malformation rates to general population levels. J Matern Fetal Med 2000;9:14–20
13. Ray JG, O'Brien TE, Chan WS. Preconception care and the risk of congenital anomalies in the offspring of women with diabetes mellitus: a meta-analysis. Q J Med 2001;94:435–444
14. Temple RC, Aldridge VJ, Murphy HR. Prepregnancy care and pregnancy outcomes in women with type 1 diabetes. Diabetes Care 2006;29:1744–1749
15. Mathiesen ER, Kinsley B, Amiel SA, Heller S, McCance D, Duran S, Bellaire S, Raben A, Insulin Aspart Pregnancy Study Group. Maternal glycemic control and hypoglycemia in type 1 diabetic pregnancy: a randomized trial of insulin aspart versus human insulin in 322 pregnant women. Diabetes Care 2007;30:771–776
16. Hod M, Damm P, Kaaja R, Visser GH, Dunne F, Demidova I, Hansen AS, Mersebach H, Insulin Aspart Pregnancy Study Group. Fetal and perinatal outcomes in type 1 diabetes pregnancy: a randomized study comparing insulin aspart with human insulin in 322 subjects. Am J Obstet Gynecol 2008;198:186.e1–7
17. McCance DR, Damm P, Mathiesen ER, Hod M, Kaaja R, Dunne F, Jensen LE, Mersebach H. Evaluation of insulin antibodies and placental transfer of insulin aspart in pregnant women with type 1 diabetes mellitus. Diabetologia 2008;51:2141–2143
18. Home PD, Lindholm A, Riis A, European Insulin Aspart Study Group. Insulin aspart vs. human insulin in the management of long-term blood glucose control in type 1 diabetes mellitus: a randomized controlled trial. Diabet Med 2000;17:762–770
19. Raskin P, Guthrie RA, Leiter L, Riis A, Jovanovic L. Use of insulin aspart, a fast-acting insulin analog, as the mealtime insulin in the management of patients with type 1 diabetes. Diabetes Care 2000;23:583–588
20. Heller SR, Colagiuri S, Vaaler S, Wolffenbuttel BH, Koelendorf K, Friberg HH, Windfeld K, Lindholm A. Hypoglycaemia with insulin aspart: a double-blind, randomised, crossover trial in subjects with type 1 diabetes. Diabet Med 2004;21:769–775
21. The Diabetes Control and Complications Trial Research Group. Hypoglycemia in the Diabetes Control and Complications Trial. Diabetes 1997;46:271–286
22. Pedersen-Bjergaard U, Pramming S, Heller SR, Wallace TM, Rasmussen AK, Jørgensen HV, Matthews DR, Hougaard P, Thorsteinsson B. Severe hypoglycaemia in 1076 adult patients with type 1 diabetes: influence of risk markers and selection. Diabetes Metab Res Rev 2004;20:479–486
23. Garg SK, Frias JP, Anil S, Gottlieb PA, MacKenzie T, Jackson WE. Insulin lispro therapy in pregnancies complicated by type 1 diabetes: glycemic control and maternal and fetal outcomes. Endocr Pract 2003;9:187–193

Modulation of β-Adrenergic Receptors in the Ventromedial Hypothalamus Influences Counterregulatory Responses to Hypoglycemia

Barbara Szepietowska,[1] Wanling Zhu,[1] Owen Chan,[1] Adam Horblitt,[1] James Dziura,[2] and Robert S. Sherwin[1]

OBJECTIVE—Norepinephrine is locally released into the ventromedial hypothalamus (VMH), a key brain glucose-sensing region in the response to hypoglycemia. As a result, this neurotransmitter may play a role in modulating counterregulatory responses. This study examines whether norepinephrine acts to promote glucose counterregulation via specific VMH β-adrenergic receptors (BAR).

RESEARCH DESIGN AND METHODS—Awake male Sprague-Dawley rats received, via implanted guide cannulae, bilateral VMH microinjections of 1) artificial extracellular fluid, 2) B2AR agonist, or 3) B2AR antagonist. Subsequently, a hyperinsulinemic-hypoglycemic clamp study was performed. The same protocol was also used to assess the effect of VMH delivery of a selective B1AR or B3AR antagonist.

RESULTS—Despite similar insulin and glucose concentrations during the clamp, activation of B2AR in the VMH significantly lowered by 32% ($P < 0.01$), whereas VMH B2AR blockade raised by 27% exogenous glucose requirements during hypoglycemia ($P < 0.05$) compared with the control study. These changes were associated with alternations in counterregulatory hormone release. Epinephrine responses throughout hypoglycemia were significantly increased by 50% when the B2AR agonist was delivered to the VMH ($P < 0.01$) and suppressed by 32% with the B2AR antagonist ($P < 0.05$). The glucagon response was also increased by B2AR activation by 63% ($P < 0.01$). Neither blockade of VMH B1AR nor B3AR suppressed counterregulatory responses to hypoglycemia. Indeed, the B1AR antagonist increased rather than decreased epinephrine release ($P < 0.05$).

CONCLUSIONS—Local catecholamine release into the VMH enhances counterregulatory responses to hypoglycemia via stimulation of B2AR. These observations suggest that B2AR agonists might have therapeutic benefit in diabetic patients with defective glucose counterregulation. *Diabetes* 60:3154–3158, 2011

Lowering glucose toward normal in patients with type 1 diabetes is well documented to reduce long-term complications (1). In clinical practice, however, intensified insulin treatment is often limited by the increased risk of severe hypoglycemia (2). In people without diabetes, a fall in blood glucose is rapidly detected by glucose-sensing neurons in the brain and periphery, and a series of compensatory responses occur to prevent or limit hypoglycemia and to restore euglycemia. Specifically, the activation of counterregulatory hormone release (e.g., glucagon and epinephrine) and the sympathetic nervous system (norepinephrine) promote endogenous glucose production, reduce tissue utilization of glucose, and generate typical warning symptoms. These protective responses against hypoglycemia are disrupted in most patients with type 1 diabetes receiving intensive insulin therapy (3,4). As a result, they display impaired neurohumoral responses to hypoglycemia and, in some cases, the loss of symptomatic awareness of hypoglycemia. The molecular mechanism(s) underlying this phenomenon are not fully understood.

Detection of hypoglycemia by glucose-sensing cells/neurons peripherally (5) and centrally (6) is critical in the defense against hypoglycemia and the prevention of brain injury. One brain region in particular, the ventromedial hypothalamus (VMH), appears to play a key role in hypoglycemia sensing (7). It contains glucose-excited and glucose-inhibited neurons that detect changes in ambient glucose levels and then alter their firing rate accordingly (8). The VMH contains glutamatergic and γ-aminobutyric acid (GABA)ergic innervations, both of which have been shown to have an effect on counterregulatory responses to hypoglycemia (9,10). In addition, monoamine neurotransmitters, such as norepinephrine, are also released into the VMH and appear to regulate VMH function during hypoglycemia. It has been reported that norepinephrine has been reported to stimulate glutamatergic neurotransmission in mechanically dissociated rat VMH neurons and that this effect is mediated via activation of β₂-adrenergic receptors (B2AR) (11). The loss of function of glutamatergic neurons in the VMH region, however, suppresses glucose counterregulation in mice (10). In addition, a rise in norepinephrine concentrations in VMH interstitial fluid has been reported during acute hypoglycemia (12), and this rise is prevented when glucose is perfused into the VMH and systemic hypoglycemia is maintained (13). Although local norepinephrine release into the VMH appears to be altered during hypoglycemia, the neuronal projection circuits coordinating this response are not fully understood. It has been suggested that the brainstem and other hypothalamic regions are important components of a glucose-sensing network coordinating defenses against hypoglycemic stress (14,15).

The current study was undertaken to assess the mechanisms by which the local release of catecholamines might act within the VMH to influence the magnitude of the counterregulatory response to hypoglycemia. Our data suggest that norepinephrine modulates VMH neurons during hypoglycemia at least in part through B2AR.

From the [1]Department of Internal Medicine and Endocrinology, Yale University School of Medicine, New Haven, Connecticut; and the [2]Department of Emergency Medicine, Yale Center for Analytical Sciences, Yale University School of Medicine, New Haven, Connecticut.
Corresponding author: Robert S. Sherwin, robert.sherwin@yale.edu.
Received 31 March 2011 and accepted 14 September 2011.
DOI: 10.2337/db11-0432

RESEARCH DESIGN AND METHODS

Male Sprague-Dawley rats (Charles River, Wilmington, MA) weighing 275–350 g were individually housed in the Yale Animal Resource Center in temperature-controlled (22–23°C) and humidity-controlled rooms. The animals were fed rat chow (Agway Prolab 3000, Syracuse, NY), given water ad libitum, and acclimatized to a 12-h light/dark cycle. The Yale University Institutional Animal Care and Use Committee approved the experimental protocols.

Surgery. Seven to 10 days before each study, all animals were anesthetized with an injection (1 mL/kg i.p.) of a mixture of xylazine (20 mg/mL AnaSed; Lloyd Laboratories, Shenandoah, IA) and ketamine (100 mg/mL Ketaset; Aveco, Fort Dodge, IA), in a ratio of 1:2 (vol/vol), before undergoing vascular surgery for the implantation of vascular catheters in a carotid artery and jugular vein. Microinjection guide cannulae were then bilaterally inserted into the VMH, targeting the ventromedial nucleus (coordinates from bregma: anteroposterior −2.6 mm, mediolateral ±0.8 mm, and dorsoventral −8.0).

Microinjection. On the morning of the study, after an overnight fast and 60 min after opening the catheters, 22-gauge microinjection needles, designed to extend 1 mm beyond the tip of the guide cannula (Plastics One, Roanoke, VA), were inserted through the guide cannula bilaterally into each VMH. The rat was then microinjected over 2 min (0.5 μL/min) using a CMA-102 infusion pump (CMA Microdialysis, North Chelmsford, MA).

The animals were microinjected immediately before the initiation of a hyperinsulinemic-hypoglycemic clamp with 1 μL of one the following pharmacologic agents: artificial extracellular fluid as a control ($n = 12$); 1 μmol/L concentration of the B2AR antagonist ICI-118,551 ($n = 12$); or 1 μmol/L concentration of the B2AR agonist formoterol ($n = 10$). The doses of B2AR agonists and antagonists selected were based on preliminary dose-ranging studies using a 1 nmol/L to 200 μmol/L concentration of the agonist and antagonist. In another set of studies, we microinjected 1 μmol/L CGP 20712 dihydrochloride, a potent, selective B1AR ($n = 7$), or 1 μmol/L SR59230A hydrochloride, a potent, selective B3AR antagonist ($n = 6$).

Hyperinsulinemic-hypoglycemic clamp. A primed-continuous intravascular infusion of 20 mU · kg^{-1} · min^{-1} regular insulin was started, and a variable infusion of 20% dextrose was adjusted in response to 10-min measurements of plasma glucose to reach a target value of 50 mg/dL within 30 min. Thereafter, plasma glucose was monitored at 10-min intervals using a glucose analyzer (Analox Instruments, Lunenburg, MA) to adjust the dextrose infusion rate to maintain a stable 50 mg/dL glucose level until the end of the study at 90 min. Blood was drawn at baseline and at 30, 60, and 90 min for measurement of plasma glucagon, epinephrine, norepinephrine, and insulin.

Probe placement. At the end of experiments, the rats were killed with an overdose of sodium pentobarbital (Sleepaway; Fort Dodge Animal Health, Fort Dodge, IA). Brains were removed, frozen, and stored at −80°C until analysis. Accuracy of microinjection needle placements was verified histologically.

Analytic procedures. Catecholamine analysis was performed by high-performance liquid chromatography using electrochemical detection (ESA, Acton, MA). Plasma insulin and glucagon were measured by radioimmunoassay (Linco, St. Charles, MO).

Data analysis. All data are expressed as means ± SEM. Baseline comparisons were performed using ANOVA. A mixed-model analysis with an unstructured covariance matrix was used to accommodate correlated responses from repeated measures. Post hoc linear contrasts were used to localize effects. Analyses were performed using SAS 9.2 software (SAS Institute, Inc., Cary, NC), with a threshold $P < 0.05$ considered as statistically significant.

RESULTS

As summarized in Table 1, the groups of rats did not differ with respect to body weight or concentrations of plasma glucose, insulin, glucagon, epinephrine, and norepinephrine at baseline. During the hyperinsulinemic-hypoglycemic clamp studies, plasma glucose and insulin in each animal group reached levels that were not significantly different (Table 2).

As shown in Fig. 1A, VMH delivery of the B2AR agonist reduced the exogenous glucose infusion rates (GIR) required to maintain target glucose concentration by 32% during the entire hypoglycemic clamp ($P < 0.01$), whereas B2AR blockade in the VMH raised exogenous glucose requirements by 27% ($P < 0.05$) compared with the control study.

These changes were accompanied by alternations in peak and in overall epinephrine responses during hypoglycemia. Delivery of B2AR agonist to the VMH increased peak epinephrine responses by 37% ($P < 0.01$) and epinephrine levels during the entire 90-min period of hypoglycemia by 50% ($P < 0.01$) compared with the control group. In contrast, VMH delivery of the B2AR antagonist suppressed the peak by 53% ($P < 0.001$) and epinephrine levels during the entire 90-min period of hypoglycemia by 32% ($P < 0.05$) compared with the control group (Fig. 1B). Peak and overall glucagon response was also increased by activation of VMH B2AR by 53 and 63%, respectively ($P < 0.01$ for both vs. control) (Fig. 1C). However, administration of the B2AR antagonist had only a small inhibitory effect on the peak glucagon response, which failed to reach statistical significance ($P = 0.051$ vs. control at 30 min) (Fig. 1C). Norepinephrine levels were also slightly higher in the B2AR agonist group, but at 90 min only ($P < 0.05$ vs. control) (Fig. 1D).

Targeted blockade of VMH B1AR or B3AR failed to suppress counterregulatory hormone responses to hypoglycemia or increase the GIR needed to maintain hypoglycemia (Fig. 2). VMH B1AR blockade had no significant effect on GIR (Fig. 2A) but did produce a modest increase in the overall epinephrine response ($P < 0.05$ vs. control) (Fig. 2B). Neither glucagon (Fig. 2C) nor norepinephrine (Fig. 2D) responses were significantly affected by B1AR blockade. VMH B3AR blockade produced a small 21% decrease in the GIR required during hypoglycemia ($P < 0.05$ vs. control). However, B3AR blockade had no significant effect on the release of epinephrine, glucagon, and norepinephrine during hypoglycemia compared with controls (Fig. 2).

DISCUSSION

Previous studies have suggested a potential role for local VMH norepinephrine neurotransmission in modulating glucose counterregulation. This view is supported by data showing that 1) norepinephrine delivery into the VMH increases blood glucose and counterregulatory hormone levels (16,17); 2) glucopenia stimulates norepinephrine turnover in the mediobasal hypothalamus, including the

TABLE 1
Baseline metabolic status of animals in the morning before the study

Variable	Control ($n = 12$)	B2AR antagonist ICI-118,551 ($n = 12$)	B2AR agonist formoterol ($n = 10$)	B1AR antagonist CGP 20712 ($n = 7$)	B3AR antagonist SR59230A ($n = 6$)
Body weight (g)	320 ± 7	316 ± 7	315 ± 6	291 ± 3.1	289 ± 9
Plasma glucose (mmol/L)	6.4 ± 0.2	6.3 ± 0.1	6.5 ± 0.2	6.3 ± 0.2	6.1 ± 0.2
Insulin (μU/mL)	7.6 ± 1.8	8.2 ± 1.3	7.9 ± 1.3	10.1 ± 0.7	12.4 ± 3.5
Glucagon (ng/L)	46 ± 3	44 ± 3	50 ± 5	58 ± 6	58 ± 5
Epinephrine (pg/mL)	115 ± 40	129 ± 42	64 ± 25	94 ± 41	146 ± 33
Norepinephrine (pg/mL)	207 ± 34	174 ± 26	166 ± 33	233 ± 63	234 ± 54

Data are presented as mean ± SEM.

TABLE 2
Plasma glucose and insulin concentrations during the final 60 min of the hyperinsulinemic-hypoglycemic clamp study for rats in each study group

Variable	Control ($n = 12$)	B2AR antagonist ICI-118,551 ($n = 12$)	B2AR agonist formoterol ($n = 10$)	B1AR antagonist CGP 20712 ($n = 7$)	B3AR antagonist SR59230A ($n = 6$)
Plasma glucose (mmol/L)	3.0 ± 0.05	3.0 ± 0.03	2.8 ± 0.03	2.9 ± 0.07	3.0 ± 0.06
Insulin (μU/mL)	$1,235 \pm 112$	$1,250 \pm 164$	$1,302 \pm 156$	$1,229 \pm 162$	$1,292 \pm 160$

Data are presented as mean $\pm$ SEM.

VMH (18,19); and 3) levels of norepinephrine increase in VMH interstitial fluid during hypoglycemia (12,13). The current study was undertaken to assess whether norepinephrine acts to promote glucose counterregulation via specific VMH BARs. The data demonstrate that local VMH delivery of a specific B2AR agonist increases both epinephrine and glucagon responses to acute hypoglycemia, whereas delivery of a B2AR antagonist suppresses epinephrine release and tends to reduce the initial glucagon response. In contrast, blockade of VMH B1AR or B3AR

failed to have a significant inhibitory effect on counterregulatory responses. It should be noted that for these studies we used similar concentrations of BAR agonists and antagonists (1 μmol/L) as were used in previous in vivo (12,20) and in vitro (11) studies examining the specific receptors mediating the effects of norepinephrine on VMH neurons. Although these concentrations exceed the nanomolar norepinephrine concentrations present in the VMH interstitial fluid, if one takes into account the dilution of the agent in the VMH and in vivo clearance from the tissue

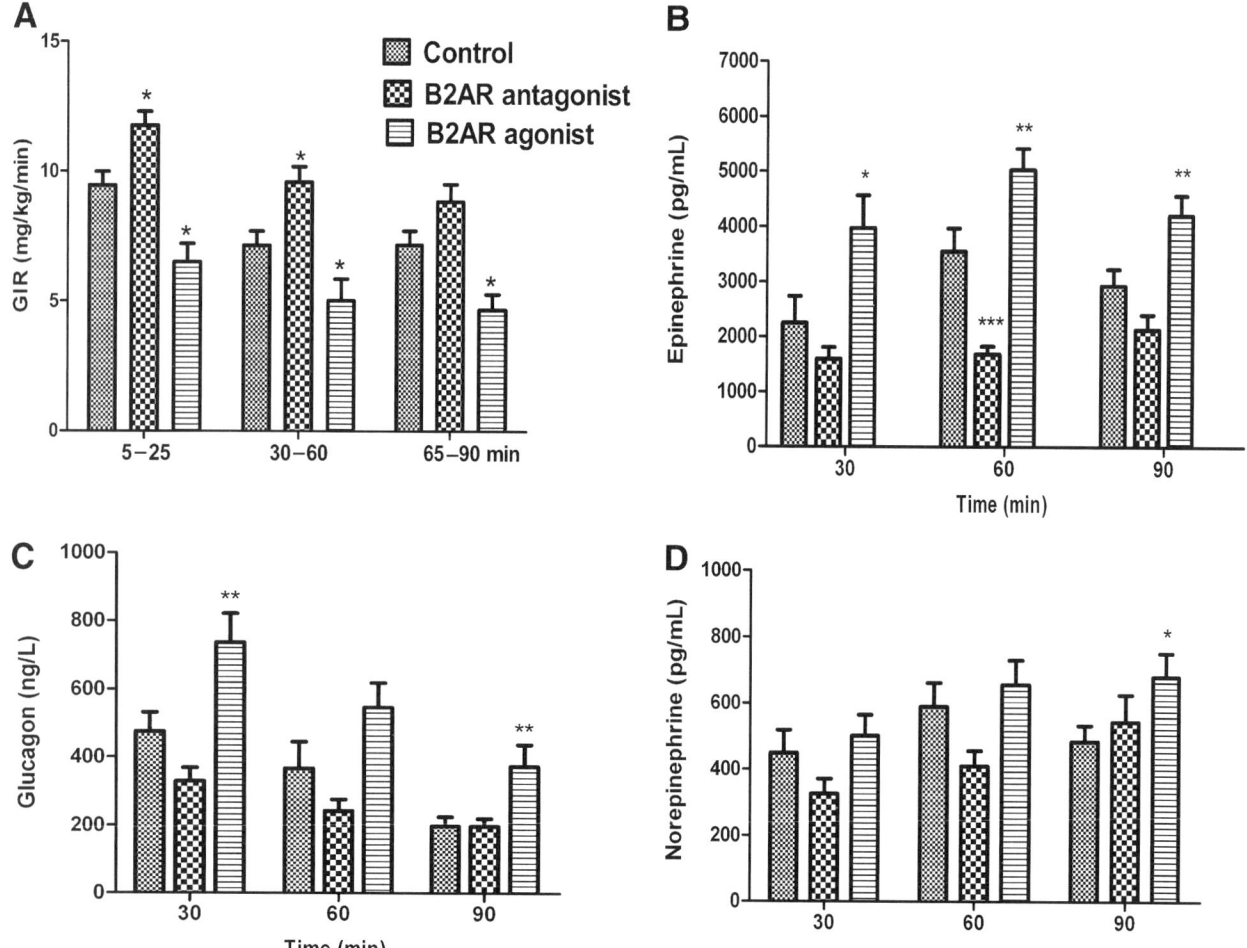

FIG. 1. B2AR modulation in the VMH and its effect on GIR and counterregulatory hormones during the hypoglycemic clamp study. GIR (*A*) and hormonal responses for plasma epinephrine (*B*), glucagon (*C*), and norepinephrine (*D*) for rats receiving microinjection of the artificial extracellular fluid vehicle (control; *n* = 12), the B2AR antagonist ICI-118,551 (*n* = 12), or the B2AR agonist formoterol (*n* = 10) during the hyperinsulinemic-hypoglycemic glucose clamp. Results are presented as mean ± SEM. Post hoc linear contrasts to localized effects; *P < 0.05, **P < 0.01, and ***P < 0.001 vs. controls.

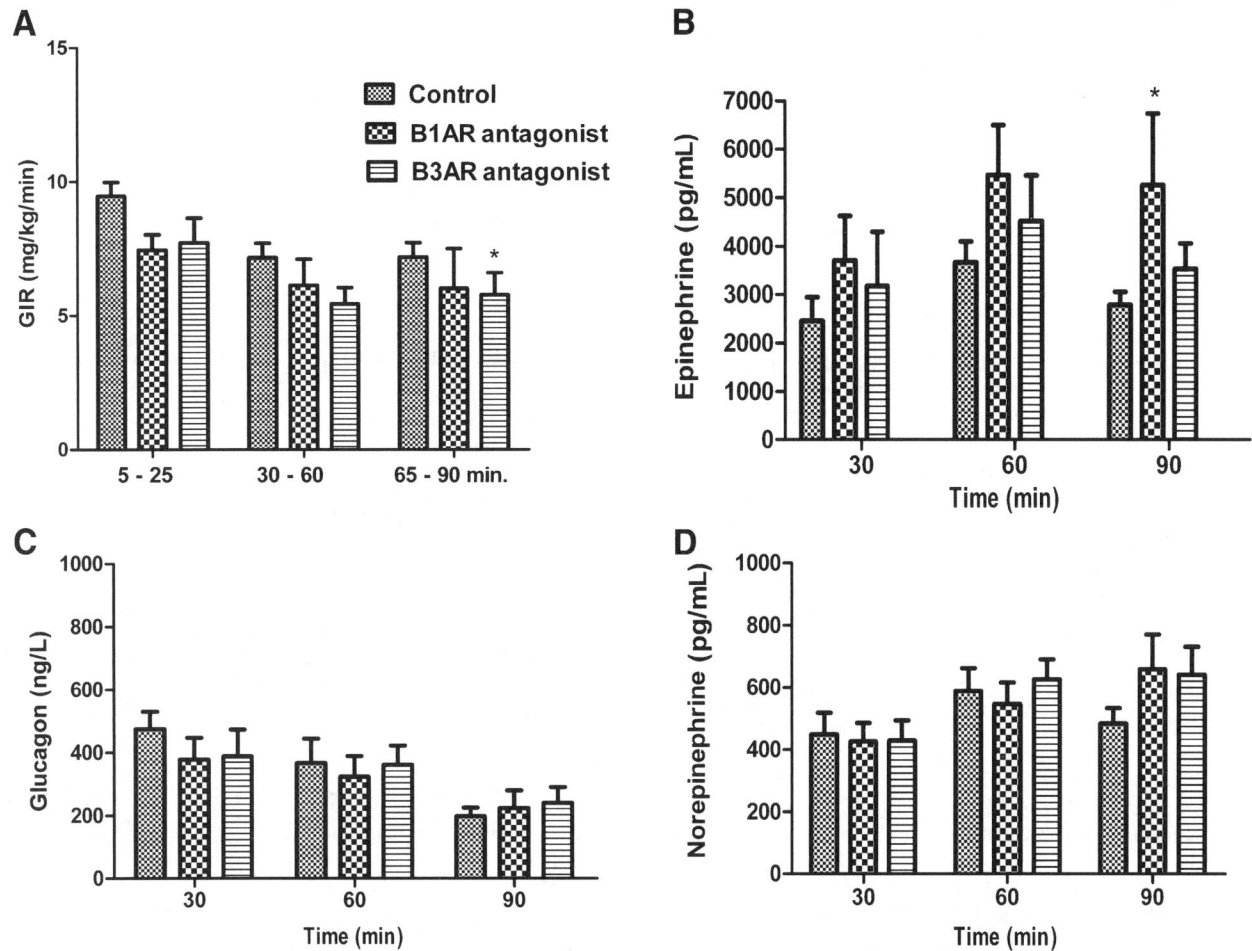

FIG. 2. Effect of VMH B1AR or B3AR blockade on GIR and counterregulatory hormones during the hypoglycemic clamp study. GIR (*A*) as well as epinephrine (*B*), glucagon (*C*), and norepinephrine (*D*) responses for rats receiving microinjection of the artificial extracellular fluid vehicle (control; *n* = 12), the B1AR antagonist CGP 20712 (*n* = 7), and the B3AR antagonist SR59230A (*n* = 6) during the hyperinsulinemic-hypoglycemic glucose clamp. Results are presented as mean ± SEM. Post hoc linear contrasts to localized effects; *$P < 0.05$ vs. controls.

during the study, the active local dose level in the VMH was considerably lower. Nevertheless, it seems unlikely that the changes we observed represent off-target effects. We have observed that if the dose of B2AR antagonist is diminished 10-fold, there is a similar degree of suppression of epinephrine responses to hypoglycemia and that if much higher doses of the compound are given, the effect on epinephrine release is less pronounced (B.S., unpublished data). Taken together, our data suggest that norepinephrine release into the VMH during hypoglycemia acts to promote glucose recovery, at least in part via stimulation of B2AR. These findings are consistent with previous studies showing that norepinephrine activates isolated glutamatergic neurons derived from the rat VMH via B2AR (11).

It is noteworthy that earlier studies suggested that norepinephrine's central actions to regulate peripheral glucose levels were mediated via α_2-receptors. Smythe et al. (18,19,21) reported that yohimbine, an α_2-receptor antagonist, markedly inhibited stress induced hyperglycemia as well as the hyperglycemic effects of 2-deoxyglucose administration. Moreover, Beverly et al. (20) reported that during hypoglycemia the norepinephrine rise within the VMH followed a bimodal pattern. The initial peaks disappeared when yohimbine was locally delivered, whereas

the second rise was suppressed in the presence of timolol, a nonselective BAR antagonist. Neither of these studies, however, examined the effect of hypothalamic adrenergic receptor modulation specifically on the responses of counterregulatory hormones to hypoglycemia. It is noteworthy in this regard that previous studies suggest that the activation of an appropriate counterregulatory response to hypoglycemia is associated with inhibition of GABA tone (9) and activation of glutamate neurons within the VMH (10). It is intriguing to speculate that norepinephrine might act via different adrenergic receptors to exert complementary effects on VMH glutamate and GABA neurotransmission to promote counterregulatory responses to hypoglycemia.

It is now recognized that hypoglycemia is detected by specialized glucose-sensing neurons located within a variety of brain regions (6,7) as well as periphery (5). Watts and Donovan, in a recent review (14), proposed that brainstem catecholaminergic neurons receive neural input from peripheral glucose sensors and then transmit this information to hypothalamic glucose-sensing neurons, including those in the VMH. Thus, these catecholaminergic projections might serve to integrate the VMH into a wide network glucose-sensing neurons.

We conclude that synaptic release of catecholamines acting via B2AR within the VMH plays an important role in modulating the magnitude of the epinephrine responses and, to lesser extent, glucagon responses to insulin-induced hypoglycemia. These observations are consistent with previous studies suggesting that administration of the B2AR agonist terbutaline may restore hypoglycemia awareness and reduce nocturnal hypoglycemia (22,23). This effect may be particularly useful in humans with homozygosity for glycine at codon 16 (GlyGly) of the B2AR who appear to show reduced B2AR sensitivity to antecedent hypoglycemia (24). Moreover, the current data are consistent with recent data indicating that repeated adrenergic receptor activation might also be involved in the generation of hypoglycemia-associated autonomic failure (25) and raise the possibility that B2AR receptor downregulation might play a role in this phenomenon. In our study we used a long-lasting, specific, commercially available β-adrenergic agonist. Given that hypoglycemia remains the major limiting factor in the use of intensified insulin therapy in the management of diabetes, our study may have potential therapeutic implications for strategies aimed at reducing the risk of severe hypoglycemia in diabetes.

ACKNOWLEDGMENTS

This work was supported by research grants from the National Institute of Diabetes and Digestive and Kidney Diseases (NIDDK; 20495), the Juvenile Diabetes Research Foundation (JDRF), and the NIDDK-supported Diabetes Endocrinology Research Center. B.S. is the recipient of a postdoctoral fellowship from the JDRF.

No potential conflicts of interest relevant to this article were reported.

B.S. researched data and wrote the manuscript. W.Z. researched data. O.C. contributed to discussion. A.H. researched data. J.D. performed statistical analysis of data. R.S.S. designed the study and reviewed and edited the manuscript.

Parts of this study were presented in abstract form at the 69th Scientific Sessions of the American Diabetes Association, New Orleans, Louisiana, 5–9 June 2009.

The authors are grateful to Aida Groszman, Maria Batsu, Codruta Todeasa, and Ralph J. Jacob, Yale Center for Clinical Investigation Core Laboratory of the Yale Medical School, for excellent technical support and assistance.

REFERENCES

1. The effect of intensive treatment of diabetes on the development and progression of long-term complications in insulin-dependent diabetes mellitus. The Diabetes Control and Complications Trial Research Group. N Engl J Med 1993;329:977–986
2. Hypoglycemia in the Diabetes Control and Complications Trial. The Diabetes Control and Complications Trial Research Group. Diabetes 1997;46: 271–286
3. Amiel SA, Tamborlane WV, Simonson DC, Sherwin RS. Defective glucose counterregulation after strict glycemic control of insulin-dependent diabetes mellitus. N Engl J Med 1987;316:1376–1383
4. Gerich JE, Langlois M, Noacco C, Karam JH, Forsham PH. Lack of glucagon response to hypoglycemia in diabetes: evidence for an intrinsic pancreatic alpha cell defect. Science 1973;182:171–173
5. Hevener AL, Bergman RN, Donovan CM. Novel glucosensor for hypoglycemic detection localized to the portal vein. Diabetes 1997;46:1521–1525
6. Frizzell RT, Jones EM, Davis SN, et al. Counterregulation during hypoglycemia is directed by widespread brain regions. Diabetes 1993;42: 1253–1261
7. Borg WP, During MJ, Sherwin RS, Borg MA, Brines ML, Shulman GI. Ventromedial hypothalamic lesions in rats suppress counterregulatory responses to hypoglycemia. J Clin Invest 1994;93:1677–1682
8. Levin BE, Dunn-Meynell AA, Routh VH. CNS sensing and regulation of peripheral glucose levels. Int Rev Neurobiol 2002;51:219–258
9. Chan O, Zhu W, Ding Y, McCrimmon RJ, Sherwin RS. Blockade of GABA(A) receptors in the ventromedial hypothalamus further stimulates glucagon and sympathoadrenal but not the hypothalamo-pituitary-adrenal response to hypoglycemia. Diabetes 2006;55:1080–1087
10. Tong Q, Ye C, McCrimmon RJ, et al. Synaptic glutamate release by ventromedial hypothalamic neurons is part of the neurocircuitry that prevents hypoglycemia. Cell Metab 2007;5:383–393
11. Lee JG, Choi IS, Park EJ, et al. beta(2)-Adrenoceptor-mediated facilitation of glutamatergic transmission in rat ventromedial hypothalamic neurons. Neuroscience 2007;144:1255–1265
12. Beverly JL, De Vries MG, Bouman SD, Arseneau LM. Noradrenergic and GABAergic systems in the medial hypothalamus are activated during hypoglycemia. Am J Physiol Regul Integr Comp Physiol 2001;280:R563– R569
13. de Vries MG, Lawson MA, Beverly JL. Hypoglycemia-induced noradrenergic activation in the VMH is a result of decreased ambient glucose. Am J Physiol Regul Integr Comp Physiol 2005;289:R977–R981
14. Watts AG, Donovan CM. Sweet talk in the brain: glucosensing, neural networks, and hypoglycemic counterregulation. Front Neuroendocrinol 2010;31:32–43
15. Marty N, Dallaporta M, Thorens B. Brain glucose sensing, counterregulation, and energy homeostasis. Physiology (Bethesda) 2007;22: 241–251
16. Chafetz MD, Parko K, Diaz S, Leibowitz SF. Relationships between medial hypothalamic alpha 2-receptor binding, norepinephrine, and circulating glucose. Brain Res 1986;384:404–408
17. Steffens AB, Scheurink AJ, Luiten PG, Bohus B. Hypothalamic food intake regulating areas are involved in the homeostasis of blood glucose and plasma FFA levels. Physiol Behav 1988;44:581–589
18. Smythe GA, Edwards SR. Suppression of central noradrenergic neuronal activity inhibits hyperglycemia. Am J Physiol 1992;263:E823–E827
19. Smythe GA, Grunstein HS, Bradshaw JE, Nicholson MV, Compton PJ. Relationships between brain noradrenergic activity and blood glucose. Nature 1984;308:65–67
20. Beverly JL, de Vries MG, Beverly MF, Arseneau LM. Norepinephrine mediates glucoprivic-induced increase in GABA in the ventromedial hypothalamus of rats. Am J Physiol Regul Integr Comp Physiol 2000;279: R990–R996
21. Smythe GA, Edwards SR. A role for central postsynaptic alpha 2-adrenoceptors in glucoregulation. Brain Res 1991;562:225–229
22. Raju B, Arbelaez AM, Breckenridge SM, Cryer PE. Nocturnal hypoglycemia in type 1 diabetes: an assessment of preventive bedtime treatments. J Clin Endocrinol Metab 2006;91:2087–2092
23. Fritsche A, Tschritter O, Häring H, Gerich J, Stumvoll M. The role of beta-adrenergic sensitivity in the pathogenesis of hypoglycaemia unawareness. Diabetes Nutr Metab 2002;15:357–361; discussion 361–362
24. Schouwenberg BJ, Smits P, Tack CJ, de Galan BE. The effect of antecedent hypoglycaemia on β2-adrenergic sensitivity in healthy participants with the Arg16Gly polymorphism of the β2-adrenergic receptor. Diabetologia 2011;54:1212–1218
25. Ramanathan R, Cryer PE. Adrenergic mediation of hypoglycemia-associated autonomic failure. Diabetes 2011;60:602–606

Brain Activation During Working Memory Is Altered in Patients With Type 1 Diabetes During Hypoglycemia

Nicolas R. Bolo,[1,2,3] Gail Musen,[3,4] Alan M. Jacobson,[3,4,5] Katie Weinger,[3,4] Richard L. McCartney,[4] Veronica Flores,[4] Perry F. Renshaw,[1,3,6] and Donald C. Simonson[7,8]

OBJECTIVE—To investigate the effects of acute hypoglycemia on working memory and brain function in patients with type 1 diabetes.

RESEARCH DESIGN AND METHODS—Using blood oxygen level–dependent (BOLD) functional magnetic resonance imaging during euglycemic (5.0 mmol/L) and hypoglycemic (2.8 mmol/L) hyperinsulinemic clamps, we compared brain activation response to a working-memory task (WMT) in type 1 diabetic subjects ($n = 16$) with that in age-matched nondiabetic control subjects ($n = 16$). Behavioral performance was assessed by percent correct responses.

RESULTS—During euglycemia, the WMT activated the bilateral frontal and parietal cortices, insula, thalamus, and cerebellum in both groups. During hypoglycemia, activation decreased in both groups but remained 80% larger in type 1 diabetic versus control subjects ($P < 0.05$). In type 1 diabetic subjects, higher HbA_{1c} was associated with lower activation in the right parahippocampal gyrus and amygdala ($R^2 = 0.45$, $P < 0.002$). Deactivation of the default-mode network (DMN) also was seen in both groups during euglycemia. However, during hypoglycemia, type 1 diabetic patients deactivated the DMN 70% less than control subjects ($P < 0.05$). Behavioral performance did not differ between glycemic conditions or groups.

CONCLUSIONS—BOLD activation was increased and deactivation was decreased in type 1 diabetic versus control subjects during hypoglycemia. This higher level of brain activation required by type 1 diabetic subjects to attain the same level of cognitive performance as control subjects suggests reduced cerebral efficiency in type 1 diabetes. *Diabetes* **60:3256–3264, 2011**

A cute episodes of hypoglycemia are a rate-limiting adverse effect in the treatment of type 1 diabetes. When severe, they can lead to seizures and coma (1). Even mild to moderate hypoglycemia is known to impair cognitive functions, such as working memory (2,3). Working memory is used to actively maintain and manipulate information over a brief period of time and to allocate attentional resources among competing subtasks (4,5). Traditionally, working-memory performance

is thought to depend primarily on a network of brain regions, including portions of the frontal and parietal lobes, thalamus, precuneus, cerebellum, and insula (6,7).

Using blood oxygen level–dependent (BOLD) functional magnetic resonance imaging (fMRI), we evaluated how diabetes impacts these neural processes under euglycemic and hypoglycemic conditions when subjects were presented with a working-memory task (WMT). Diabetes is known to negatively affect working memory (8). This task evaluates functional effects that might reflect changes in brain structure and/or presage decreases in cognitive performance. A better understanding of the brain's metabolic and physiological mechanisms underlying the cognitive functions implicated in working memory could lead to improved treatment strategies to help maintain cortical function in patients with diabetes during hypoglycemia (9).

BOLD fMRI is a well-established method for examining regional brain activation in response to physiological, pharmacological, sensory, or cognitive tasks (10). Studies that have examined brain activation in response to sensory stimulation or cognitive challenges using BOLD fMRI during hypoglycemic conditions in nondiabetic subjects (11–13) have shown that hypoglycemia reduces regional brain BOLD activation. This reduction in BOLD response during hypoglycemia has been attributed to low glucose levels causing decreases in neuronal activity, glucose oxidative metabolism, cerebral blood flow, neurovascular coupling, and/or neuronal recruitment (12).

Whether cognitive function in patients with type 1 diabetes is affected by hypoglycemia in the same manner as in nondiabetic individuals remains unclear because few studies using functional neural imaging have directly compared diabetic and nondiabetic subjects during the performance of cognitive tasks (14,15). If brain glucose transport or metabolism are altered in type 1 diabetes, as has been suggested in recent studies by our group (16) and others (17), then one would expect that the BOLD activation response during hypoglycemia may differ between diabetic patients compared with nondiabetic control subjects. On the basis of these findings, we hypothesized that *1*) patients with type 1 diabetes would have greater BOLD activation during the performance of a WMT during hypoglycemia when compared with nondiabetic control subjects, *2*) cognitive performance would deteriorate during hypoglycemia in both groups, and *3*) among type 1 diabetic patients, better glycemic control (lower HbA_{1c}) would correlate with BOLD activation responses to the WMT during hypoglycemia. We also conducted exploratory analyses to examine deactivation patterns in the default-mode network (DMN), the regions of the brain that are more active during rest (18), because of other research by our group examining the effects of diabetes on deactivation patterns during cognitive tasks and previous research suggesting that DMN function may

From the [1]Brain Imaging Center, McLean Hospital, Belmont, Massachusetts; the [2]Department of Psychiatry, Beth Israel Deaconess Medical Center, Boston, Massachusetts; the [3]Department of Psychiatry, Harvard Medical School, Boston, Massachusetts; the [4]Research Division, Joslin Diabetes Center, Boston, Massachusetts; the [5]Research Institute, Winthrop-University Hospital, Mineola, New York; the [6]Department of Psychiatry, University of Utah, Salt Lake City, Utah; the [7]Division of Endocrinology, Diabetes, and Hypertension, Brigham and Women's Hospital, Boston, Massachusetts; and the [8]Department of Medicine, Harvard Medical School, Boston, Massachusetts.
Corresponding author: Nicolas R. Bolo, nbolo@bidmc.harvard.edu.
Received 14 April 2011 and accepted 25 August 2011.
DOI: 10.2337/db11-0506

be altered in diseases that affect cognition, such as Alzheimer's disease (19).

RESEARCH DESIGN AND METHODS

The study sample consisted of 16 patients with type 1 diabetes and 16 healthy control subjects from an ongoing study of brain function during hypoglycemia in type 1 diabetes. Data from five type 1 diabetic and five control subjects were included in a previous publication (20). Demographic and clinical characteristics of the subjects are presented in Table 1. The patients' number of self-reported hypoglycemic episodes (plasma glucose <3.9 mmol/L with concomitant symptoms) in the month preceding the initial visit averaged eight episodes (range 2–28). Patients with autonomic neuropathy (assessed by standard criteria) (21), painful peripheral neuropathy, urinary albumin levels >300 mg/day, or proliferative retinopathy by review of medical records, physical exam, or self-report were excluded from the study. Other exclusion criteria were a history of psychosis or schizophrenia; cocaine, heroin, or alcohol dependence; and any contraindications to MRI, such as metallic implants, pregnancy, or claustrophobia.

Following approval from the institutional review boards of both the Joslin Diabetes Center (where patients were recruited) and the McLean Hospital (where the MRI was performed), patients provided the following information during screening: self-report of their lifetime experience of severe hypoglycemic events leading to unconsciousness (22); psychiatric history; handedness; medical history; and current medications.

Of 18 control participants who were eligible for the study, 2 were excluded from analysis because of excessive head motion during the fMRI by applying exclusion criteria of translations in excess of 3 mm in x, y, or z directions or rotations in excess of 3° around the x, y, or z axes. No diabetic subjects were excluded for head motion.

Experimental protocol. The experimental protocol is described elsewhere (20) and briefly reviewed below. On the day before the study, patients with type 1 diabetes had a continuous glucose monitor (CGM System Gold; Medtronic, Northridge, CA) inserted. If the continuous glucose monitor showed glucose <3.3 mmol/L, the study was postponed to a later date. The experiment used the insulin clamp technique with four successive time periods corresponding to different plasma glucose levels: baseline (30 min); euglycemic clamp (40 min, target glucose 5.0 mmol/L); declining glycemia (40 min, plasma glucose reduced from 5.0 to 2.8 mmol/L); and hypoglycemic clamp (30 min, target glucose 2.8 mmol/L). Anatomical MRI was performed during baseline, and fMRI was performed during the euglycemic and hypoglycemic periods while the WMT was administered (Fig. 1).

Insulin clamp technique. An intravenous catheter was inserted into an antecubital vein for the administration of insulin and glucose, and a second catheter was inserted into a distal forearm or hand vein for the withdrawal of blood samples. A heated gel pack was used to warm the hand to arterialize the venous blood. After the baseline period, regular human insulin was infused at 12

TABLE 1
Demographic and clinical characteristics of study subjects

	Type 1 diabetic subjects	Control subjects
n	16	16
Age (years)	33.8 ± 9.9 (19–50)	31.3 ± 10.0 (19–50)
Sex (men/women)	8/8	13/3
Diabetes duration (years)	16.7 ± 4.9 (7.9–26.7)	—
BMI (kg/m^2)	24.8 ± 2.9 (20.5–30.7)	25.1 ± 3.1 (20.2–31.1)
HbA$_{1c}$ (%)	7.4 ± 1.1 (5.7–9.7)	5.2 ± 0.3 (4.4–5.5)
Fasting plasma glucose (mmol/L)	6.0 ± 1.4 (4.1–8.7)	5.0 ± 0.3 (4.4–5.6)
Education (years)	16.3 ± 1.9 (13–20)	16.8 ± 2.7 (12–21)

Data are means ± SD (range).

pmol/kg per min for 110 min. The plasma glucose levels were maintained at the desired level by infusion of 20% dextrose using a negative-feedback algorithm, as previously described (23–25). After the euglycemic clamp period (40 min), the glucose infusion rate was reduced to allow the plasma glucose level to decline by 2.2 mmol/L (from 5.0 to 2.8 mmol/L) over the next 40 min, followed by the 30-min hypoglycemic clamp period. During the entire clamp protocol, glucose levels were measured every 5 min, and counterregulatory hormones (epinephrine, cortisol, growth hormone, and glucagon) were measured every 10 min. At the end of the protocol, the insulin infusion was discontinued, the glucose infusion was increased to restore euglycemia, and the subjects were given a meal and discharged.

Hormone and substrate assays. Plasma glucose was measured using the glucose oxidase method. Serum insulin and growth hormone and plasma epinephrine were measured by enzyme-linked immunosorbent assay. Plasma glucagon and cortisol were measured by radioimmunoassay.

WMT. The task stimuli were administered using Presentation software (Neurobehavioral Systems, Albany, CA). The images were projected on a backlit screen that was visualized from within the magnet bore by a mirror mounted on the head coil. Response times and errors were collected using a magnetic resonance–compatible hand-held four-button fiberoptic response pad (FORP; Current Designs, Philadelphia, PA) connected to the PC by an optical cable interface. The stimulus presentation was synchronized with the fMRI acquisition sequence at the beginning of each trial by the interface that responded to scanner-generated trigger signals. The WMT was administered 15–20 min after the beginning of the euglycemic period and again at 15–20 min after the

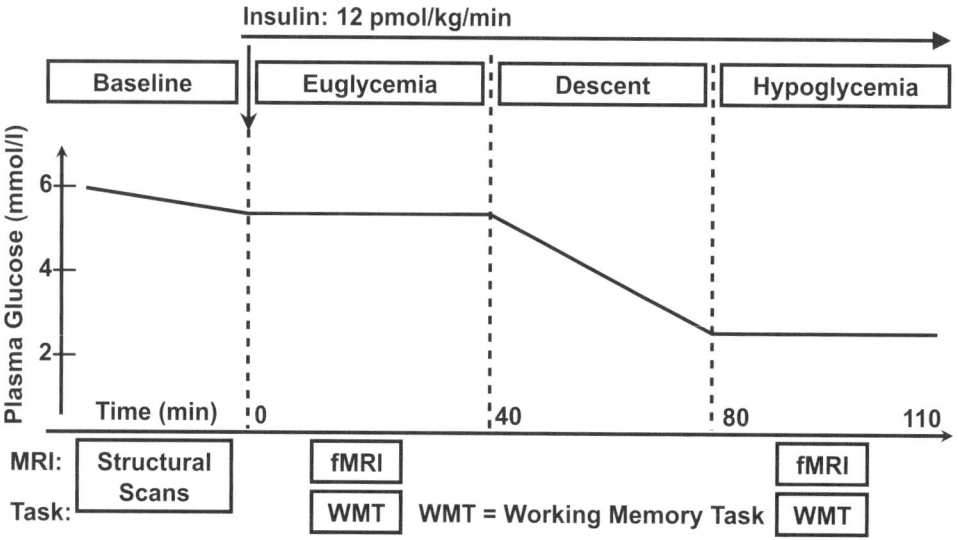

FIG. 1. Study protocol. Time line of structural and functional scans, WMTs, and periods of euglycemia (nominal 5.0 mmol/L), glucose descent, and hypoglycemia (nominal 2.8 mmol/L).

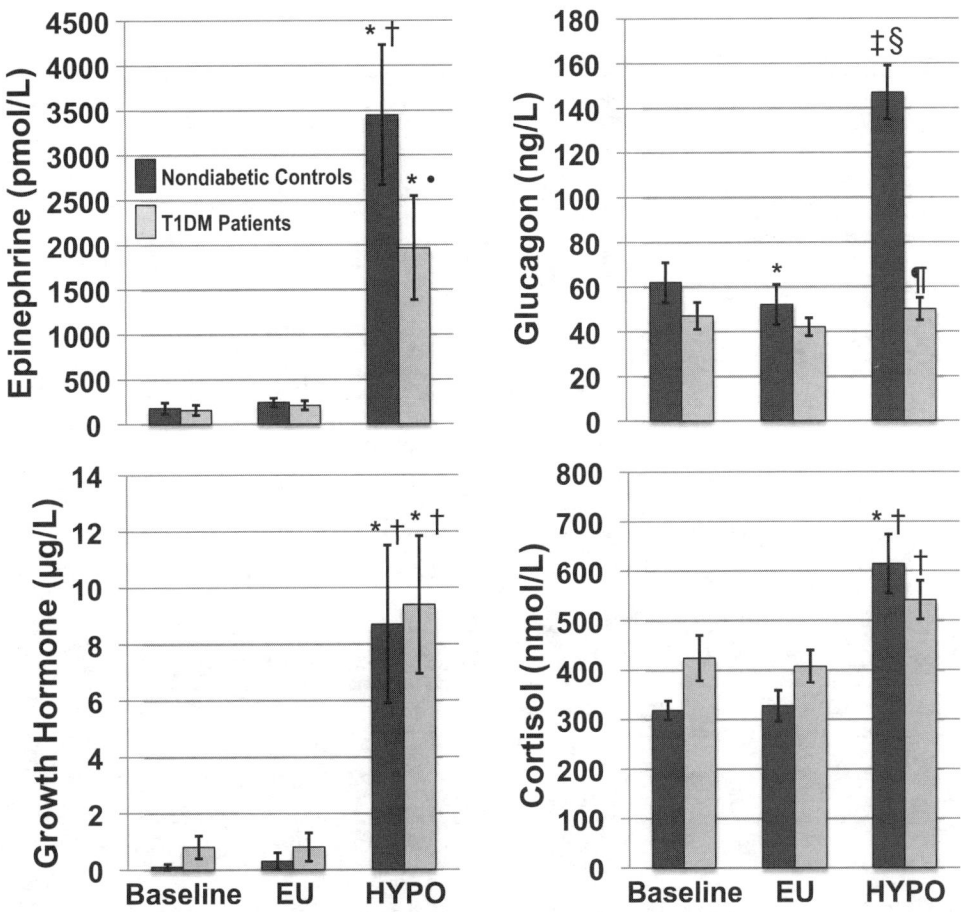

FIG. 2. Plasma levels of counterregulatory hormones (error bars ± SE) during the baseline and euglycemic periods and at the end of the hypo-glycemic period in control subjects and patients with type 1 diabetes (T1DM). EU, euglycemia; HYPO, hypoglycemia. P values for statistically significant comparisons: *$P < 0.05$ vs. baseline; †$P < 0.05$ vs. euglycemia; ‡$P < 0.01$ vs. baseline; §$P < 0.01$ vs. euglycemia; •$P < 0.05$ vs. control subjects; ¶$P < 0.001$ vs. control subjects.

beginning of the hypoglycemic period (Fig. 1). Subjects performed practice tests before the study to achieve familiarity with the test procedure, and we used randomly assigned counterbalanced forms of the test during euglycemia and hypoglycemia to minimize learning.

During the WMT, adapted from Rypma et al. (26), participants viewed a string of six digits for 1,200 ms followed by a 2,000-ms unfilled retention interval (blank screen). Then, one digit was displayed on the computer monitor for 1,500 ms, and the subject had 1,300 ms to decide whether the digit was a member of the previously seen string. Using the same timing parameters, a matched control task was used in which subjects viewed six percent symbols (%) on the screen, followed by the unfilled retention interval, followed by a right- or a left-pointing arrow. The participants were asked to press the re-sponse key corresponding to the direction of the arrow. In the rest task, par-ticipants fixated on a plus (+) sign for 30 s. Each of these three tasks (WMT, matched control, and rest) was presented four times in a block design for a total of 6 min of testing. There were 5 memory-scanning trials per block for a total of 20 memory-scanning trials.

MRI acquisition methods. All magnetic resonance images were acquired with a 3.0 Tesla Siemens Trio scanner (Siemens, Erlangen, Germany), using a cir-cularly polarized birdcage radiofrequency head coil tuned to the proton fre-quency. Global field uniformity was adjusted at the beginning of each scanning session using Siemens' automated shimming routines. A three-dimensional, T1-weighted anatomical image was acquired using a magnetization-prepared, rapid-acquisition gradient echo sequence (TR/TE = 2,100/2.74 ms; spatial reso-lution = $1 \times 1 \times 1.3$ mm^3; matrix size = $256 \times 256 \times 128$) and used for functional image registration. BOLD fMRI images covering the whole brain were acquired in the axial plane using an echo planar imaging (EPI) sequence (TR/TE = 3,000/30 ms; 26 slices acquired in interleaved scanning order; slice thickness = 5 mm; field of view = 200×200 mm^2; matrix size = 64×64), with an in-plane resolution of 3.125×3.125 mm^2. One multislice EPI volume covering the whole brain was acquired every 3 s for a total of 120 volumes for the 6-min fMRI run.

Image processing. Image processing and analyses were performed using the FSL software package (Analysis Group, FMRIB, Oxford, U.K.) running on a Mac-Pro Quad-Core Intel-Xeon computer (Apple, Cupertino, CA). All brain images were registered to the standard MNI-152 brain (Montreal Neurologic Institute) to allow multisubject analyses in standardized space and identification of all regions of interest. The first two EPI volumes of each functional run were discarded to allow for T1 equilibration. Prestatistical processing of EPI time series consisted of motion correction, slice scan-time correction, nonbrain removal, spatial smoothing with a 6-mm full-width at half-maximum three-dimensional Gaussian filter, linear trend removal, and a temporal high-pass filter with a cutoff of 120 s. Functional data were overlaid on the MNI-152 brain.

Data analyses. Regional brain activations and deactivations in response to the WMT were examined by performing a first-level general linear model (GLM) multiple regression analysis for each subject and glycemic condition. Model predictors for BOLD signal time courses were the boxcar time courses for each task stimulus paradigm convolved with a γ function to account for hemodynamic response. Predictors for the temporal derivatives of the task paradigm were added to the design matrix to improve the fit to the data by allowing for potential misspecification of the hemodynamic delay (27). The model for the baseline rest condition predictor was a con-stant function.

To compare activation and deactivation patterns between groups and conditions, higher-level multisubject mixed-effects GLM analyses compared multiple regression correlation coefficients associated with each model predictor for each brain voxel for each subject under each condition. Activations were computed by contrasting the WMT task to its control task. Deactivations were computed by contrasting the WMT task to the rest period. These higher-level analyses were performed using FSL's local analysis of mixed effects stage 1. Resulting Z score (i.e., Gaussianized T/F) statistic images were thresholded using clusters determined by $Z > 2.3$ and a corrected cluster significance threshold of $P = 0.05$ (28). These statistical parametric maps yield the clusters of adjacent brain voxels of regional activation or deactivation from which we

CONTROLS

T1DM

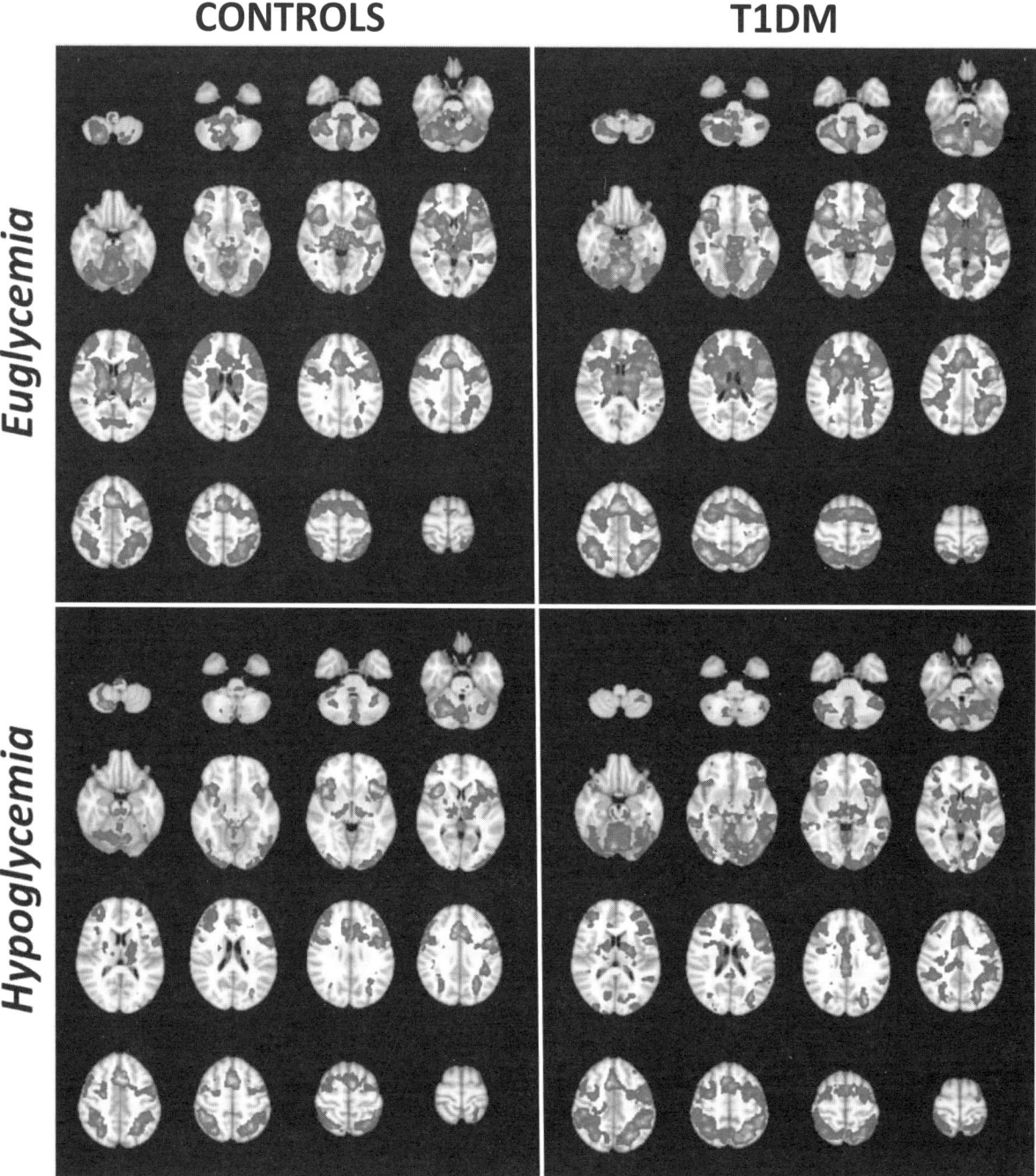

FIG. 3. BOLD activation during the WMT in control and type 1 diabetic (T1DM) subjects during euglycemia and hypoglycemia. Statistical parametric maps of regions of greatest activation during WMTs vs. control tasks for each subject group and glycemic condition. Functional activations (red-to-yellow color scale) are overlaid on the MNI-152 standard brain anatomy (gray scale). The threshold for activation was $P < 0.05$ after correction for multiple comparisons using the cluster-based threshold method (see RESEARCH DESIGN AND METHODS). During hypoglycemia, type 1 diabetic subjects exhibit greater activation than control subjects during the WMT. (A high-quality digital representation of this figure is available in the online issue.)

computed a single brain volume of activation or deactivation at the set statistical significance threshold ($P < 0.05$).

To investigate the variation of the regional percent BOLD signal change, we applied a region-of-interest (ROI) analysis in the superior parietal lobule (SPL) region, which had significant activation differences during hypoglycemia. To define the ROI, we created a binary mask of the SPL region provided by the probabilistic Harvard-Oxford Cortical Structural Atlas (29) thresholded at the 50% probability level. The ROI analysis was performed using FSL's FEATQUERY tool to extract the average time courses of parameter estimates of the percent BOLD signal change from all voxels contained in the SPL mask.

To investigate the association of WMT activation and deactivation to glycemic control in type 1 diabetes, we performed the mixed-effects GLM group analyses while including HbA$_{1c}$ values as a covariate in the design matrix. To compute the regional coefficients of correlation of activation to HbA$_{1c}$, the average percent BOLD activation values were extracted from the regions of significant correlation in type 1 diabetes during hypoglycemia using the FEATQUERY tool.

Standard statistical tests, including t tests for paired and unpaired data as appropriate, and ANOVA were used to compare glucose and counterregulatory hormone levels between diabetic and nondiabetic subjects during euglycemia and hypoglycemia. All data are presented as means ± SEM, unless

Euglycemia

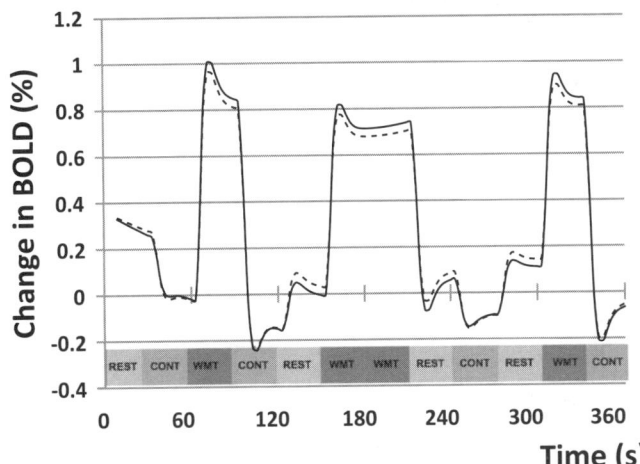

Hypoglycemia

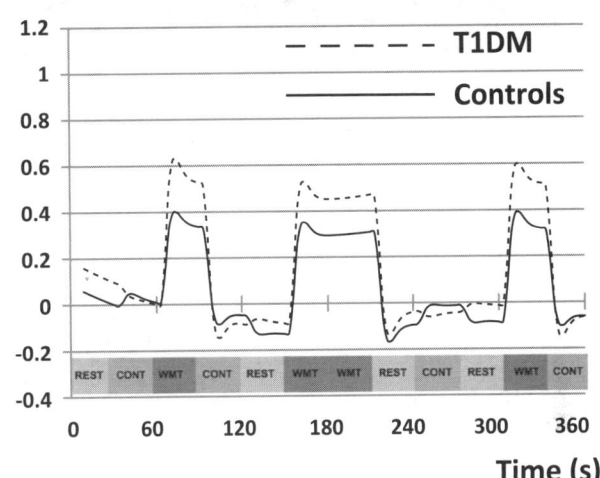

FIG. 4. Percent BOLD activation by ROI analysis during the WMT during euglycemia (*left*) and hypoglycemia (*right*). *Upper*: Location of the superior parietal lobule (SPL, association cortex including Brodmann areas 7 and 40) region used for ROI analysis is indicated at the intersection of the crosshairs on the activation maps for each subject group overlaid on the MNI-152 standard brain. *Lower*: Plots of the time courses of change in percent BOLD activation in the SPL ROI during the fMRI WMT. Percent change was measured relative to BOLD activation during the control task and averaged over all pixels in the ROI and all subjects within each subject group. The colored strip above the horizontal time axis shows the time sequence of task conditions. CONT, control task; REST, resting state task. (A high-quality digital representation of this figure is available in the online issue.)

otherwise specified, and statistical tests were conducted using a two-sided α level of 0.05.

RESULTS

Plasma glucose and counterregulatory hormones. Average plasma glucose levels during the euglycemic period for nondiabetic control and type 1 diabetic subjects were 5.0 ± 0.4 mmol/L and 5.0 ± 0.6 mmol/L, respectively. During the hypoglycemic period, average glucose levels for the two groups were 2.8 ± 0.2 mmol/L and 2.7 ± 0.1 mmol/L, respectively. There was no significant difference between groups and no significant interaction between the glycemic condition and group. Mean counterregulatory hormone levels during baseline and euglycemia and peak levels attained during hypoglycemia are shown in Fig. 2. Glucagon and epinephrine secretion were lower in the type 1 diabetic patients during hypoglycemia compared with control subjects.

Cognitive performance. Type 1 diabetic and control subjects did not differ in accuracy or reaction time during the WMT at either euglycemia or hypoglycemia. During euglycemia, control subjects achieved 85 ± 2% correct, with a reaction time of 1,133 ± 54 ms, whereas type 1 diabetic patients had 85 ± 4% correct, with a reaction time of 1,200 ± 57 ms. At hypoglycemia, control subjects had 84 ± 5% correct, with a reaction time of 1,122 ± 57 ms, whereas type 1 diabetic patients had 85 ± 4% correct, with

a reaction time of 1,204 ± 58 ms. There were no significant within-subject differences for either group when comparing the performance between glycemic conditions and no interaction between group and condition.

Functional imaging. Brain activations in response to the WMT for each subject group during each glycemic condition are shown in Fig. 3. The regions of greater BOLD activation for the WMT relative to the control task ($P < 0.05$, corrected for multiple comparisons using the cluster-based threshold method) (28) are indicated in a red-to-yellow color scale overlaid on the gray scale standard MNI-152 T1-weighted anatomical brain atlas. For both subject groups during both glycemic conditions, the WMT activated brain regions located in bilateral medial superior frontal gyrus, left precentral gyrus, bilateral SPL, bilateral middle frontal gyrus, bilateral anterior cingulate cortex, bilateral insula, left supramarginal gyrus, bilateral thalamus, bilateral inferior occipital cortex, and bilateral cerebellum.

During euglycemia, the overall extent of activation was similar in the diabetic patient and control groups, with activated brain volumes of 613 and 498 cm³, respectively. During hypoglycemia, the extent of regional BOLD activation decreased relative to euglycemia in both subject groups; however, it decreased less in patients with diabetes than in control subjects ($P < 0.05$). The regional patterns of activation also differed between groups. In type 1 diabetes, activation decreased mostly in the insula,

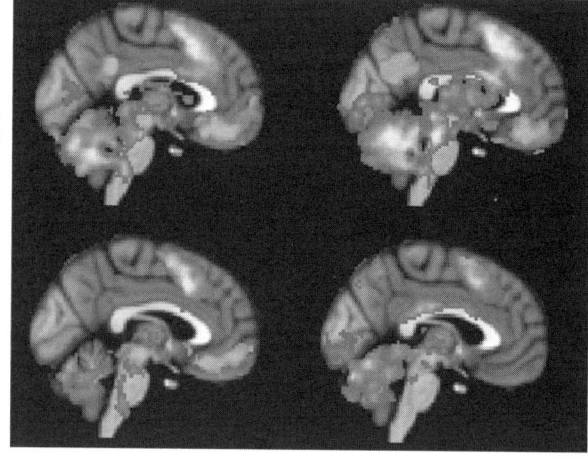

CONTROLS   T1DM

(left margin labels: Euglycemia, Hypoglycemia)

FIG. 5. BOLD activation and deactivation during the WMT in type 1 diabetic (T1DM) and control subjects during euglycemia and hypoglycemia. Statistical parametric maps of regions of greatest activation during WMTs vs. control tasks (functional activations in the red-to-yellow color scale) and regions of decreased activation during the WMTs vs. resting tasks (functional deactivations in the blue color scale) are overlaid on the MNI-152 standard brain anatomy (gray scale). The threshold for activations and deactivations was $P < 0.05$ after correction for multiple comparisons using the cluster-based threshold method (see RESEARCH DESIGN AND METHODS). During hypoglycemia, patients with type 1 diabetes exhibit less deactivation than control subjects. (A high-quality digital representation of this figure is available in the online issue.)

whereas for control subjects, activation decreased mostly in the cerebellum. Regions with higher activation in type 1 diabetes during hypoglycemia include the bilateral SPL, bilateral posterior supramarginal gyrus, bilateral anterior and posterior cingulate gyrus, left inferior frontal gyrus and posterior middle temporal gyrus, right hippocampus, and the cerebellum. Thus, during hypoglycemia, activation volumes were 80% larger in type 1 diabetic versus control subjects, with activation volumes of 431 and 239 cm³, respectively ($P < 0.05$). The extended activation volume in type 1 diabetic relative to control subjects during hypoglycemia was mainly a result of maintenance of a higher percent BOLD activation during the WMT, as illustrated in Fig. 4, which compares the time courses of the percent BOLD signal estimates averaged over the SPL region for each subject group under each glycemic condition.

Regional brain deactivations in response to the WMT for each subject group during each glycemic condition are shown in Fig. 5. Regions of lesser BOLD activation (or more deactivation) for WMT relative to the resting task ($P < 0.05$, corrected for multiple comparisons using the cluster-based threshold method) (28) are indicated in a dark blue–to–light blue color scale overlaid on the standard MNI-152 T1-weighted anatomical brain atlas in gray scale, along with activations in red to yellow. During euglycemia, WMT deactivated brain regions located in bilateral medial frontal cortex, posterior cingulate cortex, and superior lateral occipital cortex for both groups. The extent of deactivation was similar in the type 1 diabetic and control groups, with only a 10% difference between groups. Overall, deactivated brain volumes were 45 and 41 cm³, respectively. During hypoglycemia, the extent of regional BOLD deactivation decreased relative to euglycemia in both subject groups; however, it decreased more for patients with type 1 diabetes

($P < 0.05$) (i.e., they were unable to significantly deactivate these regions).

The regional patterns of decreased deactivation also differed between groups (Fig. 5). For patients with type 1 diabetes, deactivation decreased mostly in the medial frontal and posterior cingulate cortices, whereas for control subjects, deactivation decreased mostly in the posterior cingulate cortex. Control subjects also had small deactivation volumes in the cerebellum (right crus II) during hypoglycemia only. Thus, during hypoglycemia, the extent of deactivation was almost 70% smaller in type 1 diabetic relative to control subjects, with deactivation volumes of 5 cm³ located in the superior lateral occipital cortex for patients and 17 cm³ located mainly in the medial frontal and superior lateral occipital cortices for control subjects ($P < 0.05$).

Finally, we examined the relationship of HbA$_{1c}$ levels with activation patterns in type 1 diabetes by entering HbA$_{1c}$ as a covariate into the GLM. We found that lower HbA$_{1c}$ levels were associated with higher activation in the right parahippocampal gyrus and the amygdala (Fig. 6) during hypoglycemia. We also found that HbA$_{1c}$ levels were not associated with deactivation.

DISCUSSION

This study demonstrates that patients with type 1 diabetes show a different pattern of brain activation in response to a WMT than do nondiabetic control subjects during hypoglycemia. Specifically, we found that for patients with type 1 diabetes during hypoglycemia, WMT-related activation responses were increased in several cortical regions, including the parietal and frontal cortices, hippocampus, and cerebellum. Task-induced deactivations, typically observed in the DMN during cognitive effort, were significantly suppressed during hypoglycemia in bilateral medial-frontal and posterior cingulate cortices for type 1 diabetic patients compared with control subjects. Activation and deactivation patterns were similar across groups during euglycemia. Behavioral performance on the WMT was similar across groups and conditions. Finally, HbA$_{1c}$ was inversely correlated with WMT activation during hypoglycemia in the right parahippocampal gyrus and amygdala, two areas that have been reported to activate in memory-disordered populations as a form of compensatory recruitment (30–32).

The regional BOLD activations we observed in response to the WMT were compatible with those found in other fMRI studies of similar WMTs (5,26,33–35). Although the main regions that help govern working memory are the dorsolateral and medial prefrontal cortices and anterior cingulate cortex, other regions, such as the parietal lobe (36) and cerebellum (37), are known to play supplementary roles. These regions were activated more in type 1 diabetic patients than in control subjects during hypoglycemia, suggesting that supplementary brain regions may have been recruited to help preserve cognitive performance. The failure to suppress activation in the DMN also is consistent with an interpretation that type 1 diabetic patients need to recruit more brain resources for cognitive preservation (11). Similar patterns of increased activation and decreased deactivation have been observed with mild cognitive impairment (30) and in older individuals at risk for Alzheimer's disease (38), suggesting, in these cases, a compensatory response to accumulating pathology.

Cognitive performance was not altered by hypoglycemia in either subject group. Although some studies have shown similar results for less challenging WMTs (39), others have

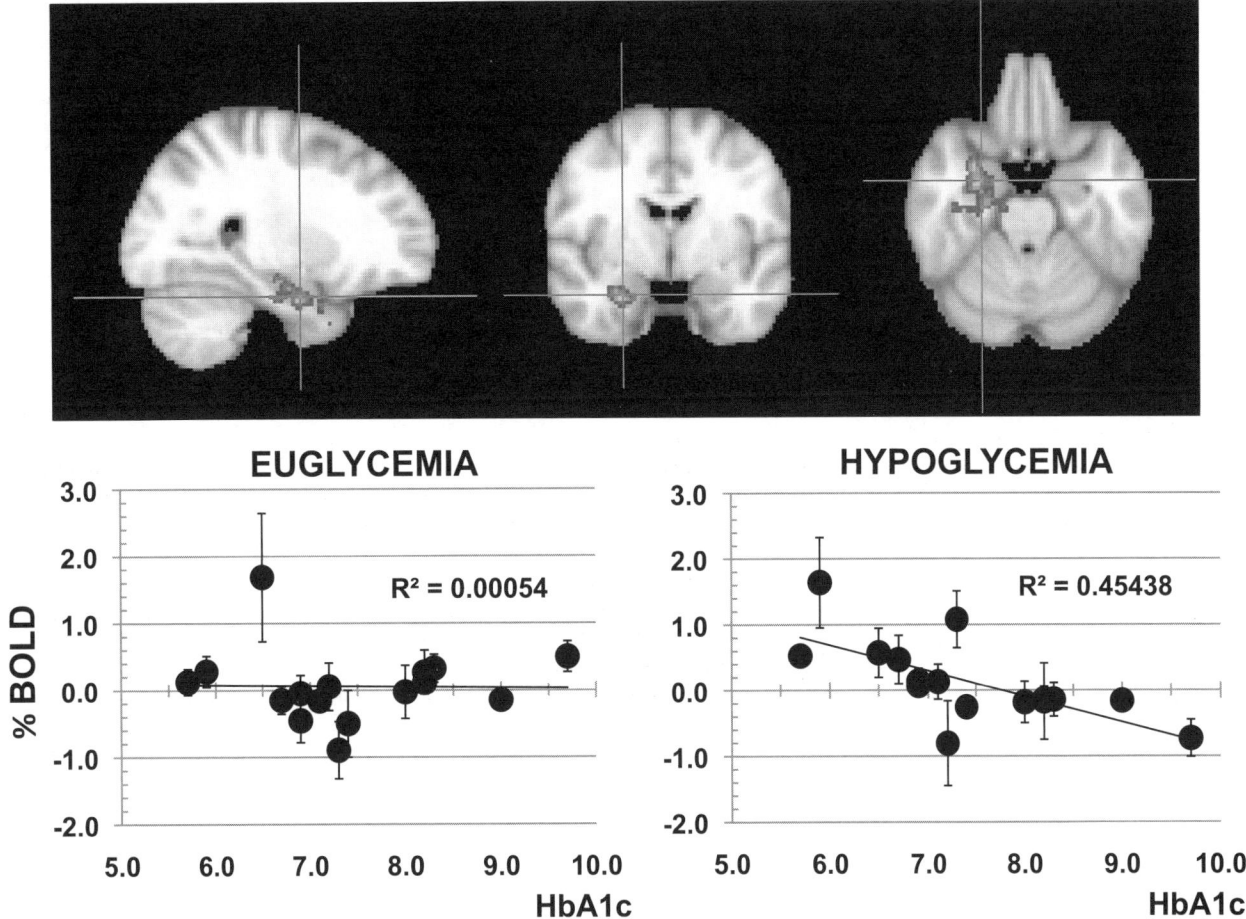

FIG. 6. Regions of BOLD activation inversely correlated with HbA$_{1c}$ in patients with type 1 diabetes. *Upper*: Statistical parametric map of the correlation of WMT activation with HbA$_{1c}$ in patients with type 1 diabetes during hypoglycemia ($P < 0.05$). Sagittal, coronal, and axial slices (from *left* to *right*) showing activation correlation in a red-to-yellow scale overlaid on the MNI-152 standard brain anatomy (gray scale). These HbA$_{1c}$-correlated activation clusters were identified in the right parahippocampal gyrus and amygdala using the Harvard-Oxford Cortical Structural Atlas. *Lower*: Plots of regional percent BOLD activation vs. HbA$_{1c}$ for patients with type 1 diabetes during euglycemia (*left*) and hypoglycemia (*right*). Filled circles with error bars: average percent BOLD activation for each patient $\pm$ SD within the region of activation. The line is the linear regression best fit of the data with its correlation coefficient R^2. (A high-quality digital representation of this figure is available in the online issue.)

shown severe impairment during hypoglycemia for highly challenging WMTs involving reasoning (2). Of importance, a number of studies have used the same Sternberg WMT used here to evaluate differences in brain activation patterns across different populations (40,41). In our study, different brain activation patterns, despite similar cognitive performance across groups, suggest unique strategies of brain recruitment used across groups to augment performance during the glycemic challenge.

Our results showing hyperactivation of brain regions in type 1 diabetic patients with low HbA$_{1c}$ and hypo-activation in patients with higher HbA$_{1c}$ could reflect upregulation of glucose transport in the brain, as seen in patients with good glycemic control (42,43). Type 1 diabetic patients may engage more brain regions to maintain the same performance to compensate for cerebral inefficiency attributed to reduced brain resources (44). These results also are consistent with the patterns observed in many physiologic systems in which a period of compensatory hyperfunction precedes functional decline and ultimate organ-system failure.

In an earlier report from our group, we demonstrated that type 1 diabetic patients showed reduced gray-matter density

in the parahippocampal gyrus associated with higher HbA$_{1c}$ (45). One possible explanation may be that gray-matter loss in this temporal region prevents its participation in the brain's response to moderate acute hypoglycemia. Wessels et al. (46) also observed abnormal brain activity patterns in patients with diabetes retinopathy, which is more likely to be associated with elevated HbA$_{1c}$ levels. However, our studies differed in both design and data analytic methodology, making a direct comparison difficult.

The differences in the hypoglycemic BOLD response between patients and control subjects found in this study may be attributed to a variety of mechanisms, including preservation of global brain glucose uptake in diabetes as a result of adaptation to hypoglycemia (12,47), differences in neurovascular coupling, resting cerebral blood flow, neuronal activity linked to oxidative metabolism, increased brain glycogen stores (48), or a tendency to use nonglucose substrates to support higher neuronal activity (49). In addition, changes in brain glucose transport or metabolism, resulting in increased brain glucose levels, might occur as a result of recurrent hypoglycemia. We reported such a finding along with accompanying increases in glutamate that were correlated with decreases in memory and executive function (16). It may follow that abnormal glutamate metabolism contributed to altered neurovascular coupling in patients in our study. Although these adaptive mechanisms in type 1 diabetes may in the short-term allow compensation for altered brain activity patterns during a hypoglycemic challenge, they may presage long-term maladaptive or adverse consequences.

Although our study demonstrates greater activation during hypoglycemia in type 1 diabetes along with reduced deactivation of the DMN, the small sample size may limit the implications of our results. However, the regional BOLD activations we observed in response to the WMT were compatible with regional activations found in other fMRI studies of similar WMTs (5,26,33–35). The reductions in BOLD response observed during hypoglycemia were also compatible with other reports showing reduced brain BOLD activation in primary or association cortex in response to sensory, motor, or cognitive tasks in nondiabetic subjects (11,12,14,47). Also, this study was unable to resolve whether the alterations in brain activation were secondary to chronic hyperglycemia or recurrent hypoglycemia. Future studies can help resolve this issue.

In summary, patients with type 1 diabetes activate more brain regions than control subjects during hypoglycemia by maintaining activity from euglycemia to hypoglycemia in task-relevant regions and by failing to suppress activation in the DMN. This suggests that type 1 diabetic patients may need to recruit more brain resources to preserve cognitive performance. The pattern of hyperactivation of both the DMN and task-relevant regions is consistent with findings in disease states with impaired cognition, such as mild cognitive impairment and Alzheimer's disease (38). There has been persistent concern about the consequences of recurrent hypoglycemia on brain structure and cognitive function. There are minimal long-term effects of recurrent hypoglycemia on cognition into middle age (50), but it is not clear whether this resiliency will last throughout the aging process. Future research should evaluate our findings as an early manifestation and warning of future clinically relevant cognitive decline. This research may guide the development of treatment regimens to enhance symptom recognition or to stabilize the neurochemical response to hypoglycemia to reduce the impact of glucodeprivation on cognitive function.

ACKNOWLEDGMENTS

This study was supported in part by National Institutes of Health grants 5R01-DK073843-03, DK-60754, DK-62218-01A1, and P30-DK-36836 (Joslin Diabetes and Endocrinology Research Center); the Herbert Graetz Fund; and grant 5M01-RR001032-32 to the Beth Israel Deaconess General Clinical Research Center.

No potential conflicts of interest relevant to this article were reported.

N.R.B., G.M., A.M.J., and K.W. researched data, contributed to discussion, and wrote, reviewed, and edited the manuscript. R.L.M. researched data, contributed to discussion, and reviewed and edited the manuscript. V.F. researched data and reviewed and edited the manuscript. P.F.R. contributed to discussion and reviewed and edited the manuscript. D.C.S. researched data, contributed to discussion, and wrote, reviewed, and edited the manuscript.

Parts of this article were presented in abstract form at the 70th Scientific Sessions of the American Diabetes Association, Orlando Florida, 25–29 June 2010, and at the 71st Scientific Sessions of the American Diabetes Association, San Diego, California, 24–28 June 2011.

The authors thank Judi Lauerman, RN, Brigham and Women's Hospital, Boston, Massachusetts, and Karen Branch, RN, Joslin Diabetes Center, Boston, Massachusetts, for their expert nursing assistance.

REFERENCES

1. Cryer PE. Hypoglycaemia: the limiting factor in the glycaemic management of type I and type II diabetes. Diabetologia 2002;45:937–948
2. Deary IJ, Sommerfield AJ, McAulay V, Frier BM. Moderate hypoglycaemia obliterates working memory in humans with and without insulin treated diabetes. J Neurol Neurosurg Psychiatry 2003;74:278–279
3. Sommerfield AJ, Deary IJ, McAulay V, Frier BM. Moderate hypoglycemia impairs multiple memory functions in healthy adults. Neuropsychology 2003;17:125–132
4. Wager TD, Smith EE. Neuroimaging studies of working memory: a meta-analysis. Cogn Affect Behav Neurosci 2003;3:255–274
5. Baddeley A. Working memory: looking back and looking forward. Nat Rev Neurosci 2003;4:829–839
6. LaBar KS, Gitelman DR, Parrish TB, Mesulam M-M. Neuroanatomic overlap of working memory and spatial attention networks: a functional MRI comparison within subjects. Neuroimage 1999;10:695–704
7. Smith EE, Jonides J. Working memory: a view from neuroimaging. Cognit Psychol 1997;33:5–42
8. Brands AM, Biessels GJ, de Haan EH, Kappelle LJ, Kessels RP. The effects of type 1 diabetes on cognitive performance: a meta-analysis. Diabetes Care 2005;28:726–735
9. Bingham E, Rosenthal JM, Amiel SA. Cognitive function in acute hypoglycaemia 2. Diabetes Nutr Metab 2002;15:363–367
10. Ogawa S, Tank DW, Menon R, et al. Intrinsic signal changes accompanying sensory stimulation: functional brain mapping with magnetic resonance imaging. Proc Natl Acad Sci USA 1992;89:5951–5955
11. Rosenthal JM, Amiel SA, Yágüez L, et al. The effect of acute hypoglycemia on brain function and activation: a functional magnetic resonance imaging study. Diabetes 2001;50:1618–1626
12. Anderson AW, Heptulla RA, Driesen N, et al. Effects of hypoglycemia on human brain activation measured with fMRI. Magn Reson Imaging 2006;24:693–697
13. Warren RE, Sommerfield AJ, Greve A, Allen KV, Deary IJ, Frier BM. Moderate hypoglycaemia after learning does not affect memory consolidation and brain activation during recognition in non-diabetic adults. Diabetes Metab Res Rev 2008;24:247–252
14. Driesen NR, Goldberg PA, Anderson AW, et al. Hypoglycemia reduces the blood-oxygenation level dependent signal in primary auditory and visual cortex: a functional magnetic resonance imaging study. J Neurosci Res 2007;85:575–582
15. Wessels AM, Rombouts SA, Simsek S, et al. Microvascular disease in type 1 diabetes alters brain activation: a functional magnetic resonance imaging study. Diabetes 2006;55:334–340
16. Lyoo IK, Yoon SJ, Musen G, et al. Altered prefrontal glutamate-glutamine-γ-aminobutyric acid levels and relation to low cognitive performance and depressive symptoms in type 1 diabetes mellitus. Arch Gen Psychiatry 2009;66:878–887
17. Criego AB, Tkac I, Kumar A, Thomas W, Gruetter R, Seaquist ER. Brain glucose concentrations in patients with type 1 diabetes and hypoglycemia unawareness. J Neurosci Res 2005;79:42–47
18. Raichle ME, MacLeod AM, Snyder AZ, Powers WJ, Gusnard DA, Shulman GL. A default mode of brain function. Proc Natl Acad Sci USA 2001;98:676–682
19. Celone KA, Calhoun VD, Dickerson BC, et al. Alterations in memory networks in mild cognitive impairment and Alzheimer's disease: an independent component analysis. J Neurosci 2006;26:10222–10231
20. Musen G, Simonson DC, Bolo NR, et al. Regional brain activation during hypoglycemia in type 1 diabetes. J Clin Endocrinol Metab 2008;93:1450–1457
21. American Diabetes Association, American Academy of Neurology. Proceedings of a consensus development conference on standardized measures in diabetic neuropathy: summary and recommendations. Diabetes Care 1992;15:1104–1107
22. The Diabetes Control and Complications Trial Research Group. Hypoglycemia in the Diabetes Control and Complications Trial. Diabetes 1997;46:271–286

23. Amiel SA, Sherwin RS, Simonson DC, Tamborlane WV. Effect of intensive insulin therapy on glycemic thresholds for counterregulatory hormone release. Diabetes 1988;37:901–907

24. DeFronzo RA, Tobin JD, Andres R. Glucose clamp technique: a method for quantifying insulin secretion and resistance. Am J Physiol 1979;237:E214–E223

25. Widom B, Simonson DC. Glycemic control and neuropsychologic function during hypoglycemia in patients with insulin-dependent diabetes mellitus. Ann Intern Med 1990;112:904–912

26. Rypma B, Prabhakaran V, Desmond JE, Glover GH, Gabrieli JD. Load-dependent roles of frontal brain regions in the maintenance of working memory. Neuroimage 1999;9:216–226

27. Beckmann CF, Jenkinson M, Woolrich MW, et al. Applying FSL to the FIAC data: model-based and model-free analysis of voice and sentence repetition priming. Hum Brain Mapp 2006;27:380–391

28. Friston KJ. Testing for anatomically specified regional effects. Hum Brain Mapp 1997;5:133–136

29. Desikan RS, Ségonne F, Fischl B, et al. An automated labeling system for subdividing the human cerebral cortex on MRI scans into gyral based regions of interest. Neuroimage 2006;31:968–980

30. Dickerson BC, Salat DH, Bates JF, et al. Medial temporal lobe function and structure in mild cognitive impairment. Ann Neurol 2004;56:27–35

31. Rosenbaum RS, Furey ML, Horwitz B, Grady CL. Altered connectivity among emotion-related brain regions during short-term memory in Alzheimer's disease. Neurobiol Aging 2010;31:780–786

32. Yetkin FZ, Rosenberg RN, Weiner MF, Purdy PD, Cullum CM. FMRI of working memory in patients with mild cognitive impairment and probable Alzheimer's disease. Eur Radiol 2006;16:193–206

33. Smith EE, Jonides J. Neuroimaging analyses of human working memory. Proc Natl Acad Sci USA 1998;95:12061–12068

34. Smith EE, Jonides J. Storage and executive processes in the frontal lobes. Science 1999;283:1657–1661

35. Duncan J, Owen AM. Common regions of the human frontal lobe recruited by diverse cognitive demands. Trends Neurosci 2000;23:475–483

36. Jonides J, Schumacher EH, Smith EE, et al. The role of parietal cortex in verbal working memory. J Neurosci 1998;18:5026–5034

37. Schmahmann JD, Sherman JC. The cerebellar cognitive affective syndrome. Brain 1998;121:561–579

38. Pihlajamäki M, Sperling RA. Functional MRI assessment of task-induced deactivation of the default mode network in Alzheimer's disease and at-risk older individuals. Behav Neurol 2009;21:77–91

39. Hvidberg A, Fanelli CG, Hershey T, Terkamp C, Craft S, Cryer PE. Impact of recent antecedent hypoglycemia on hypoglycemic cognitive dysfunction in nondiabetic humans. Diabetes 1996;45:1030–1036

40. Kim MA, Tura E, Potkin SG, et al.; FBIRN. Working memory circuitry in schizophrenia shows widespread cortical inefficiency and compensation. Schizophr Res 2010;117:42–51

41. Meda SA, Stevens MC, Folley BS, Calhoun VD, Pearlson GD. Evidence for anomalous network connectivity during working memory encoding in schizophrenia: an ICA based analysis. PLoS ONE 2009;4:e7911

42. Boyle PJ, Kempers SF, O'Connor AM, Nagy RJ. Brain glucose uptake and unawareness of hypoglycemia in patients with insulin-dependent diabetes mellitus. N Engl J Med 1995;333:1726–1731

43. McCall AL. Cerebral glucose metabolism in diabetes mellitus. Eur J Pharmacol 2004;490:147–158

44. Stern Y. What is cognitive reserve? Theory and research application of the reserve concept. J Int Neuropsychol Soc 2002;8:448–460

45. Musen G, Lyoo IK, Sparks CR, et al. Effects of type 1 diabetes on gray matter density as measured by voxel-based morphometry. Diabetes 2006; 55:326–333

46. Wessels AM, Simsek S, Remijnse PL, et al. Voxel-based morphometry demonstrates reduced grey matter density on brain MRI in patients with diabetic retinopathy. Diabetologia 2006;49:2474–2480

47. Kennan RP, Takahashi K, Pan C, Shamoon H, Pan JW. Human cerebral blood flow and metabolism in acute insulin-induced hypoglycemia. J Cereb Blood Flow Metab 2005;25:527–534

48. Choi IY, Seaquist ER, Gruetter R. Effect of hypoglycemia on brain glycogen metabolism in vivo. J Neurosci Res 2003;72:25–32

49. Mason GF, Petersen KF, Lebon V, Rothman DL, Shulman GI. Increased brain monocarboxylic acid transport and utilization in type 1 diabetes. Diabetes 2006;55:929–934

50. Jacobson AM, Ryan CM, Cleary P, et al.; Diabetes Control and Complications Trial/Epidemiology of Diabetes Interventions and Complications Study Research Group. Long-term effect of diabetes and its treatment on cognitive function. N Engl J Med 2007;356:1842–1852

Effect of Acute Hypoglycemia on Human Cerebral Glucose Metabolism Measured by ^{13}C Magnetic Resonance Spectroscopy

Kim C.C. van de Ven,[1] Bastiaan E. de Galan,[2] Marinette van der Graaf,[1,3] Alexander A. Shestov,[4] Pierre-Gilles Henry,[4] Cees J.J. Tack,[2] and Arend Heerschap[1]

OBJECTIVE—To investigate the effect of acute insulin-induced hypoglycemia on cerebral glucose metabolism in healthy humans, measured by ^{13}C magnetic resonance spectroscopy (MRS).

RESEARCH DESIGN AND METHODS—Hyperinsulinemic glucose clamps were performed at plasma glucose levels of 5 mmol/L (euglycemia) or 3 mmol/L (hypoglycemia) in random order in eight healthy subjects (four women) on two occasions, separated by at least 3 weeks. Enriched [1-^{13}C]glucose 20% w/w was used for the clamps to maintain stable plasma glucose labeling. The levels of the ^{13}C-labeled glucose metabolites glutamate C4 and C3 were measured over time in the occipital cortex during the clamp by continuous ^{13}C MRS in a 3T magnetic resonance scanner. Time courses of glutamate C4 and C3 labeling were fitted using a one-compartment model to calculate metabolic rates in the brain.

RESULTS—Plasma glucose ^{13}C isotopic enrichment was stable at 35.1 ± 1.8% during euglycemia and at 30.2 ± 5.5% during hypoglycemia. Hypoglycemia stimulated release of counterregulatory hormones (all $P < 0.05$) and tended to increase plasma lactate levels ($P = 0.07$). After correction for the ambient ^{13}C enrichment values, label incorporation into glucose metabolites was virtually identical under both glycemic conditions. Calculated tricarboxylic acid cycle rates (V_{TCA}) were 0.48 ± 0.03 μmol/g/min during euglycemia and 0.43 ± 0.08 μmol/g/min during hypoglycemia ($P = 0.42$).

CONCLUSIONS—These results indicate that acute moderate hypoglycemia does not affect fluxes through the main pathways of glucose metabolism in the brain of healthy nondiabetic subjects.
Diabetes **60:1467–1473, 2011**

H ypoglycemia is a major threat for brain function because the brain depends on a continuous glucose supply as principal source of energy. Thus, glucose counterregulatory responses are usually initiated when glucose levels fall below ~3.8 mmol/L to quickly restore euglycemia and maintain sufficient glucose delivery to the brain (1). The glucose level at which cognitive function declines is not fixed but depends on the complexity of the cognitive task and the cognitive domain that is tested. Nevertheless, although simple motor functions may be sustained despite even quite severe degrees of hypoglycemia, many aspects of cognitive performance become impaired at glucose levels between 3.1 and 3.4 mmol/L (2). During complex cognitive tasks, such as with motor vehicle driving, deterioration can already be observed at glucose levels as high as ~3.8 mmol/L (3).

Although the importance of maintaining sufficient glucose supply to the brain has been known for long, it is still unclear how hypoglycemia affects subsequent cerebral glucose metabolism. Various studies have indicated altered cerebral glucose handling during even mild symptomatic hypoglycemia. When the brain is supplied with an alternative energy source during hypoglycemia, such as lactate, the threshold level for initiation of glucose counterregulation shifts to lower glucose levels (4) and performance on cognitive function tests is maintained better (5). In accordance, upregulation of lactate transport into the brain during hypoglycemia has been associated with glucose counterregulatory defects (6). Using ^{1}H magnetic resonance spectroscopy (MRS), Bischof et al. (7) reported discrete effects of moderate hypoglycemia (~3.1 mmol/L glucose) on cerebral glucose-derived metabolite levels in healthy volunteers. Finally, positron emission tomography (PET) studies with fluor-18-fluorodeoxyglucose (FDG) and [^{11}C]-O-methyl-D-glucose (CMG) have demonstrated regional, but not global, changes in cerebral glucose metabolism based on tracer uptake in the brain during hypoglycemia in patients with diabetes (8,9). Thus, many reports suggest that human brain glucose metabolism changes under hypoglycemic conditions, but the exact changes are unclear (10). In addition, neither with ^{1}H MRS nor with PET can the cerebral metabolic rate of glucose conversion into its metabolites be determined.

With ^{13}C MRS, it is possible to study the dynamics of glucose metabolism in vivo in the human brain. Because the natural abundance of ^{13}C is only 1.1%, it can be applied as a nonradioactive magnetic resonance tracer. For this purpose, often ^{13}C enriched glucose labeled at the C-1 position is used (11). With this method, the uptake of glucose in brain tissue, as well as its conversion into several downstream metabolites, can be followed over time. To optimize the intensity of the ^{13}C signals of these metabolites, which occur at rather low concentration, most studies applying dynamic ^{13}C MRS to the human brain have been performed under hyperglycemic conditions. We previously developed a specific protocol that has enabled us to apply ^{13}C MRS with infusion of ^{13}C-labeled glucose under both euglycemic and hypoglycemic conditions in human volunteers (12). This allows for mathematical

From the [1]Department of Radiology, Radboud University Nijmegen Medical Centre, Nijmegen, the Netherlands; the [2]Department of General Internal Medicine, Radboud University Nijmegen Medical Centre, Nijmegen, the Netherlands; the [3]Department of Pediatrics, Radboud University Nijmegen Medical Centre, Nijmegen, the Netherlands; and the [4]Center for Magnetic Resonance Research, University of Minnesota, Minneapolis, Minnesota.
Corresponding author: Kim C.C. van de Ven, k.vandeven@rad.umcn.nl.
Received 16 November 2010 and accepted 28 February 2011.
DOI: 10.2337/db10-1592
This article contains Supplementary Data online at http://diabetes.diabetesjournals.org/lookup/suppl/doi:10.2337/db10-1592/-/DC1.

modeling and calculation of metabolic fluxes of glucose metabolism (13,14). The aim of the current study was to compare human in vivo brain glucose metabolism under euglycemic and hypoglycemic conditions using ^{13}C MRS.

RESEARCH DESIGN AND METHODS

Eight healthy nondiabetic volunteers (four men and four women aged 23.2 ± 2.5 years with BMI 23.9 ± 4.5 kg/m²) were enrolled for this study. The study was approved by the institutional review board of the Radboud University Nijmegen Medical Centre, and all volunteers gave written informed consent before participation. All participants were examined on two occasions: once under euglycemic conditions and once under hypoglycemic conditions, scheduled in random order and separated by at least 3 weeks. Female subjects were tested at 4- or 8-week intervals to ensure that experiments took place during corresponding periods of the menstrual cycle.

Hyperinsulinemic glucose clamps. Subjects came to the magnetic resonance research facility at 8:00 A.M. after an overnight fast and after having abstained from alcohol and caffeine-containing substances for 24 h. The brachial artery of the nondominant arm was cannulated under local anesthesia for frequent blood sampling. An intravenous catheter was inserted in the antecubital vein of the contralateral arm for administration of ^{13}C-glucose and insulin. After a 30-min equilibration period, subjects were placed on the scanner bed in supine position with their heads positioned in the magnetic resonance coil. Arterial blood was sampled to obtain baseline variables, and reference spectra were obtained without administration of exogenous ^{13}C-labeled material during the next 30 min. Subsequently, a hyperinsulinemic (60 mU/min/m², equaling approximately 1.5 mU/min/kg) euglycemic (5.0 mmol/L) or hypoglycemic (3.0 mmol/L) glucose clamp was initiated with [1-^{13}C] glucose 20% w/w, as described previously (12). Briefly, a bolus of 30 mL of 100% enriched [1-^{13}C] glucose 20% w/w was infused over 10 min at the initiation of the clamp to rapidly increase plasma ^{13}C enrichment. For the remainder of the experiments, variable infusions of 40 or 50% enriched [1-^{13}C]glucose 20% w/w were infused during the euglycemic and hypoglycemic experiments, respectively, in order to maintain plasma glucose levels at predetermined target levels. Blood was sampled every 5 min for immediate determination of plasma glucose by the glucose oxidation method (Beckmann Glucose Analyzer II; Beckman Coulter, Fullerton, CA) and later determination of plasma ^{13}C isotopic enrichment of glucose and lactate by high-resolution proton nuclear magnetic resonance (^{1}H NMR) at 500 MHz (15,16). Plasma lactate concentration was also determined by ^{1}H NMR spectra. Every 30 min, additional blood was sampled for measurement of insulin and counterregulatory hormones as previously described (12).

MRS. All studies were performed on a 3T magnetic resonance system (Magnetom Trio; Siemens, Erlangen, Germany) with a ^{1}H volume coil and a circularly polarized ^{13}C surface coil inserted into the ^{1}H coil (17). A distortionless enhanced polarization transfer (DEPT) sequence for ^{1}H to ^{13}C polarization transfer combined with proton image-selected in vivo spectroscopy (^{1}H ISIS) localization (18) was used for acquisition of ^{13}C magnetic resonance spectra. Adiabatic ^{13}C radiofrequency pulses were used in all sequences to ensure homogeneous excitation using the ^{13}C surface coil, as well as wideband alternating phase low-power technique for zero residue splitting (WALTZ-16) proton decoupling (19) to simplify the spectra and enhance signal-to-noise ratio (SNR). A voxel of ~125 mL was placed in occipital brain tissue. In all experiments, one spectrum consisted of 72 repetitions of 2 s, allowing for a time resolution of 2.5 min. Eight reference spectra were obtained before the start of [1-^{13}C]glucose infusion, during which ^{13}C MR spectra were acquired continuously. Visual stimulation was avoided by dimming the lights in the magnet room during the experiments.

^{13}C MRS data processing and quantification. The eight ^{13}C MR reference spectra were averaged and subtracted from the dynamic spectra acquired during the ^{13}C glucose clamp to correct for natural abundance ^{13}C magnetic resonance signals. To enhance the SNR, the corrected spectra were added in running averages of 15 min. The resulting spectra were fitted with the advance magnetic resonance (AMARES) algorithm (20) in the java-based MR user interface (jMRUI) software package (21). The natural abundance signal of *myo*-inositol (mI) was used to quantify glutamate C4 and glutamate C3 in the spectra based on the premise that mI has a stable concentration of 6 μmol/g and is not labeled with ^{13}C in the time frame of the experiment (22). The natural abundance signal of mI was quantified in jMRUI from the spectra obtained by adding all dynamic spectra before correction with reference spectra. DEPT ^{13}C magnetic resonance spectra measured from a phantom were used to eliminate effects of the pulse sequence profile on the experimental spectra.

Metabolic modeling. Rates of metabolic fluxes were determined using a standard one-compartment metabolic model (14,23,24) as depicted in Fig. 1.

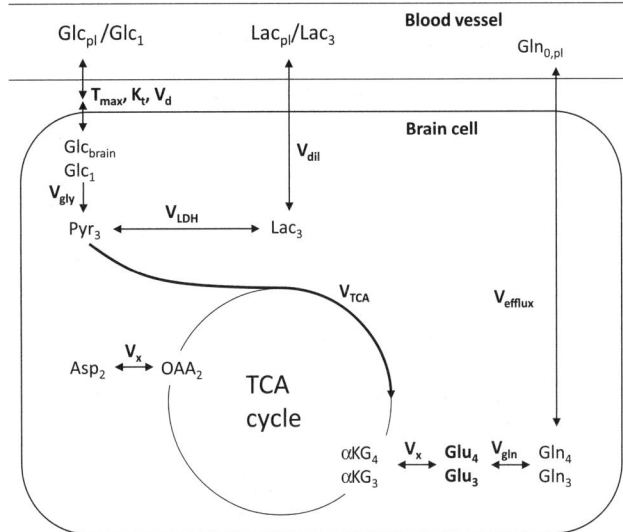

FIG. 1. One-compartment model for uptake of [1-^{13}C]glucose and its conversion into labeled metabolites. Brain glucose uptake from the blood was modeled by reversible Michaelis-Menten kinetics (40). V_{gly} represents the glycolysis rate and has a value of $0.5 × V_{TCA}$. The cycling of glutamate and glutamine between neurons and astroglia is approached by the parameter V_{gln} and assumed equal to V_{TCA}. V_{TCA}, V_{dil}, and V_{efflux} are the free parameters of the model, representing TCA cycle flux, exchange of plasma, and brain lactate and efflux of labeled glutamine, respectively. V_{LDH} represents lactate dehydrogenase and was assumed to be 3 μmol/g/min; V_X represents the exchange between α-ketoglutarate and glutamate over the mitochondrial membrane and was assumed to be 5 μmol/g/min. Furthermore, the following assumptions were made for total pool concentrations: [Glu]: 10 mmol/L; [Gln]: 2.5 mmol/L; [OAA]: 0.3 mmol/L; [αKG]: 0.25 mmol/L; [Asp]: 1.5 mmol/L; and [Pyr]: 0.15 mmol/L.

These rates (V) were assessed from the time courses of incorporation of ^{13}C isotopes into different metabolites. Time courses of glutamate C4 and glutamate C3 concentrations and plasma values and isotopic enrichments of glucose were used as input factors for the model. In this specific situation, it was also decided to take plasma lactate values and isotopic enrichment into account as input variables for the modeling process. The model was implemented in Matlab R2008b (MathWorks, Natick, MA) and consisted of differential equations describing the inflow and outflow of label from each metabolite pool. These equations were solved numerically, and a nonlinear least-squares approach was used to fit the model to the experimental data by varying free flux parameters representing V_{TCA}, the loss of label through exchange with unlabeled glutamine (V_{efflux}), and the exchange of intracellular lactate with plasma lactate (V_{dil}). V_X, representing the exchange between α-ketoglutarate and glutamate, was assumed to be 5 μmol/g/min. This value was fixed to ensure stable fitting. In literature, there is no consensus on the value of V_X; it is either determined to be much higher compared with V_{TCA} (25) or to be in the same order of V_{TCA} (23,26). However, for this study comparing two datasets, the choice of V_X is not critical; it will influence absolute values but equally for both datasets and therefore will not compromise the comparison of the two glycemic conditions. Data of all individual volunteers were fitted separately and inspected for the goodness of fit by the cost value, a parameter that represents the difference between the measured concentrations and the corresponding estimates by the model. From these fits, flux parameters were calculated.

Statistical analysis. All data are expressed as means ± SD unless otherwise indicated. Serial data (e.g., plasma hormone and lactate levels) were compared by repeated-measures ANOVA, and differences in means were tested by paired, two-tailed Student t tests. Graphpad Prism 4 (Graphpad, La Jolla, CA) was used for statistical analysis, and a P value < 0.05 was considered statistically significant.

RESULTS

As a consequence of the [1-^{13}C]glucose bolus, plasma glucose levels transiently increased to maximally 7.1 ± 0.4 mmol/L during the euglycemic experiment and to 6.6 ± 1.0 mmol/L during the hypoglycemic experiment. Thereafter, plasma glucose levels were allowed to fall and were maintained stable at 5.1 ± 0.3 mmol/L with a coefficient of variation (CV) of 4.1 ± 1.0% during the euglycemic clamp and at 3.0 ± 0.4 mmol/L (CV 5.9 ± 2.2%) during the hypoglycemic clamp (Fig. 2A). In response to hypoglycemia, plasma levels of glucagon, adrenaline, noradrenaline, cortisol, and growth hormone all significantly increased compared with baseline and compared with similar time points during the euglycemic clamp (Table 1). As expected, glucose infusion rates were approximately threefold lower during hypoglycemia than during euglycemia (2.2 ± 0.4 vs. 6.6 ± 0.9 μmol/kg/min; P < 0.001).

Isotopic enrichment of plasma glucose also peaked immediately after the bolus infusion. From t = 20 min onward, plasma ^{13}C glucose labeling was stable during both the euglycemic and the hypoglycemic clamps, although the level was slightly lower during hypoglycemia (35.1 ± 1.8% [CV 3.6 ± 2.1] vs. 30.2 ± 5.5% [CV 6.8 ± 2.4]) (Fig. 2B).

After an initial rise, plasma lactate levels remained stable during euglycemia at 1.1 ± 0.3 mmol/L, but tended to increase further in response to hypoglycemia (from 1.1 ± 0.4 to 1.5 ± 0.6 mmol/L, P = 0.07 vs. euglycemia). Conversely, plasma lactate isotopic enrichment remained constant (after an initial increase) during hypoglycemia, whereas it

increased further during euglycemia (from 6.1 ± 3.2 at t = 20 min to 8.9 ± 2.7% at t = 100 min), P < 0.0001, versus hypoglycemia (Fig. 2C and D).

All ^{13}C MR spectra were of similar spectral quality with sufficient SNR to analyze the signals of the metabolites of interest under both euglycemic and hypoglycemic conditions (Fig. 3). Under either condition, the ^{13}C label was progressively incorporated into glutamate C4, C3, and C2; glutamine C4, C3, and C2; aspartate C3 and C2; and lactate C3. Figure 4A shows the time courses of glutamate C4 labeling, which appears during the first turn of the TCA cycle, and of glutamate C3 labeling, which appears during the second turn of the TCA cycle. The isotopic enrichment of the glutamate pool was lower under hypoglycemic conditions than under euglycemic conditions. However, after correction for the lower plasma glucose ^{13}C enrichment level during hypoglycemia, the time courses for both these metabolites were virtually superimposable for the two glycemic conditions (Fig. 4B).

The time courses of ^{13}C label incorporation into glutamate C4 and C3 were fitted with a one-compartment metabolic model (Fig. 1) to compare metabolic fluxes under euglycemic and hypoglycemic conditions. The average of individually calculated TCA cycle rates (V_{TCA}) under

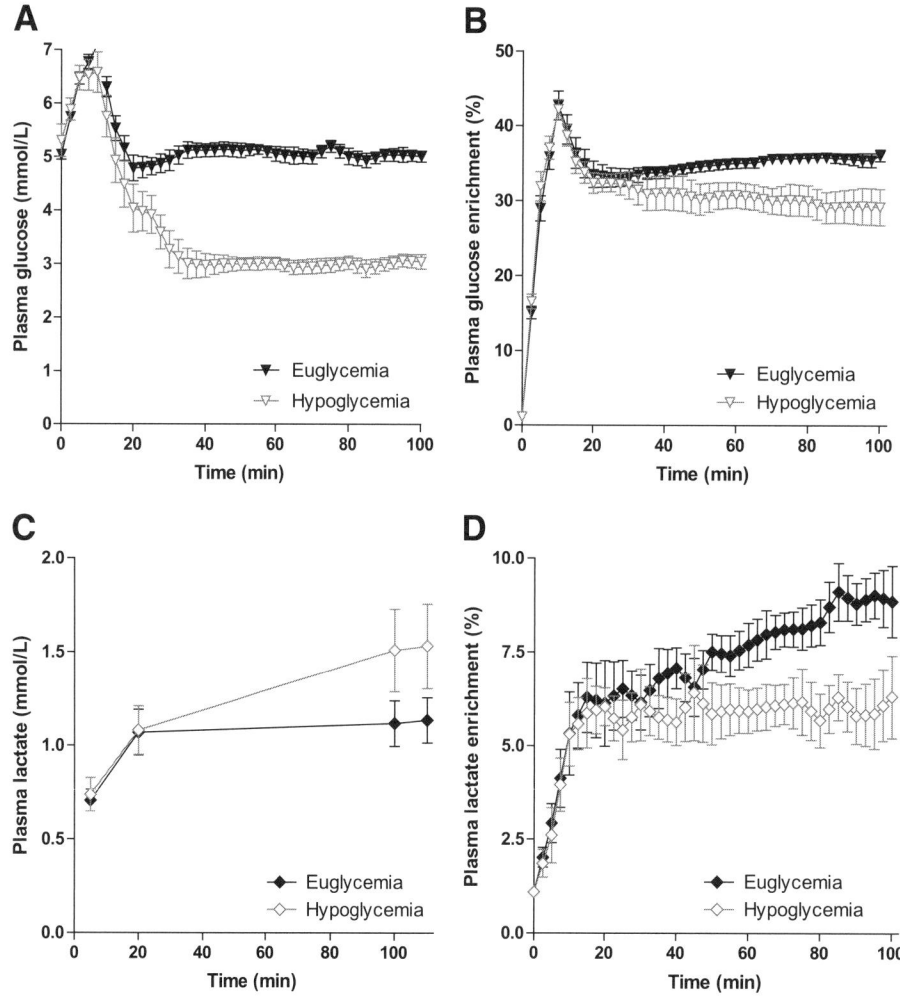

FIG. 2. Plasma glucose concentration (A), plasma glucose ^{13}C enrichment (B), plasma lactate concentration (C), and plasma lactate ^{13}C enrichment (D) as a function of time during the euglycemic and hypoglycemic clamps. Data are shown as means ± SEM.

TABLE 1
Counterregulatory hormone and insulin values during the euglycemic and hypoglycemic clamps

	Time after start of glucose infusion (min)				
	Baseline	30	90	120	P
Glucagon (pmol/L)					
Euglycemic clamp	35.5 ± 6.9	30.5 ± 7.2	28.4 ± 7.3	41.4 ± 11.1	
Hypoglycemic clamp	27.6 ± 5.1	41.9 ± 19.8	53.6 ± 16.4	77.0 ± 41.9	0.0080
Adrenaline (nmol/L)					
Euglycemic clamp	0.22 ± 0.09	0.24 ± 0.08	0.42 ± 0.20	0.41 ± 0.12	
Hypoglycemic clamp	0.20 ± 0.10	0.82 ± 1.22	3.96 ± 2.10	4.84 ± 2.51	<0.0001
Noradrenaline (nmol/L)					
Euglycemic clamp	0.91 ± 0.22	0.97 ± 0.21	1.07 ± 0.26	1.14 ± 0.31	
Hypoglycemic clamp	0.94 ± 0.4	1.15 ± 0.39	1.98 ± 1.06	1.96 ± 0.64	0.0316
Cortisol (μmol/L)					
Euglycemic clamp	0.44 ± 0.29	0.53 ± 0.13	0.42 ± 0.15	0.42 ± 0.13	
Hypoglycemic clamp	0.47 ± 0.18	0.47 ± 0.17	0.64 ± 0.33	0.89 ± 0.21	0.0048
Growth hormone (mU/L)					
Euglycemic clamp	5.91 ± 7.45	6.14 ± 7.84	14.86 ± 14.43	19.30 ± 18.34	
Hypoglycemic clamp	6.17 ± 7.16	14.44 ± 33.19	46.38 ± 47.96	74.09 ± 55.55	0.0462
Insulin (pmol/L)					
Euglycemic clamp	76.6 ± 44.1	777.8 ± 190.7	685.9 ± 114.9	694.1 ± 114.9	
Hypoglycemic clamp	63.4 ± 29.5	943.7 ± 548.11	493.7 ± 349.3	685.8 ± 107.1	0.6824

Data are means ± SD. Statistical tests performed with two-way ANOVA.

hypoglycemic clamp conditions was similar to the average values obtained under euglycemic conditions (Table 2). When the TCA cycle rates were calculated from averaged datasets (Fig. 4C; individual datasets of all participants can be found in Supplementary Fig. 1), similar values were obtained (0.48 and 0.43 μmol/g/min for euglycemia and hypoglycemia, respectively). There were also no differences between the two glycemic conditions with regard to other flux parameters. The absence of an effect of hypoglycemia on metabolic fluxes was similar among men and women in the study (data not shown).

DISCUSSION

In this study, we used ^{13}C MRS to investigate the effect of moderate hypoglycemia on glucose handling by the human brain in vivo. Despite the fact that hypoglycemia considerably stimulated glucose counterregulation, which is under control of the central nervous system, metabolism of glucose in the occipital tissue of the brain was remarkably similar under hypoglycemic and euglycemic conditions. Indeed, the time courses of ^{13}C labeling of both glutamate C4 and glutamate C3 during hypoglycemia and during euglycemia were superimposable, when corrected for plasma isotopic enrichment, and the rate of TCA cycle flux was ~0.5 μmol/g/min on both occasions. These calculated fluxes are in line with previously reported values for V_{TCA} under hyperglycemic conditions (27–29).

This is the first study to investigate and quantify cerebral glucose metabolism under hypoglycemic conditions in humans using ^{13}C MRS. The lack of a difference in cerebral glucose metabolism between hypo- and euglycemia contrasts with a ^{1}H MRS study, which suggested slowing of the TCA cycle rate during hypoglycemia based on a reduction of the glutamate-to-creatine ratio (7). However, snapshot ^{1}H magnetic resonance spectra provide steady-state levels of metabolites and cannot be used to quantify cerebral glucose metabolic fluxes, as is possible with dynamic ^{13}C MRS. Moreover, our findings are in line with a ^{13}C MRS study in rats (30) in which overall cerebral metabolism in control animals was not affected by hypoglycemia.

Mathematical modeling of the data was performed to quantify and compare metabolic processes under the two glycemic conditions. Our model showed that the rates for free flux parameters (V_{TCA}, V_{dil}, and V_{efflux}) were about similar during hypoglycemia and euglycemia. The V_{TCA} values were within the published range (27–29), but V_{dil} and V_{efflux} were higher than previously reported (31,32). Because several assumptions for V_{gln}, V_{LDH}, and V_X had to be made to derive the rates for free flux parameters, these data need to be interpreted with caution. There is ongoing debate as to which estimated values are appropriate. In the literature, for V_X values below 1 and as high as 57 μmol/g/min have been used (23,25). In the current study, the data were fitted assuming V_X = 5 μmol/g/min to optimize the fitting. Refitting the data with V_X = 1 μmol/g/min resulted in slightly lower values for V_{TCA} of 0.43 μmol/g/min during euglycemia and 0.38 μmol/g/min during hypoglycemia, but the difference between the two groups remained nonsignificant. We cannot completely exclude the possibility

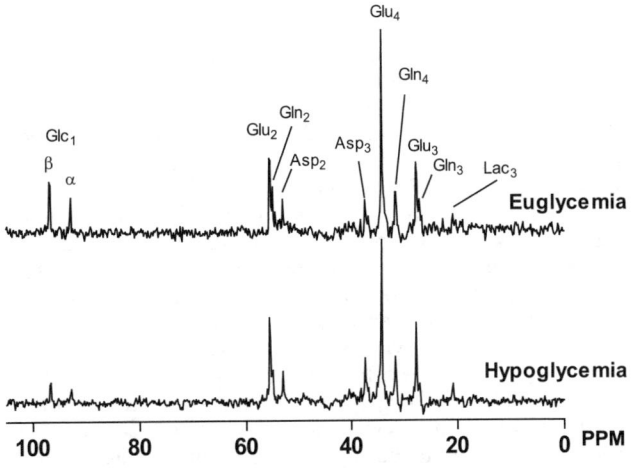

FIG. 3. Representative ^{13}C magnetic resonance spectra of the human brain measured at the end of a euglycemic experiment and a hypoglycemic experiment. PPM, parts per million.

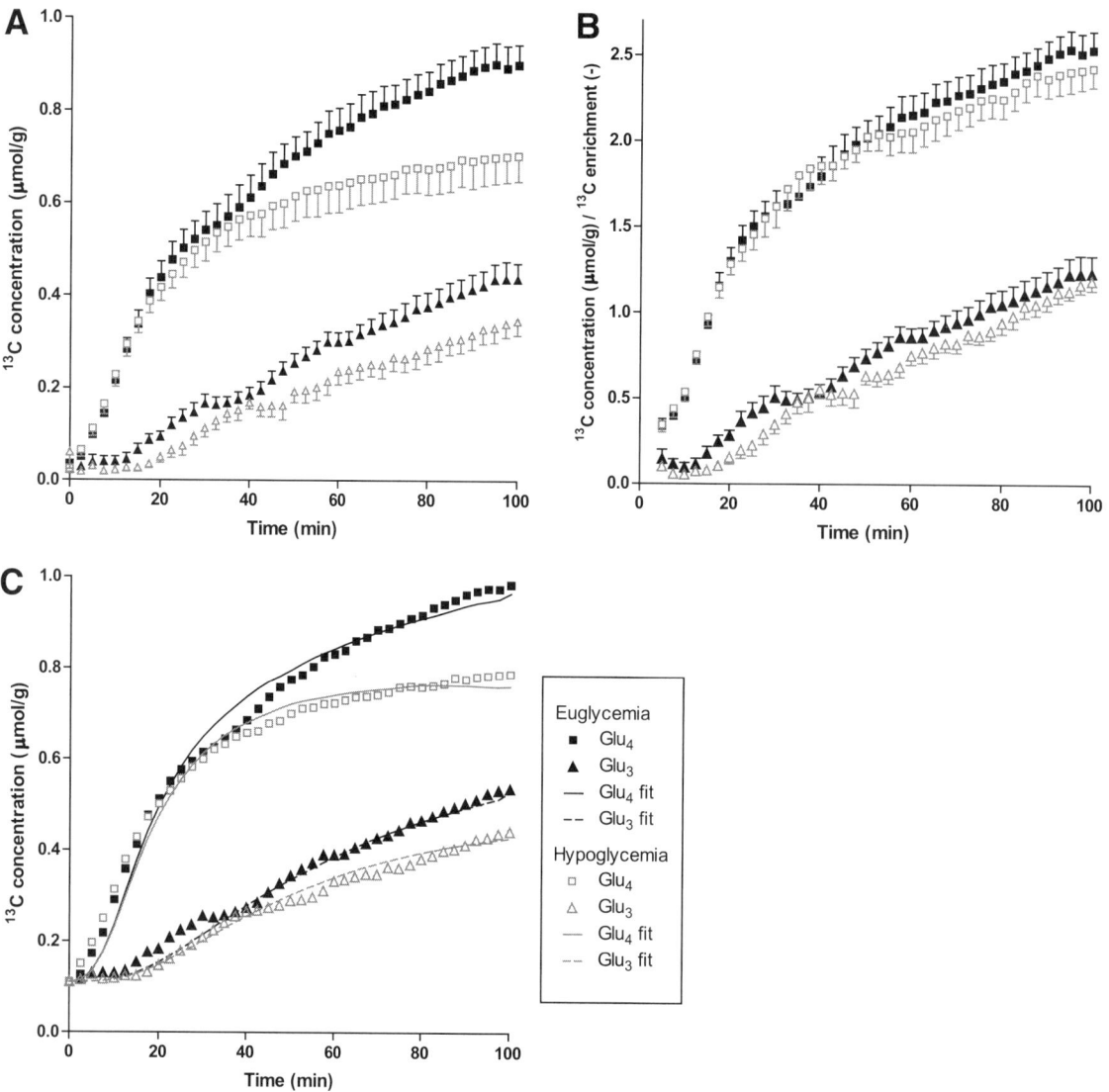

FIG. 4. *A*: Time courses of glutamate C4 and C3 labeling in brain tissue during euglycemic and hypoglycemic clamps. *B*: Time courses of glutamate C4 and C3 labeling in brain tissue corrected by plasma glucose ^{13}C enrichment. *C*: Averaged time courses of glutamate C4 and C3 labeling in brain tissue with natural abundance signal added for modeling purposes together with averaged best fits of individual datasets.

that V_{gln}, V_{LDH}, and V_X are modulated by the level of glycemia itself, but there are no data available to support such a notion. Thus, identical assumptions for the fixed model parameters were used for both glycemic conditions.

There are several potential mechanisms that could maintain normal cerebral glucose metabolism during hypoglycemia. A plausible explanation would be a compensatory increase in cerebral uptake of lactate. In agreement with previous observations (33), plasma lactate increased by approximately 50% in response to hypoglycemia. Lactate can be used by the brain as an alternative energy source and may reduce the cerebral need for glucose (34–36). After conversion to pyruvate, lactate carbons may enter the TCA cycle as the carbons of glucose do (37). A study by Mason et al. (6) has indicated that brain transporter activity for monocarboxylic substrates such as lactate can be increased twofold during hypoglycemia, which would support the hypothesis of increased lactate consumption during hypoglycemia. Moreover, even under resting conditions, increases in lactate availability stimulate consumption

of lactate by the brain at the cost of reductions in glucose utilization (34). Our model does not include net lactate uptake because this flux is small and can be neglected under physiological conditions. However, it is possible that the increased plasma lactate level during hypoglycemia could result in increased net lactate uptake in the brain. Therefore, to assess the potential contribution of net lactate uptake, we performed additional modeling incorporating net lactate uptake (0.2 μmol/g/min, estimated from lactate Michaelis-Menten kinetics through the blood-brain barrier) into the

TABLE 2
Metabolic flux values during euglycemia and hypoglycemia

	Euglycemia	Hypoglycemia	P*
V_{TCA} (μmol/g/min)	0.48 ± 0.03	0.43 ± 0.08	0.42
V_{dil} (μmol/g/min)	0.61 ± 0.25	0.61 ± 0.39	0.89
V_{efflux} (μmol/g/min)	0.41 ± 0.26	0.41 ± 0.20	0.83

Data are means ± SD. *Student *t* test.

model during hypoglycemia and found that it did not affect the values of V_{TCA} significantly (<5% change). Thus, this is unlikely to explain our findings.

Alternatively, we cannot exclude the entrance of unlabeled carbons into the TCA cycle via glycogen breakdown as was suggested by an in vivo study by Oz et al. (38). Breakdown of glycogen located in astrocytes can then provide neurons with lactate to maintain energy metabolism (39).

This study provides no evidence for a link between a decline in cognitive function and moderate hypoglycemia. As ^{13}C MRS of the brain was usually performed in a limited area of the occipital cortex, we cannot exclude the possibility that regional variation in cerebral glucose metabolism occurs. It is also possible that increased cortical activation in response to hypoglycemia stimulated glucose uptake so that any fall in glucose metabolism was sufficiently compensated for. PET studies have demonstrated increased cortical activation during hypoglycemia (~2.6 mmol/L) in various regions of the brain in diabetic men (8,9) but not in the occipital cortex, where reduced rather than increased activation was observed.

It is possible that the relatively mild hypoglycemic condition imposed during this study was only strong enough to stimulate hormonal counterregulation but that deeper hypoglycemia is required to induce impairments in cerebral glucose metabolism. However, a clamp at much lower glucose levels may be hard to achieve while maintaining stable glucose infusion at a sufficient rate, which is required for administration of the ^{13}C isotope. In addition, more severe hypoglycemia would expose participants to significantly more discomfort and risk.

In conclusion, our results indicate that acute moderate hypoglycemia does not affect cerebral glucose metabolism in healthy human volunteers. Thus, the healthy human brain appears sufficiently resilient to withstand moderate drops in plasma glucose, potentially as a consequence of increased lactate availability. Our study provides new insights into mechanisms that protect the brain from substrate deprivation, which may have important clinical implications if this finding can be reproduced in patients with type 1 diabetes, especially those suffering from repeated hypoglycemic episodes.

ACKNOWLEDGMENTS

This work was financially supported by the Dutch Diabetes Research Foundation (grant 2004.00.012), the National Institutes of Health (grants DK-069881, P41-RR-08079, and R01-NS-38672), the framework of the Center for Translational Molecular Medicine (www.ctmm.nl), project PREDICCt grant 01C-104, and the Netherlands Heart Foundation and Dutch Kidney Foundation.

No potential conflicts of interest relevant to this article were reported.

K.C.C.v.d.V. analyzed data, drafted the manuscript, contributed to interpreting data and to editing the content, and approved the final version of the paper. B.E.d.G. analyzed data, drafted the manuscript, designed the study, contributed to interpreting data and to editing the content, and approved the final version of the paper. M.v.d.G. analyzed data, designed the study, contributed to interpreting data and to editing the content, and approved the final version of the paper. A.A.S. and P.-G.H. contributed to interpreting data and to editing the content and approved the final version of the paper. C.J.J.T. and A.H. designed the study, contributed to interpreting data and to editing the content, and approved the final version of the paper.

The authors are indebted to Karin Saini, Radboud University Nijmegen Medical Centre, for assistance during the hyperinsulinemic clamps and to Dennis Klomp, Radboud University Nijmegen Medical Centre, for sequence implementation, coil development, and further technical assistance.

REFERENCES

1. Cryer PE. The barrier of hypoglycemia in diabetes. Diabetes 2008;57:3169–3176
2. Friers BM, Fisher BM (Eds.). Hypoglycemia in Clinical Diabetes. New York, Wiley, 1999
3. Cox DJ, Gonder-Frederick LA, Kovatchev BP, Julian DM, Clarke WL. Progressive hypoglycemia's impact on driving simulation performance: occurrence, awareness and correction. Diabetes Care 2000;23:163–170
4. Veneman T, Mitrakou A, Mokan M, Cryer P, Gerich J. Induction of hypoglycemia unawareness by asymptomatic nocturnal hypoglycemia. Diabetes 1993;42:1233–1237
5. Maran A, Crepaldi C, Trupiani S, et al. Brain function rescue effect of lactate following hypoglycaemia is not an adaptation process in both normal and type I diabetic subjects. Diabetologia 2000;43:733–741
6. Mason GF, Petersen KF, Lebon V, Rothman DL, Shulman GI. Increased brain monocarboxylic acid transport and utilization in type 1 diabetes. Diabetes 2006;55:929–934
7. Bischof MG, Brehm A, Bernroider E, et al. Cerebral glutamate metabolism during hypoglycaemia in healthy and type 1 diabetic humans. Eur J Clin Invest 2006;36:164–169
8. Bingham EM, Dunn JT, Smith D, et al. Differential changes in brain glucose metabolism during hypoglycaemia accompany loss of hypoglycaemia awareness in men with type 1 diabetes mellitus. An ^{11}C]-3-O-methyl-D-glucose PET study. Diabetologia 2005;48:2080–2089
9. Cranston I, Reed LJ, Marsden PK, Amiel SA. Changes in regional brain (18)F-fluorodeoxyglucose uptake at hypoglycemia in type 1 diabetic men associated with hypoglycemia unawareness and counter-regulatory failure. Diabetes 2001;50:2329–2336
10. McCrimmon RJ, Sherwin RS. Hypoglycemia in type 1 diabetes. Diabetes 2010;59:2333–2339
11. de Graaf RA, Mason GF, Patel AB, Behar KL, Rothman DL. In vivo ^{1}H-^{13}C]-NMR spectroscopy of cerebral metabolism. NMR Biomed 2003;16:339–357
12. van de Ven KC, van der Graaf M, Tack CJ, Klomp DW, Heerschap A, de Galan BE. Optimized [1-(13)C]glucose infusion protocol for ^{13}C magnetic resonance spectroscopy at 3T of human brain glucose metabolism under euglycemic and hypoglycemic conditions. J Neurosci Methods 2010;186:68–71
13. Mason GF, Rothman DL. Basic principles of metabolic modeling of NMR (13)C isotopic turnover to determine rates of brain metabolism in vivo. Metab Eng 2004;6:75–84
14. Henry PG, Adriany G, Deelchand D, et al. In vivo ^{13}C NMR spectroscopy and metabolic modeling in the brain: a practical perspective. Magn Reson Imaging 2006;24:527–539
15. Serlie MJ, de Haan JH, Tack CJ, et al. Glycogen synthesis in human gastrocnemius muscle is not representative of whole-body muscle glycogen synthesis. Diabetes 2005;54:1277–1282
16. Van Den Bergh AJ, Tack CJ, Van Den Boogert HJ, Vervoort G, Smits P, Heerschap A. Assessment of human muscle glycogen synthesis and total glucose content in vivo by ^{13}C MRS. Eur J Clin Invest 2000;30:122–128
17. Klomp DW, Renema WK, van der Graaf M, de Galan BE, Kentgens AP, Heerschap A. Sensitivity-enhanced ^{13}C MR spectroscopy of the human brain at 3 Tesla. Magn Reson Med 2006;55:271–278
18. Klomp DW, Kentgens AP, Heerschap A. Polarization transfer for sensitivity-enhanced MRS using a single radio frequency transmit channel. NMR Biomed 2008;21:444–452
19. Shaka AJ, Keeler J, Frenkiel T, Freeman R. An improved sequence for broadband decoupling: WALTZ-16. J Magn Reson 1983;52:335–338
20. Vanhamme L, van den Boogaart A, Van Huffel S, van den Boogaart A, Van Huffel S. Improved method for accurate and efficient quantification of MRS data with use of prior knowledge. J Magn Reson 1997;129:35–43
21. Naressi A, Couturier C, Devos JM, et al. Java-based graphical user interface for the MRUI quantitation package. MAGMA 2001;12:141–152
22. Ross B, Lin A, Harris K, Bhattacharya P, Schweinsburg B. Clinical experience with ^{13}C MRS in vivo. NMR Biomed 2003;16:358–369
23. Henry PG, Lebon V, Vaufrey F, Brouillet E, Hantraye P, Bloch G. Decreased TCA cycle rate in the rat brain after acute 3-NP treatment measured by in vivo ^{1}H-^{13}C] NMR spectroscopy. J Neurochem 2002;82:857–866

24. Henry PG, Criego AB, Kumar A, Seaquist ER. Measurement of cerebral oxidative glucose consumption in patients with type 1 diabetes mellitus and hypoglycemia unawareness using (13)C nuclear magnetic resonance spectroscopy. Metabolism 2010;59:100–106

25. Mason GF, Gruetter R, Rothman DL, Behar KL, Shulman RG, Novotny EJ. Simultaneous determination of the rates of the TCA cycle, glucose utilization, alpha-ketoglutarate/glutamate exchange, and glutamine synthesis in human brain by NMR. J Cereb Blood Flow Metab 1995;15:12–25

26. Choi IY, Lei H, Gruetter R. Effect of deep pentobarbital anesthesia on neurotransmitter metabolism in vivo: on the correlation of total glucose consumption with glutamatergic action. J Cereb Blood Flow Metab 2002; 22:1343–1351

27. Mason GF, Falk Petersen K, de Graaf RA, et al. A comparison of (13)C NMR measurements of the rates of glutamine synthesis and the tricarboxylic acid cycle during oral and intravenous administration of [1-(13)C]glucose. Brain Res Brain Res Protoc 2003;10:181–190

28. Gruetter R, Seaquist ER, Ugurbil K. A mathematical model of compartmentalized neurotransmitter metabolism in the human brain. Am J Physiol Endocrinol Metab 2001;281:E100–E112

29. Boumezbeur F, Mason GF, de Graaf RA, et al. Altered brain mitochondrial metabolism in healthy aging as assessed by in vivo magnetic resonance spectroscopy. J Cereb Blood Flow Metab 2010;30:211–221

30. Jiang L, Herzog RI, Mason GF, et al. Recurrent antecedent hypoglycemia alters neuronal oxidative metabolism in vivo. Diabetes 2009;58:1266–1274

31. Pan JW, Stein DT, Telang F, et al. Spectroscopic imaging of glutamate C4 turnover in human brain. Magn Reson Med 2000;44:673–679

32. Shen J, Petersen KF, Behar KL, et al. Determination of the rate of the glutamate/glutamine cycle in the human brain by in vivo ^{13}C NMR. Proc Natl Acad Sci USA 1999;96:8235–8240

33. Abi-Saab WM, Maggs DG, Jones T, et al. Striking differences in glucose and lactate levels between brain extracellular fluid and plasma in conscious human subjects: effects of hyperglycemia and hypoglycemia. J Cereb Blood Flow Metab 2002;22:271–279

34. van Hall G, Strømstad M, Rasmussen P, et al. Blood lactate is an important energy source for the human brain. J Cereb Blood Flow Metab 2009;29: 1121–1129

35. Smith D, Pernet A, Hallett WA, Bingham E, Marsden PK, Amiel SA. Lactate: a preferred fuel for human brain metabolism in vivo. J Cereb Blood Flow Metab 2003;23:658–664

36. Boumezbeur F, Petersen KF, Cline GW, et al. The contribution of blood lactate to brain energy metabolism in humans measured by dynamic ^{13}C nuclear magnetic resonance spectroscopy. J Neurosci 2010;30:13983–13991

37. Gallagher CN, Carpenter KL, Grice P, et al. The human brain utilizes lactate via the tricarboxylic acid cycle: a ^{13}C-labelled microdialysis and high-resolution nuclear magnetic resonance study. Brain 2009;132:2839–2849

38. Oz G, Kumar A, Rao JP, et al. Human brain glycogen metabolism during and after hypoglycemia. Diabetes 2009;58:1978–1985

39. Brown AM, Ransom BR. Astrocyte glycogen and brain energy metabolism. Glia 2007;55:1263–1271

40. Gruetter R, Ugurbil K, Seaquist ER. Steady-state cerebral glucose concentrations and transport in the human brain. J Neurochem 1998;70:397–408

Adrenergic Mediation of Hypoglycemia-Associated Autonomic Failure

Ranjani Ramanathan and Philip E. Cryer

OBJECTIVE—We tested the hypothesis that adrenergic activation, cholinergic activation, or both, mediate the effect of recent antecedent hypoglycemia to reduce the sympathoadrenal response to subsequent hypoglycemia, the key feature of hypoglycemia-associated autonomic failure in diabetes, in humans.

RESEARCH DESIGN AND METHODS—Seventeen healthy adults were studied on 2 consecutive days on three occasions. Day 1 involved hyperinsulinemic euglycemic (90 mg/dL × 1 h), then hypoglycemic (54 mg/dL × 2 h) clamps, in the morning and afternoon on all three occasions with *1*) saline infusion, *2*) adrenergic blockade with the nonselective α-adrenergic and β-adrenergic antagonists phentolamine and propranolol, or *3*) adrenergic blockade plus cholinergic blockade with the muscarinic cholinergic antagonist atropine in random sequence. Day 2 involved similar morning euglycemic and hypoglycemic clamps, with saline infusion, on all three occasions.

RESULTS—Compared with the responses to hypoglycemia during saline infusion on day 1, the plasma epinephrine and norepinephrine responses to hypoglycemia were reduced on day 2 (351 ± 13 vs. 214 ± 22 pg/mL for epinephrine and 252 ± 4 vs. 226 ± 7 pg/mL for norepinephrine during the last hour; both $P < 0.0001$). However, the plasma epinephrine and norepinephrine responses to hypoglycemia were not reduced on day 2 when adrenergic or adrenergic plus cholinergic blockade was produced during hypoglycemia on day 1.

CONCLUSIONS—Adrenergic blockade prevents the effect of hypoglycemia to reduce the plasma catecholamine responses to subsequent hypoglycemia. Thus, adrenergic activation mediates the effect of recent antecedent hypoglycemia to reduce the sympathoadrenal response to subsequent hypoglycemia, the key feature of hypoglycemia-associated autonomic failure in diabetes, in humans. *Diabetes* **60:602–606, 2011**

I atrogenic hypoglycemia is the limiting factor in the glycemic management of diabetes (1). It causes recurrent morbidity in most people with type 1 diabetes and in many with type 2 diabetes, and is sometimes fatal, impairs physiologic and behavioral defenses against subsequent hypoglycemia, and generally precludes maintenance of euglycemia over a lifetime of diabetes. The concept of hypoglycemia-associated autonomic failure (HAAF) in diabetes posits that recent antecedent hypoglycemia, as well as prior exercise or sleep,

From the Division of Endocrinology, Metabolism and Lipid Research, Washington University School of Medicine, St. Louis, Missouri.
Corresponding author: Philip E. Cryer, pcryer@wustl.edu.
Received 27 September 2010 and accepted 8 November 2010.
DOI: 10.2337/db10-1374
The contents of this article are solely the responsibility of the authors and do not necessarily represent the official view of the National Institutes of Health or the American Diabetes Association.

causes both the syndrome of defective glucose counterregulation (by reducing the adrenomedullary epinephrine response to subsequent hypoglycemia in the setting of absent decrements in insulin and absent increments in glucagon) and of hypoglycemia unawareness (by reducing the sympathoadrenal and resulting neurogenic symptom responses to subsequent hypoglycemia) (1–4). These two components of HAAF are both associated with a substantially increased incidence of hypoglycemia during intensive therapy for diabetes (1). Perhaps the most compelling evidence of the clinical effect of HAAF is the finding, originally in three independent laboratories (5–8), that as little as 2 to 3 weeks of scrupulous avoidance of hypoglycemia reverses hypoglycemia unawareness and improves the attenuated epinephrine component of defective glucose counterregulation in most affected patients.

The mechanisms of the attenuated sympathoadrenal response to hypoglycemia, the key feature of the pathogenesis of HAAF in diabetes (1–8), are unknown (1). Although much of the neuroscience research into this issue has focused on the hypothalamus (9), recent translational research has raised the possibility that a complex cerebral network normally regulates the hypothalamic (and thus the systemic sympathoadrenal) response to falling plasma glucose concentrations (10–12) and that an inhibitory signal mediated through the thalamus might be involved in the pathogenesis of HAAF (12).

Hypoglycemia activates the sympathoadrenal system (1,13,14). This includes the release of catecholamines that interact with α-adrenergic and β-adrenergic receptors—norepinephrine from sympathetic postganglionic neurons and epinephrine and norepinephrine from the adrenal medullae—and acetylcholine that interacts with muscarinic cholinergic receptors—from sympathetic postganglionic neurons. Hypoglycemia also activates central nervous system circuits, including those that involve adrenergic and cholinergic neurotransmission. There are, of course, an array of other neurotransmitters released in the peripheral and the central nervous systems.

We used the original model of HAAF (2) and the nonselective α-adrenergic and β-adrenergic antagonists phentolamine and propranolol as well as the muscarinic cholinergic antagonist atropine in doses shown previously to be both safe and effective (15) to test the hypothesis that adrenergic activation, cholinergic activation, or both, mediate the effect of recent antecedent hypoglycemia to reduce the sympathoadrenal response to subsequent hypoglycemia, the key feature of HAAF in diabetes (1–8), in humans.

RESEARCH DESIGN AND METHODS

This study was approved by the Washington University Human Research Protection Office and was conducted at the Washington University Clinical Research Unit (CRU).
Participants. Study participants comprised 17 adults (7 women, 10 men), with a mean (± SD) age of 29 ± 5 years and a BMI of 26.5 ± 4.6 kg/m^2, who gave

their written consent. They were in good health as determined by medical history, physical examination, and fasting plasma glucose and creatinine concentrations, hematocrits, and electrocardiograms that were within normal reference ranges.

Experimental design. Participants were studied on 2 consecutive days on three occasions, separated by at least 2 weeks, after overnight fasts. Intravenous catheters were inserted into a hand vein, with that hand kept in a ~55°C plexiglas box for arterialized venous blood sampling, and into a contralateral antecubital vein for insulin, glucose, and drug infusions and injections.

Day 1 involved hyperinsulinemic (2.0 mU/kg/min), euglycemic (90 mg/dL [5.0 mmol/L] × 1 h), and then hypoglycemic (54 mg/dL [3.0 mmol/L] × 2 h) clamps in the morning and again in the afternoon on all three occasions. Intravenous infusions during these day 1 glucose clamps were *1)* saline, *2)* the nonselective α-adrenergic receptor antagonist phentolamine mesylate (70 μg/kg, followed by 7.0 μg/kg/min) and the nonselective β-adrenergic antagonist propranolol hydrochloride (14 μg/kg, followed by 1.4 μg/kg/min), or *3)* phentolamine plus propranolol and the muscarinic cholinergic antagonist atropine (1.0 mg injected intravenously at the end of each euglycemic clamp and 60 min into each hypoglycemic clamp) in random sequence. This experimental design is illustrated, with the actual plasma glucose concentration data, in Fig. 1.

Plasma glucose concentrations were measured every 5 min at the bedside (YSI Glucose Analyzer, Yellow Springs Instruments, Yellow Springs, OH) to guide 20% glucose infusions. Heart rates and blood pressures (GE Dash 3000, Fairfield, CT) were recorded at 15-min intervals, and the electrocardiogram was monitored throughout. Arterialized venous samples for the additional analytes detailed below were drawn at 15-min intervals during the morning euglycemic and hypoglycemic clamps on both days. This model of morning and afternoon hypoglycemia reduces the sympathoadrenal response to hypoglycemia the following day (1–4), and these doses of phentolamine, propranolol, and atropine are safe and hemodynamically, metabolically, and symptomatically effective (15).

Day 2 involved identical hyperinsulinemic euglycemic and then hypoglycemic clamps, with saline infusion, in the morning on all three occasions. Arterialized venous samples were again used to measure plasma glucose concentrations every 5 min and were drawn for the analytes detailed subsequently every 15 min.

Analytic methods. Plasma glucose concentrations were measured with a glucose oxidase method (YSI Glucose Analyzer). Plasma insulin, C-peptide, growth hormone, and cortisol concentrations were measured with two site chemiluminescent assays (Immulite 1000, Siemens Corp., Los Angeles, CA). Plasma glucagon and pancreatic polypeptide concentrations were measured with Linco radioimmunoassays (Millipore, Temecula, CA). Plasma epinephrine and norepinephrine concentrations were measured with a single isotope-derivative (radioenzymatic) method (16).

Statistical methods. Time and condition related variables were analyzed by repeated measures mixed model ANOVA. Values of $P < 0.05$ were considered to indicate statistically significant differences. Data are expressed as the mean ± SE, except where the SD is indicated.

RESULTS

Plasma glucose concentrations, day 1 and day 2. Plasma glucose concentrations were clamped at euglycemic (~90 mg/dL [5.0 mmol/L]) and then hypoglycemic (~54 mg/dL [3.0 mmol/L]) levels in the morning and again in the afternoon—with intravenous infusions of saline, phentolamine plus propranolol (adrenergic blockade), or phentolamine plus propranolol with injection of atropine (adrenergic plus cholinergic blockade)—on day 1 and on the morning of day 2—with intravenous infusion of saline—after saline, phentolamine plus propranolol, or phentolamine plus propranolol with atropine on day 1 on three separate occasions (Fig. 1). The glucose infusion rates required to maintain the clamps were similar on all occasions (data not shown).

Responses on day 1. Compared with those during saline, increments in plasma epinephrine and norepinephrine concentrations during hypoglycemia were increased about threefold during adrenergic blockade and during adrenergic plus cholinergic blockade (both $P < 0.0001$; Fig. 2). The final epinephrine values were 352 ± 46 pg/mL (1,920 ± 251 pmol/L), 1,040 ± 160 pg/mL (5,680 ± 873 pmol/L), and 1,130 ± 193 pg/mL (6,170 ± 1,050 pmol/L), respectively. The final norepinephrine values were 257 ± 19 pg/mL (1.52 ± 0.11 nmol/L), 809 ± 84 pg/mL (4.78 ± 0.50 nmol/L), and 786 ± 100 pg/mL (4.65 ± 0.59 nmol/L), respectively. Increments in plasma pancreatic polypeptide concentrations during hypoglycemia were similar during saline and during adrenergic blockade but were prevented during adrenergic plus cholinergic blockade. The final pancreatic polypeptide values were 356 ± 45 pg/mL (85 ± 11 pmol/L), 374 ± 42 pg/mL (89 ± 10 pmol/L), and 75 ± 9 pg/mL (18 ± 2 pmol/L), respectively.

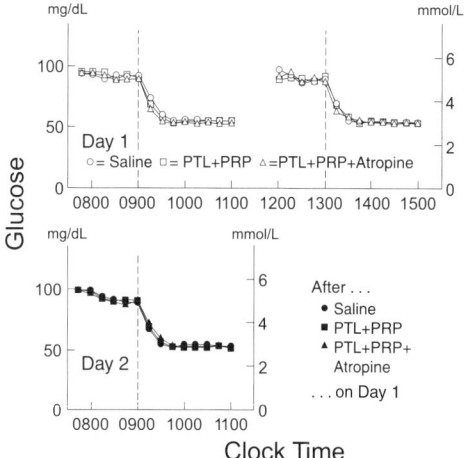

FIG. 1. Mean (SEs within the symbols) plasma glucose concentrations are shown during morning and afternoon hyperinsulinemic euglycemic and hypoglycemic clamps with intravenous infusions of saline (○), phentolamine plus propranolol (PTL + PRP, □) or phentolamine plus propranolol with injection of atropine (PTL + PRP + Atropine, △) on day 1 and during morning hyperinsulinemic euglycemic and hypoglycemic clamps with intravenous infusion of saline on day 2 after saline (●), PTL + PRP (■) or PTL + PRP + Atropine (▲) on day 1 on three separate occasions.

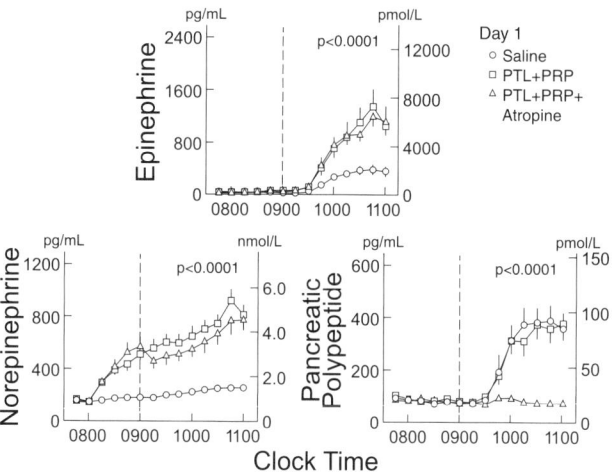

FIG. 2. Mean (± SE) plasma epinephrine, norepinephrine, and pancreatic polypeptide concentrations are shown during morning hyperinsulinemic euglycemic and hypoglycemic clamps with intravenous infusions of saline (○), phentolamine plus propranolol (PTL + PRP, □), or phentolamine plus propranolol with atropine (△) on day 1. The P values represent comparisons with the values during saline infusion (both $P < 0.0001$) for epinephrine and norepinephrine and comparisons with values during phentolamine plus propranolol with atropine ($P < 0.0001$) for pancreatic polypeptide.

Plasma concentrations of infused insulin stabilized at ~95 µU/mL (570 pmol/L) during infusion of saline but rose to ~120 µU/mL (720 pmol/L) during adrenergic blockade and during adrenergic plus cholinergic blockade (both $P <$ 0.0001; Fig. 3). The final insulin values were 96 ± 8 µU/mL (576 ± 48 pmol/L), 122 ± 12 µU/mL (732 ± 72 pmol/L), and 123 ± 9 µU/mL (738 ± 54 pmol/L), respectively. Increments in plasma glucagon concentrations during hypoglycemia were similar on all three occasions (Fig. 3). The final glucagon values were 98 ± 11 pg/mL (28 ± 3 pmol/L), 110 ± 10 pg/mL (32 ± 3 pmol/L), and 104 ± 7 pg/mL (30 ± 2 pmol/L), respectively.

Compared with those during saline, increments in plasma growth hormone and cortisol concentrations during hypoglycemia were increased during adrenergic blockade and adrenergic plus cholinergic blockade ($P < 0.0001$ under both conditions for both hormones; Fig. 3). The final growth hormone values were 13.3 ± 2.2 ng/mL (587 ± 97 pmol/L), 25.2 ± 3.2 ng/mL (1,110 ± 141 pmol/L), and 20.7 ± 2.8 ng/mL (914 ± 124 pmol/L), respectively. The final cortisol values were 18.4 ± 1.5 µg/dL (508 ± 41 nmol/L), 22.1 ± 1.4 µg/dL (610 ± 39 nmol/L), and 23.7 ± 1.6 µg/dL (654 ± 44 nmol/L), respectively.

Heart rate responses to hypoglycemia were decreased during adrenergic blockade and increased during adrenergic plus cholinergic blockade compared with those during saline (both $P < 0.0001$; Table 1). Systolic and diastolic blood pressures were reduced during adrenergic blockade and during adrenergic plus cholinergic blockade (both $P < 0.0001$; Table 1).

Responses on day 2 compared with those during saline on day 1. Compared with that during saline on day 1, the increment in the plasma epinephrine concentration during hypoglycemia was attenuated by ~50% on day 2 ($P < 0.0001$; Fig. 4). The epinephrine values during the last hour of hypoglycemia were 351 ± 13 pg/mL (1920 ± 71 pmol/L) and 214 ± 22 pg/mL (1170 ± 120 pmol/L), respectively. In contrast, the increments in plasma epinephrine during hypoglycemia were not reduced on day 2 after adrenergic blockade or adrenergic plus cholinergic

blockade on day 1 (Fig. 4). The epinephrine values during the last hour of hypoglycemia were 359 ± 26 pg/mL (1,960 ± 142 pmol/L) and 375 ± 11 pg/mL (2,050 ± 60 pmol/L), respectively.

Similarly, the increment in the plasma norepinephrine concentration during hypoglycemia was attenuated on day 2 compared with that during saline on day 1 ($P < 0.0001$; Fig. 4). The norepinephrine values during the last hour of hypoglycemia were 252 ± 4 pg/mL (1.49 ± 0.02 nmol/L) and 226 ± 7 pg/mL (1.34 ± 0.04 nmol/L), respectively. The increments in plasma norepinephrine during hypoglycemia were not reduced on day 2 after adrenergic blockade or adrenergic plus cholinergic blockade on day 1 (Fig. 4). The norepinephrine values during the last hour of hypoglycemia were 284 ± 11 pg/mL (1.68 ± 0.06 nmol/L) and 256 ± 11 pg/mL (1.51 ± 0.06 nmol/L), respectively. Compared with that during saline on day 1, the increment in the plasma pancreatic polypeptide concentration during hypoglycemia was attenuated by ~50% on day 2 under all three study conditions ($P < 0.0001$; Fig. 4). The pancreatic polypeptide values during the last hour of hypoglycemia were 373 ± 6 pg/mL (89 ± 1 pmol/L) on day 1 and 216 ± 7 pg/mL (52 ± 2 pmol/L), 214 ± 17 pg/mL (51 ± 4 pmol/L), and 239 ± 10 pg/mL (57 ± 2 pmol/L), respectively, on day 2.

Plasma concentrations of infused insulin were stable and comparable to those during saline on day 1 during all three hyperinsulinemic euglycemic and hypoglycemic clamps on day 2 (Fig. 5). Compared with that during saline on day 1, the increments in the plasma glucagon concentrations during hypoglycemia were reduced under all three conditions on day 2 ($P = 0.0263$, 0.0008 and <0.0001, respectively; Fig. 5). The glucagon values during the last hour of hypoglycemia during saline infusion on day 1 were 99 ± 1 pg/mL (28 ± 0 pmol/L). The glucagon values during the last hour of hypoglycemia on day 2 were 89 ± 3 pg/mL (26 ± 1 pmol/L), 83 ± 2 pg/mL (24 ± 1 pmol/L), and 86 ± 2 pg/mL (25 ± 1 pmol/L) after saline, adrenergic blockade, and adrenergic plus cholinergic blockade on day 1, respectively.

This was also the case for increments in the plasma cortisol concentrations during hypoglycemia on day 2 ($P = 0.0001$, <0.0001 and 0.0030) (Fig. 5). The cortisol values during the last hour of hypoglycemia during saline infusion on day 1 were 17.3 ± 0.7 µg/dL (480 ± 19 nmol/L). Cortisol values during the last hour of hypoglycemia on day 2 were 14.2 ± 0.6 µg/dL (390 ± 17 nmol/L), 13.5 ± 1.0 µg/dL (370 ± 28 nmol/L), and 15.0 ± 1.1 µg/dL (410 ± 30 nmol/L) after saline, adrenergic blockade, and adrenergic plus cholinergic blockade on day 1, respectively. Compared with that during saline on day 1, the increment in the plasma growth hormone concentration during hypoglycemia was reduced on day 2 ($P = 0.0028$; Fig. 5). The growth hormone values during the last hour of hypoglycemia were 12.6 ± 0.5 ng/mL (560 ± 22 pmol/L) on day 1 and 7.7 ± 0.2 ng/mL (340 ± 9 pmol/L) on day 2. In contrast, growth hormone values during the last hour of hypoglycemia on day 2 were not reduced after adrenergic blockade or adrenergic plus cholinergic blockade on day 1 −10.8 ± 0.8 ng/mL (480 ± 35 pmol/L) and 14.0 ± 1.4 ng/mL (620 ± 62 pmol/L), respectively.

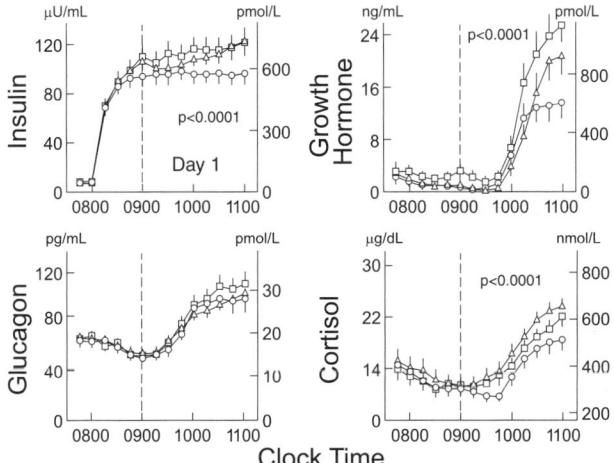

FIG. 3. Mean (± SE) plasma insulin, glucagon, growth hormone, and cortisol concentrations are shown during morning hyperinsulinemic euglycemic and hypoglycemic clamps with intravenous infusions of saline (○), phentolamine plus propranolol (□), or phentolamine plus propranolol with atropine (△) on day 1. The P values represent comparisons with the values during saline, both $P < 0.0001$ for insulin, growth hormone, and cortisol.

DISCUSSION

We used a well-documented model of HAAF in diabetes (hypoglycemia attenuates the sympathoadrenal response to hypoglycemia the following day) (1–4) and the classic adrenergic and cholinergic antagonists phentolamine,

TABLE 1
Heart rate and blood pressure responses on day 1 during clamped hyperinsulinemic euglycemia (0800–0900 h) and hypoglycemia (0900–1100 h)

	Saline			PTL + PRP			PTL + PRP + Atropine		
Clock time	HR (bpm)	sBP (mmHg)	dBP (mmHg)	HR (bpm)	sBP (mmHg)	dBP (mmHg)	HR (bpm)	sBP (mmHg)	dBP (mmHg)
0745 h	69 ± 3	125 ± 3	72 ± 2	69 ± 2	120 ± 3	68 ± 2	67 ± 3	119 ± 3	67 ± 2
0800 h	68 ± 2	125 ± 3	71 ± 2	70 ± 2	118 ± 4	66 ± 2	69 ± 3	118 ± 3	68 ± 2
0815 h	70 ± 2	124 ± 3	70 ± 3	71 ± 2	117 ± 3	63 ± 2	71 ± 3	114 ± 3	64 ± 2
0830 h	71 ± 3	125 ± 3	70 ± 2	72 ± 2	115 ± 3	60 ± 1	69 ± 3	112 ± 3	64 ± 2
0845 h	70 ± 2	124 ± 3	70 ± 2	69 ± 2	112 ± 3	60 ± 2	69 ± 2	111 ± 3	60 ± 2
0900 h	71 ± 2	124 ± 3	68 ± 2	68 ± 2	113 ± 3	58 ± 1	77 ± 4	112 ± 3	59 ± 2
0915 h	71 ± 2	125 ± 4	69 ± 3	69 ± 2	111 ± 3	57 ± 2	90 ± 3	111 ± 3	62 ± 2
0930 h	72 ± 3	124 ± 4	68 ± 2	67 ± 2	110 ± 3	57 ± 2	86 ± 3	113 ± 3	60 ± 2
0945 h	74 ± 3	123 ± 4	65 ± 3	67 ± 2	110 ± 3	55 ± 2	82 ± 3	110 ± 3	58 ± 2
1000 h	76 ± 3	126 ± 4	64 ± 2	66 ± 2	108 ± 2	53 ± 1	82 ± 2	109 ± 3	57 ± 2
1015 h	73 ± 2	125 ± 3	63 ± 3	66 ± 2	109 ± 3	52 ± 2	86 ± 2	109 ± 3	55 ± 2
1030 h	73 ± 2	122 ± 4	61 ± 3	63 ± 2	105 ± 3	52 ± 1	84 ± 2	106 ± 3	53 ± 2
1045 h	72 ± 3	122 ± 4	60 ± 2	60 ± 2	106 ± 3	51 ± 1	80 ± 2	106 ± 3	51 ± 2
1145 h	73 ± 3	119 ± 4	60 ± 2	60 ± 2	106 ± 3	51 ± 1	77 ± 2	105 ± 3	51 ± 2
P vs. saline	—	—	—	<0.0001	<0.0001	<0.0001	<0.0001	<0.0001	<0.0001

Values are mean ± SE. dBP, diastolic blood pressure; HR, heart rate; sBP, systolic blood pressure; PTL, phentolamine; PRP, propranolol.

propranolol and atropine (13–15) to test the hypothesis that adrenergic activation, cholinergic activation, or both, mediate the effect of recent antecedent hypoglycemia to reduce the sympathoadrenal response to subsequent hypoglycemia, the key feature of HAAF in diabetes (1–8), in humans.

The data indicate that adrenergic mechanisms mediate the effect of recent antecedent hypoglycemia to reduce the sympathoadrenal response to subsequent hypoglycemia. Morning and afternoon hypoglycemia with saline infusion on day 1 led to attenuated increments in plasma epinephrine and norepinephrine concentrations, markers of the

sympathoadrenal, primarily adrenomedullary, response to hypoglycemia (17), during hypoglycemia on day 2. Thus, the phenomenon that we sought to explore mechanistically— recent antecedent hypoglycemia reduces the sympathoadrenal response to subsequent hypoglycemia (1–8)—was reproduced.

However, when adrenergic blockade (without or with cholinergic blockade) was produced during hypoglycemia on day 1, the increments in plasma epinephrine and norepinephrine concentrations during hypoglycemia on day 2 were not attenuated. Thus, combined adrenergic blockade with the nonselective α-adrenergic antagonist phentolamine and the nonselective β-adrenergic antagonist propranolol prevented the effect of hypoglycemia to reduce the

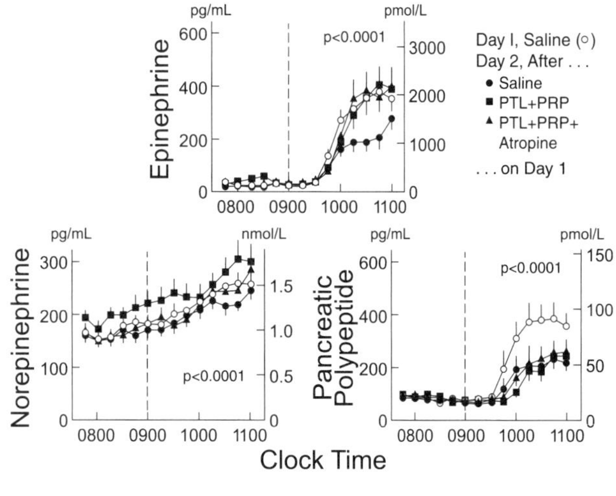

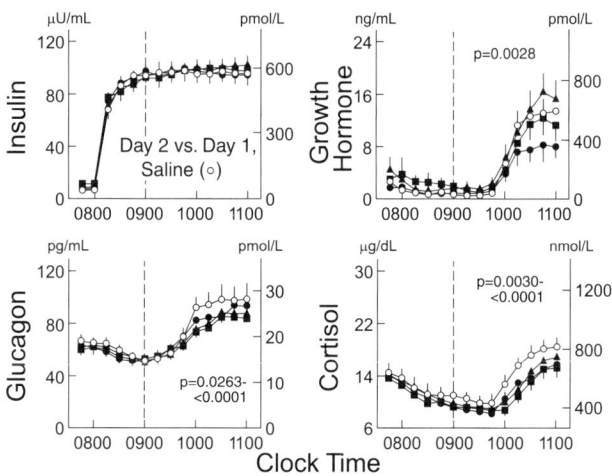

FIG. 4. Mean (± SE) plasma epinephrine, norepinephrine, and pancreatic polypeptide concentrations are shown during morning hyperinsulinemic euglycemic and hypoglycemic clamps on day 1 with saline infusion (○) and on day 2 after saline (●), phentolamine plus propranolol (PTL + PRP, ■), or phentolamine plus propranolol with atropine (PTL + PRP + Atropine, ▲) during the clamps on day 1. The P values represent comparisons with the values during saline infusion on day 1 (○), P < 0.0001 for epinephrine and norepinephrine on day 2 (●), and P < 0.0001 for pancreatic polypeptide under all three conditions on day 2 (●, ■, and ▲).

FIG. 5. Mean (± SE) plasma insulin, glucagon, growth hormone, and cortisol concentrations are shown during morning hyperinsulinemic euglycemic and hypoglycemic clamps on day 1 with saline infusion (○) and on day 2 after saline (●), phentolamine plus propranolol (■), or phentolamine plus propranolol with atropine (▲) during the clamps on day 1. The P values represent comparisons with the values during saline on day 1 (○); see text for details.

sympathoadrenal response to subsequent hypoglycemia. The latter is the key feature of HAAF in diabetes (1–8).

The data do not disclose—but do not categorically exclude—an additional cholinergic mechanism. The sympathoadrenal response to hypoglycemia on day 2 was similar whether the muscarinic cholinergic antagonist atropine was or was not administered with phentolamine and propranolol during hypoglycemia on day 1.

Morning and afternoon hypoglycemia with saline infusion on day 1 also led to attenuated increments in the plasma pancreatic polypeptide concentration, a marker of the parasympathetic response to hypoglycemia (18), during hypoglycemia on day 2. In contrast to the effect on the sympathoadrenal response, adrenergic blockade (without or with cholinergic blockade) during hypoglycemia on day 1 did not prevent the attenuated pancreatic polypeptide response to hypoglycemia on day 2. An altered parasympathetic response is not known to be involved in the pathogenesis of HAAF in diabetes (1).

To the extent the drugs used enter the central nervous system (propranolol and atropine are known to do so), the data do not distinguish between central and peripheral (autonomic) nervous system mediation of the effect of antecedent hypoglycemia to reduce the sympathoadrenal response to subsequent hypoglycemia. However, because the adrenergic antagonists block the heart rate and pressor responses to hypoglycemia, which are normally mediated by the autonomic response, one might speculate that it was blockade of adrenergic sympathoadrenal actions during hypoglycemia on day 1 that prevented an attenuated plasma catecholamine response to hypoglycemia on day 2.

The data confirm substantially higher plasma epinephrine and norepinephrine concentrations in response to hypoglycemia during adrenergic blockade on day 1 (15). That is expected because both catecholamines are cleared through β-adrenergic mechanisms in humans (19). (Given the short half-times of the antagonists and the catecholamines, a carry-over effect to the next day is unlikely.) The current findings of higher plasma concentrations of infused insulin and of endogenous growth hormone and cortisol during hypoglycemia during adrenergic blockade suggest that adrenergic mechanisms are also involved in the clearance of these hormones. The growth hormone responses to hypoglycemia, like the epinephrine and norepinephrine responses, were reduced after hypoglycemia with saline infusion but not after hypoglycemia with adrenergic blockade (without or with cholinergic blockade). An interesting finding was that the pancreatic polypeptide, glucagon, and cortisol responses to hypoglycemia were reduced on day 2 regardless of the day 1 conditions. Among these, a reduced glucagon response is a feature of HAAF (1). Thus, the data further support the view that the mechanisms of the reduced glucagon and epinephrine responses to hypoglycemia in HAAF are different (1).

In conclusion, the data indicate that adrenergic mechanisms mediate the effect of recent antecedent hypoglycemia to reduce the sympathoadrenal response to subsequent hypoglycemia, the key feature of HAAF in diabetes, in humans.

ACKNOWLEDGMENTS

This study was partly supported by National Institutes of Health Grants R37-DK-27085 and UL1-RR-24992 and by a fellowship award from the American Diabetes Association.

P.E.C. has served as a consultant to Bristol-Myers Squibb/AstraZeneca, MannKind Corp., Merck & Co., and Novo Nordisk in the past year. No other potential conflicts of interest relevant to this article were reported.

R.R. and P.E.C. designed the study, R.R. conducted it, and R.R. and P.E.C. analyzed the data and wrote the manuscript.

The authors acknowledge the assistance of the following Washington University staff: Licia Rowe, Laura Karsteter, Nilima Parikh, Tanya Eden, Shirley Frei, Janice Bathon, Paula Blood, and David Gibson of the Clinical Research Unit and of the Core Laboratory for Clinical Studies; the technical assistance of Krishan Jethi, MS; and the statistical assistance of Ling Chen, PhD, MPH. Janet Dedeke prepared this manuscript.

REFERENCES

1. Cryer PE. The barrier of hypoglycemia in diabetes. Diabetes 2008;57:3169–3176
2. Heller SR, Cryer PE. Reduced neuroendocrine and symptomatic responses to subsequent hypoglycemia after 1 episode of hypoglycemia in nondiabetic humans. Diabetes 1991;40:223–226
3. Dagogo-Jack SE, Craft S, Cryer PE. Hypoglycemia-associated autonomic failure in insulin-dependent diabetes mellitus. Recent antecedent hypoglycemia reduces autonomic responses to, symptoms of, and defense against subsequent hypoglycemia. J Clin Invest 1993;91:819–828
4. Segel SA, Paramore DS, Cryer PE. Hypoglycemia-associated autonomic failure in advanced type 2 diabetes. Diabetes 2002;51:724–733
5. Fanelli CG, Epifano L, Rambotti AM, et al. Meticulous prevention of hypoglycemia normalizes the glycemic thresholds and magnitude of most of neuroendocrine responses to, symptoms of, and cognitive function during hypoglycemia in intensively treated patients with short-term IDDM. Diabetes 1993;42:1683–1689
6. Fanelli C, Pampanelli S, Epifano L, et al. Long-term recovery from unawareness, deficient counterregulation and lack of cognitive dysfunction during hypoglycaemia, following institution of rational, intensive insulin therapy in IDDM. Diabetologia 1994;37:1265–1276
7. Cranston I, Lomas J, Maran A, Macdonald I, Amiel SA. Restoration of hypoglycaemia awareness in patients with long-duration insulin-dependent diabetes. Lancet 1994;344:283–287
8. Dagogo-Jack S, Rattarasarn C, Cryer PE. Reversal of hypoglycemia unawareness, but not defective glucose counterregulation, in IDDM. Diabetes 1994;43:1426–1434
9. Sherwin RS. Bringing light to the dark side of insulin: a journey across the blood-brain barrier. Diabetes 2008;57:2259–2268
10. Dunn JT, Cranston I, Marsden PK, Amiel SA, Reed LJ. Attenuation of amygdala and frontal cortical responses to low blood glucose concentration in asymptomatic hypoglycemia in type 1 diabetes: a new player in hypoglycemia unawareness? Diabetes 2007;56:2766–2773
11. Teves D, Videen TO, Cryer PE, Powers WJ. Activation of human medial prefrontal cortex during autonomic responses to hypoglycemia. Proc Natl Acad Sci USA 2004;101:6217–6221
12. Arbelaez AM, Powers WJ, Videen TO, Price JL, Cryer PE. Attenuation of counterregulatory responses to recurrent hypoglycemia by active thalamic inhibition: a mechanism for hypoglycemia-associated autonomic failure. Diabetes 2008;57:470–475
13. Stjärne L. Catecholaminergic neurotransmission: flagship of all neurobiology. Acta Physiol Scand 1999;166:251–259
14. Bloom FE. The catecholamine neuron: historical and future perspectives. Prog Neurobiol 2010;90:75–81
15. Towler DA, Havlin CE, Craft S, Cryer PE. Mechanism of awareness of hypoglycemia. Perception of neurogenic (predominantly cholinergic) rather than neuroglycopenic symptoms. Diabetes 1993;42:1791–1798
16. Shah SD, Clutter WE, Cryer PE. External and internal standards in the single-isotope derivative (radioenzymatic) measurement of plasma norepinephrine and epinephrine. J Lab Clin Med 1985;106:624–629
17. DeRosa MA, Cryer PE. Hypoglycemia and the sympathoadrenal system: neurogenic symptoms are largely the result of sympathetic neural, rather than adrenomedullary, activation. Am J Physiol Endocrinol Metab 2004;287:E32–E41
18. Schwartz TW. Pancreatic polypeptide: a hormone under vagal control. Gastroenterology 1983;85:1411–1425
19. Cryer PE, Rizza RA, Haymond MW, Gerich JE. Epinephrine and norepinephrine are cleared through beta-adrenergic, but not alpha-adrenergic, mechanisms in man. Metabolism 1980;29(Suppl. 1):1114–1118

Factors Predictive of Severe Hypoglycemia in Type 1 Diabetes

Analysis from the Juvenile Diabetes Research Foundation continuous glucose monitoring randomized control trial dataset

JUVENILE DIABETES RESEARCH FOUNDATION
CONTINUOUS GLUCOSE MONITORING
STUDY GROUP*

OBJECTIVE—Identify factors predictive of severe hypoglycemia (SH) and assess the clinical utility of continuous glucose monitoring (CGM) to warn of impending SH.

RESEARCH DESIGN AND METHODS—In a multicenter randomized clinical trial, 436 children and adults with type 1 diabetes were randomized to a treatment group that used CGM ($N = 224$), or a control group that used standard home blood glucose monitoring ($N = 212$) and completed 12 months of follow-up. After 6 months, the original control group initiated CGM while the treatment group continued use of CGM for 6 months. Baseline risk factors for SH were evaluated over 12 months of follow-up using proportional hazards regression. CGM-derived indices of hypoglycemia were used to predict episodes of SH over a 24-h time horizon.

RESULTS—The SH rate was 17.9 per 100 person-years, and a higher rate was associated with the occurrence of SH in the prior 6 months and female sex. SH frequency increased eightfold when 30% of CGM values were ≤ 70 mg/dL on the prior day (4.5 vs. 0.5%; $P < 0.001$), but the positive predictive value (PPV) was low ($<5\%$). Results were similar for hypoglycemic area under the curve and the low blood glucose index calculated by CGM.

CONCLUSIONS—SH in the 6 months prior to the study was the strongest predictor of SH during the study. CGM-measured hypoglycemia over a 24-h span is highly associated with SH the following day ($P < 0.001$), but the PPV is low.

Diabetes Care 34:586–590, 2011

Current constraints in blood glucose monitoring and insulin delivery technologies limit the ability of most individuals with type 1 diabetes to safely achieve and maintain recommended glucose and hemoglobin A$_{1c}$ (HbA$_{1c}$) targets. Severe hypoglycemia (SH) remains a common side effect of intensive treatment and a major barrier to achieving normoglycemia in type 1 diabetes. Several prior studies have evaluated factors associated with an increased risk of SH. In a study of 1,190 children and adolescents with type 1 diabetes, Craig et al. (1) reported that younger age, male sex, longer duration of diabetes, and intensive insulin therapy (≥ 3 injections/day) were associated with an increased risk of SH. In a study of 60 individuals, mainly adults, with insulin-dependent diabetes, Gold et al. (2) reported that the occurrence of SH was associated with prior SH, hypoglycemia unawareness, older age, and autonomic dysfunction. In the Diabetes Control and Complications Trial (DCCT) (3), an analysis of the first 424 intensively treated subjects found that predictors of SH in the intensive group included prior SH, longer duration of diabetes, higher baseline HbA$_{1c}$, lower recent HbA$_{1c}$, and higher baseline insulin doses. A later analysis of all 1,441 subjects found that a higher SH rate in both treatment groups occurred in subjects with prior SH, longer duration of diabetes, absent residual C-peptide secretion, younger age (adolescents compared with adults), and higher baseline insulin doses; the rate was higher in females than males in the conventional group but not in the intensive group and higher in those with lower baseline HbA$_{1c}$ in the conventional group but not the intensive group (4).

Recurrent episodes of mild hypoglycemia appear to cause defects in counterregulatory hormone responses to subsequent hypoglycemia placing patients with type 1 diabetes at increased risk of severe hypoglycemia. This sequence of events has been termed hypoglycemia-associated autonomic failure. The evidence supporting the development of hypoglycemia-associated autonomic failure was initially demonstrated in clinical research center–based hypoglycemic clamp studies, and a relationship between the risk of SH and antecedent biochemical hypoglycemia in the free living condition also has been reported (5).

The Juvenile Diabetes Research Foundation (JDRF) Continuous Glucose Monitoring Study Group recently reported the results of a 6-month randomized clinical trial and a 6-month extension study that evaluated the effectiveness of real-time continuous glucose monitoring (CGM) in 451 intensively treated type 1 diabetes subjects who had baseline HbA$_{1c}$ levels both within and above the target range (6–11). These studies provided a large dataset to evaluate the association of clinical and demographic factors with the development of SH. In addition, longitudinal CGM glucose data were available to evaluate the relationship between biochemical hypoglycemia detected by CGM and subsequent SH.

RESEARCH DESIGN AND METHODS—The study protocol and clinical characteristics of enrolled subjects have been described in detail (7–9). Major eligibility criteria included age ≥ 8 years, type 1 diabetes for at least 1 year, use of

• •

Corresponding author: Roy W. Beck, jdrfapp@jaeb.org.
Received 11 June 2010 and accepted 29 November 2010.
DOI: 10.2337/dc10-1111. Clinical trial reg. no. NCT00406133, clinicaltrials.gov.
This article contains Supplementary Data online at http://care.diabetesjournals.org/lookup/suppl/doi:10.2337/dc10-1111/-/DC1.
*Members of the writing committee are listed in APPENDIX, and a full group listing is available in the Supplementary Data online.

either an insulin pump or multiple (at least three) daily insulin injections, and HbA$_{1c}$ level <10.0%. Prior SH was not an exclusion and 8% of subjects in both treatment groups self-reported at least one SH event in the 6 months prior to study entry. The study consisted of a 6-month randomized trial in which subjects were randomized to either a control group that used standard home blood glucose monitoring or a CGM group that used one of the following three CGM devices: the FreeStyle Navigator (Abbott Diabetes Care, Inc., Alameda, CA), the MiniMed Paradigm REAL-Time Insulin Pump and Continuous Glucose Monitoring System (Medtronic MiniMed, Inc., Northridge, CA), or the DexCom SEVEN (DexCom, Inc., San Diego, CA). The randomized trial was followed by a 6-month extension study in which CGM was initiated in the control group and continued in the CGM group.

Analysis was limited to 436 (97%) of 451 randomized subjects who completed 12 months of follow-up. The 15 subjects with incomplete follow-up included one subject who was believed to be factitiously producing SH by intentional insulin overdose and 14 others who did not experience SH before dropping out of the study.

SH was defined as an event that required assistance from another person to administer carbohydrate, glucagon, or other resuscitative actions (3). The proportional hazards model was used to evaluate the association of baseline demographic and clinical factors with the occurrence of SH events in univariate models. Factors in the univariate models with a P value < 0.20 were included in an initial multivariate model and then a backward elimination procedure was used to remove variables with a P value > 0.05. However, because of multiple statistical comparisons, only P values < 0.01 were considered significant.

A forward selection process resulted in a similar model. To avoid colinearity in the model building, only one baseline CGM measure of hypoglycemia (percentage of values ≤70 mg/dL) was included in the models. Results were similar for the highly correlated hypoglycemic area under the curve (AUC) and the low blood glucose index (LBGI) (12) calculated from CGM data (data not shown). CGM measures of glycemic variation such as SD, coefficient of variation (defined as SD divided by the mean glucose), and the absolute rate of change (13) were also confounded with percentage of CGM values

≤70 mg/dL and were excluded from the models. Subjects with missing values for covariates were excluded from the corresponding univariate models. For the multivariate models, missing values were treated as a separate category for discrete covariates, and an indicator for missing values was added to the model for continuous covariates.

The SH rates in the control group and CGM group during their first 6 months of usage were compared using a Wilcoxon rank sum test. A paired signed rank test was used to compare the SH rate of the CGM group between the first and second 6 months. A repeated-measures logistic regression with generalized estimating equations was used to compare the SH rate between days with and without CGM use.

A second analysis evaluated the association of four CGM hypoglycemia indices (% ≤70 mg/dL, hypoglycemic AUC, LBGI, and at least 30 consecutive min ≤54 mg/dL) during 1 day with the occurrence of SH on the following day using repeated-measures logistic regression with generalized estimating equations to account for correlated data. Inclusion in this analysis was limited to those subjects who had at least one SH event for which there was at least 12 h of CGM glucose data available from the preceding day. When an additional hypoglycemic event occurred within 3 days after a prior hypoglycemic event, the event was not considered as a new event and was not counted (N = 1). Operating characteristics (sensitivity, specificity, false alarm rate, and positive predictive value [PPV]) are given for various cut points for the four CGM hypoglycemic indices.

RESULTS—One or more SH events occurred in 54 (12%) of the 436 subjects; 36 (8%) subjects experienced one event, 13 (3%) subjects had two events, 4 (0.9%) subjects had three events, and 1 (0.2%) subject had four events. The overall incidence rate of SH was 17.9 events per 100 person-years, being 21.3 in the 160 subjects ≥25 years of age, 16.0 in the 138 subjects 15–24 years of age, and 15.9 in the 138 subjects 8–14 years of age. The rate was 21.5 in the first 6 months of use by the CGM group and 15.0 during the 6 months of CGM use in the control group (which followed the 6-month randomized trial) (P = 0.56). Within the CGM group, there was a trend toward less SH during the second 6 months

compared with the first 6 months (8.0 vs. 21.5 events per 100 person-years, respectively; P = 0.02). The clinical characteristics of the 436 subjects are shown in Supplementary Table 1 according to whether or not an SH event occurred during the study.

In a univariate analysis, SH was more likely to occur in subjects who had experienced SH in the 6 months prior to study entry (P < 0.001), and there were suggestive trends for more frequent SH in adults (P = 0.06), females (P = 0.05), subjects with higher scores on the Hypoglycemia Fear Questionnaire (P = 0.02), those with a higher percentage of baseline CGM values ≤70 mg/dL (P = 0.02), and those who had higher glucose variability as assessed with the coefficient of variation (P = 0.08). In general, these factors also were associated with previous SH; consequently, in multivariate analysis only SH during the prior 6 months (hazard ratio [HR] 6.2 [95% CI 3.4–11.6]; P < 0.001) and female sex (2.3 [1.3–4.1]; P = 0.006) (Table 1) were independent predictors of SH during the study. Although the associations of SH during the prior 6 months and female sex with the occurrence of SH were highly statistically significant, the PPV for each was low (42 and 15%, respectively). The occurrence of SH was not associated with baseline HbA$_{1c}$ level. SH occurred in similar proportions of subjects who used an insulin pump and those who used multiple daily injections of insulin.

The second analysis evaluated the predictive value of CGM-measured hypoglycemia during 1 day with the occurrence of SH on the following day. During the full 12 months of follow-up of the CGM group and the last 6 months of follow-up of the control group (the time period during which CGM was used), 48 SH events occurred in 40 subjects. For 31 of the 48 events (65%), CGM was used on the day of the event, which was comparable with a usage rate of 71% on the 11,994 days without an SH event (P = 0.40). For 27 of the 48 events (N = 24 subjects), a sensor was used on the day prior to the event (for at least 12 h). Median percentage of time with glucose levels ≤70 mg/dL was 3% during the 24 h of the calendar day prior to SH compared with 2% of the time on other days (P < 0.001). Although this association was strong statistically, the PPV was extremely low (~5%), and the false alarm rate was extremely high (~95%) even when 30% or more of the glucose values were

Table 1—*Proportional hazards models of baseline factors predictive of SH (N = 436 subjects who completed the 52-week visit)***

	N	% SH‡	Univariate			Initial multivariate*			Final multivariate†		
			HR	95% CI	P value	HR	95% CI	P value	HR	95% CI	P value
Overall	436	12									
Age (years)					0.06§			0.29§			
8–14	138	10	1.0			1.0					
15–24	138	12	1.2	(0.6–2.5)		0.8	(0.4–1.7)				
≥25	160	14	1.4	(0.7–2.8)		1.0	(0.5–2.0)				
Sex					0.05			0.02			0.006
Male	199	9	1.0			1.0			1.0		
Female	237	15	1.8	(1.0–3.1)		2.2	(1.2–4.1)		2.3	(1.3–4.1)	
n SH events in 6 months prior to study					<0.001			<0.001			<0.001
None	400	10	1.0			1.0			1.0		
≥1	36	42	5.0	(2.8–9.2)		5.5	(2.8–10.6)		6.2	(3.4–11.6)	
Fingersticks per day‖					0.65§						
≤5	135	17	1.0								
6–8	179	8	0.5	(0.2–0.9)							
≥9	69	13	0.8	(0.4–1.7)							
Insulin delivery					0.70						
Injections	80	14	1.0								
Pump	356	12	0.9	(0.5–1.7)							
HbA$_{1c}$ (%)					0.32§						
<7.0	127	13	1.0								
7.0 to <8.0	197	14	1.1	(0.6–2.1)							
≥8.0	112	9	0.7	(0.3–1.5)							
Hypo Fear Score¶					0.02§			0.46§			
<20	151	8	1.0			1.0					
20 to <30	96	15	1.9	(0.9–4.2)		1.5	(0.7–3.3)				
≥30	184	15	2.0	(1.0–3.9)		1.4	(0.7–2.9)				
% CGM values ≤70 mg/dL (%)#					0.02§			0.75§			
None	25	8	1.0			1.0					
<5	207	9	1.2	(0.3–5.0)		0.9	(0.2–3.8)				
5 to <15	160	16	2.1	(0.5–8.9)		1.2	(0.2–5.6)				
≥15	44	16	2.1	(0.4–10.2)		1.3	(0.2–8.3)				
Glucose coefficient of variation (%)††					0.088§			0.54§			
<35	116	7	1.0			1.0					
35 to <40	115	13	2.0	(0.8–4.6)		1.9	(0.8–4.5)				
40 to <45	88	16	2.5	(1.0–5.9)		2.4	(0.9–6.2)				
≥45	117	15	2.2	(0.9–5.0)		1.5	(0.5–4.3)				

*Factors with P value ≤ 0.20 in univariate model are included in the initial multivariate model. †Factors with P value ≤ 0.05 in the initial multivariate model are kept in the final multivariate model. ‡Percentage of subjects with at least one SH event during the study. §P value calculated as a continuous variable. Categories are for display purposes in this table. ‖Self-reported number of home glucose meter tests per day. Data collected after study initialization and are therefore missing for 53 subjects. ¶Hypoglycemia Fear Questionnaire (20) consists of 15 5-point Likert scale items, with scores scaled to a 0–100 range. Higher score denotes more fear of hypoglycemia. Missing for five subjects. #CGM data based on blinded use at baseline for approximately 1 week prior to randomization. Results were similar for hypoglycemic AUC and LBGI (12) (data not shown). **Diabetes duration was not associated with SH. Data not shown because this factor was highly confounded with age. ††Coefficient of variation is the SD divided by the mean glucose from the CGM expressed as a percentage.

≤70 mg/dL on the day prior to a SH event (Table 2). Findings were similar for hypoglycemic AUC (0.2 on the day prior to SH vs. 0.1 on other days, P = 0.002) and LBGI (1.1 vs. 0.8, P = 0.003), with PPVs being low and false-positive rates being high for each (Supplementary Table 2). Results also were similar when assessing the predictive value of 30 consecutive min below 54 mg/dL (Supplementary Table 2). Median glucose was 131 mg/dL on the day prior to an SH event and 141 mg/dL on other days (P = 0.86).

CONCLUSIONS—We found the rate of occurrence of SH during the study to be most strongly associated with a history of SH in the 6 months prior to entry into the study. In addition, the rate was higher in females than males. Both of these findings are consistent with prior findings in the DCCT (3,4). As in our study, multivariate analyses conducted on the DCCT data did not identify a predictive model with high sensitivity (3). The incidence rate of SH in this study (17.9 events per 100 person-years) was similar to that of the

conventional therapy group in the DCCT (18.7 events per 100 person-years), but significantly lower than the rate in the intensive treatment group (61.2 events per 100 person-years) in the DCCT (Supplementary Fig. 1) (4). A similar SH rate was found in the Sensor-Augmented Pump Therapy for A1c Reduction (STAR) 3 trial (~13 events per 100 person-years in both the CGM group and control group) (14). Our results need to be viewed in the context of the study participants who were well-versed in self-management, were receiving

Table 2—*Sensitivity, specificity, false alarm rates, and PPV of CGM-measured hypoglycemia on 1 day for the occurrence of SH on the following day*

CGM glucose readings ≤70 mg/dL on prior day (%)	Total	No SH	SH	Sensitivity*	Specificity†	False alarm‡	PPV§
0	2,009	1,999	10				
>0	3,286	3,269	17	63%	38%	99.5%	0.5%
≤5	3,292	3,278	14				
>5	2,003	1,990	13	48%	62%	99.4%	0.7%
≤15	4,613	4,596	17				
>15	682	672	10	37%	87%	98.5%	1.5%
≤30	5,184	5,162	22				
>30	111	106	5	19%	98%	95.5%	4.5%
All	5,295	5,268	27				

*Sensitivity, Proportion of true SH events where the CGM indices correctly predicted the prior days as positive. †Specificity, Proportion of days without SH where the CGM indices correctly predicted the prior days as negative. ‡False alarm, Proportion of days with CGM indices predicted as positive where there were no SH in the following days. §PPV, Proportion of days with CGM indices predicted as positive where there were SH events in the following days (this is 100% minus the false alarm rate).

intensive insulin management with either an insulin pump or multiple daily injections of insulin, and were performing frequent home blood glucose monitoring.

We also found that CGM-measured hypoglycemia occurred more often on days prior to SH than on other days. However, although the statistical association was strong, the predictive value of biochemical hypoglycemia for subsequent SH was very low. This is because on any given day, SH is a rare event (<1% probability). This probability increases eightfold when more than 30% of CGM values the day prior are in the hypoglycemic range, but there is still less than a 5% chance of SH on the following day. Thus, if a CGM were programmed to sound a warning whenever 30% of values over a 24-h period were ≤70 mg/dL, more than 95% of alarms would be false. The four CGM measures of hypoglycemia studied here (% ≤70 mg/dL, AUC, LBGI, and ≤54 mg/dL for at least 30 consecutive min) are all highly correlated, and results were similar regardless which was used.

One possibility to in part explain the low predictive value could be that subjects modified their diabetes management based on the presence of CGM-measured hypoglycemia, and this reduced their risk of an SH event on the next day. Evidence against this explanation, however, is that during the randomized trial phase of the study, the SH rate in the CGM group was similar to that in the control group (8,9). Another possible factor contributing to the low PPV is measurement error from CGM. Studies of CGM accuracy have

shown that the median error during hypoglycemia ranges from 13 to 24 mg/dL (15,16) so that some episodes of true biochemical hypoglycemia are missed by CGM, and some CGM readings in the hypoglycemic range occur when the true glucose concentration is >70 mg/dL.

Kovatchev et al. (17) studied 96 adults with insulin-dependent diabetes and found that history of SH and LBGI calculated from 1 month of home glucose meter data accounted for 40% of the variance of SH episodes over the following 6 months. In another study of 85 adults with type 1 diabetes, Kovatchev et al. (18) reported that LBGI values from home glucose meter data were significantly higher in the 24 h prior to and immediately following an SH episode compared with other days in the same subjects. Cox et al. (19) reported that LBGI was predictive of SH with a sensitivity rate of 58–60% among 100 adults with type 1 diabetes, but did not report the false-positive rate. Our results with CGM data were similar to these studies in that hypoglycemic indices were significantly higher on the day prior to an SH event and that over 50% of SH events could be predicted from these measures depending on the threshold used. However, our data also show a very large false alarm rate (≥95%) when these indices are used to predict SH events. The SH rates in these previous studies, ranging from 192 to 803 events per 100 person-years (17–19), were much larger than that observed in the current study (17.9 events per 100 person-years) and in the DCCT.

In conclusion, the ability to predict the likelihood that SH will occur in the near future remains elusive. The strongest predictor is the occurrence of prior SH. Although biochemical hypoglycemia substantially increases the risk of the occurrence of SH on the next day, SH only occurs in about 1 in 20 days after preceding biochemical hypoglycemia, and thus this is a poor predictor.

Acknowledgments—The study funding was provided by JDRF (grant numbers 22-2006-1107, 22-2006-1117, 22-2006-1112, 22-2006-1123, and 01-2006-8031).

Continuous glucose monitors and sensors were purchased at a bulk discount price from DexCom, Inc. (San Diego, CA), Medtronic MiniMed, Inc. (Northridge, CA), and Abbott Diabetes Care, Inc. (Alameda, CA). Home glucose meters and test strips were provided to the study by LifeScan, Inc. and Abbott Diabetes Care, Inc. The companies had no involvement in the design, conduct, or analysis of the trial or the manuscript preparation.

Below is a listing of relationships of the investigators with companies that make products relevant to the manuscript. Research funds where listed below were provided to the legal entity that employs the individual and not directly to the individual.

B.B. reports having received consulting fees, honoraria, travel reimbursement, and research funds from Medtronic MiniMed, Inc. and grant support from DexCom, Inc. B.A.B. reports having received grant support and serving on the Medical Advisory Board for Medtronic MiniMed, Inc., grant support and a speaker honorarium from Abbott Diabetes Care, Inc., and grant support from DexCom, Inc. C.K. reports having received consulting fees from Medtronic MiniMed, Inc. L.L. reports having received consulting fees and a speaker honorarium from Abbott Diabetes Care, Inc., and consulting fees and research funding from Medtronic MiniMed, Inc. W.V.T. reports having received consulting fees from Medtronic MiniMed, Inc. S.W. reports having received research support, a speaker honorarium and travel reimbursement from Medtronic MiniMed, Inc., and a speaker honorarium from Animas Corp/LifeScan, Inc. No other potential conflicts of interest relevant to this article were reported.

The study was designed and conducted by the investigators. The writing group collectively wrote the manuscript and vouches for the data. The investigators had complete autonomy to analyze and report the trial results. There were no agreements concerning confidentiality of the data between JDRF, the authors, or their institutions. The Jaeb Center for Health Research had full access to all of the data in the study and takes responsibility for the integrity of the data and the accuracy of the data analysis.

R.F.-S. researched data, contributed to discussion, wrote the manuscript, and reviewed and edited the manuscript. J.C. contributed to discussion, wrote the manuscript, and reviewed and edited the manuscript. R.W.B. contributed to discussion and reviewed and edited the manuscript. B.B. researched data, contributed to discussion, and reviewed and edited the manuscript. B.A.B. researched data, contributed to discussion, and reviewed and edited the manuscript. H.P.C. researched data, contributed to discussion, and reviewed and edited the manuscript. L.L. researched data, contributed to discussion, and reviewed and edited the manuscript. J.M.L. researched data, contributed to discussion, and reviewed and edited the manuscript. C.K. contributed to discussion and reviewed and edited the manuscript. N.M. researched data, contributed to discussion, and reviewed and edited the manuscript. K.J.R. researched data, contributed to discussion, and reviewed and edited the manuscript. W.V.T. researched data, contributed to discussion, and reviewed and edited the manuscript. S.W. researched data, contributed to discussion, and reviewed and edited the manuscript. D.M.W. researched data, contributed to discussion, and reviewed and edited the manuscript. H.W. researched data, contributed to discussion, and reviewed and edited the manuscript. D.X. contributed to discussion and reviewed and edited the manuscript.

The JDRF CGM Study Group would like to recognize the efforts of the subjects and their families and thanks them for their participation.

APPENDIX

APPENDIX—Co-authors: Rosanna Fiallo-Scharer, MD[1]; Jing Cheng, MS[2]. Additional authors (in alphabetical order): Roy W. Beck, MD, PHD[2]; Bruce A. Buckingham, MD[3]; H. Peter Chase, MD[1]; Craig Kollman, PHD[2]; Lori Laffel, MD, MPH[4]; Jean M. Lawrence, SCD, MPH, MSSA[5]; Nelly Mauras, MD[6]; William V. Tamborlane, MD[7]; Darrell M. Wilson, MD[3]; Howard Wolpert, MD[4], of the JDRF Continuous Glucose Monitoring Study Group.

[1]Barbara Davis Center for Childhood Diabetes, Aurora, Colorado; the [2]Jaeb Center for Health Research, Tampa, Florida; [3]Stanford University, Stanford, California; the [4]Joslin Diabetes Center, Boston, Massachusetts; [5]Kaiser Permanente, San Diego, California; the [6]Nemours Children's Clinic, Jacksonville, Florida; and [7]Yale University, New Haven, Connecticut.

Additional writing committee members include Bruce Bode, MD[1]; Katrina J. Ruedy, MSPH[2]; Stuart Weinzimer, MD[3]; Dongyuan Xing, MPH[2].

[1]Atlanta Diabetes Associates, Atlanta, Georgia; the [2]Jaeb Center for Health Research, Tampa, Florida; and [3]Yale University, New Haven, Connecticut.

References

1. Craig ME, Handelsman P, Donaghue KC, et al.; NSW/ACT HbA(1c) Study Group. Predictors of glycaemic control and hypoglycaemia in children and adolescents with type 1 diabetes from NSW and the ACT. Med J Aust 2002;177:235–238
2. Gold AE, Frier BM, MacLeod KM, Deary IJ. A structural equation model for predictors of severe hypoglycaemia in patients with insulin-dependent diabetes mellitus. Diabet Med 1997;14:309–315
3. The DCCT Research Group. Epidemiology of severe hypoglycemia in the Diabetes Control and Complications Trial. Am J Med 1991;90:450–459
4. The Diabetes Control and Complications Trial Research Group. Hypoglycemia in the Diabetes Control and Complications Trial. Diabetes 1997;46:271–286
5. White NH, Skor DA, Cryer PE, Levandoski LA, Bier DM, Santiago JV. Identification of type I diabetic patients at increased risk for hypoglycemia during intensive therapy. N Engl J Med 1983;308:485–491
6. Chase HP, Beck RW, Xing D, et al. Continuous glucose monitoring in youth with type 1 diabetes: 12-month follow-up of the Juvenile Diabetes Research Foundation continuous glucose monitoring randomized trial. Diabetes Technol Ther 2010;12:507–515
7. JDRF CGM Study Group. JDRF randomized clinical trial to assess the efficacy of real-time continuous glucose monitoring in the management of type 1 diabetes: research design and methods. Diabetes Technol Ther 2008;10:310–321
8. Tamborlane WV, Beck RW, Bode BW, et al.; Juvenile Diabetes Research Foundation Continuous Glucose Monitoring Study Group. Continuous glucose monitoring and intensive treatment of type 1 diabetes. N Engl J Med 2008;359:1464–1476
9. Juvenile Diabetes Research Foundation Continuous Glucose Monitoring Study Group. The effect of continuous glucose monitoring in well-controlled type 1 diabetes. Diabetes Care 2009;32:1378–1383
10. Bode B, Beck RW, Xing D, et al.; Juvenile Diabetes Research Foundation Continuous Glucose Monitoring Study Group. Sustained benefit of continuous glucose monitoring on A1C, glucose profiles, and hypoglycemia in adults with type 1 diabetes. Diabetes Care 2009;32:2047–2049
11. Juvenile Diabetes Research Foundation Continuous Glucose Monitoring Study Group. Effectiveness of continuous glucose monitoring in a clinical care environment: evidence from the Juvenile Diabetes Research Foundation Continuous Glucose Monitoring (JDRF-CGM) trial. Diabetes Care 2010;33:17–22
12. Kovatchev BP, Cox DJ, Gonder-Frederick LA, Clarke W. Symmetrization of the blood glucose measurement scale and its applications. Diabetes Care 1997;20:1655–1658
13. Kovatchev BP, Clarke WL, Breton M, Brayman K, McCall A. Quantifying temporal glucose variability in diabetes via continuous glucose monitoring: mathematical methods and clinical application. Diabetes Technol Ther 2005;7:849–862
14. Bergenstal RM, Tamborlane WV, Ahmann A, et al.; STAR 3 Study Group. Effectiveness of sensor-augmented insulin-pump therapy in type 1 diabetes. N Engl J Med 2010;363:311–320
15. Diabetes Research in Children Network (DirecNet) Study Group. The accuracy of the Guardian RT continuous glucose monitor in children with type 1 diabetes. Diabetes Technol Ther 2008;10:266–272
16. Wilson DM, Beck RW, Tamborlane WV, et al.; DirecNet Study Group. The accuracy of the FreeStyle Navigator continuous glucose monitoring system in children with type 1 diabetes. Diabetes Care 2007;30:59–64
17. Kovatchev BP, Cox DJ, Gonder-Frederick LA, Young-Hyman D, Schlundt D, Clarke W. Assessment of risk for severe hypoglycemia among adults with IDDM: validation of the low blood glucose index. Diabetes Care 1998;21:1870–1875
18. Kovatchev BP, Cox DJ, Farhy LS, Straume M, Gonder-Frederick L, Clarke WL. Episodes of severe hypoglycemia in type 1 diabetes are preceded and followed within 48 hours by measurable disturbances in blood glucose. J Clin Endocrinol Metab 2000;85:4287–4292
19. Cox DJ, Gonder-Frederick L, Ritterband L, Clarke W, Kovatchev BP. Prediction of severe hypoglycemia. Diabetes Care 2007;30:1370–1373
20. Cox DJ, Irvine A, Gonder-Frederick L, Nowacek G, Butterfield J. Fear of hypoglycemia: quantification, validation, and utilization. Diabetes Care 1987;10:617–621

Real-Time Hypoglycemia Prediction Suite Using Continuous Glucose Monitoring

A safety net for the artificial pancreas

Eyal Dassau, phd[1,2]
Fraser Cameron, ms[3]
Hyunjin Lee, phd[4]
B. Wayne Bequette, phd[4]
Howard Zisser, md[1,2]

Lois Jovanovič, md[1,2]
H. Peter Chase, md[5]
Darrell M. Wilson, md[6]
Bruce A. Buckingham, md[6]
Francis J. Doyle III, phd[1,2]

OBJECTIVE — The purpose of this study was to develop an advanced algorithm that detects pending hypoglycemia and then suspends basal insulin delivery. This approach can provide a solution to the problem of nocturnal hypoglycemia, a major concern of patients with diabetes.

RESEARCH DESIGN AND METHODS — This real-time hypoglycemia prediction algorithm (HPA) combines five individual algorithms, all based on continuous glucose monitoring 1-min data. A predictive alarm is issued by a voting algorithm when a hypoglycemic event is predicted to occur in the next 35 min. The HPA system was developed using data derived from 21 Navigator studies that assessed Navigator function over 24 h in children with type 1 diabetes. We confirmed the function of the HPA using a separate dataset from 22 admissions of type 1 diabetic subjects. During these admissions, hypoglycemia was induced by gradual increases in the basal insulin infusion rate up to 180% from the subject's own baseline infusion rate.

RESULTS — Using a prediction horizon of 35 min, a glucose threshold of 80 mg/dl, and a voting threshold of three of five algorithms to predict hypoglycemia (defined as a FreeStyle plasma glucose readings <60 mg/dl), the HPA predicted 91% of the hypoglycemic events. When four of five algorithms were required to be positive, then 82% of the events were predicted.

CONCLUSIONS — The HPA will enable automated insulin-pump suspension in response to a pending event that has been detected prior to severe immediate complications.

Diabetes Care 33:1249–1254, 2010

The Diabetes Control and Complications Trial (DCCT) proved that glucose control in the closer-to-normal range (tight glycemic control) reduced the likelihood of eye, kidney, nerve, and cardiovascular complications of diabetes (1,2). Unfortunately, the DCCT also showed that the incidence of severe hypoglycemia was three times higher in the intensively treated group compared with the standard treatment group (1). In the DCCT, 55% of the severe lows occurred during sleep hours (1). Further, in the ad-

olescent portion of the DCCT, the risk for severe hypoglycemia was even greater, with one episode every 1.17 years (85.7 per 100 patient-years) (2). One report in children found 75% of severe lows to occur during the nighttime hours (3). The high frequency and duration of nocturnal hypoglycemia has been confirmed in clinical research center (CRC) studies, in which frequent laboratory reference glucose values were obtained. For example, in a DirecNet study of exercise-induced nocturnal hypoglycemia, children who

did not exercise had a 28% incidence of nocturnal hypoglycemia (glucose <60 mg/dl), and those who exercised had a 48% incidence of nocturnal hypoglycemia (4). In a recent study (5) of bedtime snacks and nocturnal hypoglycemia, on nights when adult subjects did not have a snack, 57% became hypoglycemic (<70 mg/dl), with an average duration of hypoglycemia of over 2.5 h. In this study, the duration of hypoglycemia was as long as 8.75 h.

Real-time continuous glucose monitoring (CGM) is becoming available with the Food and Drug Administration (FDA) approval of the MiniMed Guardian, the DexCom STS, and the Abbott Navigator. One of the major perceived benefits of real-time glucose monitoring is the ability of these devices to have alarms for hypoglycemia. For a real-time alarm to be effective, it must awaken a sleeping subject. The first FDA-approved real-time glucose monitor was the GlucoWatch™. To determine whether the alarm function on the GlucoWatch was effective in awakening children while they were sleeping, an infrared camera was used to videotape them throughout the night in the CRCs. During this admission, reference glucose values were obtained every half hour to document hypoglycemia. In this study, 71% of youths wearing the watch did not respond to nighttime alarms (6), placing these patients at a risk for nocturnal hypoglycemia despite wearing a real-time continuous glucose sensor. One possible correction of this problem would be to have the sensor send a signal to the pump so that it will stop infusing insulin when pending or real hypoglycemia has been reached and the patient has not responded to alarms. This is the primary focus of the hypoglycemia prediction algorithm.

Previous studies (7–9) have shown that when insulin infusion is stopped for 2 h or when an infusion set is disconnected for up to 30 min (7), there is essentially no risk of the patient developing significant ketones or acidosis. Three previous studies (8–10) have demonstrated that turning off an insulin pump for 2 h

From the [1]Department of Chemical Engineering, University of California Santa Barbara, Santa Barbara, California; the [2]Sansum Diabetes Research Institute, Santa Barbara, California; the [3]Department of Aeronautics and Astronautics, Stanford University, Palo Alto, California; the [4]Department of Chemical and Biological Engineering, Rensselaer Polytechnic Institute, Troy, New York; the [5]Barbara Davis Center for Childhood Diabetes, University of Colorado Health Sciences Center, Aurora, Colorado; and the [6]Department of Pediatrics, Division of Pediatric Endocrinology, Stanford Medical Center, Palo Alto, California.
Corresponding author: Eyal Dassau, dassau@engineering.ucsb.edu.
Received 10 August 2009 and accepted 18 January 2010. DOI: 10.2337/dc09-1487.

did not result in diabetic ketoacidosis (DKA). In all three studies, blood β-hydroxybutyrate concentrations were determined using both a meter (Precision Xtra™) and the hospital laboratory. In two of the studies (9,10), the continuous subcutaneous insulin infusion pumps were purposely turned off for periods of 4 and 5 h, with a gradual increase in β-hydroxybutyratek concentrations after 2 h to the upper normal range. No cases of DKA occurred in these studies.

RESEARCH DESIGN AND METHODS

The hypoglycemia prediction algorithm (HPA) was developed using data derived from 21 Navigator studies, which assessed Navigator function over 24 h in children with type 1 diabetes, aged 3–18 years, conducted in clinical research centers (CRCs) (11). Then the HPA functionality was confirmed using a separate dataset from 22 CRC admissions of type 1 diabetic subjects with a mean age of 20 years (range 6–38). In this study, hypoglycemia was induced by gradual increases in the basal insulin infusion rate by a mean of 180%, 18 of 22 subjects (82%) reached a glucose value of ≤60 mg/dl (12,13). Promising results were reported by Buckingham et al. (12), where when two different algorithms were used 60% of the pending hypoglycemic events were predicted and prevented.

CGM data were introduced to the HPA as if it were a real-time measurement; the different algorithms analyzed the data and an alarm was produced if a quorum was reached by the voting algorithm. Three hypoglycemia thresholds of 70, 80, and 90 mg/dl were evaluated, each with three different prediction horizons (V) of 35, 45, and 55 min and with three voting thresholds of 3, 4, and 5.

Hypoglycemia Prediction Algorithm

The core of the HPA is a set of individual alarms that are combined through a voting system into one combined alarm. With each new CGM datum, each individual alarm will run independently and will indicate hypoglycemia or euglycemia. Then, if the number of individual alarms that have gone off in the last 10 min is above a preset voting threshold (V), the voting alarm will trigger. A low voting threshold will generate more alarms, giving more warning but less accuracy. Finally, the combined alarm will trigger if either the voting alarm or the threshold alarm goes off. Figure 1 shows the flow

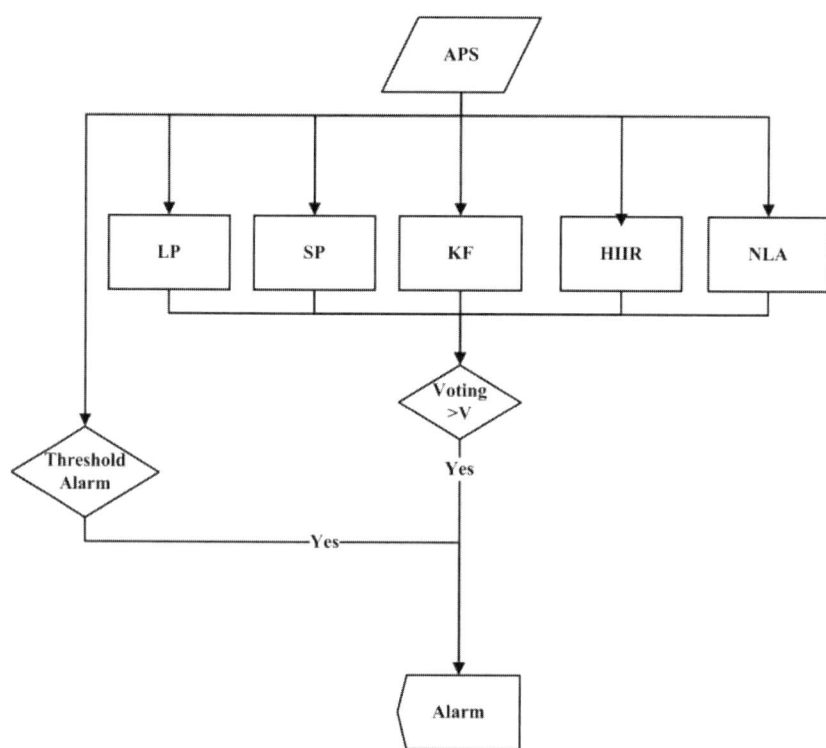

Figure 1—*Hypoglycemia alarm flowchart. The overall alarming algorithm combines multiple independent alarms into one single alarm using a voting system, where APS is the artificial Pancreas Software (24) feeding the data to the algorithms, LP is the linear prediction algorithm, SP is statistical prediction algorithm, KF is the Kalman filter algorithm, HIIR is the hybrid impulse response filter, and NLA is the numerical logical algorithm.*

of the combined hypoglycemic detection algorithm (14). Glucose predictions and analysis from CGM data can be performed in more than one way by applying different mathematical methods such as optimal estimation techniques (15,16), time series (17), and other methods. The HPA system consists of five prediction algorithms:

1. Linear projection: This alarm uses a 15-min linear extrapolation and uncertainty threshold based on the SD of the glucose measurements in the previous 15 min.
2. Kalman filtering: A Kalman filter is used to estimate glucose and its rate of change, which are then used to make predictions about future glucose levels. The filter is tuned to trade off the probability that a measured glucose change is real versus the result of sensor noise. The approach is presented in more detail in simulation studies by Palerm et al. (16) and applied to clinical hypoglycemic clamp data in Palerm and Bequette (18) and as part of a meal detection algorithm in Dassau et al. (19).

3. Hybrid infinite impulse response filter: The infinite impulse response filter takes advantage of a linear discrete-time signal-processing method (20) that generates output predictions using previous output (measured glucose concentration) without input (insulin infusion). Predicted outputs are recursively applied to the filter coefficients for a prediction horizon. The filter coefficients are updated when prediction and parameter errors are larger than user-specified bounds. The hybrid filter prediction with a factor (α) between fixed and adaptive filter coefficients is considered for safe and accurate glucose predictions. It is flexible to tune the filter performance by adjusting the data window length (WL), prediction horizon (p), and error criteria (ε_1 and ε_2).
4. Statistical prediction: Multiple empirical, statistical models are used to estimate future blood glucose values and their error bounds. From these, a probability of hypoglycemia is generated and thresholded to produce an alarm. The statistical prediction algorithm is divided into three compo-

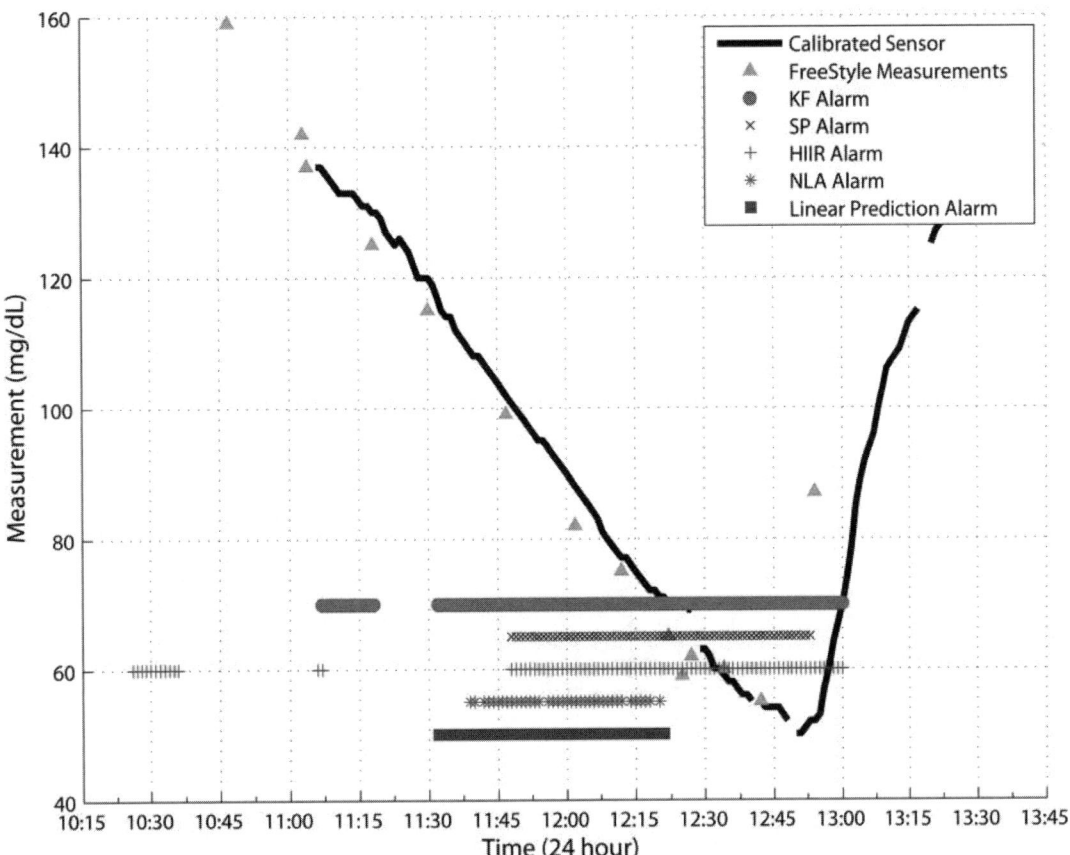

Figure 2—*An example hypoglycemic event and successful detection using an alarm threshold of 70 mg/dl and a prediction horizon of 55 min. A high-quality digital representation of this figure is available in the online issue.*

nents: *1*) calibration, which converts raw CGM and capillary blood glucose measurements into a physiologically consistent, accurate blood glucose history; *2*) prediction, which uses training data and the recent calibrated blood glucose history to generate predictions and associated accuracy estimates; and *3*) hypoglycemic alarming, which transforms the predictions and accuracy estimates into a probability of the patient becoming hypoglycemic, which is then thresholded into a binary alarm (12,21).

5. Numerical logical algorithm: Numerical logical algorithm feeds a three-point calculated rate of change using backward difference approximation and the current glucose value into logical expressions to detect impending hypoglycemia. The logical expressions verify that the rate of change is both negative and within an acceptable range as well as that the CGM glucose values are within predefined boundaries and that a pending hypoglycemic event is predicted within the threshold time window. Numerical

logical algorithm provides insensitivity to sensor signal dropouts and easy tuning.

Voting system
The voting system, as described in Fig. 1, polls each algorithm to determine whether it should alarm. If the number of algorithms that predict hypoglycemia is above the voting threshold (V) more than twice in a time window of 10 min (first crossing will prime the alarm and the second will fire the alarm) or the sensor blood glucose is below the hypoglycemic threshold, then the alarm sounds. Therefore, an alarm sounds if one of the following is true:

- The number of individual alarms meets or exceeds the voting threshold;
- The sensor interstitial glucose value is below the hypoglycemic threshold.

RESULTS — The five hypoglycemic prediction alarms were run for all proposed parameter combinations on 18 sets of data from 18 admissions. It should be noted that the reported results are based

solely on the predictive part of the method.

As can be seen from Fig. 2, hypoglycemia was reached at around noon (defined as glucose ≤70 mg/dl). This event has been predicted by the different algorithms 55, 45, and 35 min ahead of the event, and an alarm could have been issued at this time depending on the quorum threshold (e.g., 55-min warning time if two different algorithms were to issue a positive vote twice in a 10 min window). If the number of positive alarms required was three or four, a warning time would have been 40 and 35 min, respectively, sufficient time for a suspension of the pump to have prevented the event.

Table 1 shows the results from running the individual and combined algorithms against the historical pump shut-off data. The numbered columns (e.g., 1, 2, 3, 4, and 5) indicate the voting threshold for the case. The data also show that the prediction rate declines as the voting threshold increases. This can be seen in the range of prediction times obtained by varying the settings of the tuning param-

Table 1—*HPA ability to predict hypoglycemia events based on historical datasets with different voting thresholds*

Prediction horizon (min)	Alarm threshold (mg/dl)	Percent predicted hypoglycemic events for the given alarm scenario									
		1	2	3	4	5	KF	SP	HIIR	NLA	LP
35	70	91	64	55	36	18	82	55	45	91	55
45	70	100	82	73	64	36	100	64	64	91	73
55	70	100	100	100	82	36	100	100	82	91	100
35	80	100	100	91	82	45	100	100	82	91	82
45	80	100	100	100	91	64	100	100	91	91	91
55	80	100	100	100	100	82	100	100	100	91	91
35	90	100	100	82	73	55	100	100	91	64	73
45	90	100	100	82	82	55	100	100	100	64	73
55	90	100	100	82	82	55	100	100	100	64	73

LP, linear prediction algorithm; KF, Kalman filter algorithm; HIIR, hybrid impulse response filter; NLA, numerical logical algorithm; SP, statistical prediction algorithm.

eters, namely, hypoglycemia prediction time, hypoglycemia threshold value, and the voting threshold. As an example, 91% of the events were predicted 35 min prior to the event using a voting threshold of three, where voting of four of five predicted 82% of the events 35–55 min ahead with glucose threshold of 80 mg/dl. However, in theory, a higher success rate could be obtained by allowing any one of five to issue an alarm. This balance between aggressiveness of the HPA and ef-

fectiveness is an important factor since too many false alarms are a detriment to safety systems will result in disconnecting of the system by the user, rendering the system useless. HPA tuning knobs (prediction horizon, alarm threshold, and voting threshold, as seen in Table 1) allows the algorithm to be adjusted to meet the subject preferences as far as defining the hypoglycemia threshold, time to alarm prior to the event, and aggressiveness of the algorithm. These settings

could vary between day and night and be tuned to meet individual insulin sensitivity, allowing the user to enhance specificity that would prevent false alarms resulting in pump suspension, where during the day a more aggressive tuning can be set that can alert the user to take corrective action prior to the need to suspend the pump. The use of a CGM in clinical decision making is the first step toward the artificial pancreas. The prevention of nocturnal hypoglycemia based on glucose predictions as well as missed-meal alarms will reduce glucose variability and clinical complications resulting from extreme blood glucose concentrations. CGM technology, together with telemedicine applications such as E911 (22), can provide remote glucose monitoring and triangulation as well as pump suspension. This technology will help in improving the well-being of people with diabetes and peace of mind to families of children with diabetes.

When a safety algorithm is suggested, the false-positive rate is equally as important as the true-positive rate. The evaluation of the true positive has been addressed based on retrospective analysis of clinical data. The specificity of the algorithm was further evaluated

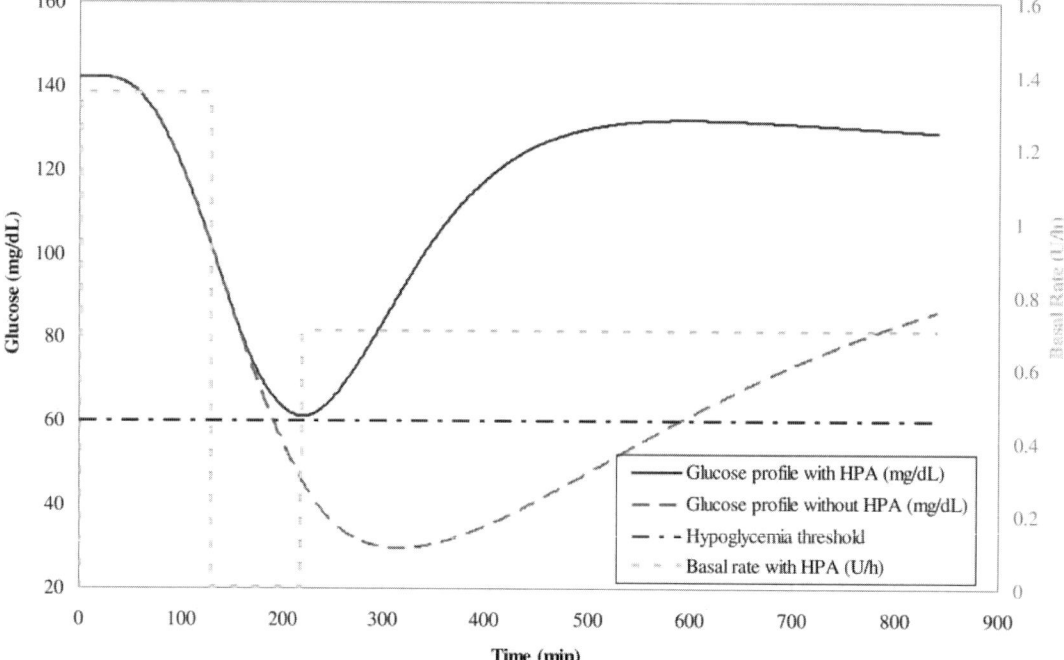

Figure 3—*HPA evaluation using the UVa/Padova Metabolic Simulator following a clinical scenario in which an erroneous basal delivery, twice the usual one, was set by the user. As can be seen in the plot, without the use of HPA the subject experienced severe hypoglycemia (red dashed line) and with the algorithm this event was prevented (blue line) by suspending the basal rate for 90 min and restoring the correct basal (green dotted line). The black dashed-dotted line denotes the hypoglycemia threshold as defined by blood glucose. A high-quality digital representation of this figure is available in the online issue.*

prospectively using the UVa/Padova FDA-accepted (23) Metabolic Simulator and is currently under clinical evaluation that will be reported in a subsequent publication. The frequency of false-positive alarms of the HPA has been assessed by running the simulator under standard conditions with a meal at 5:00 P.M., starting the hypoglycemia prediction algorithms at 9:00 P.M. and running it until 7:00 A.M. the following morning before a breakfast meal. Furthermore, the HPA was evaluated overnight using twice the usual basal insulin in order to induce hypoglycemia. The prospective analysis of the algorithm with tuning of 80 mg/dl, 45 min, and two for hypoglycemia threshold, prediction horizon and voting threshold, respectively, is provided below. This simulation supported the clinical results with only four in silico subjects crossing the 60 mg/dl blood glucose threshold out of 100 in silico adult subjects, where the glucose nadir is marginally <60 mg/dl. As can be seen from Fig. 3, the HPA predicted a pending hypoglycemic event when glucose concentration was ~104 mg/dl and suspended the pump for 90 min. This resulted in prevention of the event where, in successive simulation without the use of the algorithm, the glucose dropped to extremely low values. The false-positive rate of the algorithm with the same tuning was 9% based on a population of 100 different in silico subjects and noisy sensor. However, only three out of the nine cases where a false alarm was issued resulted in a glucose elevation of >20 mg/dl from the baseline that resulted in hyperglycemic event. It should be noted that this needs to be further evaluated by extensive clinical trials to better assess the algorithm.

The use of a sophisticated voting algorithm allows an extra degree of safety prior to issuing an alarm. In addition, voting enables the use of five different individual algorithms to predict pending hypoglycemia and not to rely on one algorithm that may or may not be the most suitable to address the variability among type 1 diabetic subjects. Furthermore, the use of a suite of algorithms allows a more robust system that can cope with glucose variability and the different glucose drop patterns that may affect rate of change and the ability to detect a pending event by a single algorithm.

CONCLUSIONS — The use of the HPA would allow for triggering of a warning alarm and/or suspension of an insulin

pump, which should decrease the risk of severe hypoglycemia. Based on clinical evaluation, insulin delivery will most likely need to be suspended 30–50 min before a projected hypoglycemic event in order to prevent most hypoglycemic events (12). On one hand, longer prediction time may provide greater ability to prevent hypoglycemia events; on the other hand, it may be impractical to suspend a pump too far from an event that may not happen due to human factors (e.g., a planned meal). The Hypoglycemia Prediction Algorithm (HPA) tuning allows flexibility in the aggressiveness of the alarm and can be set to meet user preferences. Furthermore, this technology can be easily implemented in current CGM systems and as a safety net to further artificial pancreas development.

Acknowledgments— We acknowledge the Juvenile Diabetes Research Foundation (grants 22-2006-1115, 22-2006-1108, and 22-2007-479) and the Otis Williams Fund at the Santa Barbara Foundation for their financial support.

H.P.C. has received supplies/devices for research purposes from Abbott Diabetes Care. B.A.B. was given honorarium from Abbott Diabetes Care for a lecture in February 2009. No other potential conflicts of interest relevant to this article were reported.

References

1. Nathan DM, Cleary PA, Backlund JY, Genuth SM, Lachin JM, Orchard TJ, Raskin P, Zinman B. Intensive diabetes treatment and cardiovascular disease in patients with type 1 diabetes. N Engl J Med 2005; 353:2643–2653
2. The Diabetes Control and Complications Trial Research Group. Epidemiology of severe hypoglycemia in the diabetes control and complications trial. Am J Med 1991;90:450–459
3. The Diabetes Control and Complications Trial Research Group. Effect of intensive diabetes treatment on the development and progression of long-term complications in adolescents with insulin-dependent diabetes mellitus: Diabetes Control and Complications Trial. J Pediatr 1994; 125:177–188
4. Tsalikian E, Mauras N, Beck RW, Tamborlane WV, Janz KF, Chase HP, Wysocki T, Weinzimer SA, Buckingham BA, Kollman C, Xing D, Ruedy KJ. Impact of exercise on overnight glycemic control in children with type 1 diabetes mellitus. J Pediatr 2005;147:528–534
5. Raju B, Arbelaez AM, Breckenridge SM, Cryer PE. Nocturnal hypoglycemia in type 1 diabetes: an assessment of preventive bedtime treatments. J Clin Endocri-

nol Metab 2006;91:2087–2092
6. Buckingham B, Block J, Burdick J, Kalajian A, Kollman C, Choy M, Wilson DM, Chase P. Response to nocturnal alarms using a real-time glucose sensor. Diabetes Technol Ther 2005;7:440–447
7. Zisser H. Quantifying the impact of a short-interval interruption of insulin-pump infusion sets on glycemic excursions. Diabetes Care 2008;31:238–239
8. Gandrud LM, Xing D, Kollman C, Block JM, Kunselman B, Wilson DM, Buckingham BA. The Medtronic Minimed Gold continuous glucose monitoring system: an effective means to discover hypo- and hyperglycemia in children under 7 years of age. Diabetes Technol Ther 2007; 9:307–316
9. Guerci B, Benichou M, Floriot M, Bohme P, Fougnot S, Franck P, Drouin P. Accuracy of an electrochemical sensor for measuring capillary blood ketones by fingerstick samples during metabolic deterioration after continuous subcutaneous insulin infusion interruption in type 1 diabetic patients. Diabetes Care 2003;26: 1137–1141
10. Orsini-Federici M, Akwi JA, Canonico V, Celleno R, Ferolla P, Pippi R, Tassi C, Timi A, Benedetti MM. Early detection of insulin deprivation in continuous subcutaneous insulin infusion-treated patients with type 1 diabetes. Diabetes Technol Ther 2006;8:67–75
11. Wilson DM, Beck RW, Tamborlane WV, Dontchev MJ, Kollman C, Chase P, Fox LA, Ruedy KJ, Tsalikian E, Weinzimer SA. The accuracy of the FreeStyle Navigator continuous glucose monitoring system in children with type 1 diabetes. Diabetes Care 2007;30:59–64
12. Buckingham B, Cobry E, Clinton P, Gage V, Caswell K, Kunselman E, Cameron F, Chase HP. Preventing hypoglycemia using predictive alarm algorithms and insulin pump suspension. Diabetes Technol Ther 2009;11:93–97
13. Chase HP, Buckingham BA. Pump shut off to prevent nocturnal hypoglycemia. In *2nd Conference on Advanced Technologies & Treatments for Diabetes*. Athens, Greece, 2009
14. Dassau E, Cameron FM, Lee H, Bequette BW, Doyle III FJ, Niemeyer G, Chase P, Buckingham B: Real-time hypoglycemia prediction using continuous glucose monitoring (CGM): a safety net to the artificial pancreas. Diabetes 2008; 57(Suppl. 1):A13
15. Palerm CC, Bequette BW. Hypoglycemia detection and prediction using continuous glucose monitoring: a study on hypoglycemic clamp data. J Diabetes Sci Technol 2007;1:624–629
16. Palerm CC, Willis JP, Desemone J, Bequette BW. Hypoglycemia prediction and detection using optimal estimation. Diabetes Technol Ther 2005;7:3–14

17. Sparacino G, Zanderigo F, Corazza S, Maran A, Facchinetti A, Cobelli C. Glucose concentration can be predicted ahead in time from continuous glucose monitoring sensor time-series. IEEE Trans Biomed Eng 2007;54:931–937

18. Palerm CC, Bequette BW. Hypoglycemia detection and prediction using continuous glucose monitoring: a study on hypoglycemic clamp data. J Diabetes Sci Technol 2007;1:624–629

19. Dassau E, Bequette BW, Buckingham BA, Doyle III FJ. Detection of a meal using continuous glucose monitoring (CGM): implications for an artificial β-cell. Diabetes Care 2008;31:295–300

20. Oppenheim AV, Schafer RW, Buck JR. *Discrete-Time Signal Processing.* Upper Saddle River, NJ, Prentice-Hall, 1998

21. Cameron F, Niemeyer G, Gundy-Burlet K, Buckingham B. Statistical hypoglycemia prediction. J Diabetes Sci Technol 2008;2:612–621

22. Dassau E, Jovanovič L, Doyle III FJ, Zisser H. Enhanced 911/GPS Wizard: a telemedicine application for the prevention of severe hypoglycemia: monitor, alert and locate. J Diabetes Sci Technol 2009; 3:1501–1506

23. Kovatchev BP, Breton M, Dalla Man C, Cobelli C. In silico preclinical trials: a proof of concept in closed-loop control of type 1 diabetes. J Diabetes Sci Technol 2009;3:44–55

24. Dassau E, Zisser H, Palerm CC, Buckingham BA, Jovanovič L, Doyle III FJ. Modular artificial β-cell system: a prototype for clinical research. J Diabetes Sci Technol 2008;2:863–872

Prolonged Nocturnal Hypoglycemia Is Common During 12 Months of Continuous Glucose Monitoring in Children and Adults With Type 1 Diabetes

JUVENILE DIABETES RESEARCH FOUNDATION
CONTINUOUS GLUCOSE MONITORING
STUDY GROUP*

OBJECTIVE — To characterize the amount of nocturnal hypoglycemia and evaluate factors associated with nocturnal hypoglycemia assessed with continuous glucose monitoring (CGM) in adults and children with type 1 diabetes who participated in the Juvenile Diabetes Research Foundation CGM randomized clinical trial.

RESEARCH DESIGN AND METHODS — The analysis included 36,467 nights with ≥4 h of CGM glucose readings between 12 midnight and 6:00 A.M. from 176 subjects assigned to the CGM group of the trial. The percentage of nights in which hypoglycemia occurred (two consecutive CGM readings ≤60 mg/dl in 20 min) was computed for each subject. Associations with baseline characteristics and clinical factors were evaluated using a multivariate regression model.

RESULTS — Hypoglycemic events occurred during 8.5% of nights, with the median percentage of nights with hypoglycemia per subject being 7.4% (interquartile range 3.7–12.1%). The duration of hypoglycemia was ≥2 h on 23% of nights with hypoglycemia. In a multivariate model, a higher incidence of nocturnal hypoglycemia was associated with *1*) lower baseline A1C levels ($P < 0.001$) and *2*) the occurrence of hypoglycemia on one or more nights during baseline blinded CGM ($P < 0.001$). The hypoglycemia frequency was not associated with age or with insulin modality (pump versus multiple daily injections).

CONCLUSIONS — Nocturnal hypoglycemia is frequent and often prolonged in adults and children with type 1 diabetes. Patients with low A1C levels are at an increased risk for its occurrence. One week of blinded CGM can identify patients who are at greater risk for nocturnal hypoglycemia.

Diabetes Care 33:1004–1008, 2010

Even with the use of insulin pumps and long-acting insulin analogs, severe hypoglycemia is common in patients with type 1 diabetes, especially during sleep at night. In the Diabetes Control and Complications Trial, more than half of severe hypoglycemic events occurred during sleep (1), and other studies have shown an even greater incidence of severe nocturnal hypoglycemic events in type 1 diabetes (2). Moreover, Sovik and Thordarson (3) reported that among patients aged <40 years who died over a 10-year period, 6% of the deaths were due to "dead-in-bed" syndrome, which in many instances probably was the result of severe nocturnal hypoglycemia. Delayed glucose-lowering effects of afternoon exercise (4), sleep-induced defects in counterregulatory hormone responses to hypoglycemia (5–7), and missed bedtime snacks (8) are among the contributing causes of severe nocturnal hypoglycemic events.

Studies that used retrospective and real-time continuous glucose monitoring (CGM) systems to assess glycemic control of type 1 diabetes indicate that severe hypoglycemic events are only the tip of the iceberg regarding the risk of nocturnal hypoglycemia, because many more events are unrecognized and asymptomatic (8–14). Detection of such events is important, however, because recurrent episodes of mild hypoglycemia have been shown to contribute to the development of defective counterregulatory hormone responses to subsequent reductions in blood glucose, thus setting the stage for clinically important hypoglycemic events. Buckingham et al. (15) documented four episodes of seizures occurring during the night in patients wearing CGM devices, which demonstrated that there were 2¼–4 h of low sensor glucose values preceding each seizure.

Our Juvenile Diabetes Research Foundation (JDRF) CGM Study Group recently reported the results of a 6-month randomized clinical trial and 6-month extension study that evaluated the effectiveness of real-time CGM in intensively treated type 1 diabetic subjects with baseline A1C levels ≥7.0% ($n = 322$) and <7.0% ($n = 129$) (16–18). These studies have provided a very large dataset of nighttime CGM profiles to evaluate the frequency of nocturnal hypoglycemia during 12 months of CGM use in the home environment and factors associated with greater risk.

RESEARCH DESIGN AND METHODS —
The study protocol and clinical characteristics of enrolled subjects have been described in detail elsewhere (16,17,19). Major eligibility criteria included age ≥8 years, type 1 diabetes for at least 1 year, use of either an insulin pump or multiple (at least three) daily insulin injections, and A1C level <10.0%. The dataset used for the current analyses included 180 subjects assigned to the CGM group who used either the

Corresponding author: Roy W. Beck, jdrfapp@jaeb.org.
Received 11 November 2009 and accepted 8 February 2010. Published ahead of print at http://care.diabetesjournals.org on 3 March 2010. DOI: 10.2337/dc09-2081. Clinical trial reg. no. NCT00406133, clinicaltrials.gov.
*A full listing of the members of the Juvenile Diabetes Research Foundation Continuous Glucose Monitoring Study Group is available in the online appendix at http://care.diabetesjournals.org/cgi/content/full/dc09-2081/DC1.
The costs of publication of this article were defrayed in part by the payment of page charges. This article must therefore be hereby marked "advertisement" in accordance with 18 U.S.C. Section 1734 solely to indicate this fact.

Table 1—*Baseline characteristics*

	Overall	Age-group		
		8–14 years	15–24 years	≥25 years
n	176	64	42	70
Age (years)	25.6 ± 15.6	11.6 ± 2.0	19.6 ± 3.2	42.1 ± 11.4
Diabetes duration (years)	14.7 ± 12.5	6.1 ± 3.1	10.2 ± 5.1	25.4 ± 13.2
Sex				
Female	94 (53)	34 (53)	21 (50)	39 (56)
Male	82 (47)	30 (47)	21 (50)	31 (44)
Severe hypoglycemia events in 6 months before study (self-reported)				
0	164 (93)	61 (95)	39 (93)	64 (91)
≥1	12 (7)	3 (5)	3 (7)	6 (9)
Nights with hypoglycemia during blinded use at baseline*				
0	102 (60)	42 (67)	21 (51)	39 (59)
≥1	68 (40)	21 (33)	20 (49)	27 (41)
Home blood glucose meter measurements per day (self-reported at baseline)†	6.8 ± 2.3	6.8 ± 2.0	6.0 ± 2.1	7.1 ± 2.5
≤5	43 (29)	12 (23)	16 (52)	15 (23)
6–8	78 (53)	31 (60)	12 (39)	35 (55)
>8	26 (18)	9 (17)	3 (10)	14 (22)
Insulin delivery				
Pump	163 (93)	57 (89)	38 (90)	68 (97)
Multiple daily injections	13 (7)	7 (11)	4 (10)	2 (3)
A1C	7.4 ± 0.9	7.6 ± 1.0	7.6 ± 0.8	7.1 ± 0.8
<7.0%	57 (32)	17 (27)	11 (26)	29 (41)
7.0–<8.0%	72 (41)	22 (34)	16 (38)	34 (49)
≥8.0%	47 (27)	25 (39)	15 (36)	7 (10)
Hypoglycemia Fear Scale score‡	28 ± 18	25 ± 17	29 ± 18	31 ± 18
<20	65 (37)	27 (42)	15 (36)	23 (33)
20–<30	32 (18)	14 (22)	8 (19)	10 (14)
≥30	78 (45)	22 (35)	19 (45)	37 (53)

Data are means ± SD or n (%). *From use of a blinded CGM device for 1 week at baseline, missing for 6 subjects. †Collected on randomization form, as assessed by clinic personnel over the last 7 days. A question was added to Case Report Form after study initialization, and data were missing for 29 subjects. ‡The Hypoglycemia Fear Scale consists of 15 5-point Likert scale items, with scores scaled to a 0–100 range with higher scores indicating more fear of hypoglycemia; missing for 1 subject.

FreeStyle Navigator (Abbott Diabetes Care, Alameda, CA) or the MiniMed Paradigm REAL-Time Insulin Pump and Continuous Glucose Monitoring System (Medtronic MiniMed, Northridge, CA). At baseline, a blinded CGM device was used for 1 week. Thereafter, the goal was to use the unblinded CGM device on a daily basis if possible. CGM glucose data were downloaded at each visit over 12 months of follow-up. Subjects and parents of minor subjects completed the Hypoglycemia Fear Survey (20) at baseline, 6 months, and 12 months.

The CGM data were evaluated from midnight to 6:00 A.M. Only nights having at least 4 h of glucose data were included in the analysis. Subjects needed to have at least 42 such nights to be included in the analysis (this restriction was placed because hypoglycemia rates were calculated per subject). Four subjects did not meet this criterion and were not included in the analysis. The dataset included 36,467 nights from 176 subjects with a median value of 217 nights per subject. Of the nights, 86% had the full 6 h of data without any skips from midnight to 6:00 A.M. A hypoglycemia event was defined as the occurrence of at least two CGM glucose values ≤60 mg/dl within a 20-min period. The percentage of nights with at least one hypoglycemia event was computed for each subject.

The associations between nocturnal hypoglycemia rate, defined as the percentage of nights with hypoglycemia per subject, and baseline demographic and clinical factors (listed in Table 1) were evaluated using regression models. Because of the skewed distribution of the hypoglycemia rate, a rank transformation (van der Waerden scores) was used in the models. Baseline demographic and clinical factors with $P < 0.20$ in the univariate model were included in an initial multivariate model and then a backward elimination procedure was used to remove variables with $P > 0.05$. A forward selection process resulted in a similar model. Age was evaluated as a discrete factor in three prespecified levels (8–14, 15–24, and ≥25 years). To avoid collinearity in the model building, the highly correlated baseline hypoglycemic measures (percentage of daytime, nighttime, or 24 h with hypoglycemia and number of nights with hypoglycemia) and other baseline glycemic measures (the percentage of blinded CGM values between 71 and 180 mg/dl, the percentage of values >250 mg/dl, and A1C) were included in the model one at a time. Subjects with miss-

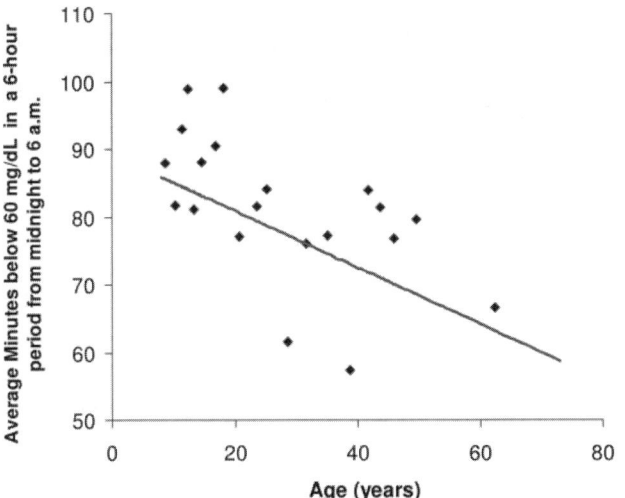

Figure 1—*Duration of hypoglycemia (≤60 mg/dl) vs. age. For presentation purposes, the hypoglycemic nights ordered by age were divided into 20 groups with an approximately equal number of nights per group. The average duration was then plotted against the average age for each group. The regression line, however, is based on all the data points, not the 20 groups.*

included in the model instead of A1C (supplementary Table 2).

There was a suggestion of an upside down U-shaped association between age and hypoglycemia rate. The median hypoglycemia rate was 6.3% in the 8- to 14-year age-group, 8.8% in the 15- to 24-year age-group, and 7.4% in the ≥25-year age-group (univariate $P = 0.05$, multivariate $P = 0.12$). The frequency of nocturnal hypoglycemia was not statistically different between pump and multiple daily injection users ($P = 0.63$). Scores on the Hypoglycemia Fear Survey completed at baseline also were not predictive of the frequency of nocturnal hypoglycemia. The factors associated with hypoglycemia appeared to be similar in the three age-groups (supplementary Table 2). The median hypoglycemia rate was 6.6% (25th and 75th interquartile range 3.5, 12.6%) in the first 6 months and 7.7% (3.7, 13.6%) in the second 6 months ($P = 0.45$).

ing values for covariates were excluded from the corresponding univariate models. For the multivariate models, missing was treated as a separate category for discrete covariates and an indicator for missing was added to the model for continuous covariates. The association of age and hypoglycemia duration during nights with a hypoglycemic event was evaluated using repeated-measures regression with rank scores. The comparison of the hypoglycemia rate in the first 6 months and in the second 6 months was based on rank scores.

Analyses were conducted using SAS (version 9.1, SAS Institute, Cary, NC). All P values are two-sided. Because of the exploratory nature of these analyses and the multiple statistical tests, the threshold for statistical significance was adjusted to $P < 0.01$.

RESULTS — The clinical characteristics of the 176 subjects who met the criteria for inclusion in these analyses are shown in Table 1. Hypoglycemic events occurred between midnight and 6:00 A.M. during 3,083 (8.5%) of the 36,467 nights, with the median percentage of nights with hypoglycemia per subject being 7.4% (interquartile range 3.7–12.1%), which is approximately twice per month. The maximum percentage of hypoglycemic nights per subject was 27.8%; six (3%) of subjects had no hypoglycemic nights (number of nights for these subjects ranged from 55 to 235, their baseline A1C ranged from 7.7 to 8.9%) (supplementary

Table 1, available in an online appendix at http://care.diabetesjournals. org/cgi/content/full/dc09-2081/DC1).

On the 3,083 nights during which hypoglycemia occurred, the median duration of hypoglycemia (≤60 mg/dl) was 53 min (interquartile range 29–110 min) and the mean was 81 ± 75 min, with 47% of nights having at least 1 h of hypoglycemia, 23% at least 2 h, and 11% at least 3 h. An exploratory plot of the duration of hypoglycemia versus age suggested a shorter mean duration of the events in subjects aged ≥25 years old than in those aged <25 years old (Fig. 1). In a statistical comparison of these two age-groups, mean duration of hypoglycemia during the nights on which hypoglycemia occurred was 73 min in subjects aged ≥25 years and 88 min in subjects aged <25 years (median 50 vs. 58 min, $P = 0.007$).

As shown in Table 2, a higher incidence of nocturnal hypoglycemia over the 12 months of follow up was associated with *1*) lower baseline A1C levels ($P < 0.001$) and *2*) the occurrence of hypoglycemia on one or more nights during baseline blinded CGM use ($P < 0.001$) in a multivariate model. Similar results were obtained when the percentage of daytime, nighttime, or 24 h with hypoglycemia during the baseline blinded CGM use was included in the model instead of the number of nights with hypoglycemia and when the percentage of blinded CGM values between 71 and 180 mg/dl or the percentage of values >250 mg/dl was

CONCLUSIONS — The >36,000 nights with ≥4 h of sensor glucose readings, totaling >2.4 million individual glucose values in 176 patients with type 1 diabetes, aged 8–72 years, provided us with a unique opportunity to determine the frequency of nocturnal hypoglycemia. During treatment aimed to lower A1C levels to ≤7.0%, as has been suggested in other smaller studies, the occurrence of nocturnal hypoglycemia in our intensively treated subjects was both frequent, occurring on 8.5% of nights during the 12 months of CGM use, and prolonged. On 23% of hypoglycemic nights, sensor glucose levels ≤60 mg/dl were present for almost 2 h and the duration of hypoglycemia was longer in those aged <25 years. It seems unlikely that the observed incidence of nocturnal hypoglycemia is an overestimate because prior outpatient studies using CGM have reported even higher rates (8,9,11–13), as have inpatient studies using blood glucose measurements (10,14). Although sensor inaccuracy could produce misclassification of some nights as to whether hypoglycemia occurred, an inpatient accuracy study conducted by the Diabetes Research in Children Network using the FreeStyle Navigator showed that the false-positive and false-negative rates for nocturnal hypoglycemia were approximately the same (21). Thus, the point estimate of nocturnal hypoglycemia from the current study is unlikely to be appreciably affected by sensor inaccuracy.

Table 2—*Association of baseline factors and nocturnal hypoglycemia*

	n	% Nights with hypoglycemia per subject	Unadjusted P value	Model 1*	Model 2†
Total	176	7.4 (3.7, 12.1)			
Age			0.05	0.12	
8–14 years	64	6.3 (2.0, 11.4)			
15–24 years	42	8.8 (3.9, 16.1)			
≥25 years	70	7.4 (4.6, 10.8)			
Sex	94	7.2 (3.7, 10.8)			
Female			0.36		
Male	82	7.8 (3.7, 14.2)			
Severe hypoglycemia events in 6 months before to study (self-reported)			0.87		
0	164	7.2 (3.7, 12.2)			
≥1	12	8.3 (4.3, 10.5)			
Nights with hypoglycemia during blinded use at baseline‡			<0.001	<0.001	<0.001
0	102	6.0 (2.8, 10.5)			
≥1	68	9.4 (5.1, 15.9)			
Home blood glucose meter measurements per day (self-reported at baseline)§‖			0.28		
≤5	43	8.1 (4.1, 13.7)			
6–8	78	8.8 (3.7, 12.2)			
>8	26	5.4 (3.2, 12.4)			
Insulin delivery					
Pump	163	7.4 (3.9, 12.0)	0.63		
Multiple daily injections	13	5.1 (1.8, 12.6)			
A1C§			<0.001	<0.001	<0.001
<7.0%	57	9.0 (5.3, 14.7)			
7.0–<8.0%	72	8.2 (4.5, 12.0)			
≥8.0%	47	3.9 (1.6, 8.7)			
Hypoglycemia Fear Scale score§¶			0.11	0.22	
<20	65	7.5 (3.3, 10.3)			
20–<30	32	7.7 (4.6, 11.0)			
≥30	78	7.0 (3.7, 13.5)			

Data are median (25th, 75th percentile). *The multivariate regression model included all variables with $P < 0.20$. †Multivariate regression model using backward selection keeping those variables with $P < 0.05$. ‡From use of a blinded CGM device for 1 week at baseline, missing for 6 subjects. §P value obtained by treating as continuous variable. ‖Collected on a randomization form, as assessed by clinic personnel over the last 7 days. A question was added to Case Report Form after study initialization, and data were missing for 29 subjects. ¶The Hypoglycemia Fear Scale consists of 15 5-point Likert scale items, with scores scaled to a 0 to 100 range with higher scores indicating more fear of hypoglycemia; missing for 1 subject.

A sensor glucose level ≤60 mg/dl rather than ≤70 mg/dl was used to define hypoglycemia because there is considerably greater concern for serious sequelae for glucose levels ≤60 mg/dl than for levels between 61 and 70 mg/dl. Moreover, in our study of sensor glucose levels in 8- to 65-year-old, healthy, nonobese subjects with normal fasting glucose and normal glucose tolerance, nighttime sensor glucose values ≤60 mg/dl were much less common than values between 61 and 70 mg/dl (median frequency 0.0 vs. 1.0%, respectively, $P < 0.001$) (22).

Not surprisingly, the frequency of nighttime hypoglycemia was greater in subjects with lower A1C values and in those who had the occurrence of nocturnal hypoglycemia during a week of blinded CGM use at baseline. The method of insulin administration was not a significant predictor, but the number of patients using multiple daily injections was small, limiting the interpretation of this finding. It also is important to note that nocturnal hypoglycemia was frequent and prolonged in our subjects even though nighttime CGM profiles were being used to adjust overnight basal rates, and long-acting insulin analog doses and sensor alarms were used to limit the duration of nocturnal hypoglycemic events.

These results support the contention that overnight insulin replacement may never be optimal in patients with type 1 diabetes until closed-loop systems that provide minute-to-minute feedback control of insulin delivery based on real-time sensor glucose sensor data are developed for home use.

Acknowledgments— The writing committee members are as follows: *Lead authors:* Nelly Mauras, MD; Dongyuan Xing, MPH; Roy W. Beck, MD, PhD; and William V. Tamborlane, MD. *Additional members (alphabetical):* Rosanna Fiallo-Scharer, MD; Irl Hirsch, MD; Craig Kollman, PhD; Lori Laffel, MD, MPH; Joyce Lee, MD, MPH; Katrina J. Ruedy, MSPH; Eva Tsalikian, MD; and Darrell Wilson, MD.

Funding for this study was provided by the Juvenile Diabetes Research Foundation (grants 22-2006-1107, 22-2006-1117, 22-2006-1112, 22-2006-1123, and 01-2006-8031). Continuous glucose monitors and sensors were purchased at a bulk discount price from DexCom (San Diego, CA), Medtronic MiniMed (Northridge, CA), and Abbott Diabetes Care (Alameda, CA). Home glucose meters and test strips were provided to the study by LifeScan and Abbott Diabetes Care. A listing of relationships of the investigators with companies that make products relevant to the manuscript between 1 July 2006 and 4 November 2009 follows. Research funds listed below were provided to the legal entity that employs the individual and not directly to the individual. C.K. received consulting fees from Medtronic MiniMed. L.L. received consulting fees from LifeScan, consulting fees and speaker honorarium from Abbott Diabetes Care, and consulting fees and research funding from Medtronic MiniMed. N.M. received grant support from Medtronic MiniMed. W.V.T. received consulting fees from Abbott Diabetes Care and LifeScan and consulting fees, speaker honorarium, and research funding from Medtronic MiniMed. No other potential conflicts of interest relevant to this article were reported.

The study was designed and conducted by the investigators listed in the online appendix, who collectively wrote the manuscript and vouch for the data. The investigators had complete autonomy to analyze and report the trial results. There were no agreements concerning confidentiality of the data between the Juvenile Diabetes Research Foundation and the authors or their institutions. The Jaeb Center for Health Research had full access to all of the data in the study and takes responsibility for the integrity of the data and the accuracy of the data analysis.

Parts of this study were presented at the Diabetes Technology Society Meeting, San Francisco, California, 5–7 November 2009.

The Juvenile Diabetes Research Foundation Continuous Glucose Monitoring Study Group recognizes the efforts of the subjects and their families and thanks them for their participation.

References

1. DCCT Research Group. Epidemiology of severe hypoglycemia in the Diabetes Control and Complications Trial. Am J Med 1991;90:450–459
2. Davis EA, Keating B, Byrne GC, Russell M, Jones TW. Hypoglycemia: incidence and clinical predictors in a large population-based sample of children and adolescents with IDDM. Diabetes Care 1997;20:22–25
3. Sovik O, Thordarson H. Dead-in-bed syndrome in young diabetic patients. Diabetes Care 1999; 22(Suppl. 2):B40–B42
4. McMahon SK, Ferreira LD, Ratnam N, Davey RJ, Youngs LM, Davis EA, Fournier PA, Jones TW. Glucose requirements to maintain euglycemia after moderate-intensity afternoon exercise in adolescents with type 1 diabetes are increased in a biphasic manner. J Clin Endocrinol Metab 2007;92:963–968
5. Diabetes Research in Children Network (DirecNet) Study Group. The effects of aerobic exercise on glucose and counterregulatory hormone concentrations in children with type 1 diabetes. Diabetes Care 2006;29:20–25
6. Diabetes Research in Children Network (DirecNet) Study Group. Impaired overnight counterregulatory hormone responses to spontaneous hypoglycemia in children with type 1 diabetes. Pediatr Diabetes 2007;8:199–205
7. Jones TW, Porter P, Sherwin RS, Davis EA, O'Leary P, Frazer F, Byrne G, Stick S, Tamborlane WV. Decreased epinephrine responses to hypoglycemia during sleep. N Engl J Med 1998;338:1657–1662
8. Wilson D, Chase HP, Kollman C, Xing D, Caswell K, Tansey M, Fox L, Weinzimer S, Beck R, Ruedy K, Tamborlane W, Diabetes Research in Children Network (DirecNet) Study Group. Low-fat vs. high-fat bedtime snacks in children and adolescents with type 1 diabetes. Pediatr Diabetes 2008;9:320–325
9. Boland E, Monsod T, Delucia M, Brandt CA, Fernando S, Tamborlane WV. Limitations of conventional methods of self-monitoring of blood glucose: lessons learned from 3 days of continuous glucose sensing in pediatric patients with type 1 diabetes. Diabetes Care 2001;24:1858–1862
10. Diabetes Research In Children Network (DirecNet) Study Group. Impact of exercise on overnight glycemic control in children with type 1 diabetes mellitus. J Pediatr 2005;147:528–534
11. Kaufman FR, Austin J, Neinstein A, Jeng L, Halvorson M, Devoe DJ, Pitukcheewanont P. Nocturnal hypoglycemia detected with the continuous glucose monitoring system in pediatric patients with type 1 diabetes. J Pediatr 2002;141:625–630
12. Wentholt IM, Maran A, Masurel N, Heine RJ, Hoekstra JB, DeVries JH. Nocturnal hypoglycaemia in type 1 diabetic patients, assessed with continuous glucose monitoring: frequency, duration and associations. Diabet Med 2007;24:527–532
13. Wiltshire EJ, Newton K, McTavish L. Unrecognised hypoglycaemia in children and adolescents with type 1 diabetes using the continuous glucose monitoring system: prevalence and contributors. J Paediatr Child Health 2006;42:758–763
14. Woodward A, Weston P, Casson IF, Gill GV. Nocturnal hypoglycaemia in type 1 diabetes—frequency and predictive factors. QJM 2009;102:603–607
15. Buckingham B, Wilson DM, Lecher T, Hanas R, Kaiserman K, Cameron F. Duration of nocturnal hypoglycemia before seizures. Diabetes Care 2008;31:2110–2112
16. Juvenile Diabetes Research Foundation Continuous Glucose Monitoring Study Group. Continuous glucose monitoring and intensive treatment of type 1 diabetes. N Engl J Med 2008;359:1464–1476
17. Juvenile Diabetes Research Foundation Continuous Glucose Monitoring Study Group. The effect of continuous glucose monitoring in well-controlled type 1 diabetes. Diabetes Care 2009;32:1378–1383
18. Juvenile Diabetes Research Foundation Continuous Glucose Monitoring Study Group. Sustained benefit of continuous glucose monitoring on HbA1c, glucose profiles, and hypoglycemia in adults with type 1 diabetes. Diabetes Care 2009;32:2047–2049
19. JDRF CGM Study Group. JDRF randomized clinical trial to assess the efficacy of real-time continuous glucose monitoring in the management of type 1 diabetes: research design and methods. Diabetes Technol Ther 2008;10:310–321
20. Cox DJ, Irvine A, Gonder-Frederick L, Nowacek G, Butterfield J. Fear of hypoglycemia: quantification, validation, and utilization. Diabetes Care 1987;10:617–621
21. Wilson DM, Beck RW, Tamborlane WV, Dontchev MJ, Kollman C, Chase P, Fox LA, Ruedy KJ, Tsalikian E, Weinzimer SA, DirecNet Study Group. The accuracy of the FreeStyle Navigator continuous glucose monitoring system in children with type 1 diabetes. Diabetes Care 2007;30:59–64
22. Fox L, Xing D, the Juvenile Diabetes Research Foundation Continuous Glucose Monitoring Study Group. Variation of interstitial measurements assessed by continuous glucose monitors in healthy, nondiabetic subjects (Abstract). Diabetes 2009;58(Suppl. 1):A112

Hypoglycemia Unawareness in Older Compared With Middle-Aged Patients With Type 2 Diabetes

Jan P. Bremer, md[1]
Kamila Jauch-Chara, md[2]
Manfred Hallschmid, phd[3]

Sebastian Schmid, md[1]
Bernd Schultes, md[1,4]

OBJECTIVE — Older patients with type 2 diabetes are at a particularly high risk for severe hypoglycemic episodes, and experimental studies in healthy subjects hint at a reduced awareness of hypoglycemia in aged humans. However, subjective responses to hypoglycemia have rarely been assessed in older type 2 diabetic patients.

RESEARCH DESIGN AND METHODS — We tested hormonal, subjective, and cognitive responses (reaction time) to 30-min steady-state hypoglycemia at a level of 2.8 mmol/l in 13 older ($\geq$65 years) and 13 middle-aged (39–64 years) type 2 diabetic patients.

RESULTS — Hormonal counterregulatory responses to hypoglycemia did not differ between older and middle-aged patients. In contrast, middle-aged patients showed a pronounced increase in autonomic and neuroglycopenic symptom scores at the end of the hypoglycemic plateau that was not observed in older patients (both $P < 0.01$). Also, seven middle-aged patients, but only one older participant, correctly estimated their blood glucose concentration to be <3.3 mmol/l during hypoglycemia ($P = 0.011$). A profound prolongation of reaction times induced by hypoglycemia in both groups persisted even after 30 min of subsequent euglycemia.

CONCLUSIONS — Our data indicate marked subjective unawareness of hypoglycemia in older type 2 diabetic patients that does not depend on altered neuroendocrine counterregulation and may contribute to the increased probability of severe hypoglycemia frequently reported in these patients. The joint occurrence of hypoglycemia unawareness and deteriorated cognitive function is a critical factor to be carefully considered in the treatment of older patients.

Diabetes Care 32:1513–1517, 2009

H ypoglycemia is the limiting factor in the glycemic management of diabetes (1). For a long time hypoglycemia was assumed a major problem only in patients suffering from type 1 diabetes (2); however, there is increasing evidence that hypoglycemic episodes are a critical factor also in type 2 diabetes (3,4). Older subjects aged >65 years, who represent the majority of type 2 diabetic patients, appear at a particularly high risk of experiencing severe hypoglycemia (3,4). Previous studies (5–7) have shown weakened perception of hypoglycemia-related symptoms in healthy older (i.e.,

nondiabetic older subjects, aged 65–80 years) as compared with younger subjects (aged 24–49 years). Of note, in aged humans, the perception of hypoglycemic symptoms was found to simultaneously occur with the impairment of cognitive functions during a stepwise reduction of blood glucose levels (7), contrasting the well-known hierarchical succession of central nervous responses to hypoglycemia in younger healthy adults who normally perceive hypoglycemic symptoms at higher glucose levels than cognitive dysfunction (4). The concurrence of glycemic thresholds for the onset of symp-

toms and of cognitive dysfunction may be expected to increase the risk for severe hypoglycemic episodes since it likely prevents behavioral counteractions (e.g., the intake of carbohydrates) (3).

To date only one study (8) has assessed subjective responses to standardized hypoglycemia in older type 2 diabetic patients (aged 72 $\pm$ 1 years), revealing an impairment in the perception of hypoglycemic symptoms that was comparable to that of age-matched healthy control subjects. Although this finding points to a decrease in hypoglycemia awareness that develops in the course of aging also in type 2 diabetic patients, this assumption has not yet been experimentally elucidated. Moreover, in the previous studies in healthy subjects (5–7), the age gap between experimental groups was rather large, raising the question as to the perception of hypoglycemia in middle-aged subjects. On this background, we examined whether older (aged $\geq$65 years) as compared with middle-aged (aged 39–64 years) type 2 diabetic patients differ in their subjective response to hypoglycemia and how hypoglycemia awareness in these age-groups relates to hormonal and cognitive effects of hypoglycemia.

RESEARCH DESIGN AND METHODS — We examined 13 older (aged $\geq$65 years) and 13 middle-aged (aged 39–64 years) type 2 diabetic patients matched for BMI, A1C, and sex in a single-step hypoglycemic clamp experiment (see Table 1 for subjects' characteristics). While type 2 diabetes therapy was comparable between groups, the older patients, as expected, displayed a longer disease duration than the middle-aged subjects. However, none of the patients displayed any clinical evidence of diabetes complications, such as neuropathy, overt nephropathy (macroproteinuria), coronary heart disease, or a history of stroke. Also, none of the patients had experienced a severe hypoglycemic episode that required help from another person during the last year before the experiments. All patients gave written informed

From the [1]Department of Internal Medicine I, University of Luebeck, Luebeck, Germany; the [2]Department of Psychiatry and Psychotherapy, University of Luebeck, Luebeck, Germany; the [3]Department of Neuroendocrinology, University of Luebeck, Luebeck, Germany; and the [4]Interdisciplinary Obesity Center, Kantonsspital St. Gallen, St. Gallen, Switzerland.
Corresponding author: Bernd Schultes, bernd.schultes@kssg.ch.
Received 21 January 2009 and accepted 18 May 2009.
Published ahead of print at http://care.diabetesjournals.org on 1 June 2009. DOI: 10.2337/dc09-0114.
The costs of publication of this article were defrayed in part by the payment of page charges. This article must therefore be hereby marked "advertisement" in accordance with 18 U.S.C. Section 1734 solely to indicate this fact.

Table 1—*Clinical characteristics of the study population*

	Middle-aged patients	Older patients	P
n	13	13	
Sex (female/male)	6/7	5/8	0.69
Age (years)	51 ± 2	70 ± 1	<0.001
Diabetes duration (years)	5 ± 1	12 ± 2	0.008
A1C (%)	7.4 ± 4	7.4 ± 2	0.97
BMI (kg/m^2)	27 ± 1	27 ± 1	1.00
Diabetes therapy			
Diet alone	3	2	0.62
Metformin	7	9	0.42
Sulfonurea	2	3	0.62
Insulin	6	7	0.70
Insulin dose (units $\cdot$ kg^{-1} $\cdot$ day^{-1})	0.20 ± 0.07	0.26 ± 0.07	0.92

Data are means ± SE and prevalences. P values derive from χ^2 or Student's t test.

consent, and the study was approved by the local ethics committee.

On the day of the experiment, patients reported to the medical research unit at 0730 h. The experiment took place in a sound-attenuated room with patients sitting on a bed with their trunk in an almost upright position (~60°) and their legs in a horizontal position. For blood sampling, a cannula was inserted into a vein on the back of a hand that was placed in a heated box (50–55°C) to obtain arterialized venous blood. A second cannula was inserted into an antecubital vein of the contralateral arm. Both cannulae were connected to long, thin tubes that enabled blood sampling and adjustment of the rate of dextrose infusion from an adjacent room without being noticed by the subject. After a 30-min baseline period starting at 0800 h, a bolus of 0.08 IU human insulin per kg body wt (Insuman Rapid; Aventis, Strasbourg, France) was administered over 4 min. Thereafter, insulin was infused at a constant rate of 2.5 mU per kg body wt per min. Blood glucose concentration was measured every 5 min and was allowed to fall to a level of 2.8 mmol/l, where it was maintained for the next 30 min by appropriately adjusted infusion of 20% dextrose solution. Immediately after the 30-min hypoglycemic plateau, the insulin infusion was stopped and blood glucose levels were normalized by increasing the rate of dextrose infusion. Blood samples were drawn once during the baseline period (i.e., before the clamp) and every 15 min during the 30-min hypoglycemic plateau.

During the baseline period, at the beginning and end of the 30-min hypoglycemic plateau, and 30 min thereafter, patients filled in a semiquantitative symptom questionnaire, rating 11 symptoms (i.e., dizziness, tingling, blurred vision, difficulty to concentrate, faintness, anxiety, palpitation, hunger, sweating, irritability, and tremor) from 0 (not at all) to 9 (severe). In accordance with previous investigators (9), the first five symptoms were considered neuroglycopenic symptoms and the latter six were considered autonomic symptoms. Immediately after filling in the questionnaires, patients were asked to estimate their current blood glucose level. Before the symptom question-

naire, reaction time to auditory stimuli was recorded during a standard vigilance task (oddball paradigm) as a measure of cognitive function. This task required the patient to discriminate target pips (pitch: 1,200 Hz, duration: 60 ms, intensity: 64 dB SPL, probability = 0.1) from randomly interspersed frequent standard pips of lower pitch (800 Hz) and to press a button with the thumb of the dominant hand as quickly as possible whenever he/she recognized a target pip. Each task sequence contained ~400 pips, presented with interstimulus intervals randomly varying between 1,000 and 3,000 ms.

Blood glucose concentration was measured using the glucose dehydrogenase method (HemoCue B-Glucose-Analyzer; Ängelholm, Sweden). Serum insulin, C-peptide, cortisol, and growth hormone concentrations were measured by commercial enzyme-linked immunoassays (all Immulite; DPC, Los Angeles, CA). Plasma ACTH and glucagon concentrations were also measured by immunoassays (ACTH: Immulite, DPC; glucagon: Adaltis, Montreal, Canada). Plasma epinephrine and norepinephrine were measured by standard high-performance liquid chromatography with electrochemical detection (Chromsystems, Munich, Germany). Data are reported as means ± SE. For statistical analyses, data were z transformed to achieve normal dis-

Table 2—*Counterregulatory hormone levels at baseline and at the end of the hypoglycemic clamp*

	Middle-aged patients	Older patients	P
n	13	13	
Epinephrine (pmol/l)			
Baseline	233 ± 62	191 ± 47	0.59
Hypoglycemia	874 ± 176	786 ± 313	0.81
Norepinephrine (μmol/l)			
Baseline	2,177 ± 324	2,021 ± 206	0.69
Hypoglycemia	2,504 ± 305	2,563 ± 250	0.88
ACTH (pmol/l)			
Baseline	4.99 ± 0.890	4.57 ± 0.643	0.70
Hypoglycemia	12.72 ± 3.217	7.10 ± 1.920	0.15
Cortisol (nmol/l)			
Baseline	387 ± 41	426 ± 35	0.47
Hypoglycemia	548 ± 58	476 ± 44	0.33
Growth hormone (pmol/l)			
Baseline	26.9 ± 11.6	50.4 ± 25.2	0.41
Hypoglycemia	250.4 ± 59.5	245.6 ± 135.7	0.98
Glucagon (pmol/l)			
Baseline	49.9 ± 9.3	38.2 ± 4.1	0.26
Hypoglycemia	41.3 ± 10.5	31.1 ± 2.6	0.36

Data are means ± SE. P values derive from Student's t test.

tribution whenever necessary. Statistical analysis was generally based on ANOVA, including the repeated-measure factor "hypo" for effects of hypoglycemia and the between-subject factor "age" for the older and middle-aged patient groups. For pairwise comparisons, unpaired Student's t tests and χ^2 tests were used. A P value <0.05 was considered significant.

RESULTS — Baseline blood glucose levels did not differ between groups (7.2 ± 0.6 vs. 7.1 ± 0.4 mmol/l; P = 0.83). The hypoglycemic plateau was reached on average 39.2 ± 5.7 min after starting the insulin infusion in the middle-aged patients and 43.8 ± 4.5 min after in the older patients (P = 0.53). During steady-state hypoglycemia, blood glucose levels were comparable between the two groups (2.7 ± 0.03 vs. 2.8 ± 0.02 mmol/l; P = 0.71), as were levels during the recovery period (P = 0.25). There were also no group differences in baseline concentrations of insulin (middle-aged 113 ± 28 vs. older 304 ± 209 pmol/l; P = 0.38) and C-peptide (middle-aged 0.62 ± 0.07 vs. older 0.51 ± 0.06 nmol/l; P = 0.27). During the hypoglycemic clamp, serum insulin levels were on average 2,159 ± 160 pmol/l in the middle-aged and 1,812 ± 215 pmol/l in the older patients (P = 0.20). In response to hypoglycemia, serum C-peptide levels decreased to comparable nadir levels in both groups (0.27 ± 0.02 vs. 0.28 ± 0.04 nmol/l; P = 0.76).

Levels of counterregulatory hormones at baseline and at the end of the hypoglycemic clamp are provided in Table 2. ANOVA indicated a significant increase in epinephrine (P = 0.002 for the hypo main effect), norepinephrine (P < 0.001), ACTH (P = 0.048), cortisol (P = 0.008), and growth hormone (P = 0.002) during hypoglycemia, but there were no difference in these increases between the two patient groups (all P > 0.18 for the respective group × hypo interaction terms). Glucagon levels did not significantly change during the clamp (P = 0.07) nor did they show any difference between groups (P = 0.57).

At baseline, scores of self-rated autonomic (3.1 ± 1.1 vs. 1.8 ± 0.8; P = 0.36) and neuroglycopenic (0.8 ± 0.5 vs. 0.7 ± 0.6; P = 0.67) symptoms did not differ between the middle-aged and older patients. Likewise, at the beginning of the hypoglycemic plateau, symptom ratings were comparable between middle-aged and older patients (autonomic symptoms,

3.2 ± 1.4 vs. 1.9 ± 0.9; P = 0.42; neuroglycopenic symptoms, 2.0 ± 1.2 vs. 1.5 ± 1.0; P = 0.61), remaining essentially unchanged in comparison to baseline scores (autonomic symptoms P > 0.82; neuroglycopenic symptoms P > 0.11, for both groups). However, at the end of the hypoglycemic interval, scores of autonomic and neuroglycopenic symptoms markedly increased in middle-aged patients, whereas symptom scores in the older patients remained almost at baseline level (P = 0.009 and P = 0.007 for the respective group × hypo interaction terms) (Fig. 1). Also, at the end of the hypoglycemic clamp, 7 of 13 middle-aged patients, but only 1 of 13 older patients, correctly estimated their blood glucose level to be <3.3 mmol/l (P = 0.011).

Older patients overall tended to show longer reaction time than middle-aged patients (P = 0.06 for the group main

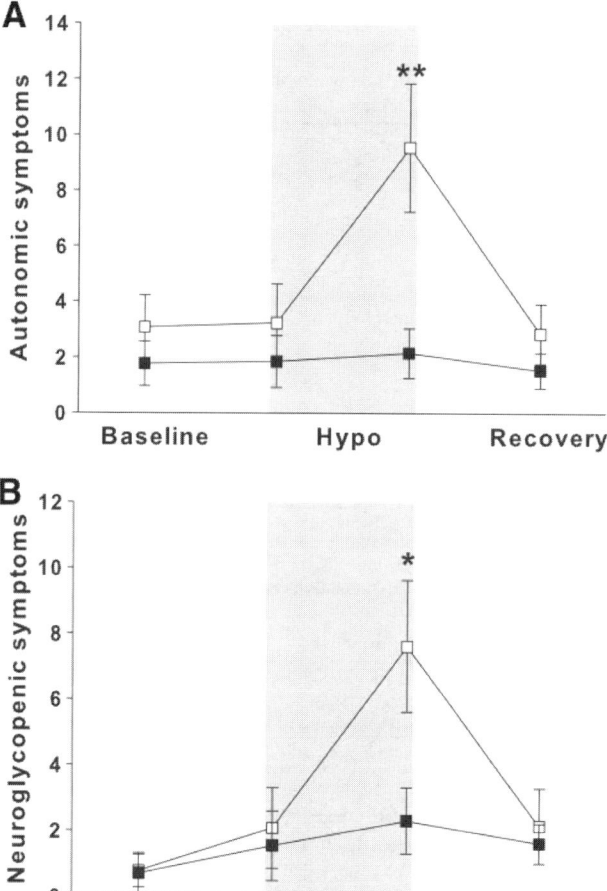

Figure 1—*Means ± SE scores of self-rated autonomic (A) and neuroglycopenic (B) symptoms during the baseline period, at the beginning and end of the 30-min hypoglycemic plateau (indicated by gray shade), and 30 min after restoration of euglycemia in 13 middle-aged (39–64 years) (□) and 13 older (≥65 years) (■) diabetic patients.* *P < 0.05; **P < 0.01.

effect) (Fig. 2). The prolongation of reaction time induced by hypoglycemia (P < 0.001 for the hypo main effect) did not differ between the two patient groups (P = 0.26 for the group × hypo interaction term). Of note, reaction time remained prolonged in both groups after euglycemia had been reestablished for 30 min (57 ± 19 ms in middle-aged and 82 ± 23 in older patients vs. respective baseline values; P = 0.012 and P = 0.003, respectively).

CONCLUSIONS — Our data indicate that type 2 diabetic patients aged ≥65 years in contrast to middle-aged patients fail to perceive neuroglycopenic and autonomic hypoglycemic symptoms even in the presence of a comparable prolongation of reaction time induced by hypoglycemia. The age-related impairment of hypoglycemia awareness was found not to depend on alterations in neuroen-

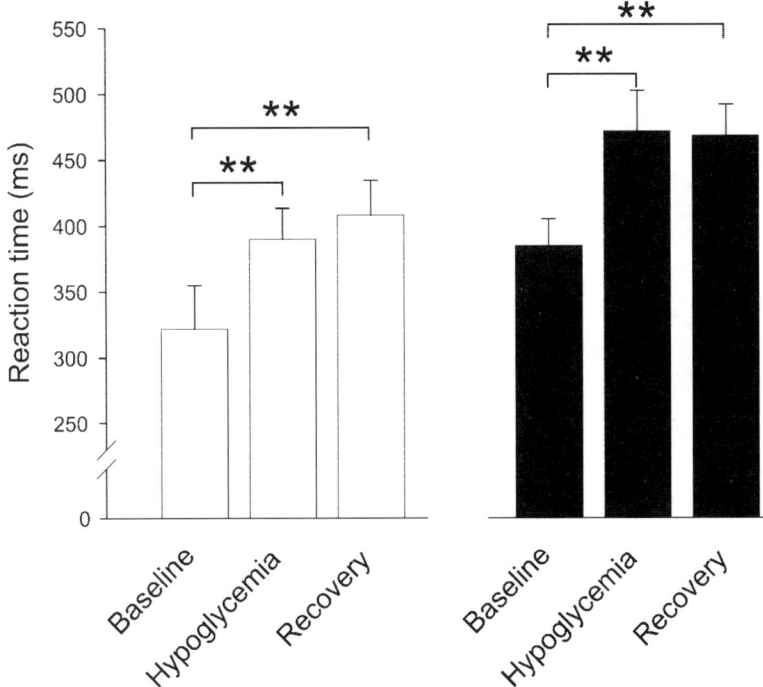

Figure 2—*Means ± SE reaction time during an auditory vigilance task at baseline, during hypoglycemia, and after restoration of euglycemia in 13 middle-aged (39–64 years) (□) and 13 older (≥65 years) (■) diabetic patients. **P < 0.01.*

docrine counterregulation because hormonal responses to hypoglycemia were similar in both age-groups. Also, the present study excludes a contribution of the quality of glycemic control as reflected by A1C levels and of diabetes medication to hypoglycemia unawareness because the two groups were comparable regarding these variables.

The markedly longer diabetes duration in the older compared with the middle-aged group may have biased our results and, in principle, may represent the critical factor determining hypoglycemia unawareness in older type 2 diabetic patients. To clarify this issue, further studies are necessary that should match type 2 diabetic patients for disease duration rather than for age. Still, from the clinical point of view, this issue appears of minor relevance because age and disease duration are highly correlated in the majority of older type 2 diabetic patients. Theoretically, asymptomatic nocturnal hypoglycemic episodes occurring in the night before the experiment, which were not systematically controlled for in our study, could have influenced our results. However, it appears rather unlikely that a possible emergence of nocturnal hypoglycemia selectively affected one of the patient groups, both of which were

comparable regarding A1C levels and medication.

The mechanisms underlying the severe impairment of hypoglycemia awareness in our older patients cannot be derived from our data. Given that the hormonal responses were pronounced and, importantly, equally strong in both age-groups, a mediation by neuroendocrine counteregulatory failure as suggested by previous studies (6) can be excluded. Rather, it might be speculated that the aged brain displays a diminished capability of perceiving physiological and cognitive alterations due to hypoglycemia. This assumption is buttressed by our finding that older patients, while being completely unaware of the hypoglycemic state, show a marked prolongation of reaction time similar to that found in middle-aged patients. In both groups, reaction time was still prolonged 30 min after restoration of euglycemia (i.e., when self-rated symptoms in the middle-aged group had already returned to baseline levels). Considering that prolonged reaction time may affect everyday life (e.g., by increasing the risk of having accidents), failure to perceive respective warning symptoms during hypoglycemia is of high relevance for patients, which underlines the clinical implications of our findings,

although they probably cannot be generalized to the effects of shorter hypoyglycemic episodes that may not elicit such prolonged deteriorating effects on reaction time. Also, reaction time is a single aspect of cognitive function, which further limits respective conclusions.

In summary, our results indicate distinct hypoglycemia unawareness in the presence of pronounced hypoglycemia-induced reaction time prolongation in older type 2 diabetic patients. This finding may, at least in part, explain why older patients are at a particularly high risk of suffering from severe hypoglycemic episodes. Given that the risk of hypoglycemia increases with the efficacy of glycemic control as reflected by low A1C levels (1,3), our results strongly support the view that glycemic targets for patients should be defined on an individual basis, thus taking into account factors such as age and probably also disease duration. This strategy appears to be of particular value considering that the recent results of the ACCORD (Action to Control Cardiovascular Risk in Diabetes) trial (10) have massively challenged the traditional "low-as-possible" dogma in diabetes care.

Acknowledgments— This study was supported in part by a grant from the Germany Diabetes Society (Deutsche Diabetes-Gesellschaft) to B.S.

No potential conflicts of interest relevant to this article were reported.

We thank Christiane Otten and Maria Baron for their expert and invaluable laboratory assistance.

References
1. Cryer PE. Hypoglycaemia: the limiting factor in the glycaemic management of type I and type II diabetes. Diabetologia 2002;45:937–948
2. Heller SR. What we know about counterregulation in type 2 diabetes. Diabetes Nutr Metab 2002;15:372–375
3. Amiel SA, Dixon T, Mann R, Jameson K. Hypoglycaemia in type 2 diabetes. Diabet Med 2008;25:245–254
4. Zammitt NN, Frier BM. Hypoglycemia in type 2 diabetes: pathophysiology, frequency, and effects of different treatment modalities. Diabetes Care 2005;28:2948–2961
5. Brierley EJ, Broughton DL, James OFW, Alberti KGMM. Reduced awareness of hypoglycaemia in the elderly despite an intact counter-regulatory response. QJMed 1995;88:439–445
6. Meneilly GS, Cheung E, Tuokko H. Altered responses to hypoglycemia of

healthy elderly people. J Clin Endocrinol Metab 1994;78:1341–1348

7. Matyka K, Evans M, Lomas J, Cranston I, Macdonald I, Amiel SA. Altered hierarchy of protective responses against severe hypoglycemia in normal aging in healthy men. Diabetes Care 1997;20:135–141

8. Meneilly GS, Cheung E, Tuokko H. Counterregulatory hormone responses to hypoglycemia in the elderly patient with diabetes. Diabetes 1994;43:403–410

9. Veneman T, Mitrakou A, Mokan M, Cryer PE, Gerich J. Induction of hypoglycemia unawareness by asymptomatic nocturnal hypoglycemia. Diabetes 1993;42:1233–1237

10. Dluhy RG, McMahon GT. Intensive glycemic control in the ACCORD and ADVANCE trials. N Engl J Med 2008;358:2630–2633

Hypoglycemia Unawareness Is Associated With Reduced Adherence to Therapeutic Decisions in Patients With Type 1 Diabetes

Evidence from a clinical audit

CHARLOTTE B. SMITH, MB
PRATIK CHOUDHARY, MB, MRCP
ANDREW PERNET, RN

DAVID HOPKINS, MB, FRCP
STEPHANIE A. AMIEL, MD, FRCP

OBJECTIVE — Hypoglycemia unawareness increases severe hypoglycemia risk. Hypoglycemia avoidance restores awareness, but it is difficult to sustain. We compared adherence to treatment changes by awareness status.

RESEARCH DESIGN AND METHODS — Case notes of 90 type 1 diabetic patients were analyzed retrospectively, identifying awareness status and insulin regimens over four visits. The proportion of patients adhering to advice and percent advice taken were calculated.

RESULTS — A total of 31 patients with hypoglycemia awareness and 19 patients with hypoglycemia unawareness were identified, with insulin regimens available in 23 and 13, respectively. Patients with hypoglycemia unawareness were older ($P = 0.001$) and had longer diabetes duration ($P = 0.002$) and lower A1C ($P = 0.007$). More patients with hypoglycemia unawareness reported severe hypoglycemia ($P = 0.002$) and fewer were adherent (53.8 vs. 87.0%, $P = 0.046$), with lower adherence scores (42.5 ± 24.7 vs. 75.3 ± 27.5%, $P = 0.001$).

CONCLUSIONS — Reduced adherence to changes in insulin regimen in hypoglycemia unawareness is compatible with habituation to hypoglycemic stress. Therapies aimed at reversing repetitive harmful behaviors may be useful to restore hypoglycemia awareness and protection from severe hypoglycemia.

Diabetes Care 32:1196–1198, 2009

H ypoglycemia unawareness in type 1 diabetes increases risk of severe hypoglycemia more than fivefold (1). Hypoglycemia awareness can be restored by hypoglycemia avoidance (2–4), which can be difficult. We hypothesized that hypoglycemia unawareness may translate into resistance to changing insulin regimens targeting hypoglycemia avoidance.

RESEARCH DESIGN AND METHODS

— We conducted retrospective case-note analysis of 90 consecutive patients with type 1 diabetes, defined by history, attending an intensified insulin therapy clinic over 3 months. This was part of a routine clinic performance audit; therefore, patient consent was not required. Patients were excluded if they had attended fewer than four visits before the audit or had incomplete notes ($n = 19$) or had undertaken major regimen change by starting pump therapy (continuous subcutaneous insulin infusion) or attending the structured type 1 diabetes education program Dose Adjustment for Normal Eating (DAFNE) ($n = 11$) (5) within the audit duration.

Visit date, weight, A1C (high-performance liquid chromatography assay, inter- and intra-assay variation of 1.9 and 1.5, respectively), DAFNE training, hypoglycemia awareness status, severe hypoglycemia episodes (requiring assistance)

since last visit, current insulin regimen, and changes made to it recorded by the clinician at each visit were collected for the last four visits. Hypoglycemia awareness was defined by the clinicians' documentation (6). Hypoglycemia-aware patients had symptomatic awareness <3.5 mmol/l as opposed to partially aware patients, who had inconsistent symptoms, and hypoglycemia-unaware patients, who had minimal or no symptoms <3.0 mmol/l. Adherence was defined using two methods. The proportion of agreed changes to insulin regimen adhered to across visits one to four was calculated for each set of consecutive visits (one to two, two to three, and three to four) and meaned to one value per patient. Patients scoring ≥50% were defined as adherent. Adherence scores (percent advice taken) were also measured. A total of 23 aware patients and 13 unaware patients had sufficient data for these assessments. Age, sex, height, psychiatric history, and exposure to cognitive behavioral therapy were collected from visit 4.

Data were analyzed using χ^2 or Mann-Whitney U test for categorical or non–normally distributed data; continuous data were tested for normality (Kolmogorov-Smirnov) and analyzed with Student's independent two-tailed t test.

RESULTS — Of the 60 patients who met the inclusion criteria, 10 were excluded for partial awareness, leaving 31 with hypoglycemia awareness and 19 with hypoglycemia unawareness (Table 1).

The mean study period for patients with hypoglycemia unawareness was shorter than for patients with hypoglycemia awareness, reflecting shorter intervals between scheduled visits. Patients with hypoglycemia unawareness were older, with longer diabetes duration. There were no significant differences between groups in sex, weight or BMI, proportion previously attending DAFNE before audit, and proportion with psychiatric morbidity or history of previous coincidental cognitive behavioral therapy.

From the Diabetes Research Group, King's College London School of Medicine, King's College, London, U.K.
Corresponding author: Charlotte Smith, charlotte.b.smith@doctors.org.uk.
Received 21 December 2008 and accepted 13 April 2009.
Published ahead of print at http://care.diabetesjournals.org on 23 April 2009. DOI: 10.2337/dc08-2259.

Table 1—*Subject characteristics*

	Hypoglycemia unaware	Hypoglycemia aware	P
n	19	31	—
Duration of observation (days)	419 ± 139	568 ± 255	0.024
Age (years)	47.5 ± 11.4	36.1 ± 10.2	0.001
Sex (% female)	52.6 (10)	71.0 (22)	0.190
Duration type 1 diabetes (years)	32.1 ± 12.9	20.5 ± 11.3	0.002
Weight (kg)	70.4 ± 16.2	73.7 ± 13.3	0.449
BMI	25.0 ± 5.0	26.1 ± 4.0	0.401
% Who did not attend	7.5 ± 11.4	12.3 ± 12.4	0.174
% Completed DAFNE	47.4 (9)	61.3 (19)	0.336
% Psychiatric history	10.5 (2)	29.2 (7)	0.282
% Cognitive behavioral therapy	10.5 (2)	24.0 (6)	0.409
% Retinopathy (any degree on retinal photography)*	55.6 (10)	61.3 (19)	0.694
% Nephropathy (microalbuminuria/ proteinuria)*	10.5 (2)	29.0 (9)	0.125
% Neuropathy (symptoms or sensory loss)*	21.1 (4)	9.7 (3)	0.261
A1C (%)	7.2 ± 0.7	8.3 ± 1.3	0.007
Insulin dose (units · kg^{-1} · day^{-1})	0.59 ± 0.16	0.77 ± 0.26	0.030

*Taken from annual review data during audit period. DAFNE, Dose Adjustment for Normal Eating, a 5-day structured education program in flexible insulin therapy for type 1 diabetic patients.

At visit 1, hypoglycemia-unaware patients had lower A1C, despite lower daily insulin doses. By visit 4, A1C in the hypoglycemia-unaware group had risen to 7.8 ± 0.8% (P < 0.001). Their insulin dose remained lower (0.54 ± 0.19 vs. 0.71 ± 0.21 units · kg^{-1} · day^{-1}, P = 0.01). Nine of 17 hypoglycemia-unaware patients (47.4%) versus three of 31 (9.6%) patients with hypoglycemia awareness reported one or more severe episode of hypoglycemia during the study (risk ratio 5.2 [95% CI 1.14–23.3], P = 0.002; median prevalence 71.4 [interquartile range 488.8] and 0.0 [0.0], P < 0.001, per 100 patient-years). No significant change occurred in awareness status over the audit (P = 0.644).

A total of 7 of 13 (53.8%) hypoglycemia-unaware patients versus 20 of 23 (87.0%) hypoglycemia-aware patients were defined as adherent (P = 0.046). A smaller percentage of advice was followed by patients with hypoglycemia unawareness (44.7 ± 19.3% vs. 70.4 ± 28.3%, P = 0.009).

More patients with previous contact with liaison psychiatry were adherent (80.7 ± 20.5% vs. 53.7 ± 28.1%, P = 0.022). Adherence was higher in patients who had experienced cognitive behavioral therapy (80.3 ± 16.5% advice taken vs. 54.6 ± 28.8%, P = 0.042).

CONCLUSIONS — Type 1 diabetic patients with hypoglycemia unawareness were older, with longer diabetes duration, more severe hypoglycemia, and lower A1C than patients with hypoglycemia awareness, consistent with published literature (7). The novel finding is that patients with hypoglycemia unawareness were significantly less adherent to agreed changes to insulin regimens than their hypoglycemia-aware counterparts, in spite of increased clinical contact. An apparent lack of benefit of this, with a rise in A1C and no change in awareness status, could relate to exclusion of 11 potentially eligible patients undertaking major changes to their diabetes management known to improve A1C and reduce hypoglycemia, group-structured education in flexible insulin therapy, or continuous subcutaneous insulin infusion (8,9).

Treatment targets in hypoglycemia unawareness focus on hypoglycemia avoidance (3,5), and the lower A1C of our hypoglycemia-unaware group at study start may have been in part related to greater exposure to hypoglycemia, a driver for unawareness. The explicit aim of treatment adjustments was impossible to assess from notes, but our data, with a rise in A1C in hypoglycemia-unaware patients, argue against benefit of relaxation of glycemic control alone (rather than hy-

poglycemia avoidance per se) to improve hypoglycemia awareness (10). Interestingly, patients who had attended coincidental cognitive behavioral therapy had a higher adherence than those who had not, although numbers were too small to analyze this by awareness status.

The audit was limited in that it was retrospective, not blinded, and did not use formal scoring to define awareness (2,11) or document discussion around insulin regimen change. Nevertheless, clinic notes were consistent in explicit documentation of the physician's assessment of awareness status. Where this was absent, the notes were excluded. Lack of clear documentation of insulin regimens across all four visits also reduced the number of records available for audit. However, these factors should not have operated differently between groups, and there were no differences in demographics between included and excluded patients. Importantly, the patients were not selected for research.

These data add a clinical dimension to neuroimaging data implicating cortical responses to hypoglycemia in generating awareness (12). Reduced adherence to changes in insulin regimens in hypoglycemia unawareness is compatible with habituation to hypoglycemic stress, with differences in central responses to it that makes further exposure to the same stimulus less stressful (13). Failure to perceive a situation as unpleasant or dangerous subjectively undermines motivation and ability to change behavior (14). About half of the patients with hypoglycemia unawareness in this audit had previously undertaken a structured education program proven both to reduce severe hypoglycemia rates (8) and restore hypoglycemia awareness in 48% of patients entering it with hypoglycemia unawareness (15). Therefore, they are likely to represent a population for whom educational strategies alone have failed. Behavioral strategies that address habituation may be useful adjuncts to educational approaches in restoring hypoglycemia awareness and protection against severe hypoglycemia.

Acknowledgments— The authors would like to thank the Diabetes Department secretaries and the Clinical Records Department at King's College Hospital, London, U.K., for their hard work and support during the study.

No potential conflicts of interest relevant to this article were reported.

Parts of this study were presented in abstract form at the 68th Scientific Sessions of the American Diabetes Association, San Francisco, California, 6–10 June 2008.

References

1. Geddes J, Schoipman JE, Zammitt NN, Frier BM. Prevalence of impaired awareness of hypoglycaemia in adults with type 1 diabetes. Diabet Med 2008;25:501–504
2. Cranston I, Lomas J, Maran A, Macdonald I, Amiel S. Restoration of hypoglycemia awareness in patients with long-duration insulin-dependent diabetes. Lancet 1994; 344:283–287
3. Dagago-Jack S, Rattarasan C, Cryer P. Reversal of hypoglycemia unawareness, but not defective glucose counterregulation, in IDDM. Diabetes 1994;43:1426–1434
4. Fanelli C, Epifano L, Rambotti A, Pampanelli S, Vincenzo A, Modarelli F, Lepore M, Annibale B, Ciofetta M, Bottini P. Meticulous prevention of hypoglycemia normalizes the glycemic thresholds and magnitude of most of neuroendocrine responses to, symptoms of, and cognitive function during hyploglycemia in intensively treated patients with short-term IDDM. Diabetes 1993;42:1983–1989
5. DAFNE Study Group. Training in flexible, intensive insulin management to enable dietary freedom in people with type 1 diabetes: Dose Adjustment for Normal Eating (DAFNE) randomised controlled trial. Br Med J 2002;325:746
6. Workgroup on Hypoglycemia, American Diabetes Association. Defining and reporting hypoglycemia in diabetes: a report from the American Diabetes Association Workgroup on Hypoglycemia. Diabetes Care 2005;28:1245–1249
7. Mokan M, Mitrakou A, Veneman T, Ryan C, Koryktowski M, Cryer P, Gerich J. Hypoglycemia unawareness in IDDM. Diabetes Care 1994;17:1397–1403
8. Bott U, Bott S, Hemmann D, Berger M. Evaluation of a holistic treatment and teaching programme for patients with type 1 diabetes who failed to achieve their therapeutic goals under intensified insulin therapy. Diabet Med 2000;17:635–643
9. Pickup JC, Sutton AJ. Severe hypoglycaemia and glycaemic control in type 1 diabetes: meta-analysis of multiple daily insulin injections compared with continuous subcutaneous insulin infusion. Diabet Med 2008;25:765–774
10. Liu D, McManus R, Ryan E. Improved counter-regulatory hormonal and symptomatic responses to hypoglycemia in patients with insulin-dependent diabetes mellitus after 3 months of less strict glycaemic control. Clin Invest Med 1996;19:71–82
11. Clarke W, Cox D, Gonder-Frederick L, Julian D, Schlundt D, Polonsky W. Reduced awareness of hypoglycemia in IDDM adults: a prospective study of hypoglycemic frequency and associated symptoms. Diabetes Care 1995;18:517–522
12. Dunn J, Cranston I, Marsden P, Amiel S, Reed L. Attenuation of amygdala and cortical responses to low blood glucose concentration in asymptomatic hypoglycemia in type 1 diabetes. Diabetes 2007;56:2766–2773
13. Armario A, Valles A, Dal-Zotto S, Marquez C, Belda X. A single exposure to severe stressors causes long-term desensitisation of the physiological response to the homotypic stressor. Stress 2004;7:157–172
14. Leventhal H, Diefenbach M, Leventhal EA. Illness cognition: using common sense to understand treatment adherence and affect cognition interactions. Cognitive Therapy and Research 1992;16:143–163
15. Hopkins D, Lawrence I, Mansell P, Thompson G, Heller S, Amiel SA. Routine structured education reduces AIC and hypoglycemia and improves psychological health in patients with type 1 diabetes (Abstract). Diabetes 2008;57 (Suppl. 1): 122–0R

Hypoglycemia and Clinical Outcomes in Patients With Diabetes Hospitalized in the General Ward

Alexander Turchin, md, ms[1,2,3]
Michael E. Matheny, md, ms, mph[4,5]
Maria Shubina, scd[1]

James V. Scanlon, pharmd[6]
Bonnie Greenwood, pharmd, bcps[1]
Merri L. Pendergrass, md, phd[1,3,7]

OBJECTIVE — Hypoglycemia is associated with adverse outcomes in mixed populations of patients in intensive care units. It is not known whether the same risks exist for diabetic patients who are less severely ill. In this study, we aimed to determine whether hypoglycemic episodes are associated with higher mortality in diabetic patients hospitalized in the general ward.

RESEARCH DESIGN AND METHODS — This retrospective cohort study analyzed 4,368 admissions of 2,582 patients with diabetes hospitalized in the general ward of a teaching hospital between January 2003 and August 2004. The associations between the number and severity of hypoglycemic (≤ 50 mg/dl) episodes and inpatient mortality, length of stay (LOS), and mortality within 1 year after discharge were evaluated.

RESULTS — Hypoglycemia was observed in 7.7% of admissions. In multivariable analysis, each additional day with hypoglycemia was associated with an increase of 85.3% in the odds of inpatient death ($P = 0.009$) and 65.8% ($P = 0.0003$) in the odds of death within 1 year from discharge. The odds of inpatient death also rose threefold for every 10 mg/dl decrease in the lowest blood glucose during hospitalization ($P = 0.0058$). LOS increased by 2.5 days for each day with hypoglycemia ($P < 0.0001$).

CONCLUSIONS — Hypoglycemia is common in diabetic patients hospitalized in the general ward. Patients with hypoglycemia have increased LOS and higher mortality both during and after admission. Measures should be undertaken to decrease the frequency of hypoglycemia in this high-risk patient population.

Diabetes Care 32:1153–1157, 2009

I n recent years, there has been an increasing focus on controlling hyperglycemia in hospitalized patients (1). Hyperglycemia is associated with adverse clinical outcomes, and randomized controlled trials in intensive care units (ICUs) have shown that aggressive treatment of elevated blood glucose improves outcomes. Tight glucose control, however, is not without risk. Studies have suggested that the benefits of tight glycemic control may be at least partially offset by the increased risk of hypoglycemia (2,3). In particular, hypoglycemia in ICUs has been linked to increased risk of mortality, seizures, and coma (4).

It remains unknown whether the risks associated with hypoglycemia found in critically ill patients can be generalized to non-ICU settings. The etiology of hypoglycemia in ICU patients may be different from that in patients hospitalized in the general ward. A number of risk factors for hypoglycemia in critically ill patients, including continuous venovenous hemofiltration, inotropic support, or sepsis are absent or less common outside of the ICU (5).

It also remains unknown whether reported risks of hypoglycemia in ICU studies, which included primarily nondiabetic patients, also apply to patients with known diabetes. Several studies have demonstrated that the relationship of elevated blood glucose with clinical outcomes may be quantitatively and qualitatively different between patients with and without a diagnosis of diabetes. Hyperglycemic patients with diabetes have been found to have lower mortality than nondiabetic hyperglycemic patients; they may also derive less or no benefit from intensive glycemic control (3,6–10). It is possible that a similar divergence exists for hypoglycemia as well.

Because the majority of hospitalized patients with diabetes are treated in the general ward, it is important to understand the relationship of hypoglycemia in diabetic patients in the general ward with clinical outcomes. To this end, we examined whether hypoglycemia in patients with diabetes hospitalized in the general ward is associated with adverse outcomes. We assessed the relationship between the number and severity of hypoglycemic episodes with in-hospital mortality and the length of hospital stay. We also evaluated the association between hypoglycemia and outpatient mortality 1 year after discharge.

RESEARCH DESIGN AND METHODS

— We conducted a retrospective cohort study to investigate whether hypoglycemia in diabetic patients hospitalized in the general ward is associated with poor clinical outcomes. We evaluated the relationship between *1*) the number of days with hypoglycemia (predictor variable) during the hospital admission and *2*) hospital mortality (primary outcome variable). We also conducted three secondary analyses: *1*) the relationship between *a*) the lowest recorded blood glucose and *b*) hospital mortality; *2*) the relationship between *a*) the number of days with hypoglycemia and *b*) outpatient mortality within 1 year from discharge; and *3*) the relationship

• •

From the [1]Brigham and Women's Hospital, Boston, Massachusetts; the [2]Clinical Informatics Research and Development, Partners HealthCare System, Boston, Massachusetts; [3]Harvard Medical School, Boston, Massachusetts; the [4]Vanderbilt Medical Center, Nashville, Tennessee; the [5]Tennessee Valley Healthcare System, Veteran's Administration, Nashville, Tennessee; the [6]Massachusetts College of Pharmacy and Health Sciences, Worcester, Massachusetts; and [7]Medco Health Solutions, Inc., Franklin Lakes, New Jersey.

Corresponding author: Alexander Turchin, aturchin@partners.org.

Received 30 November 2008 and accepted 6 April 2009.

DOI: 10.2337/dc08-2127

between *a*) the number of days with hypoglycemia and *b*) the change from the length of stay (LOS) expected based on the diagnosis-related group (DRG). The institutional review board at Partners HealthCare approved the study and waived the need for informed consent.

Study patients and settings
Patients with diabetes who were admitted to a 734-bed teaching hospital between January 2003 and August 2004 were studied. Patients with diabetes were identified through a combination of computational analysis of the text of their physician notes with billing and laboratory data using a previously validated algorithm. When compared with a manual record review, the algorithm has a sensitivity of 96.2% and a specificity of 98.0% (11). Pregnant women and newborns, patients who had stayed in an ICU during their hospitalization, patients who had received intravenous total parenteral nutrition, and patients for whom point-of-care blood glucose results were not available were excluded from the analysis.

Outcome and exposure measures
Hypoglycemia was defined as blood glucose ≤50 mg/dl. Only point-of-care blood glucose levels were used in the analysis. Changes from the expected length of hospital stay were computed as the difference between the actual LOS and the mean LOS for the patient's DRG (12). A modified Charlson Comorbidity Index was computed using administrative billing codes (13) excluding diabetes because all study subjects had this diagnosis. Patient-day weighted mean blood glucose during the hospital stay was calculated as the mean of all blood glucose readings on a single day averaged over the course of the hospital stay (14). Glomerular filtration rate (GFR) was calculated using the modification of diet in renal disease formula (15). An elevation in liver function test results was quantified as the average of the fold difference of alanine aminotransferase and aspartate aminotransferase levels over the upper limit of normal. Normal values were imputed in place of missing laboratory data. Complications of diabetes (nephropathy, neuropathy, ophthalmopathy, and peripheral vascular disease) were ascertained from the ICD-9 billing codes reported for each patient up to the end of the study period. One inpatient or two outpatient billing codes were required to confirm each diagnosis.

Data sources
Patient demographics, dates of death, admission and discharge dates, laboratory data, billing codes, discharge summaries, and outpatient physician notes were obtained from the Research Patient Data Registry, a large data warehouse that serves as a central clinical data repository for participating hospitals and clinics within the Partners HealthCare System. Computerized Physician Order Entry data were obtained from the hospital inpatient electronic health record. Point-of-care blood glucose data were obtained from the QC Manager system (Abbott Laboratories, Abbott Park, IL).

Statistical analysis
Summary statistics were constructed by using frequencies and proportions for categorical data and by using means, SDs, and medians and ranges for continuous variables. Summary statistics for patient demographics (age, sex, ethnicity, and health insurance) were calculated for individual patients. The remainder of the summary statistics were calculated for individual hospital admissions. Analysis of the outpatient mortality within 1 year from discharge was limited to the last admission during the study period for each unique patient. The univariate associations between the number of days with hypoglycemic episodes and clinical outcomes (inpatient mortality, mortality within 1 year after discharge, and length of hospital stay) were assessed using a Wilcoxon test for continuous variables and Fisher's exact test for binary variables.

To account for clustering within individual patients and to adjust for other covariates, a hierarchical (multilevel) multiple logistic regression model for the probability of inpatient death was constructed using a generalized estimated equation approach. A similar model was used for the analysis of the outpatient death within 1 year from discharge date including only the last hospital admission during the study period for each patient.

To determine the relationship between the number of days with hypoglycemic events and the length of hospital stay, we constructed a hierarchical (multilevel) multivariable mixed linear regression model with random effects to account for clustering within individual patients. Random cluster effects were used to generate the correlation structure for intracluster observations and to account for individual patient effect levels. All multivariable models included patient

age, sex, ethnicity, health insurance, patient-day weighted mean blood glucose during hospital stay, length of hospital stay expected based on the DRG, and modified Charlson Comorbidity Index as covariates. *P* values were obtained using a type III test for all multivariable analyses. Significance thresholds were adjusted for multiple hypothesis testing using the Simes-Hochberg method (16,17). All analyses were performed with SAS statistical software (version 9.1; SAS Institute, Cary, NC).

RESULTS

Hypoglycemia in hospitalized diabetic patients
We identified 5,190 admissions of patients with diabetes (excluding pregnant women and newborns) that took place between January 2003 and August 2004 and had point-of-care blood glucose testing results. Of these patients, 785 had stayed in an ICU during their hospitalization, and 37 received total parenteral nutrition. These 822 admissions were excluded from the analysis.

The final analytical dataset included 4,368 admissions of 2,582 unique patients. Median age at the time of admission was 66 years and median modified Charlson Comorbidity Index was 5 (Table 1). Most patients had sliding scale insulin ordered, and 2,700 (61.8%) received scheduled antihyperglycemic medications (either insulin or oral). Hypoglycemic events (blood glucose ≤50 mg/dl) were documented in 338 (7.7%) admissions. The average blood glucose level (measured using point-of-care testing) during a hypoglycemic episode was 41 mg/dl. Severe hyperglycemia (>300 mg/dl) was observed for 1,272 (29.1%) admissions, and in 169 (3.9%) admissions there were both severe hyperglycemia and hypoglycemia documented. In multivariable analysis the odds of a hypoglycemic episode increased by >2.5-fold for patients receiving scheduled insulin (*P* < 0.0001). Complications of diabetes and other comorbidities, GFR, liver function test abnormalities, and patient age were not associated with a change in risk for a hypoglycemic episode.

Frequency of hypoglycemia and patient mortality
In univariate analysis, inpatient mortality was 2.96% for patients who had at least one hypoglycemic episode during the hospital stay vs. 0.82% for patients who

Table 1—*Patient characteristics*

Total study admissions	4,368
Unique subjects	2,582
Mean age (years)*	63.6 ± 15.1
Female sex	1,325 (51.3)
Ethnicity	
White	1,517 (58.8)
Black	544 (21.1)
Hispanic	273 (10.6)
Other/unknown	248 (9.6)
Insurance	
Medicare	1,428 (55.3)
Medicaid	332 (12.6)
Commercial	800 (31.0)
Self-pay	22 (0.9)
Admission service	
Medical	2,702 (61.9)
Surgical	1,660 (38.0)
Unknown	6 (0.1)
Glomerular filtration rate (ml/min)	64.6 ± 38.4
Mean modified Charlson Comorbidities Index†	4.9 ± 3.3
Received sliding-scale insulin	3,479 (79.6)
Received scheduled insulin	1,427 (32.7)
Received oral antihyperglycemic agents	1,530 (35.0)
Received insulin secretagogues	1,069 (24.5)
Actual LOS (days)	4.9 ± 5.5
Deviation from DRG-based LOS (days)	−0.8 ± 5.0
Mean blood glucose (mg/dl)‡	168.8 ± 48.0
Mean days with hypoglycemia	0.1 ± 0.41
Deceased during the admission	43 (1.0)
Deceased within a year from discharge§	388 (17.9)

Data are n, n (%), or means ± SD. Aggregate patient-level characteristics (e.g., demographics) were calculated at the individual patient level, and aggregate admission-level characteristics (e.g., LOS) were calculated at the individual admission level. *At the time of the first study admission. †Diabetes was excluded from the computation of the index. ‡Patient-day weighted mean glucose level. §Calculated for the last study period admission of the 2,582 unique study patients.

had none ($P = 0.0013$). In a multivariable analysis adjusted for the patients' demographics, expected LOS, Charlson Comorbidity Index, GFR, complications of diabetes, and average blood glucose, the odds of inpatient mortality rose by 85.3% for each additional day with a hypoglycemic episode ($P = 0.009$). The odds of inpatient mortality also increased by 24.8% for each additional point of the Charlson Comorbidity Index ($P < 0.0001$). Patient age, GFR, and insulin secretagogue use during the admission had no significant relationship with inpatient mortality.

Mortality 1 year after discharge was 27.8% for patients who had at least one hypoglycemic episode vs. 14.1% for patients who had no hypoglycemic episodes ($P < 0.0001$). Univariate analysis showed a progressive increase in 1-year mortality from 14.1% for patients with no hypoglycemic episodes to 33.3% for patients with more than two hypoglycemic episodes (Fig. 1). Multivariable analysis of this dataset showed a 65.8% increase in mor-

tality 1 year after discharge for each day with a hypoglycemic episode during the admission ($P = 0.0003$) and a 41.8% decrease for patients given insulin secreta-

gogues during their hospitalization ($P = 0.0007$).

Degree of hypoglycemia and patient mortality

In univariate analysis of a subset of 338 admissions for which any hypoglycemia was documented, the mean lowest recorded blood glucose was 31.8 mg/dl for patients who died in the hospital vs. 40 mg/dl for those who did not ($P = 0.028$). Inpatient mortality rate increased progressively from 1.9% for patients whose lowest blood glucose was >39 mg/dl to 8.2% for those with lowest glucose <30 mg/dl (Fig. 2). In multivariable analysis, the odds of inpatient mortality increased threefold for every 10 mg/dl decrease in the lowest blood glucose ($P = 0.0058$). There was no significant relationship between the degree of hypoglycemia and mortality at 1 year after discharge.

Hypoglycemia and length of hospitalization

In univariate analysis, patients who had at least one episode of hypoglycemia stayed in the hospital 2.8 days longer than patients who did not have any hypoglycemic episodes ($P < 0.0001$). The difference between actual LOS and LOS expected for the DRG increased gradually from −1.0 days for patients with no hypoglycemia to 8.8 days for patients with >2 days with a hypoglycemic episode (Fig. 3).

In a multivariable analysis adjusted for the patients' demographics, expected LOS, Charlson Comorbidity Index, diabetes complications, GFR, and average blood glucose, the actual length of stay

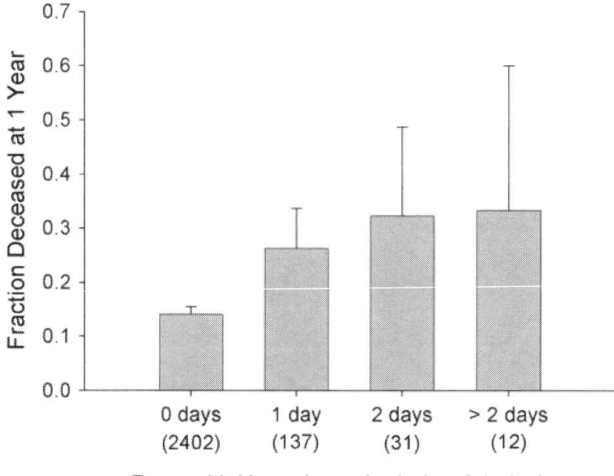

Figure 1—*Frequency of hypoglycemia and 1-year mortality. Bars indicate 95% CI. The number of admissions in each category is given in parentheses.*

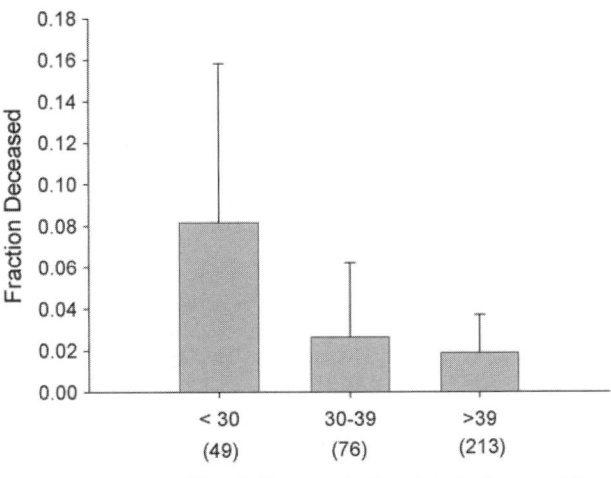

Figure 2—*Lowest blood glucose and inpatient mortality. The lowest blood glucose level recorded during the hospital stay was plotted against the fraction of patients who died during the admission for 338 patients who had at least one hypoglycemic episode documented in the hospital. Bars indicate 95% CI. The number of admissions in each category is given in parentheses.*

increased by 2.5 days compared with the average for the DRG for each additional day with a hypoglycemic episode (*P* < 0.0001). LOS also increased by 0.14 days for each additional point of the Charlson Comorbidity Index. There was no significant relationship between the lowest blood glucose level during the admission and the length of the hospital stay.

CONCLUSIONS — In this large retrospective cohort study of >4,000 admissions, we have focused on patients with known diabetes admitted to the general hospital ward. Mortality among hypoglycemic patients in this population was 3%, significantly lower than the 22–48% ob-

served in the previously published investigations that included critically ill patients (18–21). Nevertheless, we have found a similarly strong relationship between hypoglycemia and in-hospital mortality as well as LOS. Unlike in some studies of the general hospital population (18,20), this relationship was dose dependent: both LOS and inpatient mortality increased gradually as the number of hypoglycemic episodes rose. A greater degree of hypoglycemia was also associated with an increase in inpatient mortality. Furthermore, an analysis of a data subset that contained only one admission per patient revealed a strong association between the number of episodes of

hypoglycemia and outpatient mortality at 1 year after discharge from the hospital.

Although the retrospective nature of our analysis does not allow a direct inference of causality, several explanations of this relationship can be hypothesized. On the one hand, hypoglycemia could affect outcomes directly by leading to falls, seizures, or death. It could also have an indirect effect by requiring adjustments of the patients' antihyperglycemic regimen or delays of tests and procedures, consequently leading to an extension of the hospital stay.

On the other hand, hypoglycemia could be a marker for disease severity. Studies in the general hospital population, including patients in the ICU, showed that decreased caloric intake, which could be related to disease-induced anorexia, was a significant contributor to hypoglycemia (5,18). Although our study design excluded critically ill patients, malnutrition is well described in less severely ill patients as well (22). The marker hypothesis is further supported by the strong association between hypoglycemia and outpatient mortality, a finding that is difficult to explain by a direct effect of inpatient hypoglycemia on survival.

Several recommendations can be made on the basis of our results. Sicker diabetic patients in the general ward should be monitored closely for the occurrence of hypoglycemia. Extra care should be taken to prevent hypoglycemic events in this population already at high risk for adverse events, with particular attention being paid to matching the antihyperglycemic regimen to the nutritional intake. At the same time, hypoglycemia among diabetic patients in the general ward could be interpreted as a warning sign of an impending clinical deterioration. It could therefore serve as a useful indicator for the necessity of increased monitoring, more aggressive treatment of infections, transitioning to a more intensive care setting, and case management.

Our study has a number of strengths. It is the first study to focus on patients with diabetes hospitalized in the general ward, by far the largest group of inpatients at high risk for hypoglycemia. It is one of the largest analyses of the phenomenon of inpatient hypoglycemia, encompassing >4,300 admissions of 2,582 individual patients. In addition, it included both inpatient and outpatient outcomes, thus helping to differentiate

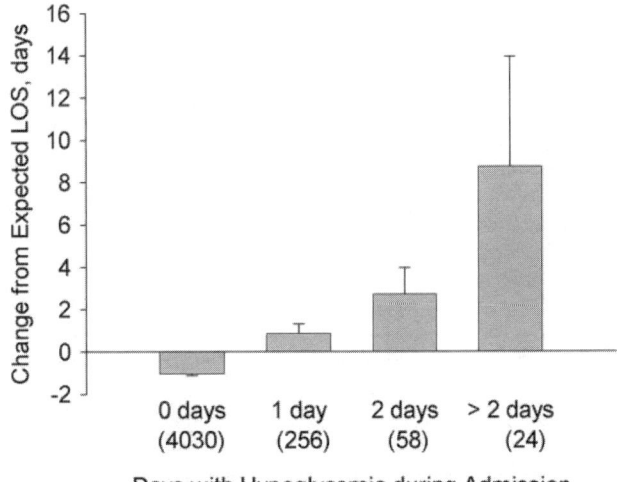

Figure 3—*Frequency of hypoglycemia and length of hospital stay. Bars indicate SEM. The number of admissions in each category is given in parentheses.*

possible immediate effects of hypoglycemia from a noncausal association.

This analysis has several limitations. The study included only patients admitted to a single academic hospital in Boston, Massachusetts, which could limit its generalizability to other geographic and health care settings. It was impossible to differentiate between type 1 and type 2 diabetes from the available data; therefore, it cannot be stated with certainty whether our findings apply to one or both conditions. However, statistically, most patients in the hospital have type 2 diabetes. Lack of nutrition information for individual patients has hindered the analysis of the causes of hypoglycemia. Furthermore, our data did not include descriptions of the types and severity of the immediate clinical sequelae (changes in mental status, loss of consciousness, or seizures) of the hypoglycemic episodes. We used point-of-care blood glucose levels in this study, the accuracy of which may have been limited, particularly at the lower glucose levels. On the other hand, central laboratory glucose levels used in many other studies are typically obtained much less frequently, possibly leading to an underestimation of the frequency and severity of hypoglycemia. In addition, unless blood samples for glucose measurement are routinely collected into tubes with a glycolysis inhibitor, the measured blood glucose level may be falsely lowered in patients with high white cell counts (23), precisely the patients at high risk for adverse outcomes. Finally, the retrospective nature of the study does not allow us to draw conclusions about causal relationships and may have led to a bias if missing data were distributed unevenly with respect to the outcomes analyzed.

In summary, hypoglycemia in diabetic patients hospitalized in the general ward was associated with increased inpatient and postdischarge mortality as well as with a prolonged LOS. Further studies are needed to establish a causal relationship. In the meantime, care should be taken to prevent hypoglycemia in this high-risk patient population.

Acknowledgments— This study was supported in part by grants from Diabetes Action Research and Education Foundation (to A.T.) and the National Library of Medicine (Grant T15-LM-07092 to M.E.M.).

No potential conflicts of interest relevant to this article were reported.

References

1. American College of Endocrinology and American Diabetes Association consensus statement on inpatient diabetes and glycemic control: a call to action. Diabetes Care 2006;29:1955–1962
2. Brunkhorst FM, Engel C, Bloos F, Meier-Hellmann A, Ragaller M, Weiler N, Moerer O, Gruendling M, Oppert M, Grond S, Olthoff D, Jaschinski U, John S, Rossaint R, Welte T, Schaefer M, Kern P, Kuhnt E, Kiehntopf M, Hartog C, Natanson C, Loeffler M, Reinhart K. Intensive insulin therapy and pentastarch resuscitation in severe sepsis. N Engl J Med 2008;358:125–139
3. Van den Berghe G, Wilmer A, Milants I, Wouters PJ, Bouckaert B, Bruyninckx F, Bouillon R, Schetz M. Intensive insulin therapy in mixed medical/surgical intensive care units: benefit versus harm. Diabetes 2006;55:3151–3159
4. Krinsley JS, Grover A. Severe hypoglycemia in critically ill patients: risk factors and outcomes. Crit Care Med 2007;35:2262–2267
5. Vriesendorp TM, van Santen S, DeVries JH, de Jonge E, Rosendaal FR, Schultz MJ, Hoekstra JB. Predisposing factors for hypoglycemia in the intensive care unit. Crit Care Med 2006;34:96–101
6. Umpierrez GE, Isaacs SD, Bazargan N, You X, Thaler LM, Kitabchi AE. Hyperglycemia: an independent marker of in-hospital mortality in patients with undiagnosed diabetes. J Clin Endocrinol Metab 2002;87:978–982
7. Van den Berghe G, Wilmer A, Hermans G, Meersseman W, Wouters PJ, Milants I, Van Wijngaerden E, Bobbaers H, Bouillon R. Intensive insulin therapy in the medical ICU. N Engl J Med 2006;354:449–461
8. Capes SE, Hunt D, Malmberg K, Gerstein HC. Stress hyperglycaemia and increased risk of death after myocardial infarction in patients with and without diabetes: a systematic overview. Lancet 2000;355:773–778
9. Kosiborod M, Rathore SS, Inzucchi SE, Masoudi FA, Wang Y, Havranek EP, Krumholz HM. Admission glucose and mortality in elderly patients hospitalized with acute myocardial infarction: implications for patients with and without recognized diabetes. Circulation 2005;111:3078–3086
10. Capes SE, Hunt D, Malmberg K, Pathak P, Gerstein HC. Stress hyperglycemia and prognosis of stroke in nondiabetic and diabetic patients: a systematic overview. Stroke 2001;32:2426–2432
11. Turchin A, Kohane IS, Pendergrass ML. Identification of patients with diabetes from the text of physician notes in the electronic medical record. Diabetes Care 2005;28:1794–1795
12. *Acute Inpatient Prospective Payment System*. Baltimore, MD, Centers for Medicare and Medicaid Services, 2006
13. Deyo RA, Cherkin DC, Ciol MA. Adapting a clinical comorbidity index for use with ICD-9-CM administrative databases. J Clin Epidemiol 1992;45:613–619
14. Goldberg PA, Bozzo JE, Thomas PG, Mesmer MM, Sakharova OV, Radford MJ, Inzucchi SE. "Glucometrics"—assessing the quality of inpatient glucose management. Diabetes Technol Ther 2006;8:560–569
15. Levey AS, Bosch JP, Lewis JB, Greene T, Rogers N, Roth D. A more accurate method to estimate glomerular filtration rate from serum creatinine: a new prediction equation: Modification of Diet in Renal Disease Study Group. Ann Intern Med 1999;130:461–470
16. Simes RJ. An improved Bonferroni procedure for multiple tests of significance. Biometrika 1986;73:751–754
17. Hochberg Y. A sharper Bonferroni procedure for multiple tests of significance. Biometrika 1988; 75:800–802
18. Fischer KF, Lees JA, Newman JH. Hypoglycemia in hospitalized patients: causes and outcomes. N Engl J Med 1986;315:1245–1250
19. Kagansky N, Levy S, Rimon E, Cojocaru L, Fridman A, Ozer Z, Knobler H. Hypoglycemia as a predictor of mortality in hospitalized elderly patients. Arch Intern Med 2003;163:1825–1829
20. Stagnaro-Green A, Barton MK, Linekin PL, Corkery E, deBeer K, Roman SH. Mortality in hospitalized patients with hypoglycemia and severe hyperglycemia. Mt Sinai J Med 1995;62:422–426
21. Shilo S, Berezovsky S, Friedlander Y, Sonnenblick M. Hypoglycemia in hospitalized nondiabetic older patients. J Am Geriatr Soc 1998;46:978–982
22. Sullivan DH, Sun S, Walls RC. Protein-energy undernutrition among elderly hospitalized patients: a prospective study. JAMA 1999;281:2013–2019
23. Schmitz HL, Glover EC. Glycolysis in leucemic blood. J Biol Chem 1927;74:761–773

Effect of Continuous Glucose Monitoring on Hypoglycemia in Type 1 Diabetes

Tadej Battelino, md, phd[1]
Moshe Phillip, md[2]
Natasa Bratina, md, phd[1]

Revital Nimri, md[2]
Per Oskarsson, md, phd[3]
Jan Bolinder, md, phd[3]

OBJECTIVE—To assess the impact of continuous glucose monitoring on hypoglycemia in people with type 1 diabetes.

RESEARCH DESIGN AND METHODS—In this randomized, controlled, multicenter study, 120 children and adults on intensive therapy for type 1 diabetes and a screening level of glycated hemoglobin A_{1c} (HbA_{1c}) <7.5% were randomly assigned to a control group performing conventional home monitoring with a blood glucose meter and wearing a masked continuous glucose monitor every second week for five days or to a group with real-time continuous glucose monitoring. The primary outcome was the time spent in hypoglycemia (interstitial glucose concentration <63 mg/dL) over a period of 26 weeks. Analysis was by intention to treat for all randomized patients.

RESULTS—The time per day spent in hypoglycemia was significantly shorter in the continuous monitoring group than in the control group (mean ± SD 0.48 ± 0.57 and 0.97 ± 1.55 h/day, respectively; ratio of means 0.49; 95% CI 0.26–0.76; $P = 0.03$). HbA_{1c} at 26 weeks was lower in the continuous monitoring group than in the control group (difference −0.27%; 95% CI −0.47 to −0.07; $P = 0.008$). Time spent in 70 to 180 mg/dL normoglycemia was significantly longer in the continuous glucose monitoring group compared with the control group (mean hours per day, 17.6 vs. 16.0, $P = 0.009$).

CONCLUSIONS—Continuous glucose monitoring was associated with reduced time spent in hypoglycemia and a concomitant decrease in HbA_{1c} in children and adults with type 1 diabetes.

Diabetes Care 34:795–800, 2011

The benefits of intensive treatment of type 1 diabetes, established almost 20 years ago (1), are difficult to achieve, despite the increased use of insulin analogs and insulin pumps, with only a minority of patients maintaining their glycated hemoglobin A_{1c} (HbA_{1c}) within the target range (2). Intensive insulin treatment and lower HbA_{1c} increase exposure to hypoglycemia (3,4). The risk of hypoglycemia is even higher in children and adolescents (5,6) and increases with the duration of diabetes (7). Frequent hypoglycemia is associated with hypoglycemia unawareness (8,9), which

may in turn lead to reduced adherence to therapeutic decisions (10). Finally, hypoglycemia may be associated with permanent damage to the central nervous system (11) and may permanently influence cognitive functions in children (12) but not in adults (13).

Recently, devices for real-time continuous glucose monitoring have been introduced to aid self-management of glycemic control and have been shown to improve HbA_{1c} levels in people with type 1 diabetes (14–17). In clinical practice recommendations, it has also been suggested that continuous glucose monitoring is

especially useful in patients with hypoglycemia unawareness and/or frequent episodes of hypoglycemia (18). However, the hypoglycemia preventive effect of continuous glucose monitoring has not been established. Therefore, we designed a randomized, controlled, multicenter clinical trial to evaluate the effect of continuous glucose monitoring on hypoglycemia in children and adults with type 1 diabetes.

RESEARCH DESIGN AND METHODS

Patients
Patients aged between 10 and 65 years with type 1 diabetes diagnosed for more than 1 year, with reasonable metabolic control assessing carbohydrate intake and self-adjusting insulin, and an HbA_{1c} level <7.5%, using intensive insulin treatment with either an insulin pump or multiple daily injections, and not using a real-time continuous glucose monitoring device for at least 4 weeks were eligible for the study. All eligible patients identified from the local diabetes registries were invited to participate and screened consecutively based on the order of their positive reply. The study protocol was designed by the researchers and approved by the institutional or national medical ethics committees from all three centers, and the conduct of the study was consistent with the Good Clinical Practice provisions of the Declaration of Helsinki with all amendments and local regulatory requirements. A written informed consent was obtained from all participants and parents of minors (under 18 years of age, who signed an assent) before enrollment.

At screening patients provided a blood sample for measurement of HbA_{1c} and entered a 4-week run-in period during which self-monitoring of blood glucose (SMBG) was conducted according to patients' standard glycemic management regimen. A FreeStyle blood glucose meter (Abbott Diabetes Care, Alameda, CA) was provided to familiarize patients with FreeStyle test strips and collect baseline SMBG frequency and glucose levels. Diaries were distributed for recording events of hypoglycemia and associated food intake, insulin doses, and exercise.

From the [1]Department of Pediatric Endocrinology, Diabetes and Metabolism, Faculty of Medicine, University Medical Centre-University Children's Hospital, University of Ljubljana, Ljubljana, Slovenia; [2]The Jesse Z. and Sara Lea Shafer Institute for Endocrinology and Diabetes, National Center for Childhood Diabetes, Schneider Children's Medical Center, Petah Tikva and Sackler Faculty of Medicine, Tel-Aviv University, Tel-Aviv, Israel; and the [3]Department of Medicine, Karolinska University Hospital Huddinge, Karolinska Institutet, Stockholm, Sweden.

Corresponding author: Tadej Battelino, tadej.battelino@mf.uni-lj.si.

Received 20 October 2010 and accepted 13 January 2011.

DOI: 10.2337/dc10-1989. Clinical trial reg. no. NCT00843609, clinicaltrials.gov.

This article contains Supplementary Data online at http://care.diabetesjournals.org/lookup/suppl/doi:10.2337/dc10-1989/-/DC1.

All patients meeting the eligibility criteria, including HbA$_{1c}$ result from the screening visit, were invited to attend the randomization visit.

Study design

Following the 1-month run-in period, patients were randomized to participate in a 6-month intervention period. Patients were assigned to home monitoring with a FreeStyle blood glucose meter and a masked continuous glucose monitor to be worn for 5 days every second week (control group) or to a group with real-time continuous glucose monitoring, wearing individual sensors for 5 days continuously for 26 weeks (continuous monitoring group). Patients and investigators were masked for the continuous glucose monitoring data in the control group. Patients were allocated to either group by permuted block randomization stratified according to age (10 to 17 years pediatric, 18 to 65 years adult) and study center. The randomization sequence was computer generated, and allocations were concealed using envelopes. Both groups were provided with the FreeStyle Navigator (Abbott Diabetes Care), a continuous glucose monitoring system that measures glucose in interstitial fluid.

All patients were trained to insert and calibrate subcutaneous sensors and to operate the continuous monitoring device. Patients in the continuous monitoring group were instructed in the use of real-time glucose readings; however, no written guidelines were given on adjustment of diabetes management based on the real-time readings. Patients also individually set their glucose alarms. All patients were encouraged to maintain their blood glucose concentration within the preprandial target range of 70 to 130 mg/dL with peak postprandial values below 180 mg/dL.

The first subcutaneous sensor was inserted upon randomization at visit 2 (day 1). The schedule of follow-up visits was identical for both groups. All patients returned for a visit 2–6 days after randomization for upload of all devices to confirm that continuous data were recorded and to replace the subcutaneous sensor under supervision. Further visits were conducted at days 60, 120, and 180 (±7 days). Data were uploaded at each visit, and adverse events including severe hypoglycemia (19), hyperglycemia resulting in ketoacidosis requiring intravenous fluids, device-related or study-related untoward events, and serious adverse events regardless of cause, were reviewed and reported.

Diabetes self-management was adjusted by patients based on the blood glucose measurements in the control group and blood glucose measurements and continuous glucose data in the continuous glucose monitoring group. Samples for HbA$_{1c}$ were collected at days 1, 60, and 180. All samples for HbA$_{1c}$ were sent to a central laboratory (Laboratorium Klinische Forschung, Kiel, Germany; measurement by Bio-Rad Variant II Turbo analyzer, Bio-Rad Laboratories, Hercules, CA).

Statistical analysis

The primary outcome was time spent in hypoglycemia (<63 mg/dL) during the 26-week study period. A sample size of 120 patients was planned to have a power of 80% to detect a difference in the time spent in hypoglycemia between study groups, assuming a population difference of 42%, a SD of 1.12, an α-level of 0.05, and a loss to follow-up of no more than 17%.

All analyses were performed according to the intent-to-treat principle, including all data collected for patients that discontinued prematurely. An excursion was defined as all consecutive recordings outside the boundary covering at least 10 min. The duration of an excursion was defined as the elapsed time from first excursion to the first reading indicating return inside the excursion boundary. Continuous glucose monitoring data in both groups were used to estimate the amount of time per day the glucose level was hypoglycemic (<63 mg/dL, <70 mg/dL, or <55 mg/dL), hyperglycemic (>180 mg/dL or >250 mg/dL), and in the target range (70 to 180 mg/dL or 90 to 180 mg/dL) for each patient. The number of hypoglycemic excursions (<55 and <63 mg/dL) per day and separately during the night period of 0000–0600 h was also calculated. The risk associated with glucose concentration outside the recommended range was assessed by calculating low blood glucose indexes (LBGIs) and high blood glucose indexes (HBGIs) (20). Comparisons between study groups were performed with the use of the Mann-Whitney U test. CIs for

Table 1—*Baseline characteristics of the patients*

	Control group	Continuous monitoring group
N	58	62
Female sex, number (%)	19 (33)	26 (42)
Age (years)*	26.0 ± 14.6	25.7 ± 14.1
Pediatric, number (%)	26 (45)	27 (44)
BMI (kg/m^2)*	22.0 ± 3.8	22.4 ± 3.8
Duration of diabetes (years)*	11.4 ± 11.4	11.6 ± 11.3
Insulin administration, number (%)		
Pump	34 (59)	47 (76)
MDI	24 (41)	15 (24)
Glycated hemoglobin at screening (%)*	6.90 ± 0.47	6.83 ± 0.44
Glycated hemoglobin at baseline (%)*	6.91 ± 0.67	6.92 ± 0.56
Record of severe hypoglycemia in last year, number (%)	7 (12)	5 (8)
Diagnosed with hypoglycemia unawareness, number (%)	4 (7)	6 (10)
Daily insulin dose (units/kg)*	0.67 ± 0.32	0.66 ± 0.25
Education, number (%)		
Pediatric patient still in education	26 (45)	29 (47)
Completed education by age 18	3 (5)	6 (10)
Completed further education	29 (50)	27 (44)
Prior use of continuous glucose monitor, number (%)	18 (31)	21 (34)
Mean blood glucose in 1-month run-in period (mg/dL)*	148 ± 28	147 ± 23
SMBG measurements per day in 1-month run-in period*	5.1 ± 2.5	5.3 ± 2.2

Differences between the control and the continuous monitoring group were not statistically significant. MDI, multiple daily injection. *Means ± SD.

the ratio of the study group means (continuous monitoring/control) were calculated using the bias-corrected accelerated (BCa) bootstrap method. A P value of less than 0.05 (two-sided test) was considered to indicate statistical significance.

Comparison between the two study groups of HbA_{1c} levels at days 60 and 180 was performed using ANCOVA on baseline HbA_{1c} level and adjusted for clinical center and adult or pediatric patient. Missing HbA_{1c} data were imputed using the last-observation-carried-forward method, including patients that discontinued prematurely.

Analyses were conducted with the use of SAS software, version 8.02 (SAS Institute, Cary, NC). All P values were two-sided.

All researchers had full access to the whole database after it was locked.

RESULTS

Patients
In the period from October 2008 to May 2009, 122 eligible patients were screened. Of these, two patients dropped out before randomization, and 58 were randomized to the control and 62 were randomized to the continuous glucose monitoring group. The study was completed by 48 patients (83%) and 53 patients (85%),

respectively. The study flowchart is depicted in Supplementary Fig. 1. Patient baseline characteristics are summarized in Table 1.

During the one-month run-in period, the mean concentration and frequency of home blood glucose monitoring was similar in the control and continuous monitoring groups (Table 1). Mean HbA_{1c} measured at the end of the run-in period before randomization was 6.9 ± 0.7 and 6.9 ± 0.6%, respectively.

In the six-month randomized study period, median sensor wear was 5.6 (pediatric 5.6, adults 4.9) and 6.1 (pediatric 6.1, adults 6.1) days per week of instructed use in the control and continuous monitoring groups, respectively. Median sensor wear in the continuous monitoring group in month 6 was 5.9 days per week. Detailed data on sensor wear are presented in Supplementary Table 1 and Supplementary Figs. 2 and 3.

Hypoglycemia
The primary outcome, time spent in hypoglycemia below 63 mg/dL, was significantly shorter in the continuous glucose monitoring group (ratio of means 0.49 [95% CI 0.26–0.76], P = 0.03) (Supplementary Fig. 4). Similarly, time spent in hypoglycemia below 70 mg/dL and below 55 mg/dL was statistically significantly shorter in the continuous

glucose monitoring group (P = 0.01 and P = 0.05, respectively; Table 2). The reduction in the primary outcome was evident from the first month and was sustained throughout the 6 months (Fig. 1).

The integrated glucose excursion index for <63 mg/dL was reduced in the continuous monitoring group (P = 0.02) as was the low blood glucose index (P = 0.02). Although not statistically significant, the number of hypoglycemic excursions (<55 and <63 mg/dL) per 24 h/day was also lower in the continuous monitoring group (P = 0.07 and P = 0.08, respectively). The number of hypoglycemic excursions <55 and <63 mg/dL during the night, however, was significantly lower in the continuous monitoring group compared with the control (0.13 ± 0.30 vs. 0.19 ± 0.19, P = 0.01; and 0.21 ± 0.32 vs. 0.30 ± 0.31, P = 0.009).

Time spent in hypoglycemia below 63 mg/dL was reduced in the continuous monitoring group by 41% (mean 0.48 vs. 0.81 h/day) in pump users and by 59% (0.49 vs. 1.20) in subjects on multiple daily injections. This end point was reduced by 48% (0.34 vs. 0.65) in pediatric subjects (10–17 years of age) and by 54% (0.59 vs. 1.27) in adults (18–65 years of age). In the post hoc per protocol analysis, where only patients that wore the sensor for >20 days (corresponding

Table 2—Glycemic outcomes

Variable	Control group	Continuous monitoring group	Ratio of means	95% CI for ratio of means	P
N	54	62			
Hours per day in hypoglycemia <63 mg/dL	0.97 ± 1.55	0.48 ± 0.57	0.49	0.26–0.76	0.03
Median (interquartile range)	0.54 (0.23–1.31)	0.26 (0.14–0.54)			
Number of hypoglycemic excursions per day					
<63 mg/dL	0.76 ± 0.94	0.53 ± 0.60	0.70	0.43–1.03	0.08
Integrated glucose excursion index (area under the curve) <63 mg/dL	11.1 ± 14.2	5.4 ± 7.6	0.49	0.29–0.79	0.02
Hours per day in hypoglycemia <55 mg/dL	0.41 ± 0.48	0.22 ± 0.34	0.55	0.34–0.91	0.05
Number of hypoglycemic excursions per day					
<55 mg/dL	0.37 ± 0.40	0.28 ± 0.54	0.76	0.47–1.43	0.07
Hours per day in hypoglycemia <70 mg/dL	1.60 ± 2.02	0.91 ± 0.81	0.57	0.36–0.80	0.01
Low blood glucose index	1.74 ± 1.62	1.18 ± 0.82	0.68	0.49–0.89	0.02
Hours per day in hyperglycemia					
>180 mg/dL	6.4 ± 3.4	5.5 ± 3.2	0.86	0.71–1.06	0.08
>250 mg/dL	1.66 ± 1.53	1.14 ± 1.46	0.69	0.48–1.07	0.06
High blood glucose index	6.0 ± 3.2	5.1 ± 3.1	0.85	0.70–1.05	0.05
Hours per day in normoglycemia					
90–180 mg/dL	13.5 ± 3.1	15.1 ± 2.7	1.12	1.04–1.21	0.003
70–180 mg/dL	16.0 ± 3.4	17.6 ± 3.2	1.10	1.02–1.18	0.009

Data are means ± SD. An excursion is defined as all consecutive recordings outside the boundary and covering at least 10 min. The duration of an excursion is defined as the elapsed time from first excursion to the first reading indicating return inside the excursion boundary.

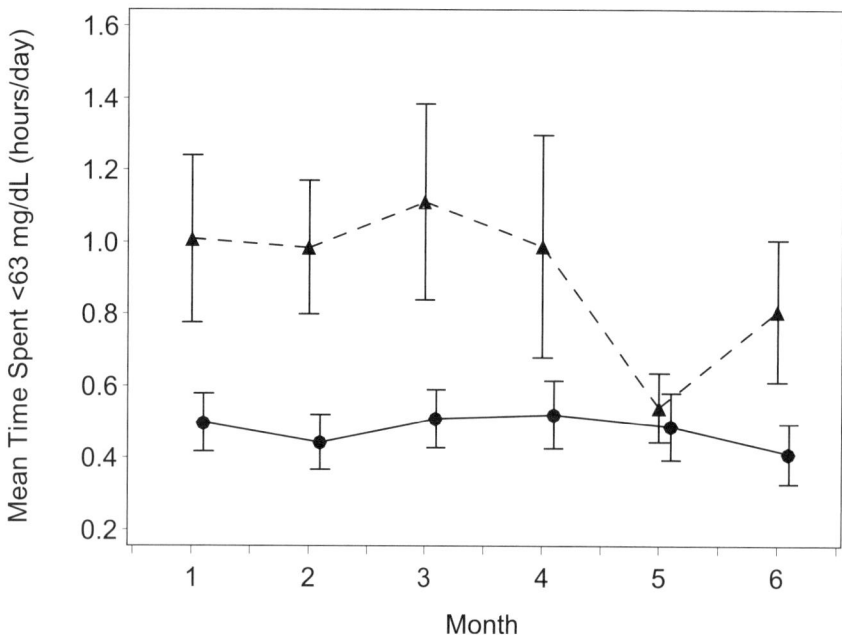

Figure 1—*Time spent below 63 mg/dL by month. Mean values ± SEs for hours per day spent <63 mg/dL over the 6-month study period in all patients. ●, continuous monitoring group; ▲, control group.*

to one third of the required time in the control group) were included (44 of 53 pediatric and 53 of 63 adult patients), the primary outcome was reduced by 64% ($P < 0.001$) and 50% ($P = 0.02$) in pediatric and adult patients, respectively.

Glycated hemoglobin and glycemic control

HbA_{1c} at 6 months, adjusted for baseline HbA_{1c} (visit 2), center and age-group was significantly lower in the continuous glucose monitoring group (mean 6.69% compared with 6.95%, difference in means −0.27, 95% CI −0.47 to −0.07, $P = 0.008$) (Fig. 2). Mean HbA_{1c} at 6 months, adjusted for baseline HbA_{1c}, center and age-group, was reduced by 0.39 in pump users (6.72 vs. 7.11). For subjects using multiple daily injections, the difference was −0.06 (6.70 vs. 6.65). Adjusted mean HbA_{1c} was reduced by 0.23 (6.92 vs. 7.15) in pediatric subjects (10–17 years of age) and by 0.31 (6.51 vs. 6.83) in adults (18–65 years of age).

Time spent in normoglycemia (70 to 180 mg/dL and 90 to 180 mg/dL) was significantly longer in the continuous glucose monitoring group (mean hours per day, 17.6 vs. 16.0, $P = 0.009$; and 15.1 vs. 13.5, $P = 0.003$). Concurrently, the time spent per day in hyperglycemia >250 mg/dL was shorter in the continuous monitoring group compared with control

group (mean hours per day, 1.14 and 1.66), although this was not statistically significant.

Adverse events

Four serious adverse events were reported although none were related to the study or device (Supplementary Table 2). There was an incident of mild diabetic ketoacidosis (DKA) in a patient in the continuous monitoring group, because of the patient disconnecting his or her insulin pump. However, this patient had stopped wearing the continuous glucose monitoring system 2 weeks before the incident. No incidents of severe hypoglycemia were reported.

CONCLUSIONS—This randomized controlled trial, designed to evaluate the effect of continuous glucose monitoring on hypoglycemia in type 1 diabetes, demonstrated a significant reduction by half in time spent in hypoglycemia in relatively well-controlled children and adults with type 1 diabetes. Notably, this finding was paralleled by a significant decrease in HbA_{1c}, contrary to the results in the Diabetes Control and Complication Trial (DCCT) study where the rate of hypoglycemia increased considerably with lower HbA_{1c} levels (21).

In the Juvenile Diabetes Research Foundation (JDRF) trial in children and

adults with $HbA_{1c} <7\%$ at randomization (15), hypoglycemia below 60 mg/dL was less pronounced in the continuous monitoring group than in the control group at the end of 6 months (median 18 vs. 35 min/day, $P = 0.05$). Moreover, combined outcomes of hypoglycemia and HbA_{1c} were significantly better in the continuous glucose monitoring patients than in the control patients, which corroborate our findings.

A recent randomized controlled trial named Sensor-Augmented Pump Therapy for A1C Reduction 3 (STAR 3) comparing sensor-augmented pump therapy with multiple-injection therapy demonstrated a significant reduction of HbA_{1c} in adults and children without an increase in hypoglycemia (22). However, the area under the curve <70 mg/dL and <50 mg/dL did not differ between the two treatment modalities. It is possible that the relatively small amount of continuous sensor data in the multiple-injection therapy group lacked sufficient power to show a difference. Additionally, the baseline HbA_{1c} was considerably higher in the STAR 3 trial as compared with the current study.

None of the participants or parents in the current study reported an event of severe hypoglycemia. Similarly, severe hypoglycemia episodes were infrequent in the JDRF trial (less than 10% of the patients) (15) and the STAR 3 trial (around 13 per 100 patient-years) (22) and did not differ between the study groups. Neither the JDRF trial nor ours was powered to detect differences in the rate of severe hypoglycemic episodes. In the open extension phase of the JDRF trial, episodes of severe hypoglycemia decreased by almost 50% in the control patients after they were switched to continuous glucose monitoring, but this was not statistically significant ($P = 0.08$) (16).

Although the number of hypoglycemic excursions below 55 mg/dL was not significantly different between the two groups per 24 h, it was significantly lower in the continuous monitoring group during the night. In the JDRF trial, a higher incidence of nocturnal hypoglycemia is associated with lower HbA_{1c} in the continuous glucose monitoring group; however, no comparison is made with the control group (23). Taken together, previous and present data may suggest that the risk of hypoglycemia is alleviated by continuous glucose monitoring. Clinically more meaningful reduction of hypoglycemic events remains to be demonstrated.

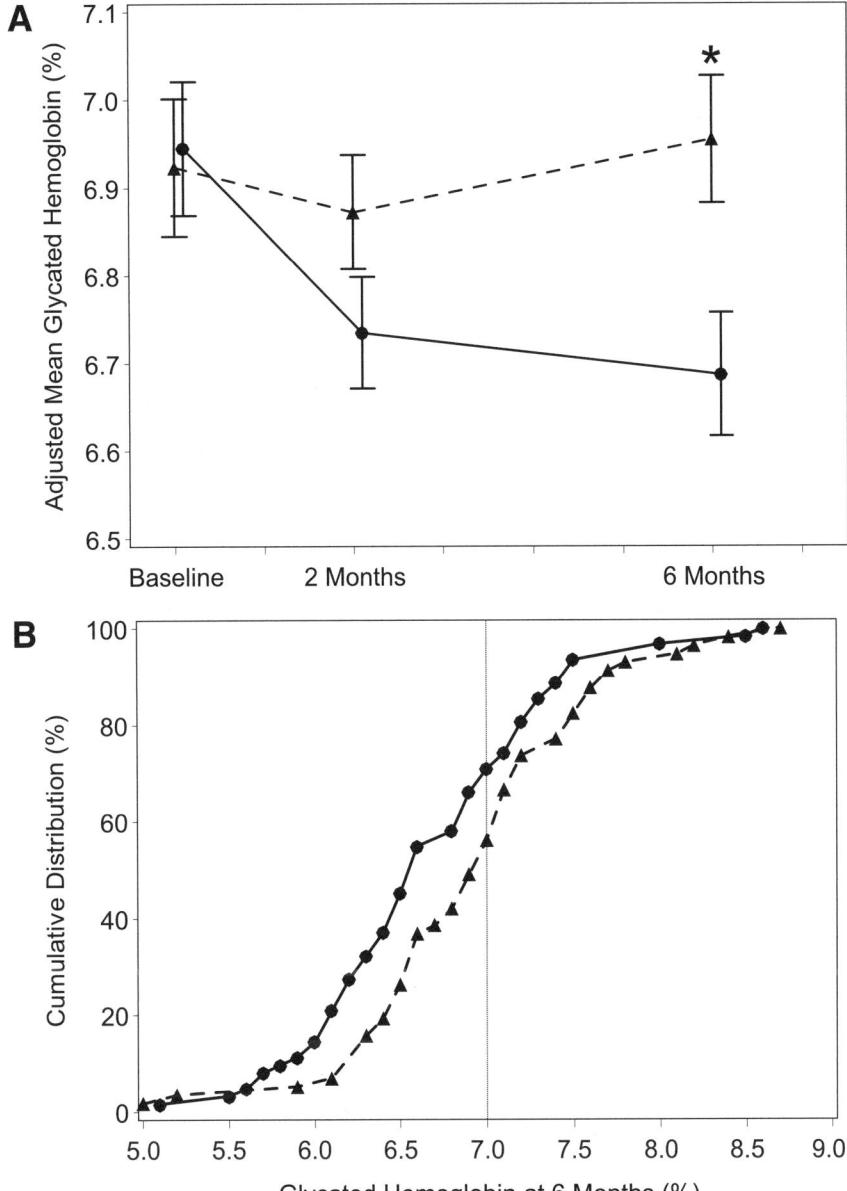

Figure 2—*Glycated HbA₁c at 2, 4, and 6 months and cumulative distribution of HbA₁c levels at 6 months. Mean values are ± SEs for HbA₁c (in %) over the 6-month study period in all patients. The means were adjusted for clinical center and adult or pediatric patient. An asterisk denotes statistical significance for comparison between the continuous monitoring and control groups with P < 0.05 (A); cumulative distribution of HbA₁c levels at 6 months among all patients is shown. The vertical line represents the American Diabetes Association target of 7.0% (B). ●, continuous monitoring group; ▲, control group.*

during the 26-week study period. In fact, compliance with the sensor wear in the control group was lower than intended (around 80%). However, when compared with previous studies, the amount of masked continuous monitoring data from the control group was substantial. Combined with the high compliance of sensor use in the continuous monitoring group, this contributed to the power of the statistical analysis.

Our results must be interpreted with caution since the patients and their families were highly motivated, demonstrating good metabolic control with an average of more than five blood glucose measurements per day before randomization, and all three participating centers were academic with high penetration of diabetes-related technology. Additionally, because of its nature, the intervention could not be blinded, rendering the results less compelling. The results may therefore not be simply generalized, and further studies are needed to evaluate the hypoglycemia-preventive effects of continuous glucose monitoring in less well-controlled and less motivated patient populations.

In conclusion, the results of the current study demonstrated significantly shorter time spent in hypoglycemia in children and adults with type 1 diabetes who used continuous glucose monitoring compared with standard SMBG, with a concomitant significant decrease of HbA₁c.

Acknowledgments—This study was supported by Abbott Diabetes Care. T.B. was supported in part by the Slovenian National Research Agency Grants J3-9663, J3-2412, and P3-0343.

T.B.'s institution received research grant support, with receipt of travel and accommodation expenses in some cases, from Abbott, Medtronic, Novo Nordisk, and Diamyd. T.B. is on the speaker's bureaux of Eli Lilly, Novo Nordisk, Bayer, and Medtronic and is a member of scientific advisory boards for Bayer, LifeScan, and Medtronic. M.P.'s institution received research grant support, with receipt of travel and accommodation expenses in some cases, from Medtronic and Dexcom. M.P. is a consultant for Animas, Medtronic, and Bayer and is a member of scientific advisory boards for CGM3, D-Medical, and Physical Logic. N.B. is on the speaker's bureau of Medtronic. R.N.'s institution received research grant support, with receipt of travel and accommodation expenses in some cases, from Medtronic and Dexcom. J.B. is on the speaker's bureau of Abbott, Medtronic, and sanofi-aventis and

Several studies have demonstrated that the use of continuous monitoring above 70% of the time is associated with significantly increased benefit and with a significant lowering of HbA₁c in all age groups (17,22,24). Compliance with the sensor wear in the current study in the continuous monitoring group was more than 6 days per week (86%) and did not decrease significantly with time, with an average of around 5.8 days/week (84%) at the end of the 26-week period (Supplementary Fig. 2B). This is roughly similar to the adult group and considerably more than the adolescent or children group of the JDRF trial (16).

This study protocol stated that the control group should wear a masked sensor for 5 days every second week, amounting to 65 days or around 9 weeks is a member of scientific advisory boards for AstraZeneca, Medtronic, and Merck Sharp & Dohme. Abbott Diabetes Care provided funding, device-related training, and analytical support. Abbott Diabetes Care was permitted to review the manuscript and suggest changes, but the final decision on content and submission of the manuscript was exclusively retained by the authors, who take responsibility for the accuracy and integrity of the data and analyses. This study was an investigator-initiated trial. The study and protocol were designed by the investigators. The manuscript was prepared by the investigators. No other potential conflicts of interest relevant to this article were reported.

T.B. contributed to the study concept and design, collected data, supervised the study, participated in data analysis and interpretation, and drafted, reviewed, and edited the manuscript. M.P. contributed to the study concept and design, collected data, supervised the study, participated in data analysis and interpretation, and reviewed and edited the manuscript. N.B., R.N., and P.O. collected data, participated in data analysis and interpretation, and reviewed and edited the manuscript. J.B. contributed to the study concept and design, collected data, supervised the study, participated in data analysis and interpretation, and reviewed and edited the manuscript.

The authors thank the following colleagues for assistance in conducting the study: Dr. Nina Bratanic and Ivica Zupancic, diabetes nurse, from the University Children's Hospital Ljubljana, Slovenia; and Ingela Bredenberg and Hilkka Lahnalampi, diabetes nurses from the Karolinska University Hospital Huddinge, Sweden. Statisticians of Abbott Diabetes Care and an independent statistician (James Gallagher, Director, Statistical Services Centre, University of Reading) worked with the investigators to prepare the statistical analysis plan and performed the analyses. Jude Douglass, a medical writer of Healthcom Partners, edited English language and style and formatted the manuscript for publication.

Parts of this study were presented at the 4th International Conference on Advanced Technologies and Treatments for Diabetes, London, U.K., 16–19 February 2011.

References

1. The Diabetes Control and Complications Trial Research Group. The effect of intensive treatment of diabetes on the development and progression of long-term complications in insulin-dependent diabetes mellitus. N Engl J Med 1993;329: 977–986

2. Hanberger L, Samuelsson U, Lindblad B, Ludvigsson J; Swedish Childhood Diabetes Registry SWEDIABKIDS. A1C in children and adolescents with diabetes in relation to certain clinical parameters: the Swedish Childhood Diabetes Registry SWEDIABKIDS. Diabetes Care 2008;31: 927–929

3. Shalitin S, Phillip M. Hypoglycemia in type 1 diabetes: a still unresolved problem in the era of insulin analogs and pump therapy. Diabetes Care 2008;31(Suppl. 2):S121–S124

4. Cryer PE. Hypoglycaemia: the limiting factor in the glycaemic management of type I and type II diabetes. Diabetologia 2002;45:937–948

5. Diabetes Control and Complications Trial Research Group. Effect of intensive diabetes treatment on the development and progression of long-term complications in adolescents with insulin-dependent diabetes mellitus: Diabetes Control and Complications Trial. J Pediatr 1994;125: 177–188

6. Bulsara MK, Holman CDJ, Davis EA, Jones TW. The impact of a decade of changing treatment on rates of severe hypoglycemia in a population-based cohort of children with type 1 diabetes. Diabetes Care 2004; 27:2293–2298

7. Cryer PE, Davis SN, Shamoon H. Hypoglycemia in diabetes. Diabetes Care 2003; 26:1902–1912

8. Daneman D. Type 1 diabetes. Lancet 2006;367:847–858

9. Cryer PE. Diverse causes of hypoglycemia-associated autonomic failure in diabetes. N Engl J Med 2004;350:2272–2279

10. Smith CB, Choudhary P, Pernet A, Hopkins D, Amiel SA. Hypoglycemia unawareness is associated with reduced adherence to therapeutic decisions in patients with type 1 diabetes: evidence from a clinical audit. Diabetes Care 2009;32:1196–1198

11. Hershey T, Perantie DC, Wu J, Weaver PM, Black KJ, White NH. Hippocampal volumes in youth with type 1 diabetes. Diabetes 2010;59:236–241

12. Gaudieri PA, Chen R, Greer TF, Holmes CS. Cognitive function in children with type 1 diabetes: a meta-analysis. Diabetes Care 2008;31:1892–1897

13. Jacobson AM, Musen G, Ryan CM, et al.; Diabetes Control and Complications Trial/ Epidemiology of Diabetes Interventions and Complications Study Research Group. Long-term effect of diabetes and its treatment on cognitive function. N Engl J Med 2007;356:1842–1852

14. Deiss D, Bolinder J, Riveline J-P, et al. Improved glycemic control in poorly controlled patients with type 1 diabetes using real-time continuous glucose monitoring. Diabetes Care 2006;29:2730–2732

15. Juvenile Diabetes Research Foundation Continuous Glucose Monitoring Study Group. The effect of continuous glucose monitoring in well-controlled type 1 diabetes. Diabetes Care 2009;32:1378–1383

16. Tamborlane WV, Beck RW, Bode BW, et al.; Juvenile Diabetes Research Foundation Continuous Glucose Monitoring Study Group. Continuous glucose monitoring and intensive treatment of type 1 diabetes. N Engl J Med 2008;359:1464–1476

17. O'Connell MA, Donath S, O'Neal DN, et al. Glycaemic impact of patient-led use of sensor-guided pump therapy in type 1 diabetes: a randomised controlled trial. Diabetologia 2009;52:1250–1257

18. American Diabetes Association. Standards of medical care in diabetes—2010. Diabetes Care 2010;33(Suppl. 1):S11–S61

19. The DCCT Research Group. Epidemiology of severe hypoglycemia in the diabetes control and complications trial. Am J Med 1991;90:450–459

20. Kovatchev BP, Clarke WL, Breton M, Brayman K, McCall A. Quantifying temporal glucose variability in diabetes via continuous glucose monitoring: mathematical methods and clinical application. Diabetes Technol Ther 2005;7: 849–862

21. The Diabetes Control and Complications Trial Research Group. Hypoglycemia in the Diabetes Control and Complications Trial. Diabetes 1997;46:271–286

22. Bergenstal RM, Tamborlane WV, Ahmann A, et al.; STAR 3 Study Group. Effectiveness of sensor-augmented insulin-pump therapy in type 1 diabetes. N Engl J Med 2010;363:311–320

23. Juvenile Diabetes Research Foundation Continuous Glucose Monitoring Study Group. Prolonged nocturnal hypoglycemia is common during 12 months of continuous glucose monitoring in children and adults with type 1 diabetes. Diabetes Care 2010;33:1004–1008

24. Beck RW, Buckingham B, Miller K, et al.; Juvenile Diabetes Research Foundation Continuous Glucose Monitoring Study Group. Factors predictive of use and of benefit from continuous glucose monitoring in type 1 diabetes. Diabetes Care 2009;32:1947–1953

Repeated Episodes of Hypoglycemia as a Potential Aggravating Factor for Preclinical Atherosclerosis in Subjects With Type 1 Diabetes

Marga Giménez, md[1,2]
Rosa Gilabert, md, phd[3]
Joan Monteagudo, md, phd[4]
Anna Alonso, bn[1]

Roser Casamitjana, md, phd[5]
Carles Paré, md, phd[6]
Ignacio Conget, md, phd[1,2]

OBJECTIVE — To evaluate through early preclinical atherosclerosis assessment whether repeated episodes of hypoglycemia represent an aggravating factor for macrovascular disease in type 1 diabetes.

RESEARCH DESIGN AND METHODS — After sample-size calculation, a case-control study of 25 patients with type 1 diabetes and repeated severe/nonsevere hypoglycemia (H-group) compared with 20 age- and sex-matched type 1 diabetes control subjects (C-group) was designed. Assessment of preclinical atherosclerosis consisted of flow-mediated brachial dilatation (FMD) and carotid and femoral intima-media thickness (IMT) studies. To consider hypoglycemia awareness, two different questionnaires and symptomatic response to an acute induction to hypoglycemia were used. Evaluation of the glycemic profile was obtained from continuous glucose monitoring. Endothelial function/inflammation markers were measured in euglycemia/hypoglycemia. A multivariate linear regression analysis was performed to test whether repeated hypoglycemia was independently associated with atherosclerosis.

RESULTS — H-group subjects displayed hypoglycemia unawareness and presented a higher percentage of continuous glucose values and area under the curve <70 mg/dl compared with the C-group (14.2 ± 8.9 vs. 6.3 ± 7.1%, $P < 0.02$ and 2.4 ± 1.8 vs. 0.6 ± 1.0 mg/dl/day, $P < 0.01$). The percentage of maximal FMD was lower in the H-group than in the C-group (6.52 ± 2.92 vs. 8.62 ± 3.13%, $P < 0.05$). A significantly higher IMT was observed at both carotid and femoral sites in the H-group (carotid 0.53 ± 0.09 vs. 0.47 ± 0.08 mm, $P < 0.05$ and femoral 0.51 ± 0.17 vs. 0.39 ± 0.09 mm, $P < 0.05$). Baseline inflammation and endothelial function markers were higher in the H-group (leukocytes 7.0 ± 1.8 vs. 5.6 ± 1.4 × 10³/ml, von Willebrand factor 119 ± 29 vs. 93 ± 26%, fibrinogen 2.82 ± 0.64 vs. 2.29 ± 0.44g/l, and soluble intercellular adhesion molecule-1 408 ± 224 vs. 296 ± 95 ng/ml; $P < 0.05$ for all).

CONCLUSIONS — In addition to the induction of hypoglycemia unawareness and an increased risk for severe hypoglycemia, repeated hypoglycemia could be related to and considered an aggravating factor for preclinical atherosclerosis in type 1 diabetes. The precise mechanisms explaining this association remain to be clarified.

Diabetes Care 34:198–203, 2011

Even though many of the cardiovascular disease (CVD) risk factors recognized in type 2 diabetes are not present in type 1 diabetic subjects, the age-adjusted relative risk for CVD in type 1 diabetes is even higher than that in type 2 diabetes (1). Since the availability of data from Diabetes Control and Compli-cations Trial (DCCT)/Epidemiology of Diabetes Interventions and Complications (EDIC) studies, there is no doubt that intensive therapy positively affects the long-term incidence of micro- and macrovascular disease in subjects with type 1 diabetes (2,3). However, because the association between glycemic control and macrovascular disease is mainly obtained from epidemiological data, the role of glycemic control in macrovascular disease is still controversial. In contrast, intensive glucose control invariably increases the risk of hypoglycemia.

Iatrogenic hypoglycemia causes recurrent morbidity in most people with type 1 diabetes. Frequent and repeated episodes of hypoglycemia almost unfailingly result in a reduced ability or failure to recognize hypoglycemia symptoms and signs. This syndrome of hypoglycemia unawareness frequently occurs in type 1 diabetes, and patients without warning symptoms are then at a high risk for severe hypoglycemia (4). In addition, hypoglycemia is a major barrier to achieving normoglycemia over a lifetime of using intensive insulin therapy and thus precludes the long-term benefits of euglycemia (4). More recently, Gill et al. (5) reported QT prolongation and cardiac and rhythm disturbances in response to nocturnal hypoglycemia in ambulatory patients with type 1 diabetes, which may support the idea of an arrhythmic basis for "death in bed syndrome."

Carotid intima-media thickness (cIMT) and the assessment of endothelial function have been shown to be markers of preclinical atherosclerosis and correlate with prevalent and incident cardiovascular disease (6). In the DCCT/EDIC, the progression of cIMT in the population of type 1 diabetic subjects was used as a measure of atherosclerosis (7).

It has also been reported that patients with type 1 diabetes presented higher cIMT and lower percentages of flow-mediated dilatation (FMD) with respect to healthy control subjects (8). Although hyperglycemia has been proven to increase the stiffness of intermediate-sized

From the [1]Endocrinology and Diabetes Unit, Hospital Clínic, Barcelona, Spain; the [2]CIBER de Diabetes y Enfermedades Metabólicas Asociadas, Barcelona, Spain; the [3]Radiology Unit, Hospital Clínic, Barcelona, Spain; the [4]Hemostasia Unit, Hospital Clínic, Barcelona, Spain; the [5]Hormonal Unit, Hospital Clínic, Barcelona, Spain; and the [6]Cardiology Unit, Hospital Clínic, Barcelona, Spain.
Corresponding author: Ignacio Conget, iconget@clinic.ub.es.
Received 16 July 2010 and accepted 28 September 2010. Published ahead of print at http://care.diabetesjournals.org on 7 October 2010. DOI: 10.2337/dc10-1371.

arteries and resistance of arteries, the analysis of discontinuous glucose profile datasets from the DCCT failed to find an association between glucose variability and the development of microvascular complications (9). Moreover, various measures for the assessment of glycemic variability have shown that there is no relationship between oxidative stress and glucose fluctuations in type 1 diabetes even though glucose variability was much higher than that in type 2 diabetes (10).

Acute hypoglycemia induces a rapid proinflammatory, platelet aggregatory, antifibrinolytic, and prothrombotic response (11,12). Recurrent hypoglycemic episodes may provoke changes in hemostatic factors and viscosity, which may reduce perfusion in diabetic microangiopathy (11,12). Rodrigues et al. (13) have recently reported that higher fibrinogen levels predict progression of coronary artery calcification in adults with type 1 diabetes. The SEARCH study has also described elevated inflammatory markers even in youth with type 1 diabetes and good metabolic control compared with control subjects, suggesting an explanation for accelerated atherosclerosis in type 1 diabetes (14). In addition, Feldman-Billard et al. (15) described hypoglycemia-induced hypertension in a group of diabetic patients. If hypoglycemia acutely provokes intense changes in hemodynamics and several hemorheological parameters, it could play a different role in atherosclerosis when chronically repeated.

Therefore, the aim of our study was to evaluate whether repeated episodes of hypoglycemia represent an aggravating factor for macrovascular disease in subjects with type 1 diabetes through early atherosclerosis-vascular assessment.

RESEARCH DESIGN AND METHODS — A total of 45 patients with type 1 diabetes were recruited for the study from 2007 to 2009. Subjects were invited to participate in the protocol if they fulfilled the following criteria: aged >18 years, type 1 diabetes duration >5 years, basal C-peptide <0.1 ng/ml, use of multiple doses of insulin in a basal-bolus schedule, and an absence of other major CVD risk factors, micro- or macrovascular complications (normal digital retinal photography results, absence of microalbuminuria, no neuropathy by clinical examination, normal ankle-brachial index, and normal stress echocardiography results), and no autonomic dysfunc-

tion (Cardionomic system; Medimatica, Milan, Italy). Patients were not taking medication chronically (including statins, antihypertensive drugs, or anti-inflammatory drugs) except insulin.

Of the 45 type 1 diabetic patients, 25 were selected as a hypoglycemic group (H-group) presenting >4 nonsevere hypoglycemia episodes per week (last 8 weeks) and >2 severe hypoglycemia episodes in the past 2 years. All episodes of capillary glycemia <70 mg/dl were considered nonsevere hypoglycemia episodes based on four to six daily capillary blood determinations. Severe hypoglycemia events were defined as those associated with neuroglycopenia severe enough to require treatment from a third party. Of the 45 type 1 diabetic patients, 20 were chosen as age- and sex-matched diabetic control subjects (C-group) presenting <2 nonsevere hypoglycemia episodes per week (last 8 weeks) and with no previous episodes of severe hypoglycemia. Anthropometric measures, general biochemical parameters, A1C values (normal range 3.5–5.5%; Menarini Diagnostici, Firenze, Italy), and lipid profile were measured at the beginning of the study.

In addition, an age- and sex-matched healthy control group (22 subjects) was selected as a comparative group for ultrasound analysis. They satisfied the criteria of being nonsmokers, having a normal fasting glycemia and lipid profile, not having hypertension, diabetes, or dyslipidemia, and not having a family history of CVD or diabetes.

The protocol included an evaluation of the frequency/awareness of hypoglycemia, an assessment of glycemic profile/glucose variability, an evaluation of endothelial function (FMD), and a carotid and femoral IMT assessment. Inflammation and endothelial function markers were evaluated.

The study protocol, conducted according to the Declaration of Helsinki, was approved by the Hospital Clínic i Universitari Ethics Committee. Informed consent was obtained from all the patients and control subjects.

Evaluation of hypoglycemia awareness
Two different questionnaires (Clarke and Gold tests [16,17]) were used to evaluate hypoglycemia awareness. To assess signs and symptoms response to a standardized situation of hypoglycemia, an acute induction to hypoglycemia with intravenous insulin was performed (18).

Subjects with type 1 diabetes answered the Hypoglycemia symptoms score questionnaire (Edinburgh scale [19]) after 30 min of euglycemia first (80–120 mg/dl) and after 30 min of hypoglycemia (45–55 mg/dl) afterward. The tests scores for the two states were compared, and the results are expressed as a percentage of increase from the baseline.

Glycemic profile and glucose variability
Immediately before vascular studies, each patient with type 1 diabetes underwent continuous glucose monitoring (CGM) for 72 h using the Medtronic Gold system. Glucose variability was evaluated by calculating mean amplitude of glucose excursions (MAGE) from continuous sensor readings. MAGE over 24 h is the mean of the absolute differences between glucose peak and nadir values in excess of at least 1 SD of the mean glucose.

Ultrasound imaging
The carotid, femoral, and brachial artery ultrasound studies were performed with an Acuson Sequoia system (Acuson Corporation, Mountain View, CA), equipped with an 8-MHz linear array transducer. The FMD studies were performed by M.G., a trained endocrinologist with experience in >150 FMD studies. The cIMT and femoral IMT (fIMT) studies were done by R.G., a radiologist with >15 years of experience. M.G. and R.G. were masked to the patient groups when they performed the FMD and IMT studies.

FMD. All patients and healthy control subjects were evaluated after 6 h of abstinence from food and caffeinated drinks. Women were examined in the follicular phase of the menstrual cycle. Capillary glycemia was always between 80 and 120 mg/dl. The brachial artery was imaged longitudinally 5–10 cm above the antecubital fossa. Baseline images were recorded continuously for 1 min. Subsequently, a blood pressure cuff positioned 4 cm below the elbow was inflated up to 250 mmHg for 5 min. The artery was continuously imaged for 4 min during the hyperemia after release of the cuff pressure to determine endothelium-dependent vasodilatation. All images were analyzed using proprietary software (Brachial Analyzer; Medical Imaging Applications, Iowa City, IA). Dilatation was calculated as maximal lumen diameter after ischemia minus lumen diameter at baseline divided by lumen diameter at baseline. Results are expressed as a percentage.

cIMT. The common carotid artery, the carotid artery bulb, and the internal carotid artery near and far wall segments were scanned bilaterally. IMT was defined as the distance between the lumen-intima and the media-adventitia interfaces. Measurements were performed offline and consisted of six manual measurements at equal distances along 1 cm on the far wall of the common carotid artery (1 cm before the bifurcation), bulb, and internal carotid artery (1 cm after the bifurcation). The mean of the 36 values for right and left sides was considered a composite measurement (cIMTcomp). Atheroma plaques (focal intrusions into the lumen with a height >50% of the nearest IMT or diffuse IMT thickening >1.2 mm) were sought by using B-mode and color Doppler imaging in all the carotid segments.

fIMT. Mean fIMT was measured in the far arterial wall along the distal 1 cm before the bifurcation. Six measurements were done manually on each side. fIMT was expressed as the mean of the 12 values.

Intraobserver variability was evaluated by comparing results from repeated examinations of 15 subjects on 2 days a week apart. The correlation coefficients for cIMT, fIMT, and percent FMD were 0.91, 0.93, and 0.74, respectively. The correlation coefficient between two different readers was 0.91 for cIMT.

Inflammation and endothelial marker evaluation

After type 1 diabetic patients had rested 30 min in euglycemia, leukocytes, high-sensitivity C-reactive protein (hs-CRP) (Behring Nephelometer analyzer; Dade Behring, Marburg, Germany), von Willebrand factor (vWF) (ELISA-based commercial kit, DG-EIA vWF; Diagnostic Grifols, Parets del Valles, Spain), fibrinogen (Thromborel S; Dade-Behring), soluble intercellular adhesion molecule-1 (sICAM-1) (ELISA-based commercial kit; BKL Diagnostics, Barcelona, Spain), soluble E-selectin (ELISA-based commercial kit; BKL Diagnostics), and interleukin-1β (1β-IL) (ELISA-based commercial kit; BioSource Europe, Nivelles, Belgium) were measured to assess inflammation and endothelial function. All of these parameters were also measured after 30 min in hypoglycemia.

Statistical analysis

Results are presented as means ± SD or percentages. Normal distribution was tested for each variable using the Kolmogorov-Smirnov test. The comparisons between groups were performed using a Student's *t* test for unpaired data for normally distributed variables or using a Mann-Whitney *U* test for nonnormally distributed variables. Proportions were compared with the use of a Fisher exact test. A multivariate linear regression analysis was performed to test whether repeated hypoglycemia was independently associated with cIMTcomp measurements. Covariates included age, sex, comorbidities (systolic blood pressure, BMI, and LDL cholesterol) and factors related to diabetes and glucose control (type 1 diabetes duration, A1C, and MAGE). $P < 0.05$ was considered statistically significant. All statistical calculations were performed with SPSS (version 14.0 for personal computers).

Sample size calculation

We planned a study of a continuous response variable from independent control subjects (C-group) and experimental subjects (H-group). Considering a true difference in the experimental and control means of 0.045 mm in cIMT, we needed to study at least 20 experimental subjects and 20 control subjects to be able to reject the null hypothesis that the population means of the experimental and control were equal with probability (power) 0.80. The type I error probability associated with this test of this null hypothesis was 0.05 (α).

RESULTS — The baseline characteristics of the H-group and C-group are shown in Table 1. There were no major differences in the whole set of clinical and laboratory parameters between type 1 diabetic subjects and healthy control subjects.

Hypoglycemia awareness and number of hypoglycemic episodes

As expected, H-group subjects had a significantly higher number of nonsevere hypoglycemia episodes per week and more severe hypoglycemia episodes than type 1 diabetic subjects in the C-group (nonsevere hypoglycemia: 5.22 ± 1.98 vs. 0.25 ± 0.50 episodes/week/subject during the previous 2 weeks, $P < 0.01$; severe hypoglycemia for 2 years before: 1.28 ± 0.45 vs. 0 episodes/patient/year).

Hypoglycemia awareness was evaluated using two different specific questionnaires. The Gold questionnaire classified 25 of 25 subjects in the H-group as having hypoglycemia unawareness but none in the C-group. On the other hand, the Clarke test classified 24 of 25 H-group subjects as having hypoglycemic unawareness and 1 of 25 as inconclusive. Again, all of the type 1 diabetic subjects from the C-group were classified as having normal awareness using the second test.

The mean score for the Edinburgh scale in euglycemia was not different between the groups (21.1 ± 2.7 vs. 20.5 ± 1.9 for the H-group and C-group, respectively). With respect to the signs/symptoms response during the acute induction of hypoglycemia, type 1 diabetic subjects in the H-group increased on average 46% on the Edinburgh scale between euglycemia and hypoglycemia, whereas those in the C-group increased 163% between both situations.

Table 1—*Characteristics of study subjects*

	H-group	C-group	P value
n	25	20	
Sex (male/female)	11/14	11/9	NS
Age (years)	34.6 ± 7.8	33.5 ± 8.7	NS
Type 1 diabetes duration (years)	16.1 ± 6.3	14.0 ± 6.5	NS
A1C (%)	6.6 ± 1.0	6.7 ± 0.7	NS
Total cholesterol (mg/dl)	171 ± 30	167 ± 34	NS
LDL cholesterol (mg/dl)	107 ± 26	101 ± 24	NS
HDL cholesterol (mg/dl)	52 ± 12	55 ± 11	NS
Triglycerides (mg/dl)	54 ± 26	47 ± 20	NS
Systolic blood pressure (mmHg)	107 ± 12	108 ± 13	NS
Diastolic blood pressure (mmHg)	71 ± 9	73 ± 10	NS
BMI (kg/m²)	23.1 ± 2.9	23.5 ± 2.3	NS
Smokers (%)	0	0	NS

Data are means ± SD.

Glycemic profile and glucose variability

With respect to the results obtained from the blinded CGM system data in type 1 diabetic patients, it was not surprising that the H-group subjects presented higher percentages of values and area under the curve <70 mg/dl with respect to the C-group (14.2 ± 8.9 vs. 6.3 ± 7.0% of values <70 mg/dl, $P < 0.02$ and 2.4 ± 1.8 vs. 0.6 ± 1.0 mg/dl area under the curve for low values, $P < 0.01$ for the H-group and C-group, respectively). Regarding glucose variability, MAGE was significantly higher in the H-group than in the C-group (136 ± 29 vs. 101 ± 28 mg/dl, $P < 0.01$).

FMD

Subjects from the H-group displayed lower percentages of FMD response to ischemia with respect to type 1 diabetic patients from the C-group (6.52 ± 2.92 vs. 8.62 ± 3.13%, $P < 0.05$) (Table 2). Both type 1 diabetic groups were compared with the Healthy-Control Group (22 subjects, 12 women, aged 32.7 ± 6.8 years), and lower percentages of dilation in the FMD test were found when compared with those obtained in the comparative group (9.41 ± 2.20% for the Healthy-Control Group).

cIMT and fIMT

As shown in Table 2, all of the measures performed in carotid and femoral sites were higher in the H-group than in the C-group. With respect to carotid arteries, both cIMT and cIMTcomp were higher in the H-group than in the C-group (cIMT 0.53 ± 0.09 vs. 0.47 ± 0.08 mm; $P < 0.05$; cIMTcomp 0.59 ± 0.13 vs. 0.47 ± 0.07 mm, $P < 0.02$). In addition, fIMT was also lower in the C-group (0.51 ± 0.17 vs. 0.39 ± 0.09 mm, $P < 0.05$). Whereas atherosclerotic plaques were detected in either the carotid or femoral area in 10 of 25 subjects from the H-group, none were detected in the C-group.

As expected, the H-group also had thicker cIMT and fIMT with respect to the healthy control group, but there were no differences between the C-group and the healthy control group (cIMT 0.47 ± 0.05 mm and fIMT 0.39 ± 0.05 mm for the healthy control group) (Table 2).

Inflammation and endothelial function markers

vWF, fibrinogen, leukocytes, and sICAM-1 were significantly higher in the H-group. In contrast, no differences between the groups

Table 2—*Mean values of carotid, femoral, and brachial ultrasound measures: FMD and IMT results and comparisons between groups*

	H-group	C-group	P value
n	25	20	
Brachial artery measures			
Baseline brachial diameter (mm)	4.13 ± 0.76	3.80 ± 0.74	NS
Maximal FMD (%)	6.52 ± 2.92	8.62 ± 3.13	<0.05
Carotid artery measures			
Mean common carotid (cIMT, mm)	0.53 ± 0.09	0.47 ± 0.08	<0.05
Mean carotid bifurcation (mm)	0.67 ± 0.18	0.50 ± 0.07	<0.02
Mean internal carotid (mm)	0.58 ± 0.20	0.45 ± 0.09	<0.02
Mean carotid composite (cIMTcomp, mm)	0.59 ± 0.13	0.47 ± 0.07	<0.01
Subjects with carotid plaques	8/25	0	
Femoral artery measures			
Mean common femoral (fIMT, mm)	0.51 ± 0.17	0.39 ± 0.09	<0.05
Subjects with femoral plaques (%)	5/25	0	
Subjects with plaques in any carotid/femoral areas	10/25	0	

Data are means ± SD.

were observed with respect to the basal determination of hs-CRP, soluble E-selectin, and 1β-IL (Table 3).

All previously mentioned parameters were also measured in the H-group and C-group after 30 min of hypoglycemia (nadir glucose concentrations: 39 ± 5 vs. 40 ± 4 mg/dl, NS for the H-group and C-group, respectively). There were no significant differences between the groups in changes evoked by hypoglycemia (Table 3).

In the multiple linear regression analysis, the allocation in the H-group determined cIMTcomp (β 0.082, $P < 0.02$) independently from the other covariates: age (β 0.008, $P < 0.001$), sex, disease

duration, BMI, systolic blood pressure, A1C, MAGE, and LDL cholesterol (β 0.001, $P < 0.03$). The complete model explained ~73% of cIMTcomp.

CONCLUSIONS — Our findings suggest that repeated hypoglycemic episodes in type 1 diabetic subjects are associated with a worse prognosis in terms of preclinical atherosclerosis profile represented not only by abnormalities in endothelial function but also by an increase in IMT in both carotid and femoral sites.

Type 1 diabetes is associated with premature arterial disease. There are some studies that have previously demonstrated endothelial dysfunction using

Table 3—*Endothelial function and inflammation biochemical markers measured in both groups in euglycemia and hypoglycemia*

	H-group	C-group	P value
n	25	20	
Euglycemia			
vWF euglycemia (%)	119 ± 29	93 ± 26	<0.02
Fibrinogen euglycemia (g/l)	2.82 ± 0.64	2.29 ± 0.44	<0.02
Leukocytes ($10^3/\mu$l)	7.0 ± 1.8	5.6 ± 1.4	<0.05
sICAM-1 euglycemia (ng/ml)	408 ± 224	296 ± 95	<0.05
hs-CRP euglycemia (mg/dl)	0.23 ± 0.30	0.15 ± 0.17	NS
E-selectin euglycemia (ng/ml)	44 ± 21	49 ± 25	NS
1β-IL euglycemia (pg/ml)	2.92 ± 6.15	1.30 ± 2.65	NS
% increase in hypoglycemia*			
vWF	3.24 ± 12.85	16.97 ± 31.91	NS
Fibrinogen	2.84 ± 12.55	10.45 ± 23.27	NS
sICAM-1	4.15 ± 11.76	6.12 ± 13.31	NS
hs-CRP	−2.35 ± 9.02	20.35 ± 61.25	NS
Soluble E-selectin	4.74 ± 10.79	0.47 ± 11.30	NS
1β-IL	41.55 ± 143.30	33.30 ± 152.75	NS

Data are means ± SD. *Expressed as percentage increased in each variable with respect to the baseline result.

FMD evaluation in type 1 diabetes (20). In addition, our article is not the first to demonstrate a higher mean cIMT in subjects with type 1 diabetes compared with a control group. In our study, the FMD response to ischemia was lower in subjects with type 1 diabetes compared with healthy control subjects, demonstrating early alteration of vascular function. In addition, in patients with repeated episodes of hypoglycemia, IMT (carotid and femoral) was higher than in the healthy control group. Hypertension, dyslipidemia, smoking, and urinary albumin excretion have been related to cIMT and atherosclerosis in type 1 diabetes (7). In our study, including patients with type 1 diabetes without CVD risk factors and microvascular and macrovascular complications, LDL cholesterol was also associated with the variation in cIMT.

The EDIC study showed that intensive insulin therapy slowed the increment of cIMT in type 1 diabetes (7). It has been found that acute hyperglycemia induces vascular changes and inflammatory response and alters myocardial ventricular repolarization in type 1 diabetes (21,22). Despite the assumption that glucose variability is greater than that in type 2 diabetes, data concerning whether glucose fluctuations are an independent risk factor for complications in type 1 diabetes are still controversial (23). However, it has been suggested that a high mean daily blood glucose, but not glucose variability, is related to arterial stiffness in patients with type 1 diabetes using CGM and a hyperglycemic clamp (24). In addition, Wentholt et al. (10) failed to demonstrate a relation between high glucose variability and elevated levels of a surrogate marker of vascular damage. In our study and considering all patients with type 1 diabetes as a whole, MAGE was not independently associated with cIMT.

Hypoglycemia is the most common and the most feared side effect of intensive insulin therapy and frequently is the major barrier to achieving glucose control as normal as possible (4). In the short term, the acute hemodynamic changes induced by hypoglycemia may precipitate and aggravate a vascular event during an acute episode (25). In the long term, especially if hypoglycemia is repeated, the abnormalities in coagulation, fibrinolysis, and inflammation associated with it could be related to the induction and progression of atherosclerosis. In our study, in addition to the induction of hypoglycemia unawareness, repeated episodes of hypoglycemia were related to a worse prognosis in terms of preclinical atherosclerosis. Considering endothelial function, FMD was significantly reduced in type 1 diabetic subjects with repeated episodes of hypoglycemia compared with that in those patients without these episodes. Accordingly, coagulation markers of endothelial damage and acute-phase inflammation markers were significantly higher in the former group.

For structural changes, a comprehensive evaluation of carotid arteries gave significant higher values of IMT in subjects having repeated episodes of hypoglycemia. The multivariate regression analysis confirmed the association of repeated episodes of hypoglycemia and cIMTcomp independently of the other CVD risk factors considered. Likewise, data on IMT from femoral arteries confirmed that preclinical atherosclerosis was aggravated by repeated episodes of hypoglycemia not only in the carotid artery but also in peripheral vascular sites. It is noteworthy that in contrast to the findings with FMD, for IMT, differences with respect to the healthy control group were only significant in patients with type 1 diabetes and repeated episodes of hypoglycemia. This observation suggests that in addition to alterations in endothelial function that occur early in type 1 diabetes, recurring episodes of hypoglycemia could be considered an aggravating or accelerating factor. There is neither complete information concerning type 1 diabetes-specific determinants of vascular damage and their interrelationships nor the minimal time of exposure required for a preclinical cardiovascular alteration. Our results point to repeated episodes of hypoglycemia being considered as a new potential risk factor. The exposure to risk factor levels throughout the life span in young people promotes the accumulation of subclinical atherosclerosis, which will be transformed into CVD events, but typically not until much later in life.

As mentioned previously, there are recent studies specifically designed to address the effects of acute hypoglycemia, confirming its proinflammatory and prothrombotic effects (11,12). For some of the inflammatory markers (leukocytes and sICAM-1). we detected significantly higher values at baseline in subjects with repeated hypoglycemia. In both group of subjects with type 1 diabetes, insulin-induced hypoglycemia elicited a heterogeneous nonsignificant rise in endothelial and inflammatory markers without any difference in the response observed with respect to the presence or absence of frequent hypoglycemia. This lack of response to provoked hypoglycemia in comparison with previous studies could be related, at least in part, to limitations of the experimental conditions of our protocol. In fact, the study of acute effects of hypoglycemia was not considered the main objective of our study, and the protocol was not designed to accurately assess mechanistic roles. As examples, we included a shorter period of hypoglycemia (30 min) before extraction and we did not control for insulin levels and the potential effect on vascular function. Moreover, and in contrast with some previous studies, we did not exclude those subjects with hypoglycemia unawareness because this clinical condition was seen in patients fulfilling our inclusion criteria. Further research is required to fully understand the link between repeated episodes of hypoglycemia and a worse prognosis in terms of preclinical atherosclerosis in type 1 diabetes. However, the putative role for endothelial and inflammatory factors in the mediation of hypoglycemia-induced vascular damage has to be taken into consideration.

In summary, in addition to the induction of hypoglycemia unawareness and an increased risk for severe hypoglycemia, repeated episodes of hypoglycemia could be related to and considered an aggravating factor for the preclinical atherosclerosis profile of type 1 diabetes.

Acknowledgments— This work was supported in part by a grant (PI060250) from the "Ministerio de Sanidad y Consumo" of Spain. M.G. is the recipient of a grant from the Hospital Clínic i Universitari of Barcelona ("Ajut a la recerca Josep Font 2006–2009").

No potential conflicts of interest relevant to this article were reported.

M.G. researched data, contributed to discussion, wrote the manuscript, and reviewed/edited the manuscript. R.G., J.M., and R.C. researched data and reviewed/edited the manuscript. A.A. and C.P. researched data. I.C. researched data, contributed to discussion, wrote the manuscript, and reviewed/edited the manuscript.

Parts of this study were presented in abstract form at the 46th annual meeting of the European Association for the Study of Diabetes, Stockholm, Sweden, 20–24 September 2010.

We thank Mercè Lara of the Endocrinology and Diabetes Unit from Hospital Clínic i Universitari (Barcelona, Spain) for her technical support during the hypoglycemia test.

References

1. Orchard TJ, Costacou T, Kretowski A, Nesto RW. Type 1 diabetes and coronary artery disease. Diabetes Care 2006;29: 2528–2538
2. The effect of intensive treatment of diabetes on the development and progression of long-term complications in insulin-dependent diabetes mellitus. The Diabetes Control and Complications Trial Research Group. N Engl J Med 1993;329: 977–986
3. Nathan DM, Cleary PA, Backlund JY, Genuth SM, Lachin JM, Orchard TJ, Raskin P, Zinman B, Diabetes Control and Complications Trial/Epidemiology of Diabetes Interventions and Complications (DCCT/EDIC) Study Research Group. Intensive diabetes treatment and cardiovascular disease in patients with type 1 diabetes. N Engl J Med 2005;353:2643–2653
4. Bolli GB. Hypoglycaemia unawareness. Diabetes Metab 1997;23(Suppl. 3):29–35
5. Gill GV, Woodward A, Casson IF, Weston PJ. Cardiac arrhythmia and nocturnal hypoglycaemia in type 1 diabetes—the 'dead in bed' syndrome revisited. Diabetologia 2009;52:42–45
6. Kastelein JJ, de Groot E. Ultrasound imaging techniques for the evaluation of cardiovascular therapies. Eur Heart J 2008; 29:849–858
7. Nathan DM, Lachin J, Cleary P, Orchard T, Brillon DJ, Backlund JY, O'Leary DH, Genuth S, Diabetes Control and Complications Trial, Epidemiology of Diabetes Interventions and Complications Research Group. Intensive diabetes therapy and carotid intima-media thickness in type 1 diabetes mellitus. N Engl J Med 2003;348:2294–2303
8. Shivalkar B, Dhondt D, Goovaerts I, Van Gaal L, Bartunek J, Van Crombrugge P, Vrints C. Flow mediated dilatation and cardiac function in type 1 diabetes mellitus. Am J Cardiol 2006;97:77–82
9. Kilpatrick ES, Rigby AS, Atkin SL. The effect of glucose variability on the risk of microvascular complications in type 1 diabetes. Diabetes Care 2006;29:1486–1490
10. Wentholt IM, Kulik W, Michels RP, Hoekstra JB, DeVries JH. Glucose fluctuations and activation of oxidative stress in patients with type 1 diabetes. Diabetologia 2008;51:183–190
11. Gogitidze Joy N, Hedrington MS, Briscoe VJ, Tate DB, Ertl AC, Davis SN. Effects of acute hypoglycemia on inflammatory and pro-atherothrombotic biomarkers in individuals with type 1 diabetes and healthy individuals. Diabetes Care 2010;33: 1529–1535
12. Wright RJ, Newby DE, Stirling D, Ludlam CA, Macdonald IA, Frier BM. Effects of acute insulin-induced hypoglycemia on indices of inflammation: putative mechanism for aggravating vascular disease in diabetes. Diabetes Care 2010;33:1591–1597
13. Rodrigues TC, Snell-Bergeon JK, Maahs DM, Kinney GL, Rewers M. Higher fibrinogen levels predict progression of coronary artery calcification in adults with type 1 diabetes. Atherosclerosis 2010; 210:671–673
14. Snell-Bergeon JK, West NA, Mayer-Davis EJ, Liese AD, Marcovina SM, D'Agostino RB, Jr, Hamman RF, Dabelea D. Inflammatory markers are increased in youth with type 1 diabetes: the SEARCH Case-Control study. J Clin Endocrinol Metab 2010;95:2868–2876
15. Feldman-Billard S, Massin P, Meas T, Guillausseau PJ, Héron E. Hypoglycemia-induced blood pressure elevation in patients with diabetes. Arch Intern Med 2010;170:829–831
16. Clarke WL, Cox DJ, Gonder-Frederick LA, Julian D, Schlundt D, Polonsky W. Reduced awareness of hypoglycemia in adults with IDDM. A prospective study of hypoglycemic frequency and associated symptoms. Diabetes Care 1995;18:517–522
17. Gold AE, MacLeod KM, Frier BM. Frequency of severe hypoglycemia in patients with type I diabetes with impaired awareness of hypoglycemia. Diabetes Care 1994;17:697–703
18. Ferrer JP, Esmatjes E, González-Clemente JM, Goday A, Conget I, Jiménez W, Gomis R, Rivera F, Vilardell E. Symptomatic and hormonal hypoglycaemic responses to human and porcine insulin in patients with type I diabetes mellitus. Diabet Med 1992;9:522–527
19. McAulay V, Deary IJ, Frier BM. Symptoms of hypoglycaemia in people with diabetes. Diabet Med 2001;18:690–705
20. Järvisalo MJ, Raitakari M, Toikka JO, Putto-Laurila A, Rontu R, Laine S, Lehtimäki T, Rönnemaa T, Viikari J, Raitakari OT. Endothelial dysfunction and increased arterial intima-media thickness in children with type 1 diabetes. Circulation 2004;109:1750–1755
21. Gordin D, Forsblom C, Rönnback M, Parkkonen M, Wadén J, Hietala K, Groop PH. Acute hyperglycaemia induces an inflammatory response in young patients with type 1 diabetes. Ann Med 2008;40: 627–633
22. Gordin D, Forsblom C, Rönnback M, Groop PH. Acute hyperglycaemia disturbs cardiac repolarization in type 1 diabetes. Diabet Med 2008;25:101–105
23. Kilpatrick ES, Rigby AS, Atkin SL. Mean blood glucose compared with HbA1c in the prediction of cardiovascular disease in patients with type 1 diabetes. Diabetologia 2008;51:365–371
24. Gordin D, Rönnback M, Forsblom C, Makinen V, Saraheimo M, Groop PH. Glucose variability, blood pressure and arterial stiffness in type 1 diabetes. Diabetes Res Clin Pract 2008;80:e4–e7
25. Desouza C, Salazar H, Cheong B, Murgo J, Fonseca V. Association of hypoglycemia and cardiac ischemia: a study based on continuous monitoring. Diabetes Care 2003;26:1485–1489

Effects of Acute Hypoglycemia on Inflammatory and Pro-atherothrombotic Biomarkers in Individuals With Type 1 Diabetes and Healthy Individuals

Nino Gogitidze Joy, md[1]
Maka S. Hedrington, md[1]
Vanessa J. Briscoe, phd, np[2]
Donna B. Tate, ms[1]
Andrew C. Ertl, phd[2]
Stephen N. Davis, md[1,2]

OBJECTIVE — Recent large randomized trials have linked adverse cardiovascular and cerebrovascular events with hypoglycemia. However, the integrated physiological and vascular biological mechanisms occurring during hypoglycemia have not been extensively examined. Therefore, the aim of this study was to determine whether 2 h of moderate clamped hypoglycemia could decrease fibrinolytic balance and activate pro-atherothrombotic mechanisms in individuals with type 1 diabetes and healthy individuals.

RESEARCH DESIGN AND METHODS — Thirty-five healthy volunteers (19 male and 16 female subjects age 32 ± 2 years, BMI 26 ± 2 kg/m^2, A1C 5.1 ± 0.1%) and twenty-four with type 1 diabetes (12 male and 12 female subjects age 33 ± 3 years, BMI 24 ± 2 kg/m^2, A1C 7.7 ± 0.2%) were studied during either a 2-h hyperinsulinemic (9 pmol · kg^{-1} · min^{-1}) euglycemic or hypoglycemic (2.9 ± 0.1 mmol/l) clamp or both protocols. Plasma glucose levels were normalized overnight in type 1 diabetic subjects prior to each study.

RESULTS — Insulin levels were similar (602 ± 44 pmol/l) in all four protocols. Glycemia was equivalent in both euglycemic protocols (5.2 ± 0.1 mmol/l), and the level of hypoglycemia was also equivalent in both type 1 diabetic subjects and healthy control subjects (2.9 ± 0.1 mmol/l). Using repeated ANOVA, it was determined that plasminogen activator inhibitor (PAI-1), vascular cell adhesion molecule (VCAM), intercellular adhesion molecule (ICAM), E-selectin, P-selectin, interleukin-6 (IL-6), vascular endothelial growth factor (VEGF), and adiponectin responses were all significantly increased ($P < 0.05$) during the 2 h of hyperinsulinemic hypoglycemia as compared with euglycemia in healthy control subjects. All measures except PAI-1 were also found to be increased during hypoglycemia compared with euglycemia in type 1 diabetes.

CONCLUSIONS — In summary, moderate hypoglycemia acutely increases circulating levels of PAI-1, VEGF, vascular adhesion molecules (VCAM, ICAM, E-selectin), IL-6, and markers of platelet activation (P-selectin) in individuals with type 1 diabetes and healthy individuals. We conclude that acute hypoglycemia can result in complex vascular effects including activation of prothrombotic, proinflammatory, and pro-atherogenic mechanisms in individuals with type 1 diabetes and healthy individuals.

Diabetes Care 33:1529–1535, 2010

Hypoglycemia occurs very commonly in individuals with type 1 diabetes. Despite this, the effects of hypoglycemia on in vivo vascular biology in type 1 diabetes have not been extensively studied. Case reports and a recent study have linked hypoglycemia with angina, myocardial infarction, and acute cerebrovascular events (1,2). More recently, a large epidemiological study has determined that hypoglycemia results in an increased risk of cardiovascular disease and all-cause mortality (3). Additionally, a recent large randomized clinical trial in type 2 diabetes has highlighted an increased risk of death when glucose levels are intensively treated (4). Whereas the role played by hypoglycemia in directly causing the increased adverse events in the Action to Control Cardiovascular Risk in Diabetes (ACCORD) trial is not established, a much stronger link between severe hypoglycemia and vascular adverse events was indicated in the Veteran's Affairs Diabetes Trial (VADT) study (also in type 2 diabetes) (5). As patients with type 1 diabetes advance into middle age, they are also likely to become more susceptible to vascular disease. Hypoglycemia has been implicated with sudden death in type 1 diabetes, although the mechanism remains speculative (6). Offsetting this risk, a previous period of intensive glucose control combined with continued moderate glycemic levels (A1C ~8.0%) has resulted in a reduction in cardiovascular disease in type 1 diabetes (7). However, information addressing any possible proinflammatory and resultant activation of pro-atherothrombotic responses in type 1 diabetes during hypoglycemia is scarce. To date, very few studies have investigated the effects of hypoglycemia on vascular physiology in type 1 diabetes (8–10). Complicating interpretation of this scarce data is the fact that insulin and glucose levels were not controlled. Thus, because it is now recognized that both insulin and hyperglycemia can have independent vascular biological effects (11), it becomes important to strictly control these two important variables. Therefore, this present study has tested the hypothesis that acute moderate hypoglycemia can activate proinflammatory mechanisms and reduce fibrinolytic balance in both individuals with type 1 diabetes and nondiabetic individuals. The hyperinsulinemic euglycemic and hypoglycemic clamp techniques were used so that insulin levels could be equated and glucose

From the [1]University of Maryland School of Medicine, Baltimore, Maryland; and the [2]Department of Diabetes, Endocrinology, and Metabolism, Vanderbilt University, Nashville, Tennessee.
Corresponding author: Stephen N. Davis, sdavis@medicine.umaryland.edu.
Received 23 February 2009 and accepted 15 March 2010. DOI: 10.2337/dc09-0354. Clinical trial reg. no. NCT00574340, clinicaltrials.gov.
The costs of publication of this article were defrayed in part by the payment of page charges. This article must therefore be hereby marked "advertisement" in accordance with 18 U.S.C. Section 1734 solely to indicate this fact.

See accompanying original article, p. 1591, and editorial, p. 1686.

values could be controlled independently during each study.

RESEARCH DESIGN AND METHODS

Thirty-five healthy subjects (19 male and 16 female subjects, age 32 years $\pm$ 2, BMI 26 $\pm$ 2 kg/m^2, A1C 5.1 $\pm$ 0.1) and twenty-four with type 1 diabetes (12 male and 12 female subjects, age 33 $\pm$ 3 years, BMI 24 $\pm$ 2 kg/m^2, A1C 7.7 $\pm$ 0.2 [normal range 4–6.5%], diabetes duration 17 $\pm$ 8 years) were studied (data can be found in online appendix Table 1, available at http://care.diabetesjournals.org/cgi/content/full/dc09-0354/DC1). Individuals with type 1 diabetes had normal bedside tests of autonomic function (12) and did not have hypoglycemia unawareness based on the methods of Gold, et al. (13). Type 1 diabetic individuals had no major macro or micro complications of diabetes. Type 1 diabetic subjects were excluded from the study if they had a history of hypoglycemia induced convulsions or a major episode of hypoglycemia in the preceding 2 years. Type 1 diabetes individuals were treated with multiple daily insulin injections or with an insulin pump. All subjects were nonsmokers and had a normal blood count, plasma lipids, plasma electrolytes, liver, and renal function, and were normotensive. No subject was taking medications known to affect neuroendocrine responses to hypoglycemia (specifically, fluoxetine) or influence platelet, clotting, or fibrinolytic balance. Some of the individuals included in the present study had served as control subjects to determine usual baseline counterregulatory responses to hypoglycemia in previous studies (14,15). Studies were approved by the Vanderbilt University human subjects Institutional Review Board, and all participants gave written informed consent.

Subjects participated in either a single hyperinsulinemic euglycemic or hypoglycemic clamp or both sets of experiments. The number of individuals participating in each arm of the study were: type 1 diabetes euglycemia ($n = 14$), type 1 diabetes hypoglycemia ($n = 17$), healthy control euglycemia ($n = 22$), healthy control hypoglycemia ($n = 25$). Ten healthy control subjects and seven individuals with type 1 diabetes participated in both euglycemic and hypoglycemic protocols in a randomized fashion. Results from this subgroup are conceptually similar to the entire cohort (data are available in online appendix Table 3, Fig. A1 and A2). All

study patients were asked to avoid any exercise and consume their usual weight-maintaining diet for 3 days before each experiment. All type 1 diabetic patients were asked to perform intensive home blood glucose monitoring (i.e., at least four glucose tests per day) and to avoid hypoglycemia for at least 5 days before a study. On the day prior to a study, intermediate or long-acting insulin was discontinued and replaced by injections of regular insulin before breakfast and lunch. Each subject was admitted to the Vanderbilt General Clinical Research Center (CRC) at ~5:00 P.M. the evening before an experiment. At this time in the individuals with type 1 diabetes, two intravenous cannulae were inserted under 1% lidocaine local anesthesia. One cannula was placed in a retrograde fashion into a vein on the back of the hand. This hand was placed in a heated box (55–60°C) during the study so that arterialized blood could be obtained. The other cannula was placed in the contralateral arm for infusions. All subjects received an evening meal, and individuals with type 1 diabetes received a continuous low-dose infusion of insulin to normalize plasma glucose. The insulin infusion was adjusted overnight to maintain blood glucose between 4.4 and 7.2 mmol/l.

Hypoglycemia experiments

All subjects were studied after an overnight, 10-h fast. Venous cannulae as described above were placed in the healthy control subjects. After this, a period of 120 min was allowed to elapse followed by a 120-min hyperinsulinemic hypoglycemic experimental period. At time 120 min, a primed constant (9.0 pmol · kg^{-1} · min^{-1}) infusion of insulin (Human Regular Insulin; Eli Lilly, Indianapolis, IN) was started and continued until 240 min. The rate of fall of glucose was controlled (~0.08 mmol/min), and the glucose nadir (2.9 mmol/l) was achieved using a modification of the glucose clamp technique. During the clamp period, plasma glucose was measured every 5 min and a 20% dextrose infusion was adjusted so that plasma glucose levels were held constant at 2.9 $\pm$ 0.1 mmol/l (16). Potassium chloride (20 mmol/l) was infused during the clamp to reduce insulin-induced hypokalemia.

Euglycemia experiments

These experiments followed the same format as the above described hypoglycemia experiments with the exception that euglycemia (5.2 $\pm$ 0.1 mmol/l) was maintained during each study.

Analytical methods

The collection of blood samples has been described elsewhere (14). Plasma glucose concentrations were measured in triplicate using the glucose oxidase method with a glucose analyzer (Beckman, Fullerton, CA). Insulin was measured as previously described with an interassay coefficient of variation (CV) of 9% (14). Catecholamines were determined by high-performacne liquid chromatography with an interassay CV of 12% for epinephrine and 8% for norepinephrine (14). Cortisol was assayed using the clinical assays γ-coat radioimmunoassay kit with an interassay CV of 6% (14). Nonesterified fatty acids (NEFAs) were measured using the WAKO kit with an interassay CV of 7%.

Blood was drawn every 60 min for soluble vascular cell adhesion molecule-1 (sVCAM-1), soluble intercellular adhesion molecule-1 (sICAM-1), E-selectin, P-selectin, interleukin-6 (IL-6), tumor necrosis factor-α (TNF-α), vascular endothelial growth factor (VEGF), plasminogen activator inhibitor 1 (PAI-1), tissue plasminogen activator (tPA), and adiponectin was drawn every 60 min and every 30 min for catecholamines, cortisol, and NEFA during the experimental period. Vascular adhesion molecules and adiponectin were assayed using LINCO Research Kits (St. Charles, Missouri) with interassay CVs of 8.5% for sVCAM, 9.7% for sICAM, 13.4% for sE-selectin, 15.9% for adiponectin), 9.02% for IL-6, 9.98% for TNF-α, and 8.2% for VEGF. P-selectin (CV 9.9%), Meso scale discovery (Gaithersburg, MD), PAI-1, and tPA antigen were determined by TintElize PAI-1 Kit with interassay CV of 3.3%.

Statistical analysis

Data are expressed as means $\pm$ SE and were analyzed using standard, parametric, one and two-way analysis of variance (ANOVA) with repeated measures where appropriate (SPSS, Chicago, IL). Data were also analyzed with paired and unpaired two tailed t test (Graph Pad Software, San Diego, CA). In all cases, a $P <$ 0.05 was accepted as statistically significant. Individual peak and nadir values during the final 60 min (at time 180 or 240 min) of hypoglycemia and euglycemia were compared for vascular biological parameters.

Glucose and insulin

Plasma glucose was maintained equivalently (5.2 ± 0.1 mmol/l) during the euglycemic clamps. Plasma glucose reached steady state by 150 min, and equivalent hypoglycemia (2.9 ± 0.1 mmol/l) was maintained during all hypoglycemia clamp procedures (online appendix Fig. A3). Insulin levels (602 ± 24 pmol/l) for both healthy and type 1 diabetes groups were similar during all four protocol clamp studies (online appendix Fig. A3).

Neuroendocrine counterregulatory hormones

Epinephrine responses were significantly higher ($P < 0.001$) during the final 30 min of hypoglycemia (5.6 ± 0.7 nmol/l, 3.14 ± 0.5 nmol/l) as compared with euglycemia (0.19 ± 0.03 nmol/l, 0.27 ± 0.04 nmol/l) in both the healthy and type 1 diabetic groups, respectively. Epinephrine values were higher during hypoglycemia in healthy control subjects ($P = 0.008$) as compared with type 1 diabetic subjects. Norepinephrine levels were also significantly higher ($P < 0.001$) during the final 30 min of hypoglycemia (1.9 ± 0.3 nmol/l, 1.8 ± 0.02 nmol/l) as compared with euglycemia (0.9 ± 0.2 nmol/l, 1.1 ± 0.01 nmol/l) in healthy control subjects and type 1 diabetic subjects, respectively. Norepinephrine levels were not different during hypoglycemia in healthy control subjects and type 1 diabetic subjects. There was a trend for plasma cortisol levels to be higher in healthy control subjects as compared with type 1 diabetic subjects (861 ± 42 vs. 725 ± 46 nmol/l, $P = 0.09$). Cortisol values were higher ($P < 0.001$) during hypoglycemia as compared with euglycemia in both healthy control subjects (861 ± 42 vs. 357 ± 24 nmol/l) and type 1 diabetic subjects (725 ± 46 vs. 302 ± 66 nmol/l), respectively.

Intermediary metabolism

Blood NEFA levels fell significantly ($P < 0.0001$) during hypoglycemic and euglycemic clamps. However, there were significantly higher levels ($P < 0.05$) of NEFA during the final 30 min of hypoglycemia as compared with euglycemia in both healthy control subjects (97 ± 11 vs. 68 ± 18 μmol/l) and type 1 diabetic patients (100 ± 18 vs. 50 ± 4 μmol/l), respectively.

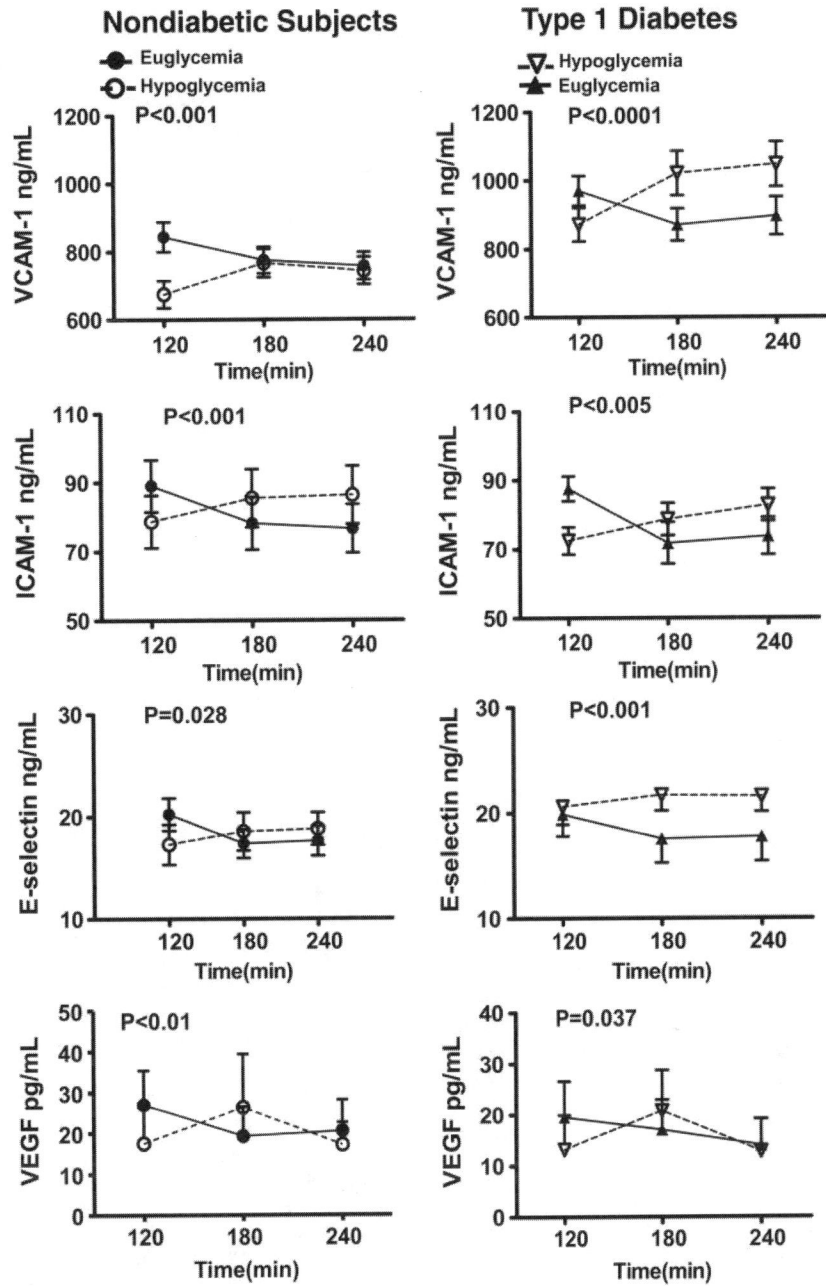

Figure 1—*Effects of hyperinsulinemic euglycemia and hypoglycemia (2.9 mmol/l) in overnight-fasted healthy control subjects (n = 35) and individuals with type 1 diabetes (n = 24) that participated in either one or both of the studies on vascular biological markers. Response of VCAM-1, ICAM-1, E-selectin, and VEGF are significantly increased during hypoglycemia as compared with euglycemia in both healthy control subjects and type 1 diabetic subjects. Statistical difference with two-way ANOVA during the 120-min clamp experiments is marked in each graph panel.*

Atherogenic vascular adhesion molecules

With the exception of VCAM-1 in healthy control subjects and ICAM-1 in subjects with type 1 diabetes, baseline values were similar at the start of euglycemic and hypoglycemic clamps (online appendix Tables 2 and 3). Plasma VCAM, ICAM, and E-selectin responses during the 120-min clamp studies were significantly different ($P < 0.05$–$P < 0.0001$ ANOVA) during hypoglycemia as compared with euglycemia in both healthy control subjects and type 1 diabetic subjects (Fig. 1). Individual peak values for VCAM, ICAM, and E-selectin were increased significantly from baseline ($P < 0.05$) during hypoglycemia (Fig. 3); mean individual nadir values of VCAM, ICAM, and E-selectin were significantly ($P < 0.05$) decreased from baseline during euglycemia in both type 1 diabetic subjects and healthy control subjects (Fig. 3). The magnitude of responses did not differ in healthy control subjects and type 1 diabetic subjects.

Platelet activation and fibrinolytic balance

Plasma P-selectin responses were significantly different ($P < 0.05$ ANOVA) during the hypoglycemic as compared with euglycemic clamp studies in both healthy control subjects and type 1 diabetic subjects (Fig. 2). Baseline PAI-1 levels were significantly different ($P < 0.05$) in the type 1 diabetes group (online appendix Table 3). Plasma PAI-1 values were significantly different during hypoglycemia as compared with euglycemia in healthy control subjects but not type 1 diabetic subjects (Fig. 2). Mean individual peak values from baseline for P-selectin and PAI-1 responses were increased ($P < 0.05$) during hypoglycemia in both healthy control subjects and type 1 diabetic subjects (Fig. 3). Nadir P-selectin and PAI-1 values were significantly ($P < 0.01$) lower from baseline during hyperinsulinemic euglycemia in both type 1 diabetic subjects and healthy control subjects (Fig. 3). Plasma concentrations of tPA did not alter during either euglycemic or hypoglycemic clamps in both normal subjects and individuals with type 1 diabetes. Responses of P-selectin, tPA and PAI-1 were similar in healthy control subjects and type 1 diabetic subjects.

Adiponectin, VEGF, and inflammatory cytokines

Baseline values for adiponectin, VEGF, IL-6, and TNFα were similar at the start of both sets of glucose clamps (online appendix Tables 2 and 3). Plasma adiponectin responses were significantly different ($P < 0.01$ ANOVA) during the 120-min hypoglycemic and euglycemic clamps in healthy control subjects and type 1 diabetic subjects (Fig. 3). Mean individual nadir values for adiponectin were significantly ($P < 0.05$) reduced from baseline during hyperinsulinemic euglycemia in both subjects with type 1 diabetes and healthy control subjects (Fig. 3). There was a trend ($P = 0.06$ ANOVA) for peak adiponectin levels to increase from baseline during hypoglycemia in type 1 diabetes (Fig. 3). VEGF and IL-6 responses

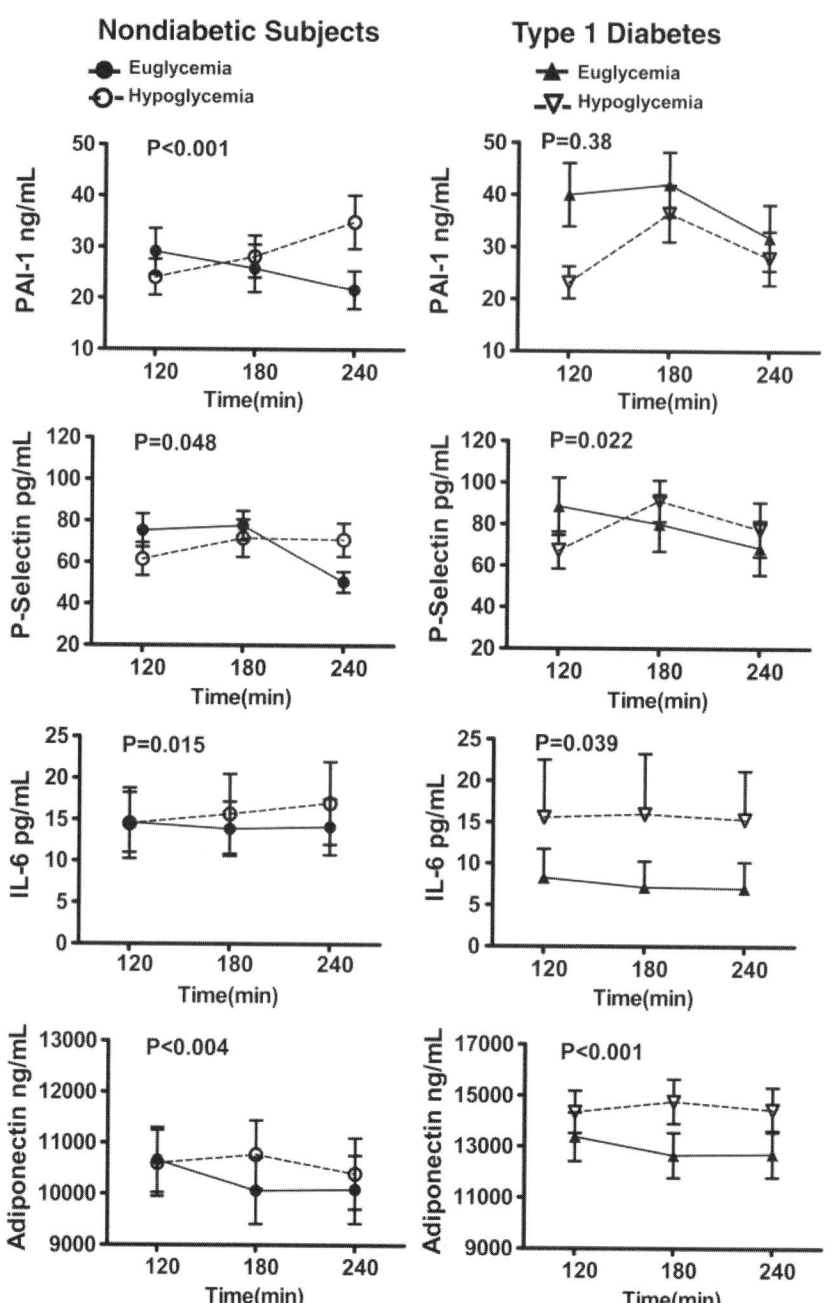

Figure 2—*Effects of hyperinsulinemic euglycemia and hypoglycemia (2.9 ± 0.1 mmol/l) in overnight-fasted healthy control subjects (n = 35) and subjects with type 1 diabetes (n = 24) that participated in either one or both of the studies on vascular biological markers. Responses of PAI-1, P-selectin, IL-6, and adiponectin are significantly increased during hypoglycemia as compared with euglycemia in healthy control subjects. Responses of P-selectin, IL-6, and adiponectin are significantly increased during hypoglycemia as compared with euglycemia in type 1 diabetes. Statistical difference with two-way ANOVA during the 120-min clamp experiments is marked in each graph panel.*

were significantly different ($P < 0.04 - P = 0.0004$ ANOVA) during hypoglycemia and euglycemia in type 1 diabetic subjects and healthy control subjects (Figs. 1 and 2). Nadir values for VEGF and IL-6 were significantly decreased ($P < 0.04 - P < 0.01$) from baseline during hyperinsulinemic euglycemia in both subjects type 1 diabetes and healthy control subjects (Fig. 3). Mean individual peak values during hypoglycemia were increased from baseline ($P < 0.05$) in both type 1 diabetic subjects and healthy control subjects. Peak values for TNF-α in-

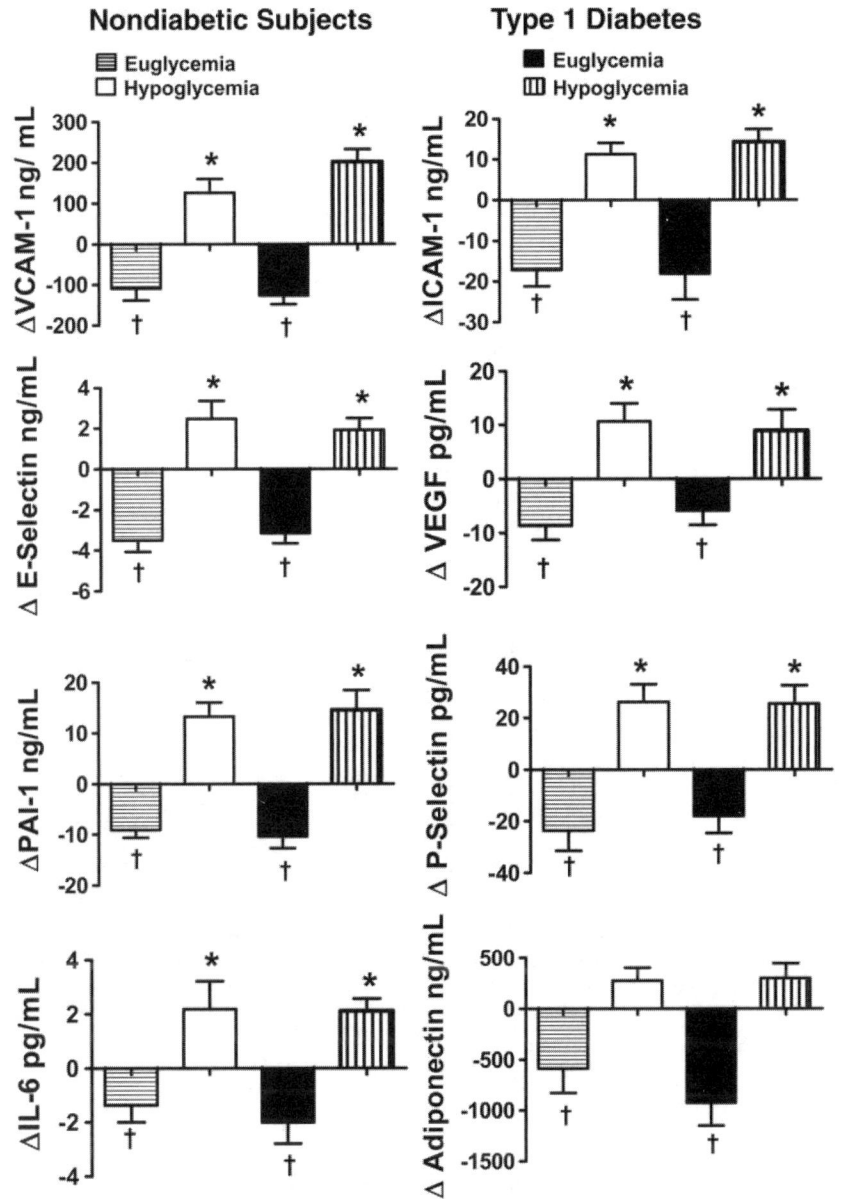

Figure 3—*Mean individual peak responses of VCAM-1, ICAM-1, E-selectin, VEGF, PAI-1, IL-6, P-selectin, and adiponectin in both healthy control subjects (n = 35) and subjects with type 1 diabetes (n = 24) that participated in either one or both of the studies are significantly increased (P <0.05) compared with baseline. †Mean individual nadir responses of VCAM-1, ICAM-1, E-selectin, VEGF, PAI-1, P-selectin, and adiponectin during hyperinsulinemic euglycemia in both healthy control subjects and type 1 diabetic subjects are significantly decreased (P <0.05) compared with baseline.*

creased from baseline (P <0.05) during hypoglycemia in type 1 diabetic subjects and nadir values were also significantly decreased (P <0.05) from baseline during hyperinsulinemic euglycemia in healthy control subjects. Adiponectin, VEGF, TNF-α and IL-6 responded similarly during hypoglycemia in healthy control subjects and type 1 diabetic subjects (Fig. 3).

CONCLUSIONS — This study has determined the effects of 2 h of clamped hyperinsulinemic euglycemia and moderate hypoglycemia on proinflammatory mechanisms and fibrinolytic balance in individuals with type 1 diabetes and healthy individuals. Our results demonstrate that hypoglycemia can have acute and widespread effects on vascular biology. Hypoglycemia can 1) activate proin-

flammatory mechanisms (ICAM, VCAM, E-selectin, VEGF, IL-6), 2) increase platelet activation (P-selectin), and 3) simultaneously decrease systemic fibrinolytic balance (increase in PAI-1, no change in tPA) in both individuals type 1 diabetes and healthy individuals. These effects were of a similar magnitude in the healthy control subjects and type 1 diabetic subjects and were in contrast to the reduced responses of the above vascular biological mechanisms that occurred during clamped euglycemia with equivalent hyperinsulinemia.

In this present study, the effects of hypoglycemia and hyperinsulinemia on different proinflammatory and potentially pro-atherothrombotic mechanisms have been determined. ICAM-1, VCAM-1 and E-selectin are cell surface proteins that are upregulated during inflammation and increase the adhesion of leukocytes to injured arterial endothelial cells, which is a primary step in plaque formation and subsequent atherosclerosis. Analysis of the responses during the hyperinsulinemic clamps demonstrates a significant effect of hypoglycemia to increase VCAM, ICAM, E-selectin, and VEGF relative to euglycemia in both healthy control subjects and type 1 diabetic subjects individuals. VEGF has been reported to be pro-atherosclerotic in animals (17). In addition, VEGF can potently increase proliferation of the endothelium leading to new blood vessels. Hypoglycemia also had similar effects, increasing plasma levels of P-selectin in both individuals with type 1 diabetes and nondiabetic individuals. P-selectin is an adhesion molecule that is activated by inflammation (18) and is expressed by both endothelial cells and platelets. Recent work has demonstrated that platelets are the major source of P-selectin, and thus this molecule has been recognized as a significant marker of platelet activation and increased thrombotic mechanisms (18). PAI-1 was increased during hypoglycemia relative to euglycemia in healthy control subjects but not subjects with type 1 diabetes. However, individual peak values of PAI-1 were increased during hypoglycemia in both healthy control subjects and subjects with type 1 diabetes, demonstrating that hypoglycemia of 2.9 mmol/l can be a stimulus for increased values of PAI-1.

Our present results demonstrate that hypoglycemia decreases systemic fibrinolytic balance by increasing PAI-1 levels while maintaining tPA values. Thus, at least two separate mechanisms for increasing thrombosis are activated by hypoglycemia in individuals with type 1 diabetes and healthy individuals. The potential in vivo causes responsible for the reduced fibrinolytic balance and increased proinflammatory mechanisms activated by hypoglycemia are not known. During hypoglycemia, a wide spectrum of physiologic responses are activated that could have potential vascular biological effects. To date, the role played by catecholamines, the sympathetic nervous system, and neuroendocrine hormones on activating adhesion molecules and influencing fibrinolytic balance is incompletely understood. One study using cultured human adipose tissue has indicated that PAI-1 levels may be suppressed by catecholamines, but increased by high dose glucocorticoids (19). Other work (20) has reported that epinephrine can play a role via α-2 adrenoceptor mechanisms in increasing platelet activation during hypoglycemia in both individuals with type 2 diabetes and healthy individuals. Therefore, it is possible that both increases in the hypothalamic-pituitary axis and the sympathetic nervous system could have effects to activate proinflammatory and pro-thrombotic mechanisms during hypoglycemia.

Circulating triglycerides and NEFA are known to decrease endothelial function and increase cellular insulin resistance via nuclear factor-κB (21). NEFAs were increased in both type 1 diabetic subjects and healthy control subjects during hypoglycemia as compared with the euglycemia studies. This occurs principally due to the increased levels of catecholamines and sympathetic nervous system drive during hypoglycemia and the unopposed suppressive effects of insulin on lipolysis during the euglycemic experiments. Thus, the elevated NEFA levels remain a possible mechanism for our findings. The cytokines, IL-6 and TNF-α, had differential responses during hypoglycemia and euglycemia in both the type 1 diabetic subjects and healthy control subjects. IL-6 was increased during hypoglycemia relative to euglycemia in both groups whereas TNF-α was increased during hypoglycemia in type 1 diabetes. The magnitude of the increase in IL-6 during hypoglycemia in the healthy control subjects was similar to that reported in two recent studies by Dotson et al. (22) and Razavi Nematollahi et al. (23) Thus, it would appear that similar to hyperglycemia, acute hypoglycemia can also mediate its pro-atherothrombotic ef-

fects via TNF-α or IL-6 pathways (21). Nitric oxide (NO) has also been implicated in the regulation of both endothelial and platelet-derived adhesion molecules (24). Although not specifically addressed in the present study, we have preliminary data indicating that hypoglycemia impairs endothelial NO function. We would therefore suggest that NO may also be a significant molecular mechanism involved in hypoglycemia's vascular effects.

Adiponectin is released from adipose tissue and is known to have powerful insulin sensitizing and antiatherogenic properties. To our knowledge, adiponectin responses have not been investigated during hypoglycemia in type 1 diabetes or healthy volunteers. We were intrigued to discover that hypoglycemia also increased (relative to euglycemia) adiponectin levels in type 1 diabetic subjects and healthy control subjects. The significance of the finding is unclear and requires further study.

We would also like to indicate that in this present study, insulin, per se, had significant, beneficial effects on vascular physiology. It is notable that in every case where hypoglycemia resulted in an activation of a pathologic process, there was an equal and opposite beneficial effect during the hyperinsulinemic euglycemic control studies in both type 1 diabetes and healthy individuals. Thus, our present results would support previous work demonstrating that insulin has anti-inflammatory and antiatherogenic properties (10,21,24,25). There are some limitations to this study. There are sizeable inter individual variations in inflammatory and pro-atherothrombotic vascular biomarkers. Thus, baseline values for VCAM-1 in healthy control subjects and ICAM-1 and PAI-1 in subjects with type 1 diabetes were significantly different at the start of the euglycemic and hypoglycemic clamps. We do not know the reason for these baseline differences. One possible explanation is that not everyone in the study participated in both euglycemic and hypoglycemic clamps. We believe this is unlikely to be the cause as there was also a significant difference in baseline PAI-1 values in the type 1 diabetic subjects who participated in both series of glucose clamps. The magnitude of the changes of the vascular biomarkers during hypoglycemia (and euglycemia) are relatively modest. Thus, maximal changes in vascular biomarkers during hypoglycemia of 50–75% is greatly reduced compared with the multiple fold

increases of neuroendocrine hormones occurring during identical hypoglycemia. However, the ability to compare the increases of the vascular biomarkers during hyperinsulinemic hypoglycemia with the similar decreases occurring during hyperinsulinemic euglycemia does demonstrate the independent effects of hypoglycemia. The clinical significance of the magnitude of the changes in the differing proinflammatory and pro-atherothrombotic vascular biomarkers is yet to be established. We only studied one level of hypoglycemia. Thus, we cannot comment on whether deeper hypoglycemia (i.e., less than 2.9 mmol/l) would have induced greater changes in vascular biological markers. Additionally, the present study was designed to study vascular physiologic changes during prolonged hypoglycemia of 2 h. Therefore, we cannot determine the effects of shorter durations of hypoglycemia (i.e., 30–45 min) on study end points.

In summary, this present study has demonstrated the complex effects of acute moderate hypoglycemia on fibrinolytic balance and proinflammatory mechanisms in type 1 diabetic subjects and healthy control subjects. Using glucose clamps to equate insulin levels, this study has demonstrated that hypoglycemia results in significant increases in proinflammatory and potentially pro-atherogenic adhesion molecules (ICAM, VCAM, E-selectin, IL-6, VEGF) platelet activation (P-selectin), and reduced fibrinolytic balance (increased PAI-1). We conclude that 1) hypoglycemia can similarly activate a broad spectrum of vascular biological mechanisms in both type 1 diabetic subjects and age- and weight-matched nondiabetic control subjects, and 2) the potentially deleterious long-term effects of hypoglycemia on pro-atherothrombotic mechanisms needs further study.

Acknowledgments— This work was supported by the following National Institutes of Health Grants: P50-HL-081009, R01-DK-069803, M01-RR-000095, P01-HL-056693, and P60-DK-020593.

N.G.J. has received a fellowship award from Takeda Pharmaceuticals. No other potential conflicts of interest relevant to this article were reported.

The authors thank Wanda Snead, Eric Allen, and the Vanderbilt Hormone Assay Core laboratory for their excellent technical assistance, and the nursing staff of the Vanderbilt Clinical Research Center for their excellent care. The authors are grateful to Jan Hicks,

Vanderbilt University, Department of Medicine, for her superb editorial assistance.

References

1. Gold AE, Marshall SM. Cortical blindness and cerebral infarction associated with severe hypoglycemia. Diabetes Care 1996; 19:1001–1003
2. Desouza C, Salazar H, Cheong B, Murgo J, Fonseca V. Association of hypoglycemia and cardiac ischemia: a study based on continuous monitoring. Diabetes Care 2003;26:1485–1489
3. Wei M, Gibbons LW, Mitchell TL, Kampert JB, Stern MP, Blair SN. Low fasting plasma glucose level as a predictor of cardiovascular disease and all-cause mortality. Circulation 2000;101:2047–2052
4. Action to Control Cardiovascular Risk in Diabetes Study Group, Gerstein HC, Miller ME, Byington RP, Goff DC Jr, Bigger JT, Buse JB, Cushman WC, Genuth S, Ismail-Beigi F, Grimm RH Jr, Probstfield JL, Simons-Morton DG, Friedewald WT Effects of intensive glucose lowering in type 2 diabetes. N Engl J Med 2008;358: 2545–2559
5. Duckworth W, Abraira C, Moritz T, Reda D, Emanuele N, Reaven PD, Zieve FJ, Marks J, Davis SN, Hayward R, Warren SR, Goldman S, McCarren M, Vitek ME, Henderson WG, Huang GD, VADT Investigators. Glucose control and vascular complications in veterans with type 2 diabetes. N Engl J Med 2009;360:129–139
6. Campbell I. Dead in bed syndrome: a new manifestation of nocturnal hypoglycemia? Diabet Med 1991;8:3–4
7. Nathan DM, Cleary PA, Backlund JY, Genuth SM, Lachin JM, Orchard TJ, Raskin P, Zinman B. Intensive diabetes treatment and cardiovascular disease in patients with type 1 diabetes. N Engl J Med 2005; 353:2643
8. Wright RJ, Frier BM. Vascular disease and diabetes: is hypoglycaemia an aggravating factor? Diabetes/Metabolism Research and Reviews 2008;24:353–363
9. Wieczorek I, Pell AC, McIver B, MacGregor IR, Ludlam CA, Frier BM. Coagulation and fibrinolytic systems in type 1 diabetes: effects of venous occlusion and insulin induced hypoglycaemia. Clin Sci (Lond) 1993;84:79–86
10. Ibbotson SH, Catto A, Davies JA, Grant PJ. The effect of insulin-induced hypoglycaemia on factor VIII:C concentrations and thrombin activity in subjects with type 1 (insulin-dependent) diabetes. Thromb Haemost 1995;73:243–246
11. Dandona P, Chaudhuri A, Ghanim H, Mohanty P. Effect of hyperglycemia and insulin in acute coronary syndromes. Am J Cardiol 2007;99:12H–18H
12. Ewing DJ, Martyn CN, Young RJ, Clarke BF. The value of cardiovascular autonomic function tests: 10 years experience in diabetes. Diabetes Care 1985;8:491–498
13. Gold AE, MacLeod KM, Frier BM. Frequency of severe hypoglycemia in patients with type 1 diabetes and impaired awareness of hypoglycemia. Diabetes Care 1994;17:697–703
14. Briscoe VJ, Ertl AC, Tate DB, Dawling S, Davis SN. Effects of a selective serotonin reuptake inhibitor, fluoxetine, on counterregulatory responses to hypoglycemia in healthy individuals. Diabetes 2008;57: 2453–2460
15. Briscoe VJ, Ertl AC, Tate DB, Davis SN. Effects of the selective serotonin reuptake inhibitor fluoxetine on counterregulatory responses to hypoglycemia in individuals with type 1 diabetes. Diabetes 2008;57: 3315–3322
16. Amiel SA, Tamborlane WV, Simonson DC, Sherwin RS. Defective glucose counterregulation after strict glycemic control of insulin-dependent diabetes mellitus. N Engl J Med 1987;316:1376–1383
17. Celletti FL, Waugh JM, Amabile PG, Brendolan A, Hilfiker PR, Dake MD. Vascular endothelial growth factor enhances atherosclerotic plaque progression.Nat Med 2001;4:425–429
18. Ferroni P, Martini F, Riondino S, La Farina F, Magnapera A, Ciatti F, Guadagni F, Soluble P-selectin as a marker of in vivo platelet activation. Clin Chim Acta 2009; 399:88–91
19. Halleux CM, Declerck PJ, Tran SL, Detry R, Brichard SM. Hormonal control of plasminogen activator inhibitor-1 gene expression and production in human adipose tissue: stimulation by glucocorticoids and inhibition by catecholamines. J Clin Endocrinol Metab 1999;84:4097–4105
20. Trovati M, Anfossi G, Cavalot F, Vitali S, Massucco P, Mularoni E, Schinco P, Tamponi G, Emanuelli G. Studies on mechanisms involved in hypoglycemia-induced platelet activation. Diabetes 1986;35: 818–825
21. Dandona P, Mohanty P, Chaudhuri A, Garg R, Aljada A. Insulin infusion in acute illness. J Clin Invest 2005;115:2069–2072
22. Dotson S, Freeman R, Failing HJ, Adler GK. Hypoglycemia increases serum interleukin-6 levels in healthy men and women. Diabetes Care 2008;31:1222–1223
23. Razavi Nematollahi L, Kitabchi AE, Kitabchi AE, Stentz FB, Wan JY, Larijani BA, Tehrani MM, Gozashti MH, Omidfar K, Taheri E. Proinflammatory cytokines in response to insulin-induced hypoglycemic stress in healthy subjects. Metabolism Clinical and Experimental 2009;58:443–448
24. Dandona P. Endothelium, inflammation, and diabetes. Curr Diab Rep 2002;2:311–315
25. Dandona P, Aljada A, Mohanty P, Ghanim H, Bandyopadhyay A, Chaudhuri A. Insulin suppresses plasma concentration of vascular endothelial growth factor and matrix metalloproteinase-9. Diabetes Care 2003;26:3310–3314

Prevention of Nocturnal Hypoglycemia Using Predictive Alarm Algorithms and Insulin Pump Suspension

Bruce Buckingham, md[1]
H. Peter Chase, md[2]
Eyal Dassau, phd[3]
Erin Cobry, bs[2]
Paula Clinton, rd[1]
Victoria Gage, rn[2]

Kimberly Caswell, aprn, bc[1]
John Wilkinson[2]
Fraser Cameron, ms[4]
Hyunjin Lee, phd[5]
B. Wayne Bequette, phd[5]
Francis J. Doyle III, phd[3]

OBJECTIVE — The aim of this study was to develop a partial closed-loop system to safely prevent nocturnal hypoglycemia by suspending insulin delivery when hypoglycemia is predicted in type 1 diabetes.

RESEARCH DESIGN AND METHODS — Forty subjects with type 1 diabetes (age range 12–39 years) were studied overnight in the hospital. For the first 14 subjects, hypoglycemia (<60 mg/dl) was induced by gradually increasing the basal insulin infusion rate (without the use of pump shutoff algorithms). During the subsequent 26 patient studies, pump shutoff occurred when either three of five ($n = 10$) or two of five ($n = 16$) algorithms predicted hypoglycemia based on the glucose levels measured with the FreeStyle Navigator (Abbott Diabetes Care).

RESULTS — The standardized protocol induced hypoglycemia on 13 (93%) of the 14 nights. With use of a voting scheme that required three algorithms to trigger insulin pump suspension, nocturnal hypoglycemia was prevented during 6 (60%) of 10 nights. When the voting scheme was changed to require only two algorithms to predict hypoglycemia to trigger pump suspension, hypoglycemia was prevented during 12 (75%) of 16 nights. In the latter study, there were 25 predictions of hypoglycemia because some subjects had multiple hypoglycemic events during a night, and hypoglycemia was prevented for 84% of these events.

CONCLUSIONS — Using algorithms to shut off the insulin pump when hypoglycemia is predicted, it is possible to prevent hypoglycemia on 75% of nights (84% of events) when it would otherwise be predicted to occur.

Diabetes Care 33:1013–1017, 2010

Continuous glucose monitoring (CGM) represents the "third era" in diabetes management after the eras of urine glucose testing and (self-monitoring) blood glucose testing. One of the important potential benefits of real-time CGM is the ability of these devices to alarm for hypoglycemia. However, a previous study showed that 71% of youth did not respond to hypoglycemia alarms during the night (1). Moreover, the most severe hypoglycemic events in the Diabetes Control and Complications Trial occurred during sleep hours (2). Davis et al. (3) found that 75% of hypoglycemic seizures in children occurred during sleep. Sovik and Thordarson (4) reported that among patients aged <40 years who died over a 10-year period, 6% of the deaths were due to "dead-in-bed" syndrome, which in many instances was probably the result of severe nocturnal hypoglycemia.

The availability of CGM systems has allowed determination of the incidence of nocturnal hypoglycemia in the home environment. In a randomized trial evaluating daily CGM use over a 6-month period in children and adults with type 1 diabetes, 216 subjects used a CGM device for a total of 25,473 nights (5). The glucose level was ≤70 mg/dl on 25% of nights, ≤60 mg/dl on 15% of nights, and ≤50 mg/dl on 8% of nights (5) (C. Kollman, unpublished data). Similar or even higher frequencies of nocturnal biochemical hypoglycemia have been found in other studies (6–9).

In a previous report, we prospectively studied the prevention of daytime hypoglycemia using CGM, hypoglycemia prediction algorithms, and temporary discontinuation of insulin via continuous subcutaneous insulin infusion (insulin pump) (10). Hypoglycemia was prevented using a 90-min pump suspension on 60–80% of days. Cengiz et al. (11) described automatic pump suspension using the proportional integral derivative algorithm during 34 h of closed-loop automated insulin delivery in 17 patients. They were successful in preventing hypoglycemia (glucose <60 mg/dl) in 14 of 18 (78%) suspension episodes. The purpose of the present study was to extend our original observations to evaluate the prevention of nocturnal hypoglycemia using hypoglycemia prediction algorithms.

RESEARCH DESIGN AND METHODS — Subjects for this study were recruited at the Barbara Davis Center (Aurora, CO) and the Stanford Medical Center (Stanford, CA). The protocol was approved by the local institutional review boards, and all subjects and parents or guardians signed an informed consent form and an assent form if necessary. Subjects in this study had had type 1 diabetes for at least 1 year and had used a downloadable insulin pump for at least 3 months.

Participants were trained on the use of the FreeStyle Navigator CGM system

From the [1]Department of Pediatric Endocrinology, Stanford University, Stanford, California; the [2]Department of Pediatrics, University of Colorado, Aurora, Colorado; the [3]Department of Chemical Engineering, University of California, Santa Barbara, Santa Barbara, California; the [4]Department of Aeronautics and Astronautics, Stanford University, Stanford, California; and the [5]Department of Chemical and Biological Engineering, Rensselaer Polytechnic Institute, Troy, New York.
Corresponding author: H. Peter Chase, peter.chase@ucdenver.edu.
Received 17 December 2009 and accepted 6 February 2010. Published ahead of print at http://care.diabetesjournals.org on 3 March 2010. DOI: 10.2337/dc09-2303.
The costs of publication of this article were defrayed in part by the payment of page charges. This article must therefore be hereby marked "advertisement" in accordance with 18 U.S.C. Section 1734 solely to indicate this fact.

(Abbott Diabetes Care, Alameda, CA) and were instructed to wear two systems for each study. The two CGM systems were usually inserted 1–2 days before admission. Subjects arrived at the Clinical Translational Research Center (CTRC) at ~7:30 P.M. after a dinner consisting of known amounts of carbohydrate, protein, and fat.

Inducing nocturnal hypoglycemia

Fourteen subjects completed the control (hypoglycemia induction) visit at the CTRC with the intent to establish a consistent method for inducing nocturnal hypoglycemia using increases in basal insulin. After admission to the CTRC and stabilization, basal insulin was increased in 5–25% increments every 90 min, depending on the current blood glucose, the glucose rate of change, and the linearly predicted glucose value to be reached by 5:00 A.M. (aim <60 mg/dl). The subject's blood glucose was monitored every 15–30 min using the FreeStyle meter built into the Navigator (the only meter used in this study). Blood was also collected for YSI (Yellow Springs, OH) glucose analysis once the FreeStyle reading was <70 mg/dl. When the hypoglycemic threshold was reached (blood glucose value <60 mg/dl), oral carbohydrates were given to return glucose levels to >70 mg/dl.

Preventing hypoglycemia

The same consistent method for inducing hypoglycemia was used in the subsequent studies to assess whether hypoglycemia prediction and insulin pump suspension could prevent nocturnal hypoglycemia. The Navigator glucose alarms, including the built-in Projected Low Alarm, were not activated during the study. For the hypoglycemia prevention studies, one of the Navigator sensors was connected to a laptop computer containing the artificial pancreas system (12) and the hypoglycemia prediction algorithm (13) composed of five separate prediction algorithms and a voting schema, explained briefly in the following.

1. Modified linear prediction alarm. This alarm uses a 15-min linear extrapolation and an uncertainty threshold based on the SD of the glucose measurements in the previous 15 min.
2. Kalman filtering. A Kalman filter is used to obtain an estimate of glucose and its rate of change, which are then used to make predictions of future glucose levels. The filter is tuned to choose between the probabilities that a measured glucose change is real versus the result of signal noise (14).
3. Adaptive hybrid infinite impulse response (HIIR) filter. An infinite impulse response filter updates parameters adaptively using the CGM signal. The HIIR filter considers a bandwidth of past data to update the filter parameters.
4. Statistical prediction. Multiple empirical, statistical models are used to estimate future glucose values and their error bounds. A probability of hypoglycemia is generated and thresholded to produce an alarm (15).
5. Numerical logical algorithm. The algorithm transmits a three-point calculated rate of change and the current value into logical expressions to detect impending hypoglycemia. The numerical logical algorithm provides insensitivity to sensor signal dropouts.

The algorithms for pump suspension were based on a 35-min prediction horizon (looking 35 min into the future) and a glucose threshold of 80 mg/dl. The glucose threshold and 35-min prediction horizon were chosen to allow time for the pump suspension to be effective in lowering insulin levels once the basal rate was suspended and was based on analysis of previous CGM data with nocturnal hypoglycemia. There is a sustained negative rate of change in glucose levels lasting a mean of 75 min after insulin pump suspension (10). In our initial 10 patient studies we required three of the hypoglycemia prediction algorithms to be simultaneously positive twice in a 10-min window before the pump was suspended. In the subsequent 16 studies we only required two alarms to be simultaneously positive twice in a 10-min window. When the hypoglycemia prediction algorithm alarmed (on a computer outside the subject's room), study staff manually suspended insulin delivery from the pump using a 90-min suspend protocol. Serum ketone levels were measured at the pump suspension, after insulin restart, and each morning on completion of the study using the Precision Xtra meter (Abbott Diabetes Care).

Criteria for restarting insulin infusion

The initial protocol involved a 90-min pump suspension when hypoglycemia was predicted. Because there were often multiple hypoglycemia events predicted each night, it was desired to limit the time insulin was suspended once the glucose was past the nadir. Thus, for the final 11 subjects, the criteria for restarting a pump suspension included 1) a minimum of 30 min of pump suspension, 2) a positive rate of change on the FreeStyle Navigator system of >0.5 mg/dl-min, and 3) a FreeStyle Navigator glucose value >80 mg/dl. When basal insulin was restarted, it was at the subject's usual rate for that time of night.

RESULTS

Inducing nocturnal hypoglycemia

Fourteen subjects, aged 12–39 years, were initially studied for the induction of nocturnal hypoglycemia in the CTRC. Many of these same subjects participated in the subsequent two hypoglycemia prevention protocols. The demographic information for subjects participating in each of the three studies is shown in Table 1. The first study was designed to develop a reliable method of producing nocturnal hypoglycemia (>80% success) and the second and third studies were designed to study the possibility of preventing nocturnal hypoglycemia using predictive algorithms and temporary insulin suspension.

With use of the protocol to generate nocturnal hypoglycemia, 13 of the 14 subjects (93%) reached glucose levels ≤60 mg/dl; 9 of 14 had levels <55 mg/dl.

Table 1—Demographic information

	Study to induce hypoglycemia	Pump shutoff requiring three predictions	Pump shutoff requiring two predictions
Age (years)	21.0 ± 7.5	22.5 ± 6.3	22.0 ± 8.9
Duration of type 1 diabetes (years)	12.1 ± 6.0	12.7 ± 5.5	11.5 ± 6.9
A1C (%)	7.8 ± 1.9	7.3 ± 0.8	7.3 ± 0.7
BMI (kg/m^2)	22.0 ± 3.1	24.6 ± 2.8	25.2 ± 3.9

Data are means ± SD.

Table 2—*Results of the three-alarm and two-alarm voting systems*

No. predictive algorithms needed to trigger pump suspension	n	Subjects without hypoglycemia	No. events*	Events without hypoglycemia
3 of 5	10	60	15	71
2 of 5	16	75	25	84

Data are % unless indicated otherwise. *An event is an episode of predicted hypoglycemia resulting in a pump suspension.

Table 3—*Distribution of algorithms that were the first, second, or third to predict hypoglycemia*

Alarm	First alarms	Second alarms	Third alarms
Statistical prediction	60	28	6
Numerical logical	30	28	24
HIIR	3	10	49
Kalman	7	31	21
Linear prediction	0	3	0

Data are %.

The mean increase in basal rate was 180%. There were no seizures or loss of consciousness.

Preventing hypoglycemia

Twenty-six subjects participated in this phase of the study. A hypoglycemia threshold of 80 mg/dl and a prediction horizon (the time the algorithm is looking into the future to predict hypoglycemia) of 35 min was used for this study. For the first 10 patient studies, the insulin pump shutoff occurred when three algorithms predicted hypoglycemia and for the last 16 patient studies only two of five prediction algorithms were required to shut off the pump. During the study with the first 10 subjects, hypoglycemia was prevented on 6 (60%) of the 10 nights. There were a total of 15 hypoglycemic events predicted during these 10 nights (three subjects having two events and one subject having three events), and hypoglycemia was prevented for 71% of the events (Table 2).

When we assessed the time between two hypoglycemia prediction algorithms voting to turn off the pump and three algorithms voting to turn off the pump, there was a mean difference of 12 min. To provide more time for the pump shutoff to be effective, we therefore conducted our next set of studies with the requirement of only two of the five algorithms to predict hypoglycemia to trigger pump suspension. This resulted in hypoglycemia being prevented on 12 of 16 nights (75%) (Table 2). Four subjects had two events during the night, one subject had three events, and one subject had four events. For the 25 hypoglycemic events, hypoglycemia was prevented 84% of the time. Figure 1 illustrates successful prevention of hypoglycemia using two insulin suspensions during the night.

We also evaluated which alarms were contributing to the first, second, and third votes to turn the pump off (Table 3). The linear prediction algorithm was the least likely to predict hypoglycemia. Other-

wise, all of the algorithms played a significant role in contributing to the vote.

Factors relating to successful hypoglycemia prevention

A comparison was done between several factors that may play a role in the success of the system. These included the accuracy of the FreeStyle Navigator system (a comparison of the FreeStyle Navigator system value with the YSI blood glucose value), the rate of change in the glucose readings at the time of pump suspension, and the YSI blood glucose value at the time of pump suspension. The difference between the FreeStyle Navigator system and the YSI glucose values at the time of pump suspension was 4 ± 9 mg/dl (mean $\pm$ SD) for successful events, and the Navigator was always reading higher than the YSI when the predictive pump shutoff failed (mean of 18 ± 10 mg/dl for failures) ($P = 0.001$). The other factors, such as rate of glucose change and YSI glucose value at the time of pump shutoff, were not significantly different between successful and unsuccessful events. The first episode of pump suspension was successful 75% of the time, and subsequent episodes were successful 80% of the time. The glucose rate of change was less with subsequent pump suspensions, because the basal rate was returned to the usual infusion rate for that time of night (mean $\pm$ SD rate of change -0.72 ± 0.42 mg/dl-min on first shutoff and -0.24 ± 0.13 mg/dl-min on subsequent shutoffs).

Early restart of basal insulin

In the last 11 patient studies, an early restart of basal insulin was permitted once the glucose was past the nadir (see RESEARCH DESIGN AND METHODS). There were 19 hypoglycemic events on these 11 nights, and the early pump restart occurred on 5 occasions. The mean peak glucose after restart of an insulin infusion in the cohort

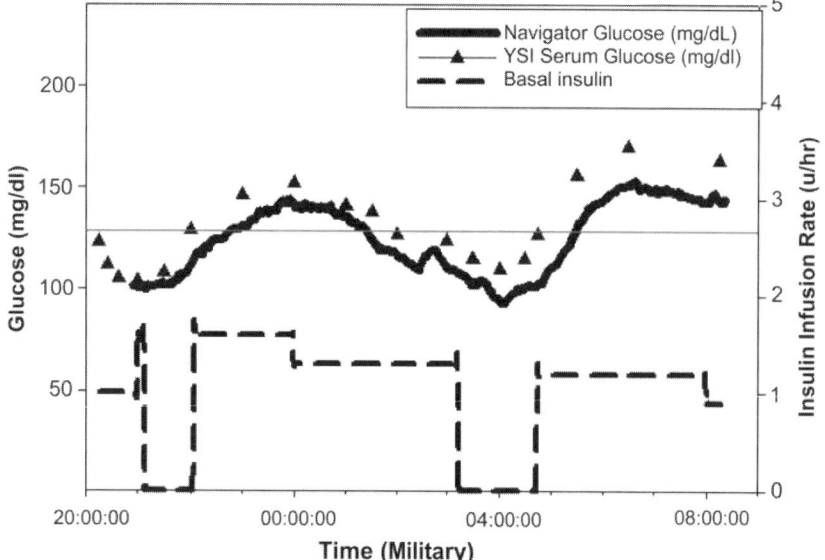

Figure 1—*Successful prevention of hypoglycemia (glucose levels by CGM or venous blood <60 mg/dl) as a result of two 90-min periods of insulin pump suspension. The hypoglycemia prediction algorithm required two (of five) alarms for pump suspension and was based on a 35-min prediction horizon and a CGM glucose threshold of 80 mg/dl.*

of 11 subjects using an early restart was 149 ± 32 mg/dl, and the maximum glucose was 210 mg/dl. In the nights in which an early restart of insulin was not permitted, the mean peak glucose after pump suspension was 158 ± 50 mg/dl and the highest glucose was 275 mg/dl. These differences were not statistically significant.

Occurrence of ketonemia

Four subjects developed ketone levels >0.3 mmol · l^{-1} · l^{-1} (range 0.4–1.5 mmol · l^{-1} · l^{-1}). In each instance, when the serum ketone levels were checked several hours later, they were <0.3 mmol · l^{-1} · l^{-1}. In two instances, the pump had been suspended for 90 min (final glucose levels 146 and 155 mg/dl), and in two instances (with more than one suspension), the pump had been suspended for a total of 180 min (final glucose levels 202 and 261 mg/dl). In each case the serum ketone levels were <0.3 mmol · l^{-1} · l^{-1} after the first suspension. There were no clinical symptoms such as upset stomach, nausea, or Kussmaul respirations, and no specific treatment was given.

CONCLUSIONS — Prevention of severe nocturnal hypoglycemic events remains one of the most challenging goals in the treatment of diabetes. With the prevention of severe hypoglycemia, it is likely that more people would be able to move toward optimal glycemic control. Because of the decrease in counterregulatory hormone secretion during sleep, even in people without diabetes (16), and the frequent loss of counterregulatory hormone secretion in people with diabetes (17,18), prevention will probably require the use of a closed-loop system. In this initial step toward a closed-loop system, we tested the use of a subcutaneous sensor signal to predict impending hypoglycemia and to trigger pump suspension. It was not possible to eliminate nocturnal hypoglycemia completely. However, hypoglycemia was prevented during 75% of the nights and for 84% of predicted events. Presumably, a hypoglycemia prediction algorithm, as used in the present study, will be combined with discontinuation of continuous subcutaneous insulin infusion at a specific glucose level. The latter currently occurs in the Medtronic MiniMed Paradigm Veo Real-Time System in Europe. The two working together may be very effective in preventing severe hypoglycemia.

In some cases for which hypoglycemia was not successfully prevented, the subjects' sensor glucose values were consistently running higher than the blood glucose values. This may have been due to CGM inaccuracy or due to the known lag time of ~8–10 min between the two compartments (19). Future investigators may be able to use a forced CGM calibration at bedtime if there is a significant discrepancy between a discrete bedtime glucose value and the sensor glucose to minimize this effect. We initially hypothesized that the rate of fall of the glucose values before a hypoglycemic event would also be a major factor in determining the success or failure of hypoglycemia prevention. However, this did not prove to be true.

To achieve a high rate of nocturnal hypoglycemia, we systematically increased nocturnal basal infusion rates until there was a >80% risk of hypoglycemia. Because of receiving higher basal insulin infusion rates than on a typical night, subjects probably experienced a more rapid rate of fall in glucose levels with a longer residual insulin effect. This may have made it more difficult for the pump suspension algorithms to prevent impending hypoglycemia. Unfortunately, even when the basal rate was at the usual infusion rate for that subject (after the first pump suspension), we still failed to prevent hypoglycemia 20% of the time.

It is known that once a person has had one hypoglycemic event, a second event is more likely (17). Thus, overall these results seem promising.

Although a rigid blood glucose cutoff of <60 mg/dl was used to define failure of prevention of hypoglycemia, it is possible that we were overly cautious. The shortest known time of prolonged hypoglycemia (<40 mg/dl while using the Medtronic Paradigm CGM system) before a seizure is currently 2.25 h (20). There were no severe hypoglycemic events in the current study. It would also be unlikely using the current protocol that the duration of hypoglycemia would be long enough to result in a severe hypoglycemic episode. Previous studies have shown that suspension of insulin delivery for up to 2 h has not resulted in significant ketosis (10,21–25). In our studies, there was mild ketosis on four occasions when the pump was suspended for 90–180 min, and in each instance serum ketone levels returned to normal with the reinstitution of basal insulin therapy.

Studies in the home setting are now needed. The initial aim will be to prevent-

ing nocturnal hypoglycemia, and studies will be randomized to include nights when the prevention system is in place and to include control nights when the system is not in use. The bedside minicomputer will randomize the nights and will also act as an intermediary (containing the prevention algorithms) between the insulin pump and the CGM. Studies will begin with adults but will then be extended to children. It is our belief that most episodes of severe nocturnal hypoglycemia will be preventable, using either this or a similar system.

Acknowledgments — This research was supported by the Juvenile Diabetes Research Foundation. B.B. was given an honorarium from Abbott Diabetes Care for a lecture in February 2009. E.D. was supported by the Otis Williams Fund at the Santa Barbara Foundation. Abbott Diabetes Care provided the FreeStyle Navigator continuous glucose monitoring systems. Karmeen Kulkarni, M.S., R.D., B.C., A.D.M., C.D.E., Marc Taub, Ph.D., and Geoff V. McGarraugh from Abbott Diabetes Care provided technical and device support. The artificial pancreas software was provided by the University of California, Santa Barbara and Sansum Diabetes Research Foundation. The Clinical Translational Research Center studies were supported in part by grants M01-RR-00070 and RR-000051 and 5M01-RR-00069 from the National Center for Research Resources, National Institutes of Health. No other potential conflicts of interest relevant to this article were reported.

We gratefully acknowledge the clinical and intellectual support and expertise provided by Darrell Wilson, M.D., and Howard Zisser, M.D.

References

1. Buckingham B, Block J, Burdick J, Kalajian A, Kollman C, Choy M, Wilson DM, Chase P, Diabetes Research in Children Network. Response to nocturnal alarms using a real-time glucose sensor. Diabetes Technol Ther 2005;7:440–447
2. The DCCT Research Group. Epidemiology of severe hypoglycemia in the Diabetes Control and Complications Trial. Am J Med 1991;90:450–459
3. Davis EA, Keating B, Byrne GC, Russell M, Jones TW. Hypoglycemia: incidence and clinical predictors in a large population-based sample of children and adolescents with IDDM. Diabetes Care 1997; 20:22–25
4. Sovik O, Thordarson H. Dead-in-bed syndrome in young diabetic patients. Diabetes Care 1999;22(Suppl. 2):B40–B42
5. Tamborlane WV, Beck RW, Bode BW, Buckingham B, Chase HP, Clemons R, Fiallo-Scharer R, Fox LA, Gilliam LK, Hirsch IB, Huang ES, Kollman C, Kowalski

AJ, Laffel L, Lawrence JM, Lee J, Mauras N, O'Grady M, Ruedy KJ, Tansey M, Tsalikian E, Weinzimer S, Wilson DM, Wolpert H, Wysocki T, Xing D. Continuous glucose monitoring and intensive treatment of type 1 diabetes. N Engl J Med 2008;359:1464–1476

6. Boland EA, DeLucia M, Brandt CA, Grey M, Tamborlane WV. Limitations of conventional methods of self blood glucose monitoring: lessons learned from three days of continuous glucose monitoring (CGMS) in pediatric patients with type 1 diabetes (Abstract). Diabetes 2000;49 (Suppl. 1):A98

7. Kaufman FR, Austin J, Neinstein A, Jeng L, Halvorson M, Devoe DJ, Pitukcheewanont P. Nocturnal hypoglycemia detected with the continuous glucose monitoring system in pediatric patients with type 1 diabetes. J Pediatr 2002;141:625–630

8. Ludvigsson J, Hanas R. Continuous subcutaneous glucose monitoring improved metabolic control in pediatric patients with type 1 diabetes: a controlled crossover study. Pediatrics 2003;111:933–938

9. Jeha GS, Karaviti LP, Anderson B, Smith EO, Donaldson S, McGirk TS, Haymond MW. Continuous glucose monitoring and the reality of metabolic control in preschool children with type 1 diabetes. Diabetes Care 2004;27:2881–2886

10. Buckingham B, Cobry E, Clinton P, Gage V, Caswell K, Kunselman E, Cameron F, Chase HP. Preventing hypoglycemia using predictive alarm algorithms and insulin pump suspension. Diabetes Technol Ther 2009;11:93–97

11. Cengiz E, Swan KL, Tamborlane WV, Steil GM, Steffen AT, Weinzimer SA. Is an automatic pump suspension feature safe for children with type 1 diabetes? An exploratory analysis with a closed-loop sys-

tem. Diabetes Technol Ther 2009;11:207–210

12. Dassau E, Zisser H, C Palerm C, A Buckingham B, Jovanovic L, J Doyle F 3rd. Modular artificial β-cell system: a prototype for clinical research. J Diabetes Sci Technol 2008;2:863–872

13. Dassau E, Cameron F, Lee H, Bequette BW, Doyle FJ, Niemeyer G, Chase HP, Buckingham B. Real-time hypoglycemia prediction using continuous glucose monitoring (CGM): a safety net to the artificial pancreas. Diabetes 2008;57 (Suppl. 1):A13

14. Palerm CC, Bequette BW. Hypoglycemia detection and prediction using continuous glucose monitoring—a study on hypoglycemic clamp data. J Diabetes Sci Technol 2007;1:624–629

15. Cameron F, Niemeyer G, Gundy-Burlet K, Buckingham B. Statistical hypoglycemia prediction. J Diabetes Sci Technol 2008;2:612–621

16. Jones TW, Porter P, Sherwin RS, Davis EA, O'Leary P, Frazer F, Byrne G, Stick S, Tamborlane WV. Decreased epinephrine responses to hypoglycemia during sleep. N Engl J Med 1998;338:1657–1662

17. Cryer PE, Davis SN, Shamoon H. Hypoglycemia in diabetes. Diabetes Care 2003; 26:1902–1912

18. Diabetes Research in Children Network (DirecNet) Study Group, Tsalikian E, Tamborlane W, Xing D, Becker DM, Mauras N, Fiallo-Scharer R, Buckingham B, Weinzimer S, Steffes M, Singh R, Beck R, Ruedy K, Kollman C. Blunted counterregulatory hormone responses to hypoglycemia in young children and adolescents with well-controlled type 1 diabetes. Diabetes Care 2009;32:1954–1959

19. Cengiz E, Tamborlane WV. A tale of two compartments: interstitial versus blood

glucose monitoring. Diabetes Technol Ther 2009;11(Suppl. 1):S11–S16

20. Buckingham B, Wilson DM, Lecher T, Hanas R, Kaiserman K, Cameron F. Duration of nocturnal hypoglycemia before seizures. Diabetes Care 2008;31:2110–2112

21. Diabetes Research in Children Network (DirecNet) Study Group, Tsalikian E, Kollman C, Tamborlane WB, Beck RW, Fiallo-Scharer R, Fox L, Janz KF, Ruedy KJ, Wilson D, Xing D, Weinzimer SA. Prevention of hypoglycemia during exercise in children with type 1 diabetes by suspending basal insulin. Diabetes Care 2006;29:2200–2204

22. Orsini-Federici M, Akwi JA, Canonico V, Celleno R, Ferolla P, Pippi R, Tassi C, Timi A, Benedetti MM. Early detection of insulin deprivation in continuous subcutaneous insulin infusion-treated patients with type 1 diabetes. Diabetes Technol Ther 2006;8:67–75

23. Castillo MJ, Scheen AJ, Lefèbvre PJ. The degree/rapidity of the metabolic deterioration following interruption of a continuous subcutaneous insulin infusion is influenced by the prevailing blood glucose level. J Clin Endocrinol Metab 1996; 81:1975–1978

24. Scheen A, Castillo M, Jandrain B, Krzentowski G, Henrivaux P, Luyckx AS, Lefèbvre PJ. Metabolic alterations after a two-hour nocturnal interruption of a continuous subcutaneous insulin infusion. Diabetes Care 1984;7:338–342

25. Scheen AJ, Krzentowski G, Castillo M, Lefèbvre PJ, Luyckx AS. A 6-hour nocturnal interruption of a continuous subcutaneous insulin infusion: 2. Marked attenuation of the metabolic deterioration by somatostatin. Diabetologia 1983;24:319–325

Antecedent Hypoglycemia Impairs Autonomic Cardiovascular Function
Implications for Rigorous Glycemic Control

Gail K. Adler,[1,2] Istvan Bonyhay,[2,3] Hannah Failing,[1,2] Elizabeth Waring,[2,3] Sarah Dotson,[1,2] and Roy Freeman[2,3]

OBJECTIVE—Glycemic control decreases the incidence and progression of diabetic complications but increases the incidence of hypoglycemia. Hypoglycemia can impair hormonal and autonomic responses to subsequent hypoglycemia. Intensive glycemic control may increase mortality in individuals with type 2 diabetes at high risk for cardiovascular complications. We tested the hypothesis that prior exposure to hypoglycemia leads to impaired cardiovascular autonomic function.

RESEARCH DESIGN AND METHODS—Twenty healthy subjects (age 28 ± 2 years; 10 men) participated in two 3-day inpatient visits, separated by 1–3 months. Autonomic testing was performed on days 1 and 3 to measure sympathetic, parasympathetic, and baroreflex function. A 2-h hyperinsulinemic [hypoglycemic (2.8 mmol/l) or euglycemic (5.0 mmol/l)] clamp was performed in the morning and in the afternoon of day 2.

RESULTS—Comparison of the day 3 autonomic measurements demonstrated that antecedent hypoglycemia leads to *1*) reduced baroreflex sensitivity (16.7 ± 1.8 vs. 13.8 ± 1.4 ms/mmHg, $P = 0.03$); *2*) decreased muscle sympathetic nerve activity response to transient nitroprusside-induced hypotension (53.3 ± 3.7 vs. 40.1 ± 2.7 bursts/min, $P < 0.01$); and *3*) reduced ($P < 0.001$) plasma norepinephrine response to lower body negative pressure (3.0 ± 0.3 vs. 2.0 ± 0.2 nmol/l at −40 mmHg).

CONCLUSIONS—Baroreflex sensitivity and the sympathetic response to hypotensive stress are attenuated after antecedent hypoglycemia. Because impaired autonomic function, including decreased cardiac vagal baroreflex sensitivity, may contribute directly to mortality in diabetes and cardiovascular disease, our findings raise new concerns regarding the consequences of hypoglycemia. *Diabetes* **58:360–366, 2009**

C ontrol of blood glucose is the cornerstone of diabetes management because glycemic control decreases the incidence and progression of diabetic microvascular (1–4) and, in some studies, macrovascular complications (2,5). However, rigorous glycemic control leads to an increased incidence of hypoglycemia (1,6). Even a single episode of hypoglycemia may impair the counterregulatory metabolic and autonomic responses to subsequent hypoglycemia (7). Recently, evidence has emerged suggesting an association between hypoglycemia and increased mortality in critically ill patients receiving insulin therapy (8). An increase in mortality was also observed in the highly intensive treated limb (targeting A1C values of <6%) of a multicenter clinical trial of individuals with type 2 diabetes at high risk for cardiovascular disease events (9). The cause of the mortality in these studies could not be directly attributed to hypoglycemia.

Cardiovascular autonomic impairment is associated with and may cause increased mortality (10–14). Autonomic neuropathy is a predictor of increased mortality in many diabetic cohort studies (10,11). In addition, impaired heart rate variability is associated with increased risk of mortality in patients after a myocardial infarct (12). More recent studies in the postmyocardial infarction population have shown that impaired baroreflex sensitivity is an independent predictor of cardiac mortality (13,14).

In an effort to extend our understanding of the effect of hypoglycemia on the autonomic nervous system, we tested the hypothesis that prior exposure to hypoglycemia would lead to impaired control of cardiovascular autonomic function. We therefore examined cardiovascular autonomic function using standardized tests measuring sympathetic, parasympathetic, and baroreflex function before and after euglycemic-hyperinsulinemic and hypoglycemic-hyperinsulinemic clamp studies.

RESEARCH DESIGN AND METHODS

We recruited healthy men and women, aged 18 to 50 years. A complete medical history, physical examination, and screening autonomic testing were performed; and blood samples for electrolytes, liver function tests, and complete blood count were obtained to determine subject eligibility. Each subject participated in two 3-day inpatient study visits, separated in time by 1–3 months (Fig. 1). On days 1 and 3 of each study visit, subjects underwent autonomic nervous system testing. On day 2, either two (morning and afternoon) hypoglycemic-hyperinsulinemic clamp studies or two euglycemic-hyperinsulinemic clamp studies were performed. Those subjects randomized to hypoglycemia on the first inpatient study visit were exposed to euglycemia on the second study visit, and vice versa. All autonomic testing was performed at Beth Israel Deaconess Medical Center by investigational staff unaware of subject condition, and subjects were transferred by wheelchair and taxi (0.4 Km) to and from Brigham and Women's Hospital General Clinical Research Center (GCRC) for overnight stays and day-2 study procedures. The institutional review boards at both institutions approved all study procedures, and all subjects gave written informed consent.

Diet and activity. Subjects refrained from vigorous exercise for 7 days before each admission. Subjects consumed an isocaloric diet provided by the GCRC containing 125 ± 10 mmol/day sodium, 100 ± 10 mmol/day potassium, and 200 ± 13 mmol/day calcium with water ad libitum for 4 days before study

From the [1]Division of Endocrinology, Diabetes, and Hypertension, Department of Medicine, Brigham and Women's Hospital, Boston, Massachusetts; [2]Harvard Medical School, Boston, Massachusetts; and the [3]Department of Neurology, Beth Israel Deaconess Medical Center, Boston, Massachusetts.
Corresponding author: Roy Freeman, rfreeman@bidmc.harvard.edu.
Received 22 August 2008 and accepted 12 November 2008.
Published ahead of print at http://diabetes.diabetesjournals.org on 3 December 2008. DOI: 10.2337/db08-1153.

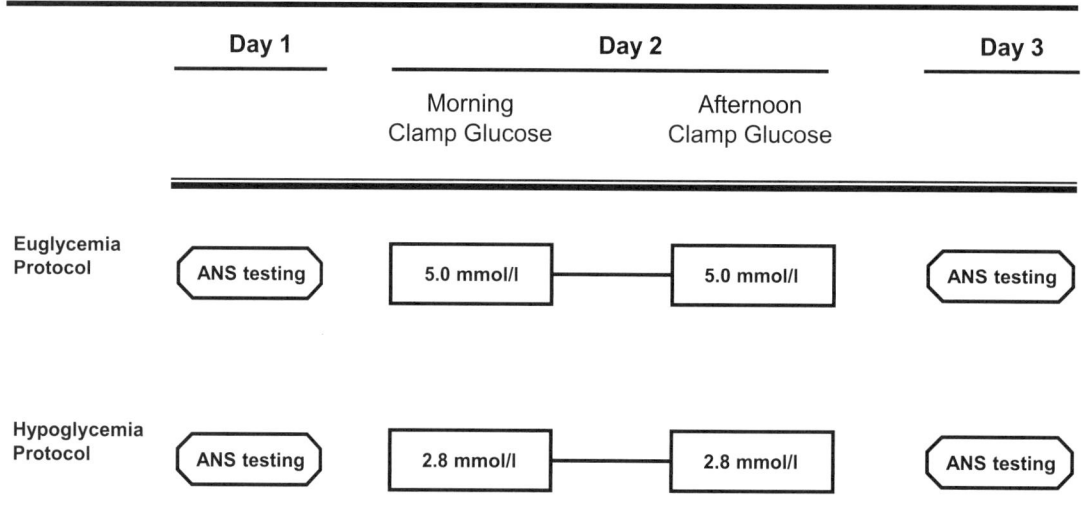

FIG. 1. Study design. Subjects participated in two, 3-day/2-night protocols separated in time by 1–3 months. Subjects were randomized by admission to participate in either euglycemic (target blood glucose 5.0 mmol/l)-hyperinsulinemic clamp studies or hypoglycemic (target blood glucose 2.8 mmol/l)-hyperinsulinemic clamp studies on day 2. Autonomic nervous system (ANS) testing was conducted on days 1 and 3 by investigators unaware of whether a subject was participating in the euglycemia or hypoglycemia protocol.

procedures and continuing through to end of day 3. Subjects received a minimum of 2,000 ml fluid orally on day 2.

Hyperinsulinemic clamp protocols. After completing day 1 autonomic testing, subjects were admitted to the Brigham and Women's Hospital GCRC. After fasting and remaining supine overnight, subjects received a primed, constant infusion of insulin (160 and 120 mU/m² body surface area/min sequentially for 5 min each, followed by 80 mU/m² body surface area/min for 125 min of Novolin R; Novo Nordisk, Princeton, NJ). At $t = -15, 0, 45, 75, 105$, and 135 min of the insulin infusion, blood was withdrawn for determination of hormone levels via an indwelling intravenous catheter that was placed in a retrograde fashion near the wrist of a hand resting in a warm box (66°C). Blood was withdrawn for glucose determination every 5 min, and the rate of a 20% dextrose infusion was adjusted to achieve target blood glucose levels of 5.0 mmol/l for the euglycemic clamps and 2.8 mmol/l for the hypoglycemic clamps. At the end of the 135-min insulin infusion, subjects received a small snack, and the dextrose infusion rate was adjusted to achieve blood glucose levels of at least 5.0 mmol/l. After a 90-min break, the hyperinsulinemic clamp procedure was repeated. Afternoon insulin infusions during hypoglycemic clamp studies were extended as necessary to achieve 90 min of hypoglycemia. In four subjects, the insulin infusion was increased by 50% to achieve the target glucose level of 2.8 mmol/l. On day 2, 24-h urine collections were obtained. The next morning, subjects returned to Beth Israel Deaconess Medical Center for the day-3 autonomic testing.

Autonomic testing. Testing was performed at 9:00 A.M. in the autonomic laboratory of the Beth Israel Deaconess Medical Center on days 1 and 3 of each study visit. All autonomic investigators were unaware as to whether subjects had been exposed to hypoglycemia or euglycemia on day 2. Subjects received a light breakfast 2 h before testing. Subjects were allowed at least a 20-min rest in the supine position in a quiet, dim lit environment to attain psychological and physiological equilibration before testing. R-R interval, beat-to-beat blood pressure (Finometer; FMS, Amsterdam, the Netherlands), and oscillometric blood pressure (Dinamap; Critikon, Tampa, FL) were measured. Muscle sympathetic nerve activity (MSNA) was recorded from the peroneal nerve with microneurography. Neural signal was filtered (bandwidth 0.7–2.0 kHz), rectified, and integrated (time constant, 0.1 s) (Nerve Traffic Analyzer model 662c-3; University of Iowa Bioengineering, Iowa City, IA). Sympathetic bursts were identified by their characteristic morphology and relationship to R waves on the electrocardiogram using an automated sympathetic neurogram analysis program (15). The number of sympathetic bursts was expressed as bursts per minute. The following tests were performed in sequential order.

Paced breathing heart rate variability. The high-frequency region of the R-R interval power spectrum during supine paced breathing was used to assess baseline cardiac vagal function. Subjects were instructed to initiate a breath with each tone of a series of computer generated auditory cues at a preset, evenly spaced rate of 12 breaths/min. The autospectra of the R-R interval were estimated for the 7-min segment using the Blackman Tukey's method. Power spectral estimates of the R-R interval heart rate were

quantified using the area (power) of the spectrum in the high-frequency region (0.15–0.50 Hz) (16).

Baroreflex assessment. The modified Oxford technique was used to assess cardiac vagal and sympathetic baroreflex function (17). After a resting period of 30 min, a 5-min baseline recording was made followed by the baroreflex test: sequential administration of bolus injections of 100 μg sodium nitroprusside and of 150 μg phenylephrine hydrochloride produced a drop in systolic blood pressure of ~15 mmHg below baseline followed by a rise of ~15 mmHg above baseline. The cardiac vagal baroreflex was assessed by the relation between R-R interval and systolic blood pressure (Fig. 2B). The muscle sympathetic nerve response to transient hypotension was determined (17).

Simulated orthostatic stress with lower body negative pressure. Graded lower-body negative pressure (LBNP) was used to simulate orthostatic stress without the confounding effects of muscle contraction. Supine subjects were sealed at the waist in a metal tank. After a 5-min baseline data collection period, pressures of −10, −20, −30, and −40 mmHg were generated sequentially. Four minutes were spent at each negative pressure level. Blood was drawn for hormone measurements via an indwelling venous catheter at baseline and after 3 min of each negative pressure level. Subjects rated their symptoms of lightheadedness, dizziness, weakness, nausea, sweating, and feelings of impending blackout or fainting on a scale of 0–10 (with 10 indicating the most severe symptom level) using a standardized questionnaire at minute 3 of each level of LBNP. A score greater than or equal to 3 was considered a clinically significant symptom.

Laboratory tests. Serum insulin levels were measured using the Insulin-Coat-A Count kit from Diagnostic Products (Los Angeles, CA), with a lower limit of detection of 18 pmol/l. Serum glucose levels were measured using the Beckman Glucose Analyzer 2 (Beckman Coulter, Chaska, MN). Plasma norepinephrine, plasma epinephrine, and 24-h urinary epinephrine levels were assayed using the 2 CAT RIA kit (Immuno Biological Laboratories, Minneapolis, MN). Using the Cortisol Diagnostic Products Coat-A-Count RIA kit, 24-h urinary collections were assayed for free cortisol levels; and using the Roche reagent (COBAS Integra 400, Roche Diagnostics, Indianapolis, IN), they were assayed for creatinine.

Statistical analysis. Data were analyzed using repeated-measures ANOVA with main effects of treatment (antecedent hypoglycemia and antecedent euglycemia) and either characteristic points on the cardiac baroreflex relation curve or LBNP level. Nonrepeated measures assessed in two conditions were analyzed using Student's two-tailed paired t test. Categorical variables were compared using Fisher's exact test. Data are expressed as means ± SE.

RESULTS

Demographics, screening, and baseline (day 1) assessments. Twenty healthy subjects (age 28 ± 2 years; 10 men) were studied. Subjects had an average BMI of 24.1 ± 0.6 kg/m², resting heart rate of 64 ± 2 bpm, systolic blood

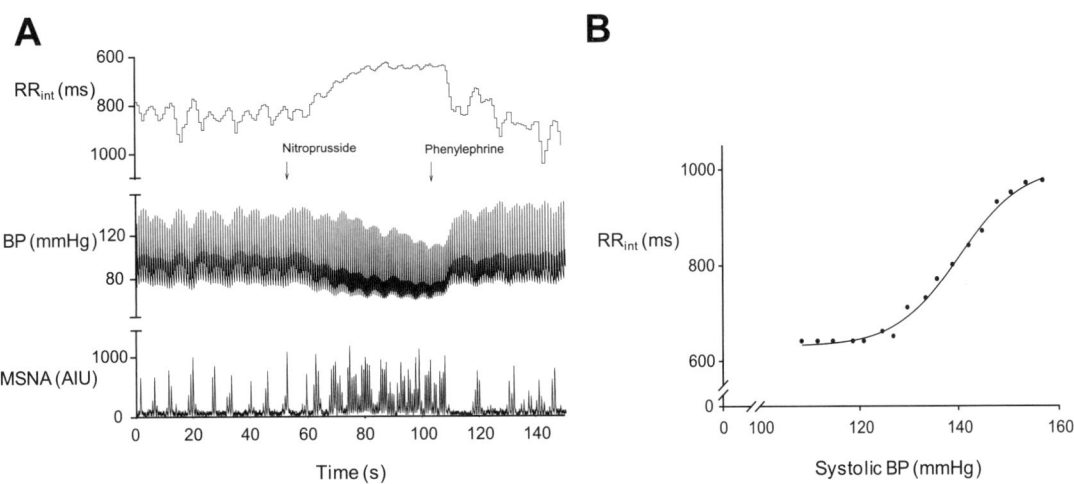

FIG. 2. *A*: R-R interval (RR$_{int}$), systolic blood pressure (BP), and muscle sympathetic neurogram (MSNA) recording from a representative subject during the modified Oxford procedure. The timing of the nitroprusside and phenylephrine administration is marked by arrows. AIU, arbitrary integration units. *B*: The relationship between systolic BP and RR$_{int}$ during the rising portion of the BP trace in this subject is shown. The slope of the linear portion of the sigmoid curve is the measure of the baroreflex sensitivity.

pressure of 107 ± 2 mmHg, and diastolic blood pressure of 69 ± 2 mmHg at screening. Autonomic testing performed at screening was within normal limits in all subjects. Baseline assessments of all autonomic measures were similar on both of the day 1 studies.

Insulin clamp. Morning baseline levels of glucose (5.3 ± 0.2 and 5.1 ± 0.1 mmol/l) and insulin (3.9 ± 0.3 and 3.8 ± 0.4 μU/ml) were similar on euglycemic and hypoglycemic clamp study days, respectively. Serum insulin levels averaged 123 ± 3 μU/ml during the clamp studies, with no significant differences between any of the four clamp studies. Blood glucose averaged 2.8 ± 0.0 mmol/l for the final 105 min of both the morning and afternoon hypoglycemic clamp procedures and 5.0 ± 0.0 mmol/l for both corresponding periods of the euglycemic clamps (Fig. 3).

Cortisol and epinephrine were elevated in 24-h urine collections obtained on the day of the hypoglycemic clamps compared with levels in urine collections on the day of the euglycemic clamps, whereas urinary creatinine levels were similar (Fig. 4). Urine sodium levels were similar on the euglycemic (119 ± 8 mmol/TV) and hypoglycemic (102 ± 7 mmol/TV) clamp study days.

Cardiac vagal and sympathetic baroreflex assessment. Cardiac vagal baroreflex sensitivity, as determined by the slope of the relation between R-R interval and blood pressure during the modified Oxford test performed on day 3, was significantly reduced after antecedent hypoglycemia compared with antecedent euglycemia (Fig. 5*A* and *B*).

Furthermore, to take into account any potential influence of the variability in baroreflex sensitivity between admissions, we determined the baroreflex sensitivity difference (ΔBRS) (baroreflex sensitivity on day 3 − baroreflex sensitivity on day 1 of the same admission). ΔBRS with antecedent hypoglycemia on day 2 (-1.6 ± 4.3 ms/mmHg) was significantly less than ΔBRS with antecedent euglycemia on day 2 (2.3 ± 6.3, $P < 0.01$).

Characteristics of the cardiac vagal baroreflex function curve (threshold, mid, and saturation points) are shown in Table 1 and demonstrate a shift toward the right after antecedent hypoglycemia compared with antecedent euglycemia. Sympathetic nerve activity during the hypotensive period of the modified Oxford test was significantly lower after antecedent hypoglycemia compared with antecedent euglycemia (Fig. 5*C*). There was no association between BMI, sex, clamp insulin levels, HOMA index, and the effect of antecedent hypoglycemia on baroreflex sensitivity.

Cardiac vagal function during paced breathing. The R-R interval high-frequency spectral power determined during paced breathing tended to be lower after the hypogly-

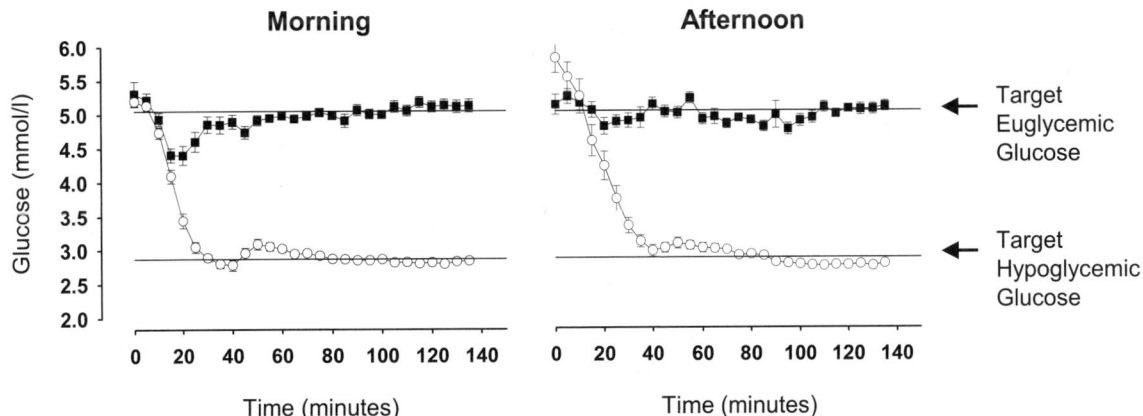

FIG. 3. Serum glucose levels during euglycemic-hyperinsulinemic clamp studies (■) and during hypoglycemic-hyperinsulinemic clamp studies (○). Arrow indicates target glucose of 5.0 mmol/l for the euglycemia protocol and 2.8 mmol/l for the hypoglycemia protocol.

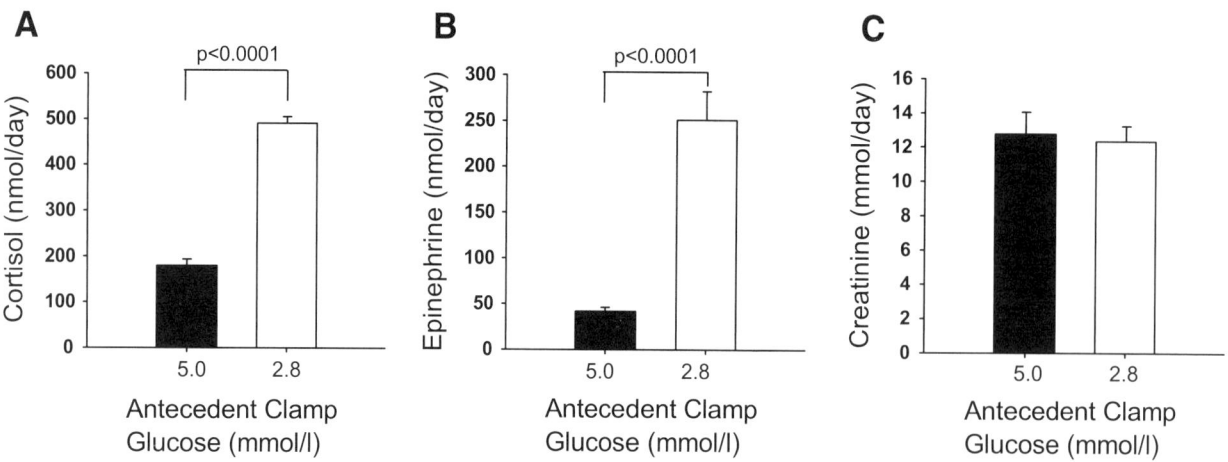

FIG. 4. Cortisol (*A*), epinephrine (*B*), and creatinine (*C*) levels in 24-h urines collected on the day of the euglycemic-hyperinsulinemic clamp studies (■) and hypoglycemic-hyperinsulinemic clamp studies (□).

cemic clamp compared with the euglycemic clamp (609 ± 103 vs. 804 ± 206 ms², $P = 0.13$). There was a positive correlation between the power spectral density and cardiac vagal baroreflex sensitivity determined after antecedent hypoglycemia ($r = 0.67, P < 0.01$) and after antecedent euglycemia ($r = 0.57, P < 0.05$).

Simulated orthostatic stress with LBNP. The R-R interval and systolic blood pressure at baseline and in response to increasing levels of LBNP were similar, irrespective of whether the study was performed after antecedent hypoglycemia or antecedent euglycemia (Fig. 6*A* and *B*). Plasma norepinephrine levels rose in response to increasing levels of negative pressure ($P < 0.0001$); however, this response was significantly blunted after antecedent hypoglycemia compared with antecedent euglycemia (Fig. 6*C*). Plasma epinephrine levels also increased during LBNP ($P < 0.05$), but this response was not significantly affected by the antecedent glucose level (Fig. 6*D*).

In the posteuglycemic condition, a total of 5 of 20 (25%) subjects experienced clinically significant symptoms or signs of impending syncope, compared with 12 of 20 (60%)

subjects in the posthypoglycemic condition ($P = 0.05$, Fisher's exact test).

DISCUSSION

Our data demonstrate that antecedent hypoglycemia results in a significant decrease in *1*) cardiac vagal baroreflex sensitivity and *2*) the sympathetic response to both a transient pharmacologically induced hypotensive stress and a graded simulated orthostatic stress using LBNP. It is well established that prior exposure to hypoglycemia attenuates the autonomic nervous system response to subsequent hypoglycemia (7,18). The present data, which show that prior hypoglycemia attenuates the autonomic response to specific cardiovascular stresses, extend those findings. Furthermore, the evidence that antecedent hypoglycemia attenuates cardiovascular autonomic control may have significant clinical implications; impaired autonomic function is associated with and may be a contributor to mortality in diabetes and cardiovascular disease (10,12–14).

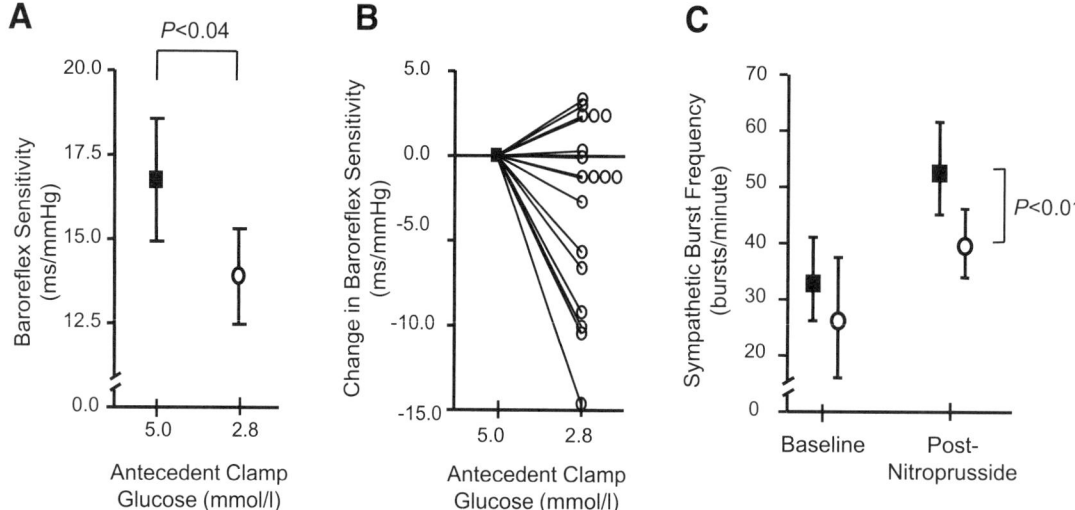

FIG. 5. *A*: Baroreflex sensitivity after antecedent euglycemic (■) or hypoglycemic (○) clamp studies. *B*: Change in baroreflex sensitivity in individual subjects after antecedent hypoglycemia versus antecedent euglycemia. *C*: MSNA assessed at baseline and after nitroprusside in subjects after antecedent euglycemia (■) or antecedent hypoglycemia (○).

TABLE 1
Baroreflex function characteristics

	After euglycemia	After hypoglycemia
Threshold		
SBP (mmHg)	120 ± 4	123 ± 4
R-R interval (ms)	790 ± 37	813 ± 33
Midpoint		
SBP (mmHg)	127 ± 4	132 ± 3*
R-R interval (ms)	966 ± 39	977 ± 39
Saturation		
SBP (mmHg)	134 ± 4	138 ± 3
R-R interval (ms)	1,142 ± 50	1140 ± 47
Baroreflex slope (mmHg/ms)	16.7 ± 1.8	13.8 ± 1.4*

Data are means ± SE. SBP, systolic blood pressure. *$P < 0.05$.

It is well established from studies in healthy and diabetic subjects that exposure to recent hypoglycemia reduces the counterregulatory hormone (e.g., epinephrine, glucagon, and adrenocorticotropic hormone) and autonomic nervous system responses to subsequent hypoglycemia. This hypoglycemia-associated autonomic failure/dysfunction leads to decreased ability to sense hypoglycemia and restore euglycemia (7). However, there are conflicting reports as to whether antecedent hypoglycemia impairs the autonomic response to nonhypoglycemic stimuli as well as hypoglycemic stimuli. In one study of type 1 diabetic subjects, the epinephrine and norepinephrine responses to exercise and upright posture were intact after antecedent hypoglycemia (19). Other studies of type 1 diabetic subjects suggested that the deficit is more generalized (20,21); the epinephrine and norepinephrine responses to a cold pressor test were reduced in well-controlled type 1 diabetic subjects (20), and antecedent hypoglycemia reduced the normal exercise-induced rise in epinephrine, norepinephrine, glucagon, growth hormone, pancreatic polypeptide, and cortisol in healthy individuals (21). Our data are consistent with these latter studies and strongly support the view that the effects of antecedent hypoglycemia on the autonomic nervous system are more generalized and not specific to subsequent hypoglycemic stimuli.

Prior studies have shown that during hypoglycemia, there is acquired prolongation of the rate corrected Q-T interval (22). Our findings show that antecedent hypoglycemia leads to impaired control of cardiovascular func-

tion, even after euglycemia is restored, and that the effects of antecedent hypoglycemia on autonomic function can last for at least 16 h. We demonstrated that antecedent hypoglycemia attenuated the sympathoadrenal and muscle sympathetic nerve activity outflow responses to simulated orthostatic stress and transient hypotension. Thus, in the clinical setting, it is possible that recent exposure to hypoglycemia could impair sympathetic nervous system responses to cardiovascular stresses.

Antecedent hypoglycemia also decreased baroreflex sensitivity, which indicates impairment in vagal cardiac modulation. Decreases in vagal autonomic function may lead to attenuation of vagal protection against sudden arrhythmic death. Impaired cardiac vagal control, as determined by reduced heart rate variability, is associated with increased risk of postmyocardial infarction mortality, even after adjusting for clinical, demographic, other Holter features, and ejection fraction (12,23–25). In addition, impairment of baroreflex sensitivity has been associated with adverse outcomes in clinical (13,14) and preclinical (26) studies.

Baroreflex sensitivity, calculated from the measurement of the heart rate–blood pressure relation after an intravenous bolus of phenylephrine, was a significant independent risk predictor of cardiac mortality in the Autonomic Tone and Reflexes After Myocardial Infarction (ATRAMI) study, an international multicenter prospective study of 1,284 patients with a recent myocardial infarction (14). The 2-year mortality for individuals with baroreflex sensitivity <3.1 ms/mmHg was 9%, versus 2% for those with preserved baroreflex sensitivity. In a 5-year follow-up study of a subset of 244 patients with ST-segment elevation myocardial infarction and normal ejection fraction, impaired baroreflex sensitivity (<3.1 ms/mmHg) 4–6 weeks after the myocardial infarction identified patients with a relative risk of cardiovascular mortality of 11.4, compared with those without impaired baroreflex sensitivity (13).

In the current study, baroreflex sensitivity in normal subjects after antecedent hypoglycemia did not reach the level of 3.1 ms/mmHg; however, given the observed reduction that was evident in our studies (6 of 20 subjects had a decrease in baroreflex sensitivity of >5 ms/mmHg, and 3 subjects had a decrease in baroreflex sensitivity of ≥10 ms/mmHg), it is possible that similar changes after hypoglycemia in individuals impaired baroreflex sensitivity at baseline would lead to baroreflex sensitivity <3.1 ms/

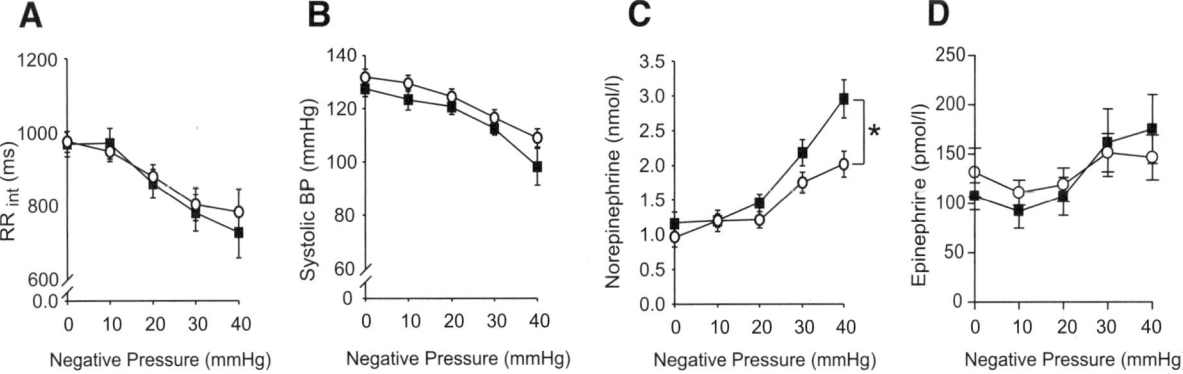

FIG. 6. Effect of antecedent euglycemia and hypoglycemia on RR interval (RR$_{int}$) (A), systolic blood pressure (BP) (B), norepinephrine (C), and epinephrine (D) responses to the stimulated orthostatic stress of LBNP. ■, measurements obtained after euglycemic-hyperinsulinemic clamp studies. ○, measurements obtained after hypoglycemic-hyperinsulinemic clamp studies. *$P < 0.001$.

mmHg. Thus, hypoglycemia-induced impairment in baroreflex sensitivity and/or sympathetic nervous system cardiovascular control (as noted above) could have clinical implications, especially in critically ill patients or in patients at high risk for cardiovascular events.

The high-frequency power of the R-R interval in response to paced breathing, also an index of cardiac vagal control, correlated positively with cardiac vagal baroreflex sensitivity in our study. There was a strong tendency toward a reduction in the high-frequency R-R interval power in the posthypoglycemic state, but this did not reach statistical significance. Several possible explanations for this finding exist. These include the following: *1*) The provocation for the cardiac vagal baroreflex assessment (transient hypotension) provided a more consistent and potent stimulus than the provocation for respiratory-mediated R-R interval variability (we did not monitor or control the depth of respiration); and *2*) there is a differential effect of hypoglycemia on the autonomic pathways involved in the two reflexes. In future studies, both frequency and amplitude of respiration should be monitored.

The present data may have implications for diabetic subjects particularly those with autonomic neuropathy who may have an increased mortality risk (10). Furthermore, it is possible that the consequences of antecedent hypoglycemia on autonomic function may be amplified in diabetic subjects, particularly those with autonomic dysfunction. For example, although the reduced counterregulatory and hormonal response to antecedent hypoglycemia occurs in the absence of diabetic autonomic neuropathy, as measured by standard tests of autonomic function (18,27), several (28–30), although not all (22), studies suggest that the presence of autonomic dysfunction further attenuates the autonomic response to hypoglycemia.

Other populations in which the consequences of antecedent hypoglycemia on autonomic function may be more apparent are critically ill patients and individuals with diabetes at risk for cardiovascular events. There is a significant increase in mortality in critically ill patients who experience hypoglycemia. The risk is similar irrespective of whether the critically ill patients received intensive or conventional insulin therapy and is not directly caused by hypoglycemia (8). Similarly, in the Action to Control Cardiovascular Risk in Diabetes (ACCORD) study, which enrolled individuals with diabetes at increased risk of cardiovascular events, intensively lowering blood glucose to a goal glycated hemoglobin (A1C) level of <6.0% increases the risk of death compared with a less intensive treatment goal of 7.0–7.9% (9). The difference does not appear to be directly due to hypoglycemia or the use of a specific drug. Furthermore, and perhaps of mechanistic importance, although the relative risk of nonfatal myocardial infarction is lower in the intensively treated group, all cause mortality and mortality from cardiovascular causes is greater. The effect of antecedent hypoglycemia on autonomic cardiovascular function in individuals with diabetes and in vulnerable diabetic subpopulations, such as critically ill patients or patients with cardiovascular disease, is an important area for additional study.

The randomized cross-over design of this study provides the advantage of each subject serving as his/her own control. Additionally, subjects were exposed to similar insulin levels during the hypoglycemic and euglycemic clamp procedures. However, this trial design also imposed a potential limitation of residual effects from exposure to hypoglycemia/euglycemia during the first study visit.

Therefore, we reevaluated subjects at least 1 and up to 3 months after the initial study visit. To ensure no interval change in autonomic function between clamps, baseline autonomic testing was performed before each clamp. Furthermore, physical activity and dietary intake (including electrolytes) were rigorously controlled.

In summary, these data suggest that cardiovascular autonomic function, specifically, baroreflex sensitivity and the sympathetic response to a hypotensive stress, is attenuated after antecedent hypoglycemia. Attenuation of cardiac vagal baroreflex sensitivity is an independent predictor of mortality in postmyocardial infarction patients. Because our findings have potential implications for rigorous glycemic control in diabetes, studies are needed to determine the effects of antecedent hypoglycemia on autonomic cardiovascular function in individuals with type 1 and type 2 diabetes.

ACKNOWLEDGMENTS

This work was supported in part by the U.S. Public Health Service, National Institutes of Health grants RO1 DK063296 and MO1 RR002635.

No potential conflicts of interest relevant to this article were reported.

The authors thank Jackson Chang, Laura Colburn, Anthony Pilowa, Marcelo Risk, J. Andrew Taylor, Peter Studinger, and the Brigham and Women's Hospital GCRC staff for contributions to this research.

REFERENCES

1. The Diabetes Control and Complications Trial Research Group: The effect of intensive treatment of diabetes on the development and progression of long-term complications in insulin-dependent diabetes mellitus. *N Engl J Med* 329:977–986, 1993
2. UK Prospective Diabetes Study (UKPDS) Group: Intensive blood-glucose control with sulphonylureas or insulin compared with conventional treatment and risk of complications in patients with type 2 diabetes (UKPDS 33). *Lancet* 352:837–853, 1998
3. Ohkubo Y, Kishikawa H, Araki E, Miyata T, Isami S, Motoyoshi S, Kojima Y, Furuyoshi N, Shichiri M: Intensive insulin therapy prevents the progression of diabetic microvascular complications in Japanese patients with non-insulin-dependent diabetes mellitus: a randomized prospective 6-year study. *Diabetes Res Clin Pract* 28:103–117, 1995
4. Gaede P, Vedel P, Larsen N, Jensen GV, Parving HH, Pedersen O: Multifactorial intervention and cardiovascular disease in patients with type 2 diabetes. *N Engl J Med* 348:383–393, 2003
5. Nathan DM, Cleary PA, Backlund JY, Genuth SM, Lachin JM, Orchard TJ, Raskin P, Zinman B: Intensive diabetes treatment and cardiovascular disease in patients with type 1 diabetes. *N Engl J Med* 353:2643–2653, 2005
6. The DCCT Research Group: Epidemiology of severe hypoglycemia in the diabetes control and complications trial. *Am J Med* 90:450–459, 1991
7. Cryer PE: Mechanisms of hypoglycemia-associated autonomic failure and its component syndromes in diabetes. *Diabetes* 54:3592–3601, 2005
8. Van den Berghe G, Wilmer A, Milants I, Wouters PJ, Bouckaert B, Bruyninckx F, Bouillon R, Schetz M: Intensive insulin therapy in mixed medical/surgical intensive care units: benefit versus harm. *Diabetes* 55:3151–3159, 2006
9. Gerstein HC, Miller ME, Byington RP, Goff DC Jr, Bigger JT, Buse JB, Cushman WC, Genuth S, Ismail-Beigi F, Grimm RH Jr, Probstfield JL, Simons-Morton DG, Friedewald WT: Effects of intensive glucose lowering in type 2 diabetes. *N Engl J Med* 358:2545–2559, 2008
10. Maser RE, Mitchell BD, Vinik AI, Freeman R: The association between cardiovascular autonomic neuropathy and mortality in individuals with diabetes: a meta-analysis. *Diabetes Care* 26:1895–1901, 2003
11. Vinik AI, Ziegler D: Diabetic cardiovascular autonomic neuropathy. *Circulation* 115:387–397, 2007
12. Bigger JT, Fleiss JL, Rolnitzky LM, Steinman RC: The ability of several short-term measures of R-R variability to predict mortality after myocardial infarction. *Circulation* 88:927–934, 1993
13. De Ferrari GM, Sanzo A, Bertoletti A, Specchia G, Vanoli E, Schwartz PJ: Baroreflex sensitivity predicts long-term cardiovascular mortality after

myocardial infarction even in patients with preserved left ventricular function. *J Am Coll Cardiol* 50:2285–2290, 2007

14. La Rovere MT, Bigger JT Jr, Marcus FI, Mortara A, Schwartz PJ: Baroreflex sensitivity and heart-rate variability in prediction of total cardiac mortality after myocardial infarction: ATRAMI (Autonomic Tone and Reflexes After Myocardial Infarction) Investigators [see comments]. *Lancet* 351:478–484, 1998

15. Hamner JW, Taylor JA: Automated quantification of sympathetic beat-by-beat activity, independent of signal quality. *J Appl Physiol* 91:1199–1206, 2001

16. Saul JP, Berger RD, Chen MH, Cohen RJ: Transfer function analysis of autonomic regulation: II. Respiratory sinus arrhythmia. *Am J Physiol* 256:H153–H161, 1989

17. Ebert TJ, Cowley AW Jr: Baroreflex modulation of sympathetic outflow during physiological increases of vasopressin in humans. *Am J Physiol* 262:H1372–H1378, 1992

18. Dagogo-Jack SE, Craft S, Cryer PE: Hypoglycemia-associated autonomic failure in insulin-dependent diabetes mellitus: recent antecedent hypoglycemia reduces autonomic responses to, symptoms of, and defense against subsequent hypoglycemia. *J Clin Invest* 91:819–828, 1993

19. Rattarasarn C, Dagogo-Jack S, Zachwieja JJ, Cryer PE: Hypoglycemia-induced autonomic failure in IDDM is specific for stimulus of hypoglycemia and is not attributable to prior autonomic activation. *Diabetes* 43:809–818, 1994

20. Kinsley BT, Widom B, Utzschneider K, Simonson DC: Stimulus specificity of defects in counterregulatory hormone secretion in insulin-dependent diabetes mellitus: effect of glycemic control. *J Clin Endocrinol Metab* 79:1383–1389, 1994

21. Davis SN, Galassetti P, Wasserman DH, Tate D: Effects of antecedent hypoglycemia on subsequent counterregulatory responses to exercise. *Diabetes* 49:73–81, 2000

22. Lee SP, Yeoh L, Harris ND, Davies CM, Robinson RT, Leathard A, Newman C, Macdonald IA, Heller SR: Influence of autonomic neuropathy on QTc interval lengthening during hypoglycemia in type 1 diabetes. *Diabetes* 53:1535–1542, 2004

23. Kleiger RE, Miller JP, Bigger JT Jr, Moss AJ: Decreased heart rate variability and its association with increased mortality after acute myocardial infarction. *Am J Cardiol* 59:256–262, 1987

24. Malik M, Camm AJ: Significance of long term components of heart rate variability for the further prognosis after acute myocardial infarction. *Cardiovasc Res* 24:793–803, 1990

25. Odemuyiwa O, Malik M, Farrell T, Bashir Y, Poloniecki J, Camm J: Comparison of the predictive characteristics of heart rate variability index and left ventricular ejection fraction for all-cause mortality, arrhythmic events and sudden death after acute myocardial infarction. *Am J Cardiol* 68:434–439, 1991

26. Schwartz PJ, Vanoli E, Stramba-Badiale M, De Ferrari GM, Billman GE, Foreman RD: Autonomic mechanisms and sudden death: new insights from analysis of baroreceptor reflexes in conscious dogs with and without a myocardial infarction. *Circulation* 78:969–979, 1988

27. Hepburn DA, Patrick AW, Eadington DW, Ewing DJ, Frier BM: Unawareness of hypoglycaemia in insulin-treated diabetic patients: prevalence and relationship to autonomic neuropathy. *Diabet Med* 7:711–717, 1990

28. Bottini P, Boschetti E, Pampanelli S, Ciofetta M, Del Sindaco P, Scionti L, Brunetti P, Bolli GB: Contribution of autonomic neuropathy to reduced plasma adrenaline responses to hypoglycemia in IDDM: evidence for a nonselective defect. *Diabetes* 46:814–823, 1997

29. Fanelli C, Pampanelli S, Lalli C, Del Sindaco P, Ciofetta M, Lepore M, Porcellati F, Bottini P, Di Vincenzo A, Brunetti P, Bolli GB: Long-term intensive therapy of IDDM patients with clinically overt autonomic neuropathy: effects on hypoglycemia awareness and counterregulation. *Diabetes* 46:1172–1181, 1997

30. Meyer C, Grossmann R, Mitrakou A, Mahler R, Veneman T, Gerich J, Bretzel RG: Effects of autonomic neuropathy on counterregulation and awareness of hypoglycemia in type 1 diabetic patients. *Diabetes Care* 21:1960–1966, 1998

Improving Epinephrine Responses in Hypoglycemia Unawareness With Real-Time Continuous Glucose Monitoring in Adolescents With Type 1 Diabetes

Trang T. Ly, fracp[1]
Jacqueline Hewitt, fracp[1]
Raymond J. Davey, bsc[2]

Ee Mun Lim, frcpa, fracp[3,4]
Elizabeth A. Davis, fracp[1,5]
Timothy W. Jones, fracp, md[1,5]

OBJECTIVE — To determine whether real-time continuous glucose monitoring (CGM) with preset alarms at specific glucose levels would prove a useful tool to achieve avoidance of hypoglycemia and improve the counterregulatory response to hypoglycemia in adolescents with type 1 diabetes with hypoglycemia unawareness.

RESEARCH DESIGN AND METHODS — Adolescents with type 1 diabetes with hypoglycemia unawareness underwent hyperinsulinemic hypoglycemic clamp studies at baseline to determine their counterregulatory hormone responses to hypoglycemia. Subjects were then randomized to either standard therapy or real-time CGM for 4 weeks. The clamp study was then repeated.

RESULTS — The epinephrine response during hypoglycemia after the intervention was greater in the CGM group than in the standard therapy group.

CONCLUSIONS — A greater epinephrine response during hypoglycemia suggests that real-time CGM is a useful clinical tool to improve hypoglycemia unawareness in adolescents with type 1 diabetes.

Diabetes Care 34:50–52, 2011

H ypoglycemia unawareness is defined as the onset of neuroglycopenia before autonomic activation (1). Patients have defective symptomatic and counterregulatory responses, in particular impaired epinephrine response to hypoglycemia. Both defective counterregulatory responses and hypoglycemia unawareness constitute the hypoglycemia-associated autonomic failure associated with recurrent iatrogenic hypoglycemia (2–4).

In adults, it has been demonstrated that as little time as 2 to 3 weeks of avoidance of hypoglycemia reverses hypoglycemia unawareness and improves the attenuated epinephrine component of defective counterregulation in affected patients (5–7). Although strict avoidance of hypoglycemia can restore autonomic symptoms of hypoglycemia and improve counterregulatory responses to hypoglycemia, this is difficult to achieve in practice. Real-time continuous glucose monitoring (CGM) allows patients to view their blood glucose levels almost instantaneously and offers potential to reduce hypoglycemia frequency.

This study was designed to determine whether real-time CGM with preset alarms at specific glucose levels would prove a useful tool to achieve avoidance of hypoglycemia and therefore improve the counterregulatory response to hypoglycemia in adolescents with type 1 diabetes with hypoglycemia unawareness.

RESEARCH DESIGN AND METHODS — Adolescents with type 1 diabetes aged 12–18 years with hypoglycemia unawareness attending Princess Margaret Hospital diabetes clinics were invited to participate. Hypoglycemia unawareness score was determined by the use of modified Clarke's questionnaire (8). This questionnaire has been shown to accurately identify patients with impaired awareness of hypoglycemia for both clinical and research purposes (9). A score of ≥8 is suggestive of hypoglycemia unawareness. Consent was obtained for all participants.

All subjects underwent a hyperinsulinemic hypoglycemic clamp study at baseline to assess hypoglycemic symptoms and hormonal responses. Subjects were then randomized to either standard therapy (standard group) or to the use of real-time (Medtronic Minimed Paradigm REAL-Time System) CGM (CGM group) for 4 weeks. At the end of the 4-week period, all patients underwent a repeat hypoglycemic clamp study.

Hyperinsulinemic hypoglycemic clamp
During this procedure, the antecubital vein was cannulated for insulin and glucose infusion, and blood was sampled from the contralateral hand vein placed in a box heated to 60°C. Regular insulin (Human Actrapid; Novo Nordisk, Crawley, U.K.) was infused at a constant rate of 80 mU/m^2/min. Target plasma glucose levels were achieved by adjusting the rate of infusion of 20% glucose in water. Plasma glucose concentrations were maintained initially at euglycemia (5–6 mmol/l) over a period of 1 h. Following this, blood glucose was lowered over 30 min to a nadir of 2.8 mmo/l. The blood glucose concentration of 2.8 mmol/l was

From the [1]Department of Endocrinology and Diabetes, Princess Margaret Hospital for Children, Perth, Western Australia, Australia; the [2]School of Sport Science, Exercise and Health, The University of Western Australia, Perth, Western Australia, Australia; [3]PathWest Laboratory Medicine, Queen Elizabeth II Medical Centre, Nedlands, Western Australia, Australia; the [4]Department of Endocrinology and Diabetes, Sir Charles Gairdner Hospital, Nedlands, Western Australia, Australia; and the [5]Telethon Institute for Child Health Research, Centre for Child Health Research, The University of Western Australia, Perth, Western Australia, Australia.
Corresponding author: Trang T. Ly, Trang.Ly@health.wa.gov.au.
Received 3 June 2010 and accepted 30 September 2010. Published ahead of print at http://care.diabetesjournals.org on 7 October 2010. DOI: 10.2337/dc10-1042.

The costs of publication of this article were defrayed in part by the payment of page charges. This article must therefore be hereby marked "advertisement" in accordance with 18 U.S.C. Section 1734 solely to indicate this fact.

maintained for 40 min for the hypoglycemia phase. Euglycemia was then restored.

For the duration of the clamp procedure, blood glucose was analyzed at the bedside using a glucose oxidase technique (YSI 2300; Yellow Springs Instruments, Yellow Springs, OH). Additional samples of arterialised venous blood were taken to measure plasma insulin, glucagon, epinephrine, norepinephrine, cortisol, and growth hormone concentrations.

Study intervention

Following the first hypoglycemic clamp study, both groups were advised to strictly avoid hypoglycemia with fingerstick testing at least four to six times daily to maintain blood glucose levels between 6 and 10 mmol/l for the 4-week period. In addition, the CGM group wore real-time CGM with subcutaneous sensor with preset low alarms at 6 mmol/l and was advised to institute standard hypoglycemia treatment for blood glucose levels below 6 mmol/l with target blood glucose level of 8 mmol/l.

The CGM group received an an additional 2 h of instructions regarding sensor insertion and usage. Sensors were changed every 3 days.

Outcome measures

The major outcome measure was the epinephrine response to hypoglycemia measured during the hypoglycemia clamp study. Plasma epinephrine levels were measured by ELISA (Diagnostika GMBH, Hamburg, Germany) and samples were analyzed in duplicate. The interassay coefficient of variation at 10 pmol/l and 5,460 pmol/l were 2% and 5.5%, respectively.

RESULTS — Eleven subjects were studied, including five subjects in the standard group (age 15.0 ± 0.8 years, A1C 7.9 ± 0.3% since diagnosis, duration 6.5 ± 1.2 years) and six subjects in the CGM group (age 13.8 ± 0.7 years, A1C 7.7 ± 0.2% since diagnosis, duration 5.2 ± 1.4 years).

At baseline, the epinephrine response to hypoglycemia was blunted, and there was no difference between subjects randomized to standard or CGM groups (percentage change 288 ± 151 vs. 214 ± 72%, standard vs. CGM group, respectively; $P = 0.688$). Following the intervention, there was a greater epinephrine response in the CGM group (percentage change 114 ± 83 vs. 604 ± 234%, standard vs. CGM group, respectively; $P =$

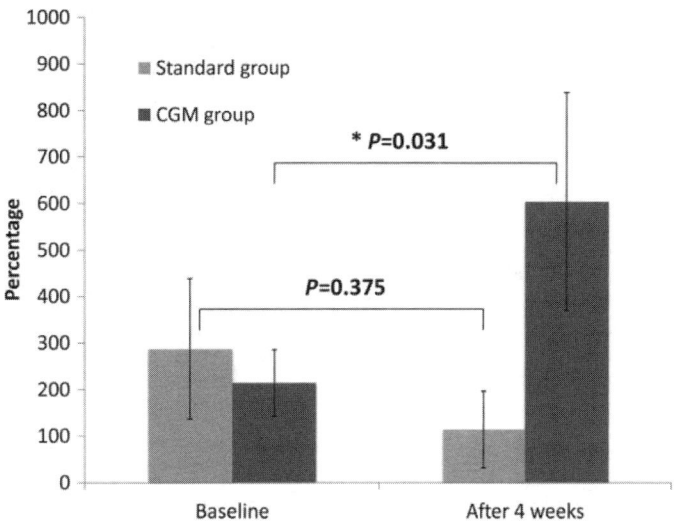

Figure 1—*Change in epinephrine response during hypoglycemia. Data are means ± SE.*

0.048). This represents a greater percentage rise in epinephrine concentrations during hypoglycemia following therapy in the CGM group ($P = 0.375$ vs. 0.031, standard vs. CGM group, respectively) as shown in Fig. 1. Peak adrenaline response during hypoglycemia after the intervention was also greater in the CGM group than in the standard group (1,093 ± 221 vs. 572 ± 162 pmol/l; $P = 0.048$). Subjects in the CGM group reported higher adrenergic symptoms scores after the intervention than the standard group (5.4 ± 0.4 vs. 3.4 ± 0.2; $P < 0.001$).

The mean A1C at baseline was 7.9 ± 0.3% for both groups. Following the intervention, there was no deterioration in glycemic control in the standard or CGM group (A1C 7.9 ± 0.4 vs. 8.3 ± 0.3%; $P = 0.587$).

The glucagon response was absent at baseline and after intervention in both groups. There was no change in cortisol and growth hormone responses to hypoglycemia for both groups.

CONCLUSIONS — The epinephrine response to hypoglycemia in patients with type 1 diabetes with hypoglycemia unawareness was greater after the use of real-time CGM with low glucose alarms than with standard medical therapy alone. The use of CGM was not associated with deterioration in A1C. This greater epinephrine response during hypoglycemia suggests that real-time CGM is a useful clinical tool to improve hypoglycemia unawareness in adolescents with type 1 diabetes. The high risk of associated severe hypoglycemia requires that hypogly-

cemia unawareness be recognized and treated.

This study demonstrates that blunted counterregulatory responses to hypoglycemia do occur in adolescents with a relatively short duration of diabetes. In addition to the blunted epinephrine response, most of these subjects reported no adrenergic symptoms during their baseline hypoglycemic clamp study.

A limitation of this study is the sample size. However, evaluating counterregulatory response with hypoglycemia clamp studies is a robust method, and this technique limits inclusion of a large number of subjects.

Acknowledgments— No potential conflicts of interest relevant to this article were reported.

T.T.L. wrote the manuscript and collected and researched data. J.H. reviewed and edited the manuscript, collected data, and contributed to the study design. R.J.D. reviewed and edited the manuscript and contributed to the study design. E.M.L. reviewed and edited the manuscript and researched data. E.A.D. contributed to discussion, researched data, and reviewed and edited the manuscript. T.W.J. contributed to the study design, researched data, and wrote the manuscript.

We thank the families and children of Princess Margaret Hospital Diabetes Clinic for participating in this study.

References

1. Cryer PE. Hypoglycaemia: the limiting factor in the glycaemic management of

Type I and Type II diabetes. Diabetologia 2002;45:937–948

2. Cryer PE. Mechanisms of hypoglycemia-associated autonomic failure and its component syndromes in diabetes. Diabetes 2005; 54:3592–3601

3. Heller SR, Cryer PE. Reduced neuroendocrine and symptomatic responses to subsequent hypoglycemia after 1 episode of hypoglycemia in nondiabetic humans. Diabetes 1991;40:223–226

4. Dagogo-Jack SE, Craft S, Cryer PE. Hypoglycemia-associated autonomic failure in insulin-dependent diabetes mellitus. Recent antecedent hypoglycemia reduces autonomic responses to, symptoms of, and defense against subsequent hypoglycemia. J Clin Invest 1993;91:819–28

5. Fanelli C, Pampanelli S, Epifano L, Rambotti AM, Di Vincenzo A, Modarelli F, Ciofetta M, Lepore M, Annibale B, Torlone E. Long-term recovery from unawareness, deficient counterregulation and lack of cognitive dysfunction during hypoglycaemia, following institution of rational, intensive insulin therapy in IDDM. Diabetologia 1994; 37:1265–1276

6. Cranston I, Lomas J, Maran A, Macdonald I, Amiel SA. Restoration of hypoglycaemia awareness in patients with long-duration insulin-dependent diabetes. Lancet 1994; 344:283–287

7. Dagogo-Jack S, Rattarasarn C, Cryer PE. Reversal of hypoglycemia unawareness, but not defective glucose counterregulation, in IDDM. Diabetes 1994;43:1426–1434

8. Clarke WL, Cox DJ, Gonder-Frederick LA, Julian D, Schlundt D, Polonsky W. Reduced awareness of hypoglycemia in adults with IDDM. A prospective study of hypoglycemic frequency and associated symptoms. Diabetes Care 1995;18:517–522

9. Geddes J, Wright RJ, Zammitt NN, Deary IJ, Frier BM. An evaluation of methods of assessing impaired awareness of hypoglycemia in type 1 diabetes. Diabetes Care 2007;30:1868–1870

Recurrent Antecedent Hypoglycemia Alters Neuronal Oxidative Metabolism In Vivo

Lihong Jiang,[1] Raimund I. Herzog,[2] Graeme F. Mason,[1,3] Robin A. de Graaf,[1] Douglas L. Rothman,[1] Robert S. Sherwin,[2] and Kevin L. Behar[3]

OBJECTIVE—The objective of this study was to characterize the changes in brain metabolism caused by antecedent recurrent hypoglycemia under euglycemic and hypoglycemic conditions in a rat model and to test the hypothesis that recurrent hypoglycemia changes the brain's capacity to utilize different energy substrates.

RESEARCH DESIGN AND METHODS—Rats exposed to recurrent insulin-induced hypoglycemia for 3 days (3dRH rats) and untreated controls were subject to the following protocols: [2-^{13}C]acetate infusion under euglycemic conditions ($n = 8$), [1-^{13}C]glucose and unlabeled acetate coinfusion under euglycemic conditions ($n = 8$), and [2-^{13}C]acetate infusion during a hyperinsulinemic-hypoglycemic clamp ($n = 8$). In vivo nuclear magnetic resonance spectroscopy was used to monitor the rise of ^{13}C-labeling in brain metabolites for the calculation of brain metabolic fluxes using a neuron-astrocyte model.

RESULTS—At euglycemia, antecedent recurrent hypoglycemia increased whole-brain glucose metabolism by $43 \pm 4\%$ ($P < 0.01$ vs. controls), largely due to higher glucose utilization in neurons. Although acetate metabolism remained the same, control and 3dRH animals showed a distinctly different response to acute hypoglycemia: controls decreased pyruvate dehydrogenase (PDH) flux in astrocytes by $64 \pm 20\%$ ($P = 0.01$), whereas it increased by $37 \pm 3\%$ in neurons ($P = 0.01$). The 3dRH animals decreased PDH flux in both compartments ($-75 \pm 20\%$ in astrocytes, $P < 0.001$, and $-36 \pm 4\%$ in neurons, $P = 0.005$). Thus, acute hypoglycemia reduced total brain tricarboxylic acid cycle activity in 3dRH animals ($-37 \pm 4\%$, $P = 0.001$), but not in controls.

CONCLUSIONS—Our findings suggest that after antecedent hypoglycemia, glucose utilization is increased at euglycemia and decreased after acute hypoglycemia, which was not the case in controls. These findings may help to identify better methods of preserving brain function and reducing injury during acute hypoglycemia. *Diabetes* **58:1266–1274, 2009**

From the [1]Department of Diagnostic Radiology, Yale University School of Medicine, The Anlyan Center, New Haven, Connecticut; the [2]Department of Internal Medicine, Yale University School of Medicine, The Anlyan Center, New Haven, Connecticut; and the [3]Department of Psychiatry, Magnetic Resonance Research Center, Yale University School of Medicine, The Anlyan Center, New Haven, Connecticut.

Corresponding author: Lihong Jiang, lihong.jiang@yale.edu.

Received 2 December 2008 and accepted 2 March 2009.

Published ahead of print at http://diabetes.diabetesjournals.org on 10 March 2009. DOI: 10.2337/db08-1664.

L.J. and R.I.H. contributed equally to this article.

Large clinical trials have established that the long-term complications of diabetes can be mitigated by tight glycemic control (1,2). Intensive insulin therapy, however, is limited by an increased risk of severe hypoglycemia, which results, in large part, from a blunting of counterregulatory responses as well as reduced awareness of hypoglycemia (3–6). Characterization of the underlying metabolic adaptations involved could lead to new therapeutic approaches aimed at improving glycemic control without compromising the risk of severe hypoglycemia.

Impaired judgment and decreased memory function during acute hypoglycemia are thought to be consequences of alterations of brain energy metabolism, in particular the absence of glucose, the primary energy substrate for the brain (7,8). The blunting of epinephrine and glucagon responses to hypoglycemia observed in type 1 diabetic patients exposed to frequent hypoglycemic episodes are reproduced in animal models of recurrent antecedent insulin-induced hypoglycemia, suggesting that such models may offer insights into the metabolic adaptations observed in the clinical setting (9–11). Studies of cognitive performance using a spatial memory task in nondiabetic and diabetic rats exposed to recurrent hypoglycemia for 3 consecutive days (3dRH rats) and in nondiabetic animals exposed to weekly bouts of hypoglycemia for nearly a year have revealed better performance at euglycemia, suggesting that adaptations of brain glucose transport and/or metabolism are similar to those reported for diabetic patients (9,10). These studies suggest that our animal models may offer insights into the metabolic adaptations observed in the clinical setting (9,11,12).

It is also possible that when the brain is repeatedly deprived of its main energy substrate, glucose, its capacity to take up and utilize alternate fuels such as monocarboxylic acids or ketone bodies is increased. This view is supported by a recent nuclear magnetic resonance (NMR) spectroscopy study that demonstrated an increase in acetate metabolism in type 1 diabetic patients with hypoglycemia unawareness (13). In contrast, 3dRH rodents under hypoglycemic conditions performed worse on a memory task than saline-injected controls (9).

The current study was undertaken to assess the effects of antecedent recurrent hypoglycemia on the brain's capacity to oxidize glucose and an alternate fuel (acetate). Three different experiments were conducted using both control and 3dRH animals. First, we measured neuronal and astroglial metabolic fluxes under euglycemic conditions using [2-^{13}C]acetate, which is primarily metabolized by astroglia-labeling neurons through the glutamate/glutamine neurotransmitter cycle. The accumulation of label in the stable metabolite pools of glutamine and glutamate

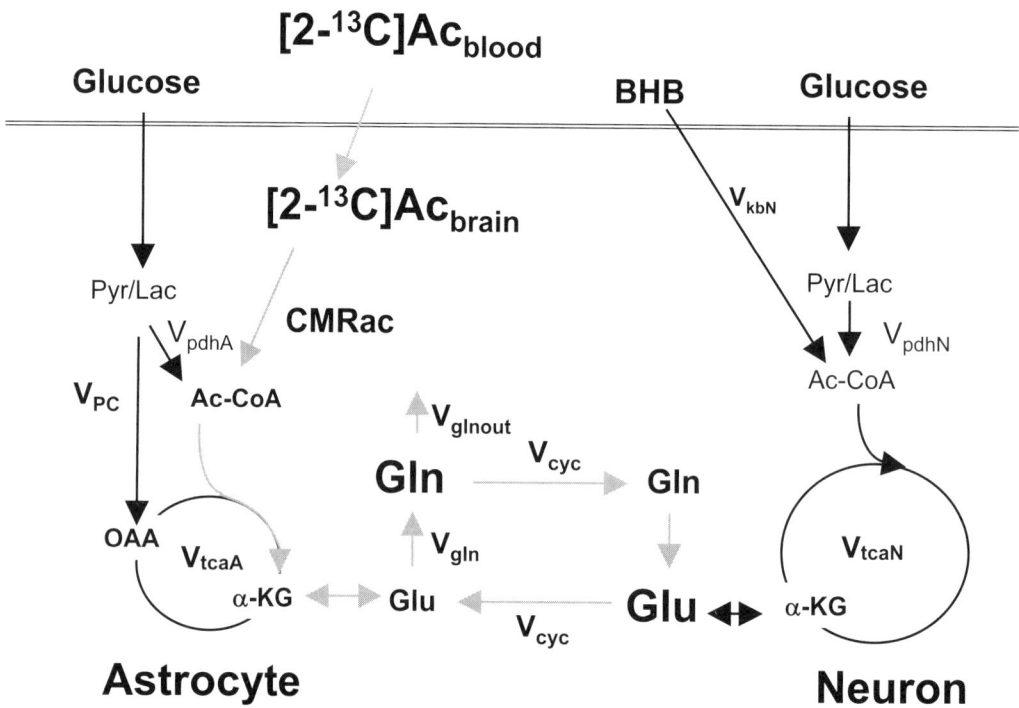

FIG. 1. Two-compartment model of the contribution of infused labeled acetate ([2-^{13}C]Ac) to astroglial and neuronal metabolism. Modified after Lebon et al. (33). Ac-CoA, acetyl-CoA; Gln, glutamine; Glu, glutamate; α-KG, α-ketoglutarate; Lac, lactate; OAA, oxaloacetate; Pyr, pyruvate.

was monitored by localized ^{1}H-observed, ^{13}C-edited (^{1}H-[^{13}C]) NMR spectroscopy. This approach, when used in conjunction with a two-compartment mathematical model of brain metabolism (Fig. 1), allows the quantitation of the rates of neuronal and glial tricarboxylic acid (TCA) cycles, glutamate/glutamine neurotransmitter cycle, and other metabolic pathways in brain (13,14). Second, to more directly assess neuronal metabolism using a substrate that is predominately metabolized in neurons, we measured metabolic fluxes during infusion of [1-^{13}C]glucose in conjunction with unlabeled acetate. Lastly, metabolic fluxes were assessed during acute hypoglycemic-hyperinsulinemic clamp and [2-^{13}C]acetate infusion to reveal the extent to which glucose and acetate contributes to brain oxidative metabolism when blood glucose is deficient.

RESEARCH DESIGN AND METHODS

Male Sprague-Dawley rats (Charles River, Wilmington, MA) of 220–250 g were housed in the Yale Animal Resource Center, fed a standard pellet diet (ProLab 3000; Agway, Syracuse, NY), and maintained on a 12-h day/night cycle. Experimental protocols were in accordance with laboratory animal care guidelines and were approved by the Yale animal care and use committee.

Recurrent hypoglycemia. Recurrent hypoglycemia was induced as previously described (15). Briefly, animals received intraperitoneal injections of regular insulin (10 U/kg Humulin R; Lilly, Indianapolis, IN) to produce 3 h of hypoglycemia on 3 consecutive days, resulting in tail vein glucose levels of 30–40 mg/dl. After 3 h, animals were given access to food and allowed to return to euglycemia. On the following day, NMR experiments were performed.

Surgical preparation. During surgical preparation for in vivo NMR experiments, animals were anesthetized with 3% halothane, underwent tracheotomy, and were ventilated with a mixture of 30% O$_2$/69% N$_2$O/1% halothane via a small-animal ventilation system (Harvard Apparatus, Holliston, MA). The left femoral artery was catheterized for continuous monitoring of blood pressure, plasma sampling, and blood gas analysis (Table 1). Core body temperature was measured and maintained at 37 ± 1°C using a water heating pad. Both femoral veins were cannulated for infusion of insulin, glucose, and acetate. Isotopically labeled substrates were infused into a separate line using com-

puter-controlled pumps (Harvard Apparatus). Animals were then placed into a plastic holder with a surface coil positioned directly on top of the scalp for NMR experiments.

Experimental groups

Euglycemia: acetate infusion. For this study, 2 mol/l [2-^{13}C]acetate (99% ^{13}C-sodium salt; Cambridge Isotopes, Andover, MA) at pH = 7 was infused into 3dRH (*n* = 8) and control (*n* = 8) animals under basal euglycemic conditions. Animals had free access to food the night before the experiment to avoid significant ketone body accumulation. A bolus continuous infusion of labeled acetate designed to produce steady-state plasma levels was given according to the following protocol: 6.25 µmol · min^{-1} · g^{-1} from 0 to 15 s, 0.875 from 15 s to 4 min, 0.5 from 4 to 8 min, and 0.25 thereafter.

Euglycemia: glucose/acetate coinfusion. Because of the uncertainty associated with this method of determining neuronal PDH flux (V_{pdhN}), we performed a coinfusion study with [1-^{13}C]glucose and unlabeled acetate to measure V_{pdhN} more directly. For this study, 1.1 mol/l [1-^{13}C]glucose (99% ^{13}C; Cambridge Isotopes, Andover, MA) was coinfused with 2 mol/l acetate into 3dRH (*n* = 8) and control (*n* = 8) animals under basal euglycemic conditions. Unlabeled acetate was infused in identical doses as in the protocol described above, and 20 min later [1-^{13}C]glucose was administered as a bolus of 4.05 µmol · g^{-1} · min^{-1} for 15 s followed by stepped exponential reduction of infusion rates every 30 s for the next 8 min, arriving at a steady rate of 0.051 µmol · g^{-1} · min^{-1} for the remainder of the experiment. Regular insulin (50 mU · kg^{-1} · min^{-1}) was used during the initial 30 min to prevent plasma glucose from increasing in association with the labeled glucose infusion.

Hypoglycemia: acetate infusion. For this study, 2 mol/l [2-^{13}C]acetate was infused into 3dRH (*n* = 8) and control (*n* = 8) animals during acute insulin-induced hypoglycemia. Animals were fasted overnight before a hyperinsulinemic-hypoglycemic clamp study (50 mU · kg^{-1} · min^{-1}) in which a variable infusion of 20% dextrose (Hospira, Lakeforest, IL) was used to maintain plasma glucose at the target level of 2.1 ± 0.2 mmol/l (Fig. 2A). Plasma glucose concentrations (Fig. 2B) were measured every 10 min in between NMR scans using a Beckman glucose analyzer 2 (Beckman Coulter, Fullerton, CA). Infusion rates of labeled acetate were reduced by 20% compared with the euglycemic studies to optimize physiological parameters, such as blood pressure, blood pH, Po$_2$, and Pco$_2$. This dose, however, was sufficient for plasma acetate levels to saturate transport.

NMR spectroscopy. After placement of the animals into the scanner, in vivo NMR spectroscopy was performed during the respective infusions in a 9.4 T horizontal bore magnet (Magnex; Scientific, Oxford, U.K.) equipped with a 9-cm-diameter gradient coil insert (490 mT/m, 175 µS; Resonance Research, Billerica, MA). The magnet was interfaced to an Avance console (Bruker,

TABLE 1
Effect of [2-13C]acetate infusions on physiological variables and substrates (concentrations and 13C-enrichments) measured in arterial plasma of control and 3dRH rats under euglycemic and hypoglycemic conditions

| | Euglycemia | | | | Hypoglycemia | | | |
| | Control | | 3dRH | | Control | | 3dRH | |
	Before	After	Before	After	Before	After	Before	After
pH	7.37 ± 0.02	7.40 ± 0.03	7.36 ± 0.01	7.35 ± 0.02	7.38 ± 0.01	7.43 ± 0.01	7.40 ± 0.01	7.47 ± 0.02*†
P_{CO_2} (mmHg)	38 ± 1	45 ± 2	41 ± 4	44 ± 4	35 ± 3	38 ± 2	35 ± 3	37 ± 4
P_{O_2} (mmHg)	130 ± 7	120 ± 5	148 ± 5	147 ± 9	130 ± 10	170 ± 15	130 ± 10	160 ± 15
Glucose								
mmol/l	9.4 ± 0.7	12.5 ± 1.1	8.1 ± 0.03	11 ± 0.3	2.3 ± 0.2	2.0 ± 0.2	2.3 ± 0.7	2.3 ± 0.7
%E	0	n.d.	0	n.d.	0	n.d.	0	n.d.
BHB								
mmol/l	0.3 ± 0.03	0.5 ± 0.1	0.3 ± 0.03	0.37 ± 0.07	1.2 ± 0.07	0.9 ± 0.06	1.2 ± 0.6	0.7 ± 0.4
%E	0	18 ± 0.7	0	17 ± 5	0	17.9 ± 1.3	0	3.3 ± 1.9
Lactate								
mmol/l	1.3 ± 0.1	1.6 ± 0.3	1.0 ± 0.07	1.20 ± 0.02	1.0 ± 0.07	0.8 ± 0.07	1.0 ± 0.2	0.8 ± 0.4
%E	0	2.6 ± 0.4	0	2.5 ± 0.7	0	n.d.	0	n.d.
Acetate								
mmol/l	0.13 ± 0.01	9.6 ± 0.9	0.14 ± 0.02	10.6 ± 1.5	0.13 ± 0.02	8.2 ± 2	0.14	11 ± 5
%E	0	90 ± 0.7	0	88 ± 1.3	0	86 ± 2	0	84 ± 6

The natural abundance of 13C (1.1%) was subtracted from the percentage enrichments (%E). *$P < 0.05$ and $P < 0.01$ for control vs. 3dRH; †$P < 0.05$ and $P < 0.01$ for euglycemia vs. hypoglycemia. n.d., non-detectable.

Billerica, MA). Spectra were obtained from a 14-mm-diameter surface radiofrequency coil tuned to 1H (400 MHz). 13C-inversion and decoupling radiofrequency pulses (100 MHz) were delivered by two orthogonally positioned coils

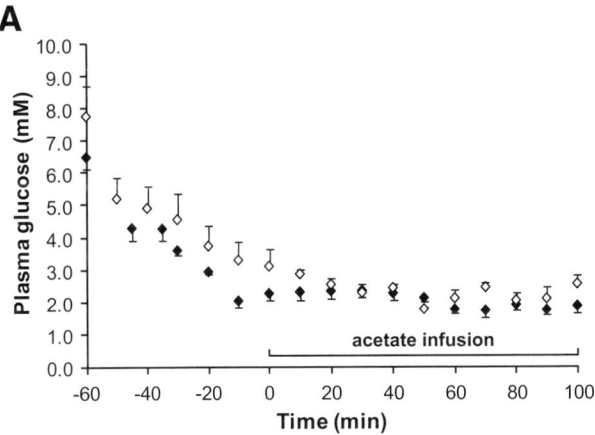

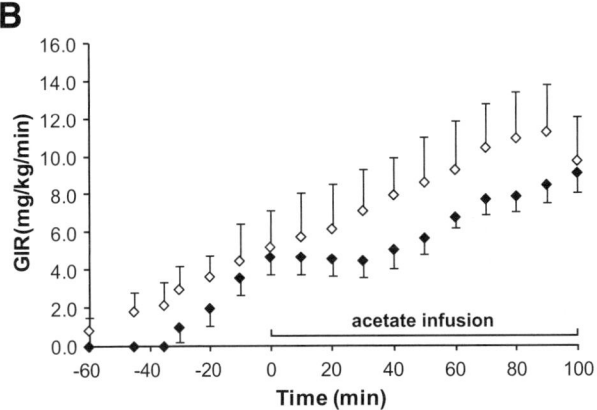

FIG. 2. Hypoglycemic-hyperinsulinemic clamp. *A*: Plasma glucose concentration. *B*: Glucose infusion rate (GIR). The time point at $t = 0$ min indicates the beginning of the 13C-labeled acetate infusion and spectral acquisition. Error bars = SE. ♦, controls; ◇, 3dRH.

driven in quadrature. Localized 1H-[13C] NMR spectra were obtained from a volume of 180 μl ($6 \times 5 \times 6$ mm³), centered in the middle of the cortex. Field homogeneity was optimized by adjustment of first- and second-order shims using the automated Fastmap algorithm (16), achieving a line-width-at-half-height of 15 Hz. Localization was achieved with the LASER (localized by adiabatic selective refocusing) pulse sequence and water suppression by CHESS 4 (chemical shift selective 4) imaging (17–19). Spectra were collected with repetition at a time of 2.5 s (20). At the end of the experiment, animals were removed from the magnet, and brains were frozen in situ using liquid nitrogen while mechanical ventilation was continued to preserve labile metabolites (21,22).

Brain extracts and plasma samples for high-resolution NMR spectroscopy were prepared using a procedure described previously (23,24). Metabolite concentrations and 13C-enrichments were measured using 1H-[13C] NMR at 11.7 T on a Bruker Avance vertical bore spectrometer.

Metabolic modeling. Metabolic fluxes were determined by fitting the two-compartment model of astrocytic and neuronal metabolism depicted in Fig. 1, which is based on the time courses of 13C-enrichment of the C4 position of glutamate and glutamine (Glu4 and Gln4) during the infusion of [2-13C]acetate (Fig. 3A) and the 13C-enrichment of Glu3 and Gln3 at the end of infusion (Fig. 3B). For a driver function, the measured time course of [2-13C]acetate in the brain was used instead of plasma acetate levels to eliminate uncertainties associated with acetate transport kinetics. Mass and isotopic flows from [2-13C]acetate to glial and neuronal glutamate and glutamine pools were expressed as coupled differential equations (see the supplementary materials, available in an online appendix at http://diabetes.diabetesjournals.org/cgi/content/full/db08-1664/DC1) within the CWave 3.0 software package (25) running in Matlab 7.0 (Mathworks, Natick, MA). The equations were solved using a first-order Runge-Kutta algorithm, and fitting optimization was achieved using simulated annealing hybridized with a Levenberg-Marquardt algorithm (26) with fixed values for V_{cyc}/V_{tcaN} and V_{kbN}, where V_{cyc} indicates the rate of the glutamate/glutamine neurotransmitter cycle, V_{tcaN} indicates the rate of neuronal tricarboxylic acid cycle, and V_{kbN} indicates the rate of neuronal β-hydroxybutyrate utilization. The V_{cyc}/V_{tcaN} ratio was calculated from the steady-state 13C percentage enrichments of Glu4 and Gln4 from [2-13C]acetate according to the following (24):

$$V_{cyc}/V_{tcaN} = (Glu4_N - c_i)/(Gln4_A - Glu4_N)$$

where "N" and "A" designate the neuronal and astroglial compartments, respectively. We assumed that glutamate was distributed between neurons (90%) and astroglia (10%) and glutamine was located entirely in astroglia. The steady-state enrichment of astroglial Glu4 was assumed to equal that of Gln4; thus, the percentage enrichment of neuronal glutamate is given by $Glu4_N = (Glu4 - Gln4 \times 0.1)/0.9$. The correction factor c_i removes contributions to $Glu4_N$ (at the level of acetyl-CoA) from metabolism of 13C-labeled plasma products derived from [2-13C]acetate metabolism in peripheral tissues, e.g., plasma glucose-C1 (and/or lactate-C3) and β-hydroxybutyrate (BHB)-C4/C2

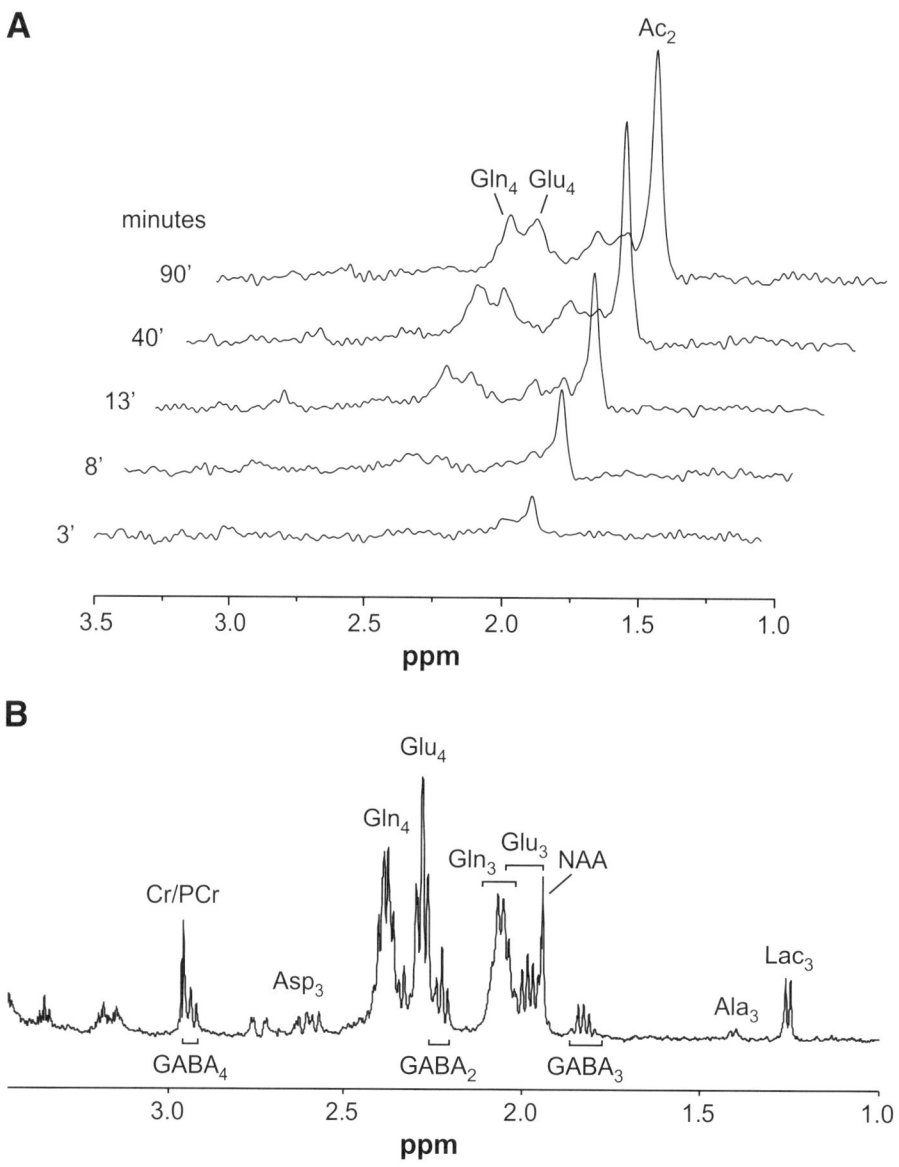

FIG. 3. NMR spectra. *A*: Representative stack of in vivo ^{1}H-[^{13}C] difference spectra acquired over time, revealing gradual accumulation of brain [2-^{13}C]acetate and its subsequent appearance in the stable metabolite pools of Glu4, Glu3, Gln4, and Gln3. *B*: Representative high-resolution ^{1}H-[^{13}C] spectra of brain tissue extracts used to further resolve the metabolite concentrations and enrichments of different carbon positions of glutamate-C4,3,2 (Glu$_{4,3,2}$); glutamine-C4,3,2 (Gln$_{4,3,2}$); GABA-C2,3,4, aspartate-C3 (Asp$_3$); alanine-C3 (Ala$_3$); and lactate-C3 (Lac$_3$). Combination of these two measurements revealed the time courses of label accumulation in these metabolite pools, which were then used in the two-compartment model of brain metabolism to determine the metabolic fluxes. Cr, creatine; NAA, N-acetylaspartate; PCr, phosphocreatine.

(for details on calculation of this correction factor, see the supplemental materials).

Statistical analysis. The error distributions were reported as the SE. P values were calculated using Student's t test using Microsoft Excel, and $P \leq 0.05$ was considered to be statistically significant. Monte-Carlo analysis of each animal's dataset was performed with CWave to assess the distribution of uncertainties in the model parameters for individual animals (27) (see supplemental materials). The uncertainties in Monte Carlo fitting were smaller than the group variabilities for each parameter reported in this study, indicating that treatment differences were not obscured by uncertainties associated with data fitting.

RESULTS

Effect of recurrent hypoglycemia on acetate metabolism under euglycemia. Within 1 min of initiating the [2-^{13}C]acetate infusion, a steady-state plasma level of ~10

mmol/l was reached and maintained throughout the 100-min experiment. There was rapid ^{13}C-labeling of plasma BHB at the C4 position (reaching ~18%) and at the C3 position of plasma lactate (~2.5%) in both control as well as 3dRH pretreated animals. A 30% increase in blood glucose concentration occurred in both groups during the acetate infusion, without any detectable ^{13}C-labeling of glucose (Table 1). Brain [2-^{13}C]acetate accumulation in the in vivo NMR spectra was immediately observed, suggesting that metabolic flux would not be limited by blood-brain barrier transport of acetate in either group (Table 2). Although animals from both groups showed similar plasma glucose levels, exposure to antecedent recurrent hypoglycemia resulted in 34% higher brain glucose concentrations (1.27 ± 0.04 and 1.72 ± 0.08 μmol/g for control

TABLE 2
Brain extract metabolite concentrations (μmol/g) and ^{13}C-percentage enrichments (%E) at the end of the [2-^{13}C]acetate infusion

	Euglycemia		Hypoglycemia	
	Control	3dRH	Control	3dRH
Acetate				
Concentration (μmol/g)	1.5 ± 0.2	1.2 ± 0.3	1.2 ± 0.1	0.8 ± 0.2
C2 (%E)	90 ± 0.7	88 ± 1.4	86 ± 2	84 ± 2
Glucose				
Concentration (μmol/g)	1.27 ± 0.04	1.72 ± 0.08*	0.35 ± 0.04	0.4 ± 0.04
C1 (%E)	n.d.	n.d.	n.d.	n.d.
Lactate				
Concentration (μmol/g)	2.2 ± 0.2	2.3 ± 0.2	1.9 ± 0.5	3.4 ± 0.3*†
C3 (%E)	2.3 ± 0.2	2.6 ± 0.2	3.4 ± 0.5	1.2 ± 0.4*†
Aspartate				
Concentration (μmol/g)	2.9 ± 0.1	2.7 ± 0.1	3.3 ± 0.5	3.9 ± 0.5*†
C3 (%E)	7.1 ± 0.8	6.5 ± 0.6	5.9 ± 0.4	6.5 ± 0.8
Glutamate				
Concentration (μmol/g)	10.8 ± 0.5	11.5 ± 0.6	11.5 ± 0.6	12.1 ± 0.8
C2 (%E)	2.8 ± 0.3	3.2 ± 0.3		
C3 (%E)	7.7 ± 0.4	7.6 ± 0.5	8.7 ± 0.6	7.7 ± 0.7
C4 (%E)	10.5 ± 0.3	10.8 ± 0.5	13.9 ± 0.6†	14.3 ± 1‡
Glutamine				
Concentration (μmol/g)	6.9 ± 0.3	6.6 ± 0.3	7.2 ± 0.4	7.2 ± 0.6
C2 (%E)	7.3 ± 0.4	6.7 ± 0.3		
C3 (%E)	11.2 ± 0.7	10.4 ± 0.2	11.5 ± 0.4	10.0 ± 0.6
C4 (%E)	23.7 ± 1.0	22.9 ± 0.8	27.8 ± 0.5†	29 ± 0.8†
GABA				
Concentration (μmol/g)	1.6 ± 0.1	1.7 ± 0.2	1.8 ± 0.2	2.7 ± 0.4‡
C2 (%E)	9.2 ± 0.4	10.3 ± 0.5	12.0 ± 0.3‡	11.3 ± 1
C3 (%E)	5.3 ± 0.7	5.9 ± 0.4	7.3 ± 0.6	5.3 ± 1.4
C4 (%E)	6.9 ± 0.7	6.1 ± 0.3	9.2 ± 1.1†	7.3 ± 1.2

The natural abundance of ^{13}C (1.1%) was subtracted from the percentage enrichments. *$P < 0.05$ 3dRH vs. control; †$P < 0.05$; ‡$P < 0.01$ hypoglycemia vs. euglycemia within a group. n.d., non-detectable.

and 3dRH, respectively; $P = 0.002$), suggesting an increased glucose transport capacity in the 3dRH group.

The V_{cyc}/V_{tcaN} ratio, representing the coupling between glutamate/glutamine cycling and the neuronal TCA cycle, had no significant change after exposure to recurrent hypoglycemia (0.58 ± 0.05) in comparison to controls (0.51 ± 0.03, $P = 0.15$). Figure 4 (*top panels*) shows the group averages for ^{13}C time courses of Glu4 and Gln4

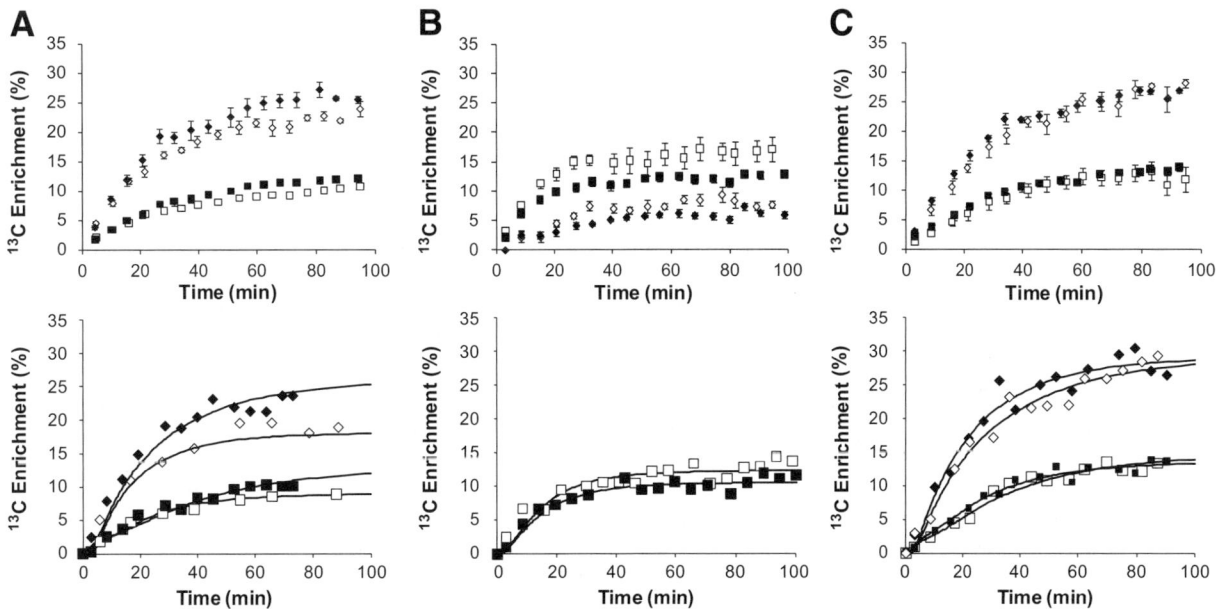

FIG. 4. Time courses of Glu4 and Gln4 labeling during labeled substrate infusions. *A*: [2-^{13}C]acetate at euglycemia. *B*: [1-^{13}C]glucose and unlabeled acetate at euglycemia. *C*: [2-^{13}C]acetate at hypoglycemia. Group-averaged data are depicted in the upper panels, whereas representative individual animals with best fits of the two-compartment metabolic model appear in lower panels. ◆, Gln4 control; ◇, Gln4 3dRH; ■, Glu4 control; □, Glu4 3dRH. Error bars = SE.

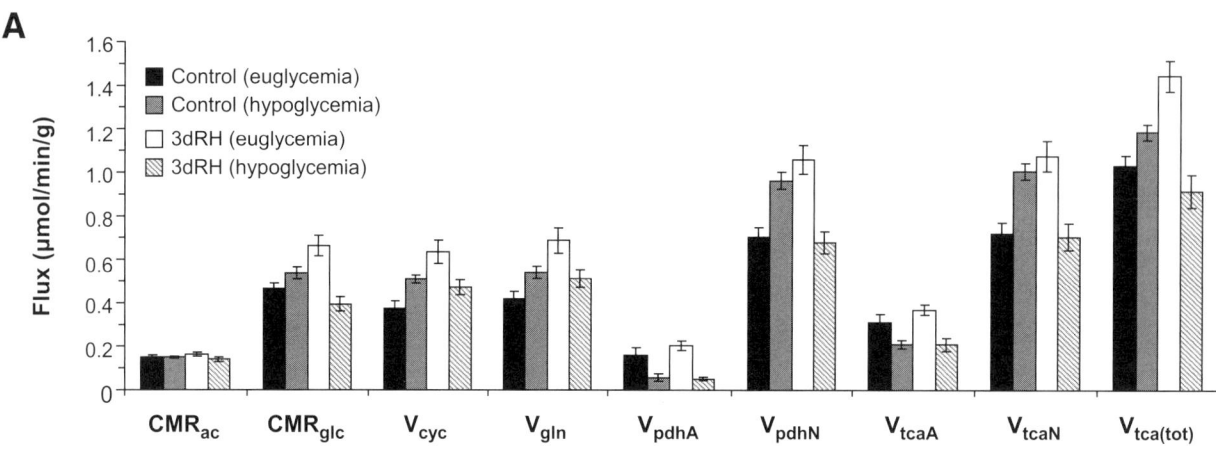

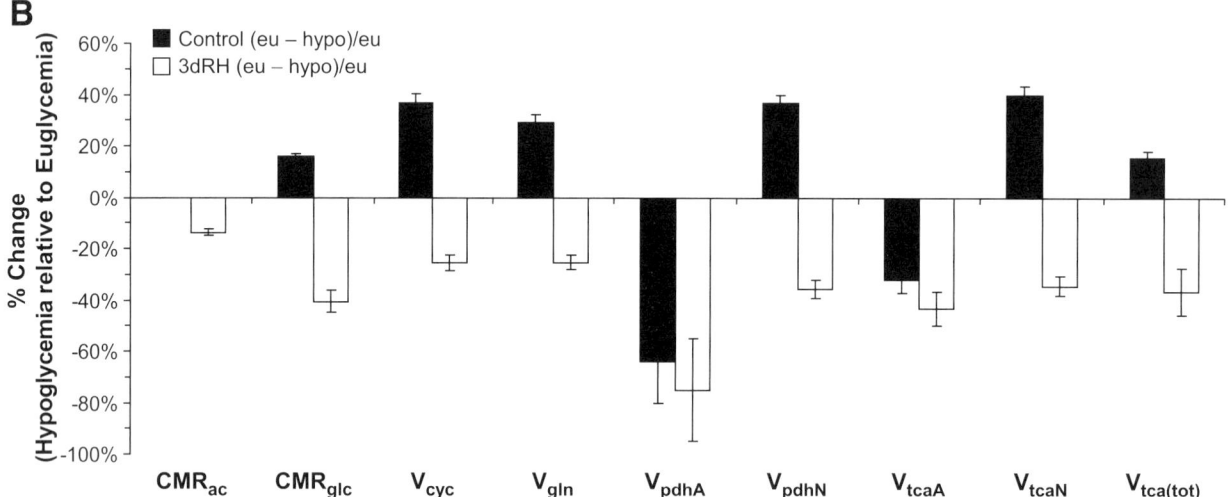

FIG. 5. Metabolic fluxes derived from two-compartment model. *A*: In control and 3DRH animals under euglycemia and hypoglycemia. *B*: Percentage change in metabolic rates from euglycemia (eu) to hypoglycemia (hypo) within groups, calculated as: [(euglycemia – hypoglycemia)/euglycemia] × 100.

during [2-^{13}C]acetate infusion in control and 3dRH animals under euglycemia. Individual time courses served as the input for the metabolic model.

Although brain acetate metabolism (cerebral metabolic rate [CMR]$_{ac}$) did not differ significantly between 3dRH and control animals (0.15 ± 0.01 vs. 0.16 ± 0.01 μmol · g^{-1} · min^{-1} for control vs. 3dRH, P = 0.2), brain glucose metabolism (CMR$_{gl}$) under euglycemia was increased in the 3dRH animals by 43 ± 4% (0.46 ± 0.3 vs. 0.66 ± 0.5 μmol · g^{-1} · min^{-1} for control vs. 3dRH, P = 0.003) (Fig. 5*A*). This increase was further reflected by a 50% increase of V_{pdhN} in the neuronal compartment (0.70 ± 0.08 vs. 1.06 ± 0.09 μmol · g^{-1} · min^{-1}, P = 0.008), suggesting an overall increased capacity to utilize glucose. Total brain TCA cycle activity increased as a consequence (1.03 ± 0.05 vs. 1.45 ± 0.07 μmol · g^{-1} · min^{-1}, P < 0.004). Because the metabolism of labeled acetate does not result in ^{13}C label flow through pyruvate dehydrogenase, V_{pdhN} is instead calculated by the metabolic model based on several dilutional fluxes, with the main contribution coming from unlabeled glucose.

Effect of recurrent hypoglycemia on neuronal PDH flux under euglycemia. The plasma glucose level during the coinfusion of [1-^{13}C]glucose and unlabeled acetate was maintained at 9 ± 1 mmol/l in the control and 8.1 ± 0.8

mmol/l in the 3dRH group (P = 0.11). Throughout, acetate concentrations were comparable between the groups as well as in comparison to the labeled acetate infusions, described above. In contrast, we did not observe labeling of BHB, but we did see a significantly higher degree of [3-^{13}C]lactate labeling in the plasma (9.5 ± 0.4 vs. 6.4 ± 0.06% fE for control vs. 3dRH, P = 0.02).

The rate of isotopic enrichment of the brain glutamate pool was considerably higher than that of glutamine (Fig. 4), a reflection of the metabolic compartmentalization and the higher contribution of glucose-derived metabolites to neuronal metabolism. Because lactate uses the same metabolic pathway as glucose in the brain, it equally contributes to V_{pdhN}. The two-compartment model, using the ^{13}C time courses of plasma glucose and lactate as well as brain Glu4 and Gln4, was therefore used to calculate V_{pdhN}. Comparing results from the [2-^{13}C]acetate infusion with this direct determination of V_{pdhN} using [1-^{13}C]glucose revealed essentially the same values (0.75 ± 0.05 and 1.09 ± 0.07 μmol · min^{-1} · g^{-1} for control and 3dRH, respectively; P = 0.003) (Fig. 5*A*), thereby confirming our finding of increased V_{pdhN} in the 3dRH group.

Effect of recurrent hypoglycemia on astrocytic and neuronal metabolism during acute hypoglycemia. In this experiment the hyperinsulinemic-hypoglycemic clamp maintained plasma glucose levels constant at 2.1 ± 0.2 mmol/l in both groups during the infusion of $[2\text{-}^{13}\text{C}]$acetate (Fig. 2). In keeping with a loss of counterregulatory responses in the 3dRH model, a 20% higher glucose infusion rate was required in these animals to maintain the same degree of glycemia. The other physiological parameters were controlled at similar levels, and plasma concentrations of acetate, lactate, and BHB were comparable between groups (Table 1). The most striking change was a decrease in BHB labeling from 17.9 ± 3.9 to $3.3 \pm 1.9\%$ ($P < 0.001$) after exposure to recurrent hypoglycemia (Table 2), consistent with the presence of reduced peripheral ketones in the context of increased peripheral acetate utilization. Furthermore, during hypoglycemia, brain concentrations of GABA in 3dRH rats were increased by 50% ($P = 0.05$) compared with controls, without significant changes of ^{13}C-enrichment of GABA. When comparing the time courses of Glu4 and Gln4 for the 3dRH and control groups, we observed no obvious differences in the rates of Gln4 labeling and only small changes in Glu4 labeling (Fig. 4C).

We constrained two parameters in fitting the metabolic model to the time course data: the ratio of glutamate neurotransmitter cycling to neuronal TCA cycle flux (V_{cyc}/V_{tcaN}) and the rate of neuronal ketone body utilization (V_{kbN}). In the current study, blood BHB enrichment was 17.9 and 3.3% at the end of the $[2\text{-}^{13}\text{C}]$acetate infusion in hypoglycemic control and 3dRH animals, respectively, which led to relatively small contributions (and corrections in Eq. 1) (supplementary materials) of 2.1% ($= 100 \times 0.179 \times 0.12$) and 0.2% ($= 100 \times 0.033 \times 0.12$). Including these corrections in Eq. 1 had only minor and insignificant ($P = 0.17$) effects on the calculated values of V_{cyc}/V_{tcaN} for the control (0.52 ± 0.07) and 3dRH (0.64 ± 0.09) animals. V_{kbN} was set to 0.04 ± 0.02 (3dRH) and 0.04 ± 0.01 (control) based on individual plasma BHB concentrations.

Together with the brain $[2\text{-}^{13}\text{C}]$acetate concentration, the time courses of label appearance in ^{13}C brain acetate, plasma BHB, brain Glu4, Gln4, and end points of Glu3 and Gln3, we determined the metabolic fluxes of 3dRH versus control animals under hypoglycemic clamp conditions (Fig. 5B). Although we observed a $24 \pm 5\%$ lower V_{pdhN} in 3dRH animals compared with controls ($P = 0.004$) and a decrease in total TCA cycle flux (1.12 ± 0.02 vs. 0.91 ± 0.08 μmol $\cdot$ min^{-1} $\cdot$ g^{-1}, $P = 0.007$), the other parameters remained similar between the groups (CMR$_{ac}$ $P = 0.2$, V_{gln} $P = 0.3$, V_{pdhA} $P = 0.4$, and V_{cyc} $P = 0.2$).

Comparing metabolic fluxes of control animals under euglycemic and hypoglycemic conditions, we found no significant changes in overall brain acetate metabolism (CMR$_{ac}$, $P = 0.5$). In controls, brain glucose consumption (CMR$_{gl}$) in response to hypoglycemia was increased by $16 \pm 1\%$ ($P < 0.05$), mostly due to an increase in glucose-related fluxes in the neuronal compartment, namely V_{pdhN} ($37 \pm 3\%$, $P < 0.01$) and V_{tcaN} ($40 \pm 3\%$, $P = 0.05$). In contrast, astroglial glucose uptake (V_{pdhA}) was decreased by $32 \pm 5\%$ ($P = 0.01$), suggesting a redistribution of glucose consumption to maintain neuronal function, as reflected by a preserved brain total TCA cycle activity (Fig. 5B).

Similar to controls, 3dRH animals showed no changes in CMR$_{ac}$. However, in a response opposite to controls, a significant $40 \pm 5\%$ decrease in CMR$_{gl}$ ($P < 0.001$) was observed in response to hypoglycemia (Fig. 5B). Glucose flux in the astrocytic compartment dropped by $75 \pm 20\%$ (V_{pdhA}, $P < 0.001$) and in neurons by $36 \pm 4\%$ (V_{pdhN}, $P =$

0.005). The combined effect of these decreases in both compartments is a resultant total brain TCA cycle activity decrease by $37 \pm 4\%$ ($P = 0.001$). Comparing the relative contributions of acetate and glucose when going from euglycemia to hypoglycemia (CMR$_{ac}$/CMR$_{gl}$), the control group showed a 12% decrease ($P = 0.06$), whereas 3dRH rats revealed a 24% increase ($P = 0.006$), indicating an increased relative contribution of acetate to brain metabolism in 3dRH animals under hypoglycemic conditions. In this context, however, it is important to note that at baseline euglycemic conditions, 3dRH animals already show a 43% higher degree of brain glucose consumption (CMR$_{gl}$) than control animals ($P = 0.004$).

DISCUSSION

In this study, we measured the rates at which glucose and an alternate fuel (acetate) is oxidized under different glycemic conditions. Measurements of brain metabolism in animals exposed to recurrent hypoglycemia resulted in two main observations. First, after antecedent recurrent hypoglycemia, basal brain glucose metabolism at euglycemia is increased in comparison to controls. This increase was mainly attributable to higher neuronal glucose oxidation, suggesting that when glucose is present in sufficient amounts, neurons are better able to use glucose. Second, under standardized relatively severe hypoglycemic conditions, 3dRH animals showed a decrease in brain glucose consumption in neurons and astroglia, which contrasts with control animals, in which neuronal glucose metabolism was preserved (Fig. 5A). Thus, there is a fundamentally different metabolic response of neurons to hypoglycemia between 3dRH and control animals: whereas acetate consumption remained comparable under euglycemia and hypoglycemia in both groups, acetate comprised a greater relative contribution to total brain oxidation.

Controversy exists regarding the relative degree of cognitive impairment caused by acute hypoglycemia in patients with type 1 diabetes compared with nondiabetic subjects (rev. in 28). This may be in part a consequence of metabolic adaptations that occur in response to different degrees of antecedent exposure to hypoglycemia (29,30). In a previous study using the same rodent model, 3dRH animals subjected to a spatial memory test under euglycemia performed better than controls, whereas they did worse during acute hypoglycemia (9). The current observation of higher total TCA cycle activity under euglycemia and lower activity under hypoglycemia in 3dRH animals parallels this biological effect. The better performance under euglycemia in 3dRH animals may be related, in part, to changes in glucose transport across the blood-brain barrier, resulting in a higher brain glucose level at comparable plasma glucose, an effect we also observed using microdialysis in previous studies of our 3dRH model (9,15). The 34% increase in brain glucose levels measured here in the 3dRH group at euglycemia is consistent with the 17% increase reported in type 1 diabetic patients with hypoglycemia unawareness at euglycemia (10). Furthermore, our data establish that the higher brain glucose concentration is not the consequence of a decrease in glucose utilization, but instead occurs despite accelerated brain glucose metabolism.

To overcome the relative uncertainty associated with using $[2\text{-}^{13}\text{C}]$acetate, a predominantly glial fuel, for the calculation of glucose consumption, we performed a confirmatory experiment with [1-^{13}C]glucose as a substrate. The measured neuronal PDH flux in 3dRH animals (1.06 ± 0.10 vs. 1.09 ± 0.07 μmol · min^{-1} · g^{-1} for [2-^{13}C]acetate vs. [1-^{13}C]glucose) was the same for both substrates, further supporting the accuracy of our metabolic model.

In this animal study, transporter kinetics were saturated by an infusion of [2-^{13}C]acetate at a level higher than is ethically and technically permissible in comparable human studies. The acetate infusion resulted in reliable brain acetate measurements, which then allowed us to accurately determine metabolic fluxes independent of potential changes in monocarboxylic acid transport transporter activity at the blood-brain barrier, which are anticipated in the context of exposure to recurrent hypoglycemia (13).

In the current study, all animal groups (euglycemic and hypoglycemic) showed ^{13}C-labeling of BHB from [2-^{13}C]acetate (Table 1), likely because of its rapid metabolism in the liver. BHB labeled with ^{13}C at C4 and C2 would contribute to ^{13}C-labeling of glutamate-C4, as well as other carbon positions. At euglycemia (control and 3dRH), plasma BHB levels were low (~0.3 mmol/l), such that labeling of glutamate-C4 would be negligible. However, during hypoglycemia, baseline BHB levels were elevated (~1 mmol/l) because animals were fasted overnight to reduce their liver glycogen content. The lower rate of brain glucose utilization in hypoglycemic 3dRH animals is not likely attributable to increased consumption of ketone bodies. BHB levels were the same in both groups, and brain levels were not detected, implying similar blood-to-brain concentration gradients—the driving force for BHB utilization in the brain. Furthermore, if BHB utilization had been greater in 3dRH compared with control animals, there would have been greater dilution of brain glutamate-C4 enrichment relative to control animals, which was not seen (14.3 vs. 13.9%, $P = 0.14$) (Table 2).

The contribution of acetate to astroglial TCA cycle flux (CMR$_{ac}$/V$_{tcaA}$) under hypoglycemia was increased by 50% in both control and 3dRH animals compared with euglycemia. A similar value for the ratio CMR$_{ac}$/V$_{tcaA}$ was reached in both groups (0.71 ± 0.19 and 0.67 ± 0.26 for control and 3dRH, respectively), suggesting that acetate metabolism was saturated in each case. This value is very similar to the maximal value predicted for CMR$_{ac}$/V$_{tcaA}$ in human subjects with type 1 diabetes (0.69 ± 0.17) (13). Assuming that our rat model of recurrent hypoglycemia mimics relevant features of glial metabolism in humans, the difference noted previously between type 1 diabetic and control subjects are likely related to an increase in transporter activity.

It is possible that reduced neuronal TCA cycle activity in the context of preserved glycolytic flux may have caused the elevated lactate levels we observed in the brains of 3dRH animals under hypoglycemia. This lactate was less enriched and could have been either derived from endogenous brain glycogen stores or derived directly from unlabeled brain glucose. However, because our model does account for labeled as well as unlabeled lactate as a contribution to neuronal PDH flux and the final labeled glutamate and glutamine pools were comparable, these possibilities are not likely explanations for the significant decrease in V_{pdhN} we observed.

3dRH animals showed higher GABA levels during acute hypoglycemia, which was not observed in control animals (Table 2). Other studies from our group have, in fact, demonstrated a threefold increase in GABA in hypotha-

lamic interstitial fluid (31) and increased long-term potentiation in hippocampal slice preparations in rats exposed to recurrent hypoglycemia (32). Because GABA is an inhibitory neurotransmitter and increased levels could reduce neuronal activity as well as metabolic demand under hypoglycemic conditions in 3dRH animals, this could be a cause of the reduced neuronal TCA cycle activity we observed in our study.

In summary, our study provides the first evidence that recurrent hypoglycemia increases neuronal glucose metabolism under euglycemia. Under hypoglycemia, glucose metabolism decreased, whereas acetate utilization remained constant, the latter supporting a greater relative fraction of total oxidative metabolism. Neuron-specific alternate fuels may therefore provide a means of reducing the risk of hypoglycemia-induced brain injury in intensively treated diabetic patients.

ACKNOWLEDGMENTS

This work was supported in part by National Institutes of Health (NIH), National Institute of Diabetes and Digestive and Kidney Diseases (NIDDK) Grant R01 DK027121 (to K.L.B.), National Institute of Neurological Disorders and Stroke (NINDS) Grant R01 NS037527, NS051854-01 (to D.L.R.), NIDDK Grant R37 DK20495, and Juvenile Diabetes Research Foundation Grant 4-2004-807 (to R.S.S.). R.I.H. was supported by a Ruth Kirschstein National Research Service Award from the NIDDK (F32 DK077461) and G.F.M. by K02 AA-13430. We also gratefully acknowledge NIH NINDS Grant 1 P30 NS052519 and the Quantitative Neuroscience with Magnetic Resonance Program for NMR spectrometer and facilities support and NIDDK Grant P30 DK45735 of the Yale Diabetes Endocrinology Research Center.

No potential conflicts of interest relevant to this article were reported.

The authors thank Terry Nixon and Scott McIntyre of the MRRC Engineering Core for maintenance of the NMR spectrometer and technical support, Peter Brown for design and fabrication of the NMR probe and transceiver coils, Bei Wang for animal surgery, and Wanling Zhu for recurrent hypoglycemia treatment.

REFERENCES

1. Diabetes Control and Complications Trial Research Group: The effect of intensive treatment of diabetes on the development and progression of long-term complications in insulin-dependent diabetes mellitus. N Engl J Med 1993;329:977–986
2. UK Prospective Diabetes Study (UKPDS) Group: Intensive blood-glucose control with sulphonylureas or insulin compared with conventional treatment and risk of complications in patients with type 2 diabetes (UKPDS 33). Lancet 1998;352:837–853
3. Amiel SA, Sherwin RS, Simonson DC, Tamborlane WV. Effect of intensive insulin therapy on glycemic thresholds for counterregulatory hormone release. Diabetes 1988;37:901–907
4. Cryer PE. Iatrogenic hypoglycemia as a cause of hypoglycemia-associated autonomic failure in IDDM: a vicious cycle. Diabetes 1992;41:255–260
5. Cryer PE. Hypoglycemia risk reduction in type 1 diabetes. Exp Clin Endocrinol Diabetes 2001;109(Suppl. 2):S412–S423
6. Cryer PE. Banting Lecture: Hypoglycemia: the limiting factor in the management of IDDM. Diabetes 1994;43:1378–1389
7. Ferguson SC, Blane A, Wardlaw J, Frier BM, Perros P, McCrimmon RJ, Deary IJ. Influence of an early-onset age of type 1 diabetes on cerebral structure and cognitive function. Diabetes Care 2005;28:1431–1437
8. Warren RE, Frier BM. Hypoglycaemia and cognitive function. Diabetes Obes Metab 2005;7:493–503
9. McNay EC, Sherwin RS. Effect of recurrent hypoglycemia on spatial cognition and cognitive metabolism in normal and diabetic rats. Diabetes 2004;53:418–425

10. Criego AB, Tkac I, Kumar A, Thomas W, Gruetter R, Seaquist ER. Brain glucose concentrations in patients with type 1 diabetes and hypoglycemia unawareness. J Neurosci Res 2005;79:42–47

11. Jacob RJ, Dziura J, Blumberg M, Morgen JP, Sherwin RS. Effects of recurrent hypoglycemia on brainstem function in diabetic BB rats: protective adaptation during acute hypoglycemia. Diabetes 1999;48:141–145

12. Powell AM, Sherwin RS, Shulman GI. Impaired hormonal responses to hypoglycemia in spontaneously diabetic and recurrently hypoglycemic rats: reversibility and stimulus specificity of the deficits. J Clin Invest 1993;92:2667–2674

13. Mason GF, Petersen KF, Lebon V, Rothman DL, Shulman GI. Increased brain monocarboxylic acid transport and utilization in type 1 diabetes. Diabetes 2006;55:929–934

14. Patel AB, De Graaf RA, Mason GF, Rothman DL, Shulman RG, Behar KL. Coupling of glutamatergic neurotransmission and neuronal glucose oxidation over the entire range of cerebral cortex activity. Ann N Y Acad Sci 2003;1003:452–453

15. Herzog RI, Chan O, Yu S, Dziura J, McNay EC, Sherwin RS: Effect of acute and recurrent hypoglycemia on changes in brain glycogen concentration. Endocrinology 2008;149:1499–1504

16. Gruetter R, Weisdorf SA, Rajanayagan V, Terpstra M, Merkle H, Truwit CL, Garwood M, Nyberg SL, Ugurbil K. Resolution improvements in in vivo 1H NMR spectra with increased magnetic field strength. J Magn Reson 1998;135:260–264

17. Garwood M, DelaBarre L. The return of the frequency sweep: designing adiabatic pulses for contemporary NMR. J Magn Reson 2001;153:155–177

18. Haase A, Frahm J, Hanicke W, Matthaei D. 1H NMR chemical shift selective (CHESS) imaging. Phys Med Biol 1985;30:341–344

19. Scheenen TW, Klomp DW, Wijnen JP, Heerschap A. Short echo time 1H-MRSI of the human brain at 3T with minimal chemical shift displacement errors using adiabatic refocusing pulses. Magn Reson Med 2008;59:1–6

20. de Graaf RA, Mason GF, Patel AB, Behar KL, Rothman DL. In vivo 1H-[13C]-NMR spectroscopy of cerebral metabolism. NMR Biomed 2003;16:339–357

21. Katsura K, Folbergrova J, Siesjo BK. Changes in labile energy metabolites, redox state and intracellular pH in postischemic brain of normo- and hyperglycemic rats. Brain Res 1996;726:57–63

22. Ponten U, Ratcheson RA, Salford LG, Siesjo BK. Optimal freezing conditions for cerebral metabolites in rats. J Neurochem 1973;21:1127–1138

23. Patel AB, Rothman DL, Cline GW, Behar KL. Glutamine is the major precursor for GABA synthesis in rat neocortex in vivo following acute GABA-transaminase inhibition. Brain Res 2001;919:207–220

24. Patel AB, de Graaf RA, Mason GF, Rothman DL, Shulman RG, Behar KL: The contribution of GABA to glutamate/glutamine cycling and energy metabolism in the rat cortex in vivo. Proc Natl Acad Sci U S A 2005;102:5588–5593

25. Mason GF, Falk Petersen K, de Graaf RA, Kanamatsu T, Otsuki T, Shulman GI, Rothman DL. A comparison of (13)C NMR measurements of the rates of glutamine synthesis and the tricarboxylic acid cycle during oral and intravenous administration of [1-(13)C]glucose. Brain Res Brain Res Protoc 2003;10:181–190

26. Alcolea A, Carrera J, Medina A. A hybrid Marquardt-Simulated Annealing method for solving the groundwater inverse problem. In *Proceedings of ModelCARE 99, Zürich, September, 1999*. Zürich, Switzerland, IAHS, 2000, p. 157–163 (IAHS publ. no. 265)

27. Mason GF, Behar KL, Rothman DL, Shulman RG. NMR determination of intracerebral glucose concentration and transport kinetics in rat brain. J Cereb Blood Flow Metab 1992;12:448–455

28. Kodl CT, Seaquist ER. Cognitive dysfunction and diabetes mellitus. Endocr Rev 2008;29:494–511

29. Sommerfield AJ, Deary IJ, McAulay V, Frier BM. Short-term, delayed, and working memory are impaired during hypoglycemia in individuals with type 1 diabetes. Diabetes Care 2003;26:390–396

30. Widom B, Simonson DC. Glycemic control and neuropsychologic function during hypoglycemia in patients with insulin-dependent diabetes mellitus. Ann Intern Med 1990;112:904–912

31. Chan O, Cheng H, Herzog R, Czyzyk D, Zhu W, Wang A, McCrimmon RJ, Seashore MR, Sherwin RS. Increased GABAergic tone in the ventromedial hypothalamus contributes to suppression of counterregulatory responses after antecedent hypoglycemia. Diabetes 2008;57:1363–1370

32. McNay EC, Williamson A, McCrimmon RJ, Sherwin RS. Cognitive and neural hippocampal effects of long-term moderate recurrent hypoglycemia. Diabetes 2006;55:1088–1095

33. Lebon V, Petersen KF, Cline GW, Shen J, Mason GF, Dufour S, Behar KL, Shulman GI, Rothman DL. Astroglial contribution to brain energy metabolism in humans revealed by 13C nuclear magnetic resonance spectroscopy: elucidation of the dominant pathway for neurotransmitter glutamate repletion and measurement of astrocytic oxidative metabolism. J Neurosci 2002;22:1523–1531

Effects of Acute Insulin-Induced Hypoglycemia on Indices of Inflammation

Putative mechanism for aggravating vascular disease in diabetes

Rohana J. Wright, mrcp[1]
David E. Newby, phd[2]
David Stirling, phd[3]
Christopher A. Ludlam, phd[3]
Ian A. Macdonald, phd[4]
Brian M. Frier, md[1]

OBJECTIVE — To examine the effects of acute insulin-induced hypoglycemia on inflammation, endothelial dysfunction, and platelet activation in adults with and without type 1 diabetes.

RESEARCH DESIGN AND METHODS — We studied 16 nondiabetic adults and 16 subjects with type 1 diabetes during euglycemia (blood glucose 4.5 mmol/l) and hypoglycemia (blood glucose 2.5 mmol/l). Markers of inflammation, thrombosis, and endothelial dysfunction (soluble P-selectin, interleukin-6, von Willebrand factor [vWF], tissue plasminogen activator [tPA], high-sensitivity C-reactive protein [hsCRP], and soluble CD40 ligand [sCD40L]) were measured; platelet-monocyte aggregation and CD40 expression on monocytes were determined using flow cytometry.

RESULTS — In nondiabetic participants, platelet activation occurred after hypoglycemia, with increments in platelet-monocyte aggregation and P-selectin ($P \le 0.02$). Inflammation was triggered with CD40 expression increasing maximally at 24 h ($3.13 \pm 2.3\%$ vs. $2.06 \pm 1.0\%$) after hypoglycemia ($P = 0.009$). Both sCD40L and hsCRP ($P = 0.02$) increased with a nonsignificant rise in vWF and tPA, indicating a possible endothelial effect. A reduction in sCD40L, tPA, and P-selectin occurred during euglycemia ($P = 0.03$, $P \le 0.006$, and $P = 0.006$, respectively). In type 1 diabetes, both CD40 expression ($5.54 \pm 4.4\%$ vs. $3.65 \pm 1.8\%$; $P = 0.006$) and plasma sCD40L concentrations increased during hypoglycemia (peak 3.41 ± 3.2 vs. 2.85 ± 2.8 ng/ml; $P = 0.03$). Platelet-monocyte aggregation also increased significantly at 24 h after hypoglycemia ($P = 0.03$). A decline in vWF and P-selectin occurred during euglycemia ($P \le 0.04$).

CONCLUSIONS — Acute hypoglycemia may provoke upregulation and release of vasoactive substances in adults with and without type 1 diabetes. This may be a putative mechanism for hypoglycemia-induced vascular injury.

Diabetes Care 33:1591–1597, 2010

I n people with type 1 diabetes the rapid institution of strict glycemic control aggravates microvascular complications, particularly retinopathy (1). Although attributed to reduced capillary blood flow causing localized ischemia (1), greater exposure to hypoglycemia may have worsened microangiopathy through its putative effects on local vasculature (2). In addition, cardiovascular stress associated with hypoglycemia may precipitate acute macrovascular events in a diseased circulation. While supported by anecdotal reports (3), the increase in cardiovascular mortality in people with type 2 diabetes in the Action to Control Cardiovascular Risk in Diabetes (ACCORD) trial (4) (and possibly in the Veterans Affairs Diabetes Trial [5]), in which intensive treatment had tripled the frequency of severe hypoglycemia, has caused concern.

Possible mechanisms by which hypoglycemia may damage blood vessels include changes in regional blood flow, mobilization and activation of neutrophils, platelet activation, and enhanced coagulation and viscosity of the blood (3,6–8). Plasma concentrations of C-reactive protein, interleukin-6 (IL-6), and endothelin-1 increase during hypoglycemia (9–11) and may promote vascular disease (12).

Investigation of processes operating at a cellular level to cause atherosclerosis has focused on the potential influences of vascular inflammation, endothelial dysfunction, coagulation, and platelet activation. The present study sought to determine the effects of acute insulin-induced hypoglycemia on inflammation, coagulation, and platelet and monocyte function in adults with and without type 1 diabetes.

RESEARCH DESIGN AND METHODS —

Participants in the study included 16 nondiabetic adult volunteers with no medical history and 16 healthy adults with type 1 diabetes (Table 1). Those with diabetes had no history of hypertension or macrovascular disease, and microvascular disease was excluded. Screening for retinopathy used digital retinal photography, absence of neuropathy was confirmed by clinical examination, and nephropathy was excluded by the absence of microalbuminuria. Subjects with a history of impaired awareness of hypoglycemia or a previous serious reaction to hypoglycemia were excluded. None had a history of head injury, seizure, blackouts, alcohol or drug abuse and psychiatric illness, and their only other medication was the contraceptive pill. Diabetes Control and Complications Trial–aligned A1C was measured using high performance liquid chromatography (nondiabetic reference range 5.0–6.05%; Bio-Rad Laboratories, Munich, Germany); the mean ± SD of the participants with diabetes was $7.91 \pm 0.92\%$. All gave written informed consent before participation, and the study was approved by the Local Medical Research Ethics Committee.

From the [1]Department of Diabetes, Royal Infirmary of Edinburgh, Edinburgh, U.K.; the [2]Centre for Cardiovascular Science, University of Edinburgh, Edinburgh, U.K.; the [3]Department of Haematology, Royal Infirmary of Edinburgh, Edinburgh, U.K.; and the [4]School of Biomedical Sciences, University of Nottingham, Nottingham, U.K.
Corresponding author: Brian M. Frier, brian.frier@luht.scot.nhs.uk.
Received 4 January 2010 and accepted 22 March 2010. DOI: 10.2337/dc10-0013.

See accompanying original article, p. 1529, and editorial, p. 1686.

Table 1—*Baseline demographic characteristics*

	Nondiabetic subjects	Subjects with diabetes
n	16	16
Age (years)	28 (26.7–35)	28 (25–37.5)
BMI (kg/m^2)	22.86 ± 2.4	26.40 ± 4.0
Male/female	6/10	7/9
Duration of diabetes (years)	N/A	10 (4.2–19)
A1C (%)	N/A	7.91 ± 0.9

Data are median (interquartile range) and means ± SD unless otherwise indicated.

A modified hyperinsulinemic glucose clamp (13) was used to maintain blood glucose at a predetermined level: euglycemia at 4.5 mmol/l and hypoglycemia at 2.5 mmol/l. Each subject underwent two laboratory sessions, separated by at least 2 weeks (mean 7.2 weeks), of a euglycemic study and a hypoglycemic study in a randomized, counterbalanced fashion.

The participants with type 1 diabetes monitored blood glucose intensively during the 48 h preceding each study, which was postponed if any blood glucose value was <3.5 mmol/l or if symptoms suggestive of hypoglycemia were experienced. After fasting overnight, morning insulin was withheld. A retrograde-intravenous cannula for blood-glucose sampling was inserted into the nondominant hand, which was heated to arterialize the venous blood (14). A cannula in the nondominant antecubital fossa was used to infuse 20% dextrose and soluble insulin (Human Actrapid; Novo Nordisk, Crawley, U.K.) at a constant rate of 1.5 mU/kg/min using a Gemini PCI pump (Alaris Medical Systems, San Diego, CA). The dextrose was infused at a variable rate depending on arterialized blood glucose concentrations, which were measured at 5 min intervals using the glucose oxidase method (2300 Stat; Yellow Springs Instruments, Yellow Springs, OH). A third cannula in the other antecubital fossa was dedicated to blood sampling for inflammatory markers.

On each study day, the arterialized blood glucose was stabilized initially at 4.5 mmol/l for 30 min and either maintained at that level (euglycemia) or lowered over 20 min to 2.5 mmol/l for 60 min (hypoglycemia), after which blood glucose was restored to 4.5 mmol/l. Subjects consumed a standardized meal after each study. Blood sample time points were: baseline, during the experimental session (+45 min), during recovery (+105 min), at +6 h, and at +24 h.

Flow cytometry

Whole blood samples were collected at the predetermined time points using D-Phenylalanyl-L-prolyl-L-arginine chloromethyl ketone, a selective thrombin inhibitor, as an anticoagulant. Samples (100 μl) of whole blood were immediately incubated with 10 μl of each monoclonal antibody (AbD Serotec, Kidlington, U.K.) for 30 min at room temperature, with subsequent red cell lysis by the addition of 1 ml of fluorescent-activated cell sorter (FACS) Lyse solution (Becton Dickinson, Oxford, U.K.). Flow cytometry using the FACS Calibur system (Becton Dickinson, Oxford, U.K.) was performed immediately after the experimental session to assess platelet-monocyte aggregation (CD14/CD42a) and CD40 expression on monocytes (CD14/CD40). Isotype controls were performed in addition to both mono- and dual-stain for each parameter assessed at each time point.

Soluble marker assays

Citrated plasma and serum samples were collected at the predetermined time points. These were separated immediately and frozen at −80°C until analysis for the soluble markers:

Von Willebrand factor (vWF) (enzyme-linked immunosorbent assay [ELISA]; coefficient of variation [CV] 7.3%), tissue plasminogen activator (tPA) antigen (Hyphen Biomed Zymutest; intra-assay CV 3.5%, inter-assay CV 4.4%), soluble CD40 ligand (sCD40L) (high sensitivity ELISA, Bender Medsystems; intra-assay CV 5.5%, inter-assay CV 7.2%), soluble P-selectin (ELISA, R&D Systems; intra-assay CV 5.1%, inter-assay CV 8.8%), IL-6 (High sensitivity ELISA, R&D Systems; intra-assay CV 5.9%, inter-assay CV 9.9%), and high sensitivity CRP (DRG Diagnostics; DRG Instruments, Marburg, Germany; intra-assay CV 4.2%, inter-assay CV 4.1%).

Catecholamine assays

Samples for epinephrine quantification were collected in EDTA tubes and immediately separated and frozen at −80°C until analysis by high-performance liquid chromatography and electrochemical detection (intra-assay CV 1.2%, inter-assay CV 3.9%).

Hypoglycemia symptom score

The Edinburgh Hypoglycemia Scale (15) was used to assess the symptoms experienced during each experimental session.

Statistical analyses

Results were analyzed using SPSS version 15.0 for Windows (SPSS, Chicago, IL). A general linear model (repeated-measures ANOVA) was used, with order of session (euglycemia-hypoglycemia or hypoglycemia-euglycemia) as a between-subjects factor, and condition (euglycemia or hypoglycemia) as a within-subjects factor, to compare hypoglycemia with euglycemia. Additional analysis using paired t tests was performed to assess the change in any given parameter from baseline. A P value <0.05 was considered to be significant. Results are reported as mean ± SD unless otherwise stated.

RESULTS — Hypoglycemia provoked a symptomatic response in all subjects with increased scores of autonomic ($P \leq 0.002$), neuroglycopenic ($P < 0.001$), and malaise ($P \leq 0.008$) symptoms compared with baseline. Comparison of baseline levels of inflammatory, endothelial and platelet markers in nondiabetic subjects and subjects with type 1 diabetes showed a significantly higher concentration of soluble P-selectin ($P = 0.01$) and of CD40 expression on monocytes ($P = 0.006$) in those with diabetes, demonstrating the chronic inflammatory response associated with diabetes.

Blood glucose

Target blood glucose concentrations were achieved (Fig. 1). In nondiabetic subjects, blood glucose concentrations were 2.58 ± 0.2 and 4.42 ± 0.5 mmol/l during hypoglycemia and euglycemia, respectively. In those with type 1 diabetes, blood glucose concentrations were 2.46 ± 0.22 and 4.53 ± 0.24 mmol/l, respectively. The blood glucose nadir was similar in both groups.

Counterregulatory response

Plasma epinephrine increased during hypoglycemia in participants with and with-

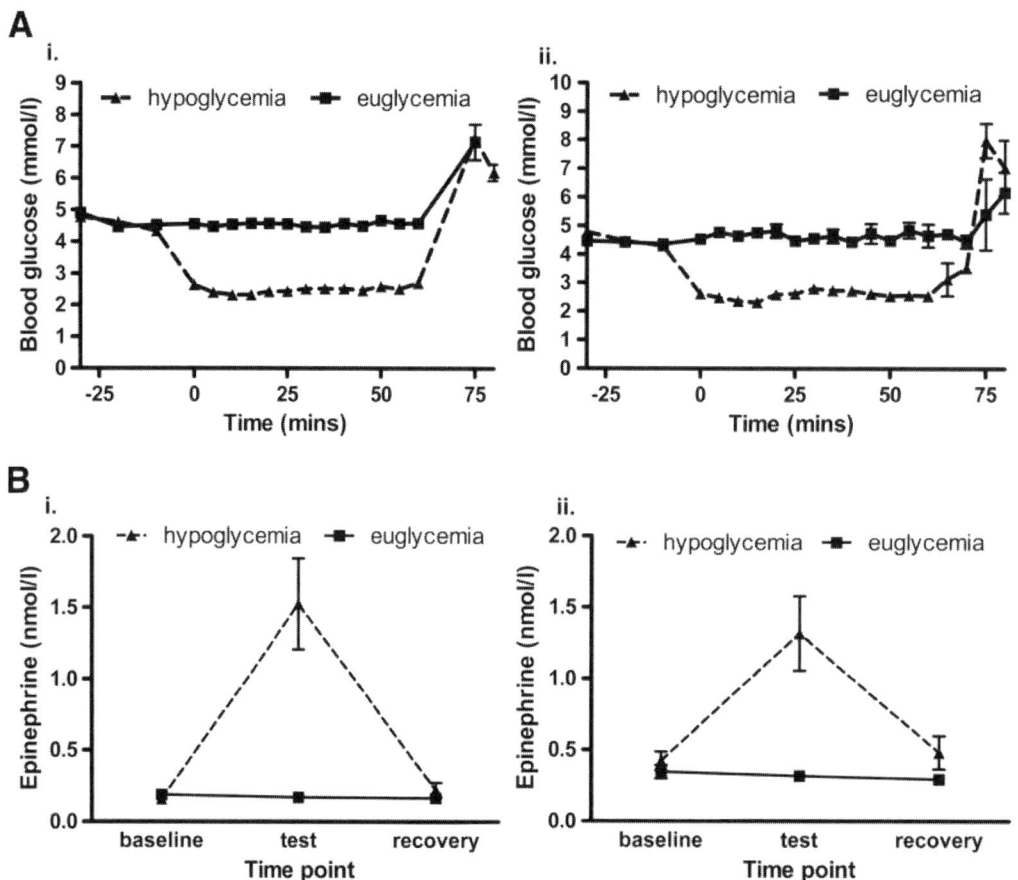

Figure 1—A: *Blood glucose concentrations during hyperinsulinemic hypoglycemic and euglycemic clamp studies.* B: *Epinephrine responses to experimental procedures.* i. *nondiabetic subjects;* ii. *subjects with type 1 diabetes.*

out type 1 diabetes ($P \leq 0.001$; Fig. 1). The epinephrine response occurred only during hypoglycemia and returned rapidly to baseline as anticipated (16).

Platelet activation

Platelet-monocyte aggregation. In nondiabetic subjects, platelet-monocyte aggregation appeared to rise, from a baseline level of 0.72 ± 0.8% to 3.09 ± 8.1% during hypoglycemia, with a peak of 3.49 ± 10.4% at 24 h (Fig. 2). Platelet-monocyte aggregation remained unchanged throughout euglycemia. The difference between conditions, and from baseline, did not achieve statistical significance.

In participants with diabetes, there was a late rise in platelet-monocyte aggregation after hypoglycemia at 24 h compared with baseline ($P = 0.03$).

Soluble P-selectin. Soluble plasma P-selectin concentrations increased after hypoglycemia in nondiabetic subjects, exhibiting a late response at 6 h ($P = 0.01$) and 24 h ($P = 0.02$; Fig. 2) but

decreasing during euglycemia ($P = 0.006$).

P-selectin also decreased during euglycemia in the diabetic group ($P = 0.04$), but did not change during hypoglycemia.

Endothelial markers

tPA. In nondiabetic subjects, plasma tPA concentrations increased during hypoglycemia, with a higher peak tPA concentration (12.55 ± 16.7 compared with 6.80 ± 7.9 ng/ml) (NS between conditions). Plasma tPA decreased significantly between baseline and test phase ($P = 0.004$) and recovery phase ($P = 0.006$), with a paradoxical rise between baseline and 24 h ($P = 0.06$) after euglycemia (Table 2). However, a diurnal variation in tPA concentration is recognized to occur, which may account for the decline observed during euglycemia (17). No significant differences occurred in the diabetic group (Table 2).

vWF. A trend toward a difference in plasma vWF concentrations was observed between hypoglycemia and euglycemia at

6 h in the nondiabetic subjects ($P = 0.07$) (Table 2).

Plasma vWF concentrations decreased between baseline and test phase ($P = 0.02$) and recovery phase ($P = 0.03$) after euglycemia in the participants with diabetes. No such decrement was observed during hypoglycemia (Table 2).

Inflammation

CD40 expression. CD40 expression on monocytes increased after hypoglycemia in nondiabetic subjects, from a baseline of 1.92 ± 2.2% to a maximum of 3.13 ± 2.3% at 24 h ($P = 0.009$). A significant difference between hypoglycemia and euglycemia conditions was present at 6 h ($P = 0.05$) and at 24 h ($P = 0.04$) (Table 2).

In participants with type 1 diabetes, monocyte CD40 expression increased from 3.69 ± 3.4% to 5.54 ± 4.4% during hypoglycemia ($P = 0.006$), compared with no change during euglycemia (3.64 ± 2.0% to 3.65 ± 1.8%, respectively; $P = $ NS). The increment during

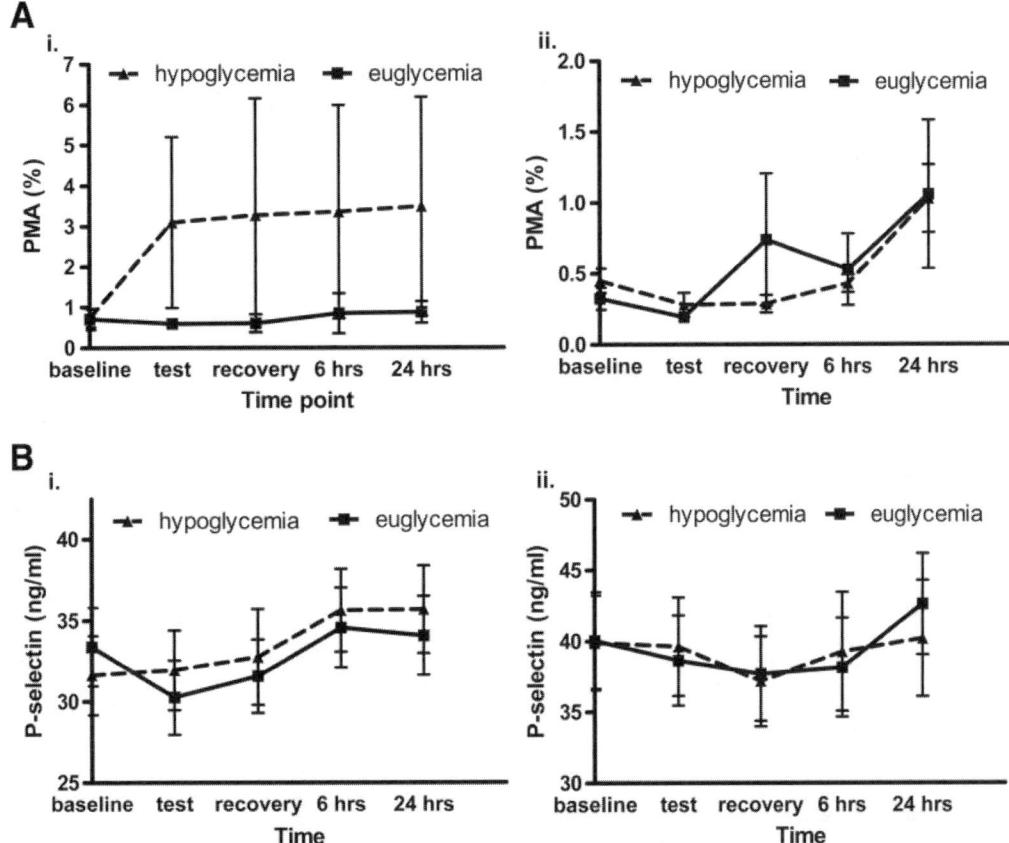

Figure 2—*Platelet activation in response to experimental hypoglycemia and euglycemia. A: Platelet-monocyte aggregation. B: Soluble P-selectin, i. Nondiabetic subjects, ii. Subjects with type 1 diabetes.*

hypoglycemia had dissipated by the time of the recovery phase and remained unchanged thereafter (Table 2).

sCD40L. In nondiabetic subjects, plasma sCD40L concentrations were higher during hypoglycemia than during euglycemia (2.80 ± 3.2 vs. 2.41 ± 2.8 ng/ml), with a trend toward significance ($P = 0.09$). A significant reduction in sCD40L concentration occurred during euglycemia between baseline and recovery phase ($P = 0.03$) (Table 2).

In those with diabetes, a significant difference was observed between the baseline levels on each study day: 3.36 ± 2.9 ng/ml on the hypoglycemia day compared with 2.86 ± 2.8 ng/ml on euglycemia day ($P = 0.03$), rendering subsequent measurements difficult to compare. A significant difference was again observed between the experimental condition levels, with a level of 3.41 ± 3.2 ng/ml during hypoglycemia and 2.85 ± 2.8 ng/ml during euglycemia ($P = 0.03$) (Table 2). Changes from baseline did not achieve significance.

IL-6. IL-6 levels rose in all experiments, maximally at 6 h, irrespective of condition, with no clear differences identifiable in either group between the study conditions (Table 2).

hsCRP. Test phase hsCRP was higher in all subjects during hypoglycemia (1.81 ± 1.9 vs. 1.22 ± 1.9 ng/ml in nondiabetic participants [$P = 0.02$]; 2.72 ± 3.1 vs. 2.20 ± 2.9 ng/ml in subjects with diabetes [$P = ns$]) (Table 2). A significant difference was observed in the baseline concentrations in the nondiabetic participants ($P = 0.01$), frustrating interpretation of subsequent responses.

CONCLUSIONS — Previous studies have demonstrated that hypercoagulability, platelet and neutrophil activation, C-reactive protein, IL-6, and Endothelin-1 are upregulated after acute hypoglycemia (3,6–11), while a euglycemic insulin infusion (for at least 2 h) was shown to reduce inflammatory markers, consistent with an anti-inflammatory effect of insulin (18). The present study sought to replicate these effects, while investigating other underlying mechanisms of vascular disease, and tests were selected to investigate the effect of acute hypo-

glycemia on important cellular processes (platelet activation, endothelial dysfunction and inflammation) underlying the development of acute and chronic vascular complications in type 1 diabetes.

The present study showed that hypoglycemia generated a response in some of these markers, suggesting that hypoglycemia-induced metabolic stress may have adverse pathophysiological consequences while the euglycemic insulin infusion caused a potentially beneficial decrement in some parameters. However, the magnitude of most observed changes was small, and not all markers changed significantly.

The present study confirmed that platelet activation is promoted by hypoglycemia (8), with increments both in platelet-monocyte aggregation and soluble P-selectin. Conversely, P-selectin decreased during euglycemia. Endothelial function, using vWF and tPA Ag as surrogate markers, may have been disrupted, as shown by the increase in vWF after hypoglycemia in nondiabetic volunteers, but this change was not replicated in those with diabetes. However, a reduction in vWF occurred after euglycemia in diabetic participants, which should confer vascular benefit. tPA Ag also appeared to increase in nondiabetic subjects during hypoglycemia, while declining during euglycemia, whereas no significant changes occurred in the diabetic group. Soluble markers of inflammation, sCD40L and hsCRP, were higher during hypoglycemia, with an elevation of hsCRP being observed in all subjects. Unfortunately, baseline differences in hsCRP in nondiabetic subjects, and in sCD40L in the diabetic subjects, frustrated interpretation of subsequent responses. sCD40L was apparently reduced during euglycemia in nondiabetic participants. Surprisingly, IL-6 increased in all experiments regardless of glycemic status, with a maximal response at 6 h. This response is inexplicable, and contrasts with a previous report (10). Monocyte CD40 expression also increased, suggesting promotion of the interaction of the CD40-CD40 ligand dyad (from the tumor necrosis factor receptor family), thus affecting another process in the pathway leading to atherosclerotic plaque rupture (19,20). This change occurred much earlier in the diabetic than the nondiabetic subjects, in whom the response was delayed, prolonged, and still present at 24 h. The persistence of these vascular changes for 24 h after the hypoglycemic stimulus, or their later emergence, suggests that the period of risk after hypoglycemia may be present long after blood glucose recovery.

For some markers, a positive trend after hypoglycemia was evident, without achieving statistical significance, or the only measurable difference between conditions was a beneficial effect associated with euglycemia. The sample size may have been insufficient to achieve significance, particularly as the magnitude of responses was small. It was not feasible to study a larger number of subjects using a procedure that is labor-intensive and costly. In a previous study, larger increments in inflammatory markers were observed during an insulin tolerance test, where hypoglycemia of <39 mg/dl (<2.2 mmol/l) was induced (21). The more rapid reduction to a lower blood glucose causing a greater hypoglycemic stimulus may have heightened the magnitude of the responses, compared with the more modest changes that occurred during a controlled glucose clamp (blood glucose 2.5 mmol/l [45 mg/dl]), as observed in the present study. A further limitation of the present study was the need to ex-

Table 2—Endothelial function and inflammation in nondiabetic subjects and subjects with type 1 diabetes

	Euglycemia					Hypoglycemia				
	Baseline	Test	Recovery	+6 h	+24 h	Baseline	Test	Recovery	+6 h	+24 h
Nondiabetic subjects										
tPA (ng/ml)	7.37 ± 8.1	6.80 ± 7.9*	6.44 ± 7.5	6.99 ± 9.3	8.51 ± 7.8†	12.55 ± 16.7	9.10 ± 10.2*	9.83 ± 12.0	11.45 ± 11.6	
vWF (iU/ml)	0.81 ± 0.3	0.76 ± 0.3	0.78 ± 0.2	0.80 ± 0.3	0.85 ± 0.3	0.82 ± 0.3	0.81 ± 0.3	0.89 ± 0.5	0.90 ± 0.3	
CD40 (%)	1.51 ± 1.4	2.23 ± 3.2†	2.40 ± 3.2†	0.84 ± 0.7	2.06 ± 1.0	1.47 ± 1.1	1.55 ± 1.5	1.98 ± 2.4‡	3.13 ± 2.3†‡	
sCD40L (ng/ml)	2.68 ± 3.1	2.41 ± 2.8	2.40 ± 2.9*	2.63 ± 2.9	3.08 ± 3.3	2.80 ± 3.2	2.55 ± 3.2	2.72 ± 3.3	2.79 ± 3.2	
IL-6 (pg/ml)	0.86 ± 0.5	1.06 ± 1.2	1.05 ± 1.0	5.98 ± 4.6†	1.23 ± 0.9	0.92 ± 0.5	1.62 ± 1.2†	4.37 ± 4.3†	1.00 ± 0.9	
hsCRP (ng/ml)	1.04 ± 1.1	1.22 ± 1.9	1.18 ± 1.9	1.24 ± 1.6	1.31 ± 1.5	1.83 ± 1.5‡	1.81 ± 1.9‡	1.56 ± 1.3*	1.90 ± 1.6	
Subjects with type 1 diabetes										
tPA (ng/ml)	15.25 ± 30.2	17.70 ± 31.1	15.99 ± 27.5	22.13 ± 46.2	20.86 ± 34.8	18.12 ± 30.1	20.55 ± 36.1	17.69 ± 31.1	18.37 ± 32.6	22.98 ± 40.3
vWF (iU/ml)	0.91 ± 0.2	0.85 ± 0.2*	0.91 ± 0.3	0.85 ± 0.2*	0.99 ± 0.2	0.93 ± 0.2	0.95 ± 0.2	0.91 ± 0.2	0.90 ± 0.2	1.02 ± 0.2
CD40 (%)	3.64 ± 2.0	3.65 ± 1.8	4.14 ± 2.5	3.97 ± 2.3	4.35 ± 2.0	3.69 ± 3.4	5.54 ± 4.4†	3.36 ± 3.0	4.88 ± 2.4	4.70 ± 2.8
sCD40L (ng/ml)	2.86 ± 2.8	2.85 ± 2.8	2.84 ± 2.8	2.91 ± 2.9	3.25 ± 3.2†	3.36 ± 2.9‡	3.41 ± 3.2†	3.10 ± 2.9*	3.05 ± 2.8*	3.44 ± 2.9
IL-6 (pg/ml)	0.69 ± 0.5	1.38 ± 1.9	1.58 ± 1.8	2.25 ± 2.8†	1.19 ± 1.2	1.21 ± 1.7	1.15 ± 1.5	1.76 ± 1.5	1.96 ± 2.2	
hsCRP (ng/ml)	2.52 ± 3.1	2.20 ± 2.9	2.32 ± 2.8	1.92 ± 1.8	3.40 ± 3.6	2.84 ± 3.2	2.72 ± 3.1	2.70 ± 3.2	2.89 ± 3.3	2.34 ± 2.8

Data are means ± SD. *Significant decrease from baseline (P < 0.05); †significant increase from baseline (P < 0.05); ‡significant difference between hypoglycemia and euglycemia (P < 0.05).

amine the experimental conditions on two separate days in a counterbalanced fashion. Because the baseline levels of many inflammatory markers can differ on separate days, as was observed with sCD40L and hsCRP, this biological variability hinders the interpretation and comparison of subsequent results. However, the present study design was necessary to allow comparison of the euglycemia and hypoglycemia conditions in individual subjects, as both time and insulin infusion per se may exert effects on biomarker levels. This study design cannot control for other day-to-day factors that could influence baseline levels of inflammatory markers. However, the effects of hypoglycemia could be evaluated, as each participant acted as their own control. This produces less variability than a comparison of results among individuals, as more inter-individual variation in inflammatory marker levels is present than intra-individual variation. In addition, it was possible to analyze each study separately, by examining changes in parameters from baseline on that particular day, enabling the detection of significant effects exerted by hypoglycemia compared with euglycemia. Baseline levels of all markers (except IL-6) were higher in the diabetic group (significant for P-selectin and CD40 expression). This could affect the magnitude of response induced by the experimental procedures. However, an analysis of the percentage change from baseline was consistent with the trends identified in the absolute results (shown as in the online appendix available at http://care.diabetesjournals.org/cgi/content/full/dc10-0013/DC1).

As anticipated, epinephrine secretion was stimulated by hypoglycemia. It is likely that hormonal changes underlie the activation and upregulation of the vascular biomarkers. Catecholamines promote platelet activation (22), while adrenoceptor blockade attenuates these effects (23,24). The participants with type 1 diabetes exhibited attenuated plasma epinephrine responses to hypoglycemia compared with the nondiabetic subjects, who were naïve to such a hypoglycemic stimulus, this being consistent with the recognized decline in the magnitude of counterregulatory hormonal responses with increasing duration of type 1 diabetes (25). This attenuated epinephrine response may explain the lower responses of vascular biomarkers to hypoglycemia.

In summary, the effects of hypogly-cemia on several vascular biomarkers that are implicated in the pathogenesis of vascular disease, would support the premise that acute hypoglycemia may be detrimental to an already diseased vasculature (2). Euglycemia may have a protective, anti-inflammatory effect. In the present study, the participants had no overt vascular disease and were unlikely to develop any demonstrable effects from a short period of exposure to hypoglycemia. However, in people with diabetes of long duration, who are likely to have underlying vascular disease, these responses may not be benign. The release of potent vasoactive substances could potentially aggravate chronic vasculopathy, and contribute to the precipitation of acute macrovascular events. This may aggravate established diabetic micro- and macrovascular disease in those who are exposed to recurrent hypoglycemia.

Acknowledgments— The cost of assays was supported by research grants from the Scottish Society of Physicians and the Edinburgh branch of Diabetes UK.

No potential conflicts of interest relevant to this article were reported.

References

1. Hanssen KF, Dahl-Jørgensen K, Lauritzen T, Feldt-Rasmussen B, Brinchmann-Hansen O, Deckert T. Diabetic control and microvascular complications: the near-normoglycaemic experience. Diabetologia 1986;29:677–684
2. Frier BM, Hilsted J. Does hypoglycaemia aggravate the complications of diabetes? Lancet 1985;2:1175–1177
3. Wright RJ, Frier BM. Vascular disease and diabetes: is hypoglycaemia an aggravating factor? Diabetes Metab Res Rev 2008;24: 353–363
4. Action to Control Cardiovascular Risk in Diabetes Study Group, Gerstein HC, Miller ME, Byington RP, Goff DC Jr, Bigger JT, Buse JB, Cushman WC, Genuth S, Ismail-Beigi F, Grimm RH Jr, Probstfield JL, Simons-Morton DG, Friedewald WT Effects of intensive glucose lowering in type 2 diabetes. N Engl J Med 2008;358: 2545–2559
5. Duckworth W, Abraira C, Moritz T, Reda D, Emanuele N, Reaven PD, Zieve FJ, Marks J, Davis SN, Hayward R, Warren SR, Goldman S, McCarren M, Vitek ME, Henderson WG, Huang GD, for the VADT Investigators. Glucose control and vascular complications in veterans with type 2 diabetes. N Engl J Med 2009;360: 129–139
6. Frier BM, Corrall RJ, Davidson NM, Weber RG, Dewar A, French EB. Peripheral blood cell changes in response to acute hypoglycaemia in man. Eur J Clin Inv 1983;13:33–39
7. Fisher BM, Quin JD, Rumley A, Lennie SE, Small M, MacCuish AC, Lowe GD. Effects of acute insulin-induced hypoglycaemia on haemostasis, fibrinolysis and haemorheology in insulin-dependent diabetic patients and control subjects. Clin Sci 1991;80:525–531
8. Trovati M, Anfossi G, Cavalot F, Vitali S, Massucco P, Mularoni E, Schinco P, Tamponi G, Emanuelli G. Studies on mechanisms involved in hypoglycemia-induced platelet activation. Diabetes 1986;35: 818–825
9. Galloway PJ, Thomson GA, Fisher BM, Semple CG. Insulin-induced hypoglycemia induces a rise in C-reactive protein (Letter). Diabetes Care 2000;23:861
10. Dotson S, Freeman R, Failing HJ, Adler GK. Hypoglycemia increases serum interleukin-6 levels in healthy men and women. Diabetes Care 2008;31:1222–1223
11. Wright RJ, Macleod KM, Perros P, Johnston N, Webb DJ, Frier BM. Plasma endothelin response to acute hypoglycemia in adults with type 1 diabetes. Diabet Med 2007;24:1039–1042
12. Libby P, Ridker PM, Maseri A. Inflammation and atherosclerosis. Circulation 2002;105:1135–1143
13. De Fronzo R, Tobin JD, Andres R. Glucose clamp technique: a method for quantifying insulin secretion and resistance. Am J Physiol 1979;273:E214–E223
14. Abumrad NN, Rabin D, Diamond MP, Lacy WW. Use of a heated superficial hand vein as an alternative site for the measurement of amino acid concentrations and for the study of glucose and alanine kinetics in man. Metabolism 1981; 30:936–940
15. Gold AE, MacLeod KM, Frier BM. Frequency of severe hypoglycemia in patients with type 1 diabetes with impaired awareness of hypoglycemia. Diabetes Care 1994;17:697–703
16. Thompson CJ, Baylis PH. Endocrine changes during insulin-induced hypoglycaemia. In *Hypoglycaemia and Diabetes: Clinical and Physiological Aspects*. Frier BM, Fisher BM, Eds. Edward Arnold, London, U.K., 1993, p.116–131
17. Rydzewski A, Urano T, Nagai N, Takada Y, Katoh-Oishi Y, Taminato T, Yoshimi T, Takada A. Diurnal variation in serum remnant-like lipoproteins, platelet aggregation and fibrinolysis in healthy volunteers. Haemostasis 1997;27:305–314
18. Dandona P, Chauduri A, Ghanim H, Mohanty P. Insulin as an anti-inflammatory and antiatherogenic modulator. J Am Coll Cardiol 2009;53 (Suppl. 5):S14–S20
19. Schönbeck U, Libby P. CD40 signaling and plaque instability. Circ Res 2001;89: 1092–1103

20. Mach F, Schönbeck U, Libby P. CD40 signaling in vascular cells: a key role in atherosclerosis? Atherosclerosis 1998; 137(Suppl.):S89–S95

21. Razavi Nematollahi L, Kitabchi AE, Kitabchi AE, Stentz FB, Wan JY, Larijani BA, Tehrani MM, Gozashti MH, Omidfar K, Taheri E. Proinflammatory cytokines in response to insulin-induced hypoglycemic stress in healthy subjects. Metabolism 2009;58:443–448

22. Steel CM, French EB, Aitchison WR. Studies on adrenaline-induced leucocytosis in normal man. I. The role of the spleen and of the thoracic duct. Br J Haematol 1971;21:413–421

23. Fisher BM, Hepburn DA, Smith JG, Frier BM. The effect of alpha-adrenergic blockade on responses of peripheral blood cells to acute insulin-induced hypoglycaemia in humans. Eur J Clin Invest 1990; 20:51–55

24. Takeda H, Kishikawa H, Shinohara M, Miyata T, Suzaki K, Fukushima H, Ichinose K, Shichiri M. Effect of alpha 2-adrenoceptor antagonist on platelet activation during insulin-induced hypoglycaemia in type 2 (noninsulin-dependent) diabetes mellitus. Diabetologia 1988;31:657–663

25. Kerr D, Richardson T. Counterregulatory deficiencies in diabetes. In *Hypoglycaemia in Clinical Diabetes.* 2nd edition. Frier BM, Fisher M, Eds. John Wiley and Sons, Chichester, U.K., 2007, p. 121–140

Impaired Awareness of Hypoglycemia in a Population-Based Sample of Children and Adolescents With Type 1 Diabetes

Trang T. Ly, mbbs[1]
Patricia H. Gallego, md, msc[1]

Elizabeth A. Davis, fracp[1,2]
Timothy W. Jones, fracp, md[1,2]

OBJECTIVE — To determine the prevalence and clinical associations of impaired awareness of hypoglycemia in a population-based sample of children and adolescents with type 1 diabetes.

RESEARCH DESIGN AND METHODS — A validated questionnaire was administered to 656 patients with type 1 diabetes over a 6-month period to determine hypoglycemia awareness status. Case ascertainment was 79% of the clinic population. The rate of severe hypoglycemia was determined by data collected prospectively in the preceding year.

RESULTS — Impaired awareness of hypoglycemia was present in 29% of patients. Patients with impaired awareness of hypoglycemia had an earlier onset of diabetes ($P < 0.001$), were younger ($P < 0.001$), and had lower mean levels of A1C since diabetes onset ($P = 0.006$) and at their last visit ($P = 0.001$). The overall rate of severe hypoglycemia was 24.5 episodes per 100 patient-years in the preceding year. The severe hypoglycemia rate was higher in those with impaired awareness of hypoglycemia (37.1 vs. 19.3 episodes per 100 patient-years, $P < 0.001$). Among patients aged <6 years ($n = 46$), 59% of care providers reported impaired awareness of hypoglycemia, and the rate of severe hypoglycemia was significantly higher in those reporting impaired awareness (33.3 vs. 52 episodes per 100 patient-years, $P = 0.02$). More patients with recurrent hypoglycemia reported impaired awareness of hypoglycemia (47 vs. 28%, $P = 0.03$).

CONCLUSIONS — A significant proportion of children and adolescents with type 1 diabetes have impaired awareness of hypoglycemia. Screening for impaired awareness is an important component of routine diabetes care and can identify patients at increased risk of a severe hypoglycemic event.

Diabetes Care 32:1802–1806, 2009

Hypoglycemia is a well-known complication of insulin therapy in children and adolescents with diabetes. The risk of recurrent and severe hypoglycemia causes significant anxiety and emotional morbidity for patients and their families and is a limiting factor in the achievement of tight glycemic control.

Hypoglycemia unawareness is defined as the onset of neuroglycopenia before autonomic activation (1). Patients have defective symptomatic and counterregulatory hormone responses to hypoglycemia and are unable to initiate self-treatment. This impaired awareness has been associated with severe hypoglycemia, accounting for 36% of the hypoglycemia that occurred while subjects were awake during the Diabetes Control and Complications Trial (2).

The neurological consequences of severe hypoglycemia are particularly important in the young child with type 1 diabetes. Hypoglycemia has been associated with a decrease in neurocognitive function in children with type 1 diabetes, particularly those in whom diabetes is diagnosed before the age of 5–6 years (3–5). Repeated hypoglycemic seizures in young children may also cause structural brain changes, as suggested by the prevalence of mesial temporal sclerosis in 16% of a cohort of children with early-onset type 1 diabetes (6). Severe hypoglycemia adds to the considerable burden of disease in families through increased anxiety, poor sleep, increased hospitalizations, excessive lowering of insulin dose, and worsening of glycemic control (7).

For clinical and research purposes, determining the presence of hypoglycemia unawareness in children and adolescents with diabetes is important. Various methods have been applied, including the use of self-reporting symptom questionnaires and inducing experimental hypoglycemia in the laboratory to determine the symptom response threshold and counterregulatory hormone response. The aim of this study was to determine the prevalence of impaired awareness of hypoglycemia in a large, population-based cohort with childhood-onset type 1 diabetes, assessed with a self-reporting questionnaire, and to study the relationship between impaired hypoglycemia awareness and severe hypoglycemia.

RESEARCH DESIGN AND METHODS — Children and adolescents with type 1 diabetes aged between 6 months and 19 years and diabetes duration of at least 6 months, attending pediatric diabetes clinics at Princess Margaret Hospital were eligible to participate in the study. Princess Margaret Hospital is the only pediatric diabetes referral center for the population of Western Australia, and almost all children with type 1 diabetes in the state are registered and treated here. Previous studies have shown that this center has a case ascertainment close to 100% (8,9). All patients have had ongoing prospective documentation from diagnosis, at 3-month intervals, of hypoglycemic events, diabetic ketoacidosis, and glycemic control measured by A1C.

Patients and care providers had undergone extensive diabetes education during their initial inpatient admission at diagnosis, including the recognition and treatment of hypoglycemic episodes. All patients were given glucagon at discharge, and care providers had been instructed on

From the [1]Department of Endocrinology and Diabetes, Princess Margaret Hospital for Children, Perth, Western Australia, Australia; and the [2]Telethon Institute for Child Health Research, Centre for Child Health Research, The University of Western Australia, Perth, Western Australia, Australia.
Corresponding author: Timothy W. Jones, tim.jones@health.wa.gov.au.
Received 19 March 2009 and accepted 1 July 2009.
Published ahead of print at http://care.diabetesjournals.org on 8 July 2009. DOI: 10.2337/dc09-0541.

its use. Insulin regimens included a combination of twice-daily injections (NPH insulin and analog) through to four injections per day with analog insulins and continuous subcutaneous insulin infusion therapy.

A validated questionnaire to characterize hypoglycemia unawareness was applied to children and adolescents and/or their care providers. This questionnaire was based on a tool used to assess reduced awareness of hypoglycemia in an adult population by Clarke et al. (10). This questionnaire has been shown to accurately identify patients with impaired awareness of hypoglycemia for both clinical and research purposes (11). In this study, patients scoring ≤3 were categorized as having normal awareness and patients scoring ≥4 were categorized as having impaired awareness. The original items for scoring severe hypoglycemia in the previous 12 months and moderate hypoglycemia in the previous 6 months were not included in our questionnaire as these data were collected prospectively in this clinic population.

For children up to the age of 10 years or those who were unable to fill out the questionnaire, parents or care providers were asked to complete it. For children aged between 10 and 12 years, both care providers and children completed the questionnaire. Children aged >12 years completed the questionnaires independently. The test-retest reliability of this questionnaire was verified by retesting the first 100 patients and/or care providers.

Definition of severe hypoglycemia
For the purposes of this study, severe hypoglycemia was defined as an event leading to loss of consciousness or seizure. This strict definition was used because it is an unequivocal end point rather than the more commonly used definition of severe hypoglycemia, which is an event requiring help from another individual. This more common definition is difficult to apply to young children, particularly those <6 years of age, because all hypoglycemic episodes may require assistance in this age-group. Patient data were collected prospectively at routine clinic visits every 3 months using a specifically designed data collection form, completed by a limited number of physicians. The details of data collection have been documented previously (9,12). In summary, both patients and parents were instructed on how to record details of the hypoglycemic event including blood glucose lev-

els and response to treatment. All care providers were instructed to obtain a blood glucose value at each event once the safety of the child was assured. In our cohort, glucose values were obtained >98% of the time. This information was subsequently reviewed by the clinician and, if validated, was recorded on the data collection form. The physician reviewed the history of the event, the glucose recording and its timing, and the recovery history before judging the event to be hypoglycemia related. In addition to the logbooks, most families phoned the diabetes management team to receive advice on event management after a hypoglycemic event of this severity. These calls were recorded. We note that there was a close correlation between recall at the clinic through logbooks and calls to the diabetes team, providing further evidence that recall was accurate over this time period.

Definition of recurrent hypoglycemia
Recurrent hypoglycemia was defined as the occurrence of ≥2 episodes of severe hypoglycemia in the preceding year.

Laboratory measurements
A1C was measured at each 3-month visit. A1C was assessed by an agglutination inhibition immunoassay (Ames DCA 2000; Bayer, Mishawaka, IN). The inter- and intra-assay coefficients of variation were 2.5 and 2.3%, respectively.

Statistical analysis
Clinical characteristics of the study groups were compared using Student's t test (mean ± SD) for variables normally distributed and the Mann-Whitney U test (median ± SD [interquartile range]) for those with a nonnormal distribution.

RESULTS — A total of 656 patients and/or care providers (317 male and 339 female) completed the questionnaire over a 6-month period. During this period, there were 829 patients attending the clinic, giving a case ascertainment of 79%. Mean ± SD age was 12.8 ± 4.0 years with A1C of 8.5 ± 1.0% since diagnosis and 8.1 ± 1.4% at the last visit. During the 12 months before the questionnaire visit, data were collected at each 3-month visit. The patients had to have had at least three visits in the preceding 12 months to be included. Of all subjects, the mean number of visits was 3.7 in the previous

year, and 92% of patients had 4 visits recorded.

The clinical characteristics of the cohort with impaired and normal awareness are shown in Table 1. Impaired awareness of hypoglycemia was present in 29% of patients. No differences were observed in sex or diabetes duration; however, patients with impaired hypoglycemia awareness had an earlier onset of diabetes ($P < 0.001$), were younger ($P < 0.001$), and had lower levels of mean A1C since diabetes onset and at their last visit ($P = 0.006$ and $P = 0.001$, respectively). Among patients aged <6 years ($n = 46$), 19 patients (41%) and 27 patients (59%) were observed in the group with impaired and normal awareness, respectively ($P < 0.001$). There was no difference observed in hypoglycemia awareness scores between patients receiving injections compared with those receiving continuous subcutaneous insulin infusion therapy.

In the preceding year, a total of 161 episodes of severe hypoglycemia were recorded among all patients, giving an overall incidence of 24.5 episodes/100 patient-years. This rate was significantly higher among patients reporting impaired hypoglycemia awareness (37.1 vs. 19.3 episodes per 100 patient-years, $P < 0.001$). Among patients aged <6 years, the rate of severe hypoglycemia was significantly higher in those with reported impaired awareness (33.3 vs. 52 episodes per 100 patient-years, $P = 0.02$).

Table 2 summarizes the clinical features of patients with recurrent and nonrecurrent hypoglycemia in the preceding year. Thirty-eight patients had recurrent hypoglycemia with no differences in sex, age of onset, diabetes duration, or A1C between the recurrent and nonrecurrent groups. More patients with recurrent hypoglycemia reported impaired awareness of hypoglycemia (47% vs. 28%, $P = 0.03$). As expected, the rate of severe hypoglycemia was much higher in the recurrent group (252.6 vs. 10.5 episodes per 100 patient-years).

Table 3 demonstrates the findings in patients with diabetes duration >5 years compared with those with diabetes duration <5 years. In the group with diabetes for >5 years, higher levels of mean A1C since diabetes onset were observed ($P < 0.001$). Even with this higher A1C, a higher rate of severe hypoglycemia (32.6 vs. 17.8 episodes per 100 patient years, $P < 0.001$) occurred among those with a diabetes duration of >5 years; however,

Table 1—*Characteristics of children and adolescents with type 1 diabetes with normal and impaired hypoglycemia awareness*

	Total	Normal awareness	Impaired awareness	P
n (%)	656	465 (71)	191 (29)	
Sex (male/female)	317/339	221/244	96/95	NS
Age at diagnosis (years)	7.4 ± 4.0	8.0 ± 4.0	5.9 ± 3.8	<0.001
Age at questionnaire (years)	12.8 ± 4.0	13.5 ± 3.6	11.0 ± 4.4	<0.001
Duration of diabetes (years)	5.4 ± 3.9	5.5 ± 3.9	5.2 ± 3.8	NS
A1C (%) since diagnosis	8.5 ± 1.0	8.6 ± 1.0	8.3 ± 1.0	0.006
A1C (%) at last visit	8.1 ± 1.4	8.2 ± 1.4	7.8 ± 1.2	0.001
Severe hypoglycemia: episodes in preceding year	161	90	71	
Rate of severe hypoglycemia (episodes/100 patient-years)	24.5	19.3	37.1	<0.001
Patients, age ≤6 years, n = 46 (%)	46	41	59	<0.001
Rate of severe hypoglycemia in patients aged ≤6 years (episodes/100 patient-years)	21.7	5.2	33.3	0.02

Data are means ± SD unless indicated otherwise.

no differences in hypoglycemia awareness were observed between the groups.

CONCLUSIONS — In this study, impaired hypoglycemia awareness assessed by a validated, self-reporting questionnaire was reported in 29% of children and adolescents. Overall, the rate of severe hypoglycemia was almost double in the group with impaired awareness. This was even more prominent in children aged <6 years with a 6-fold increase in the rate of severe hypoglycemia in the group with impaired awareness, as observed by care providers. Care providers of children in this age-group have difficulty recognizing hypoglycemia in their children. This group of care providers reported a change in the pattern of symptoms associated with hypoglycemia in their children. These results suggest that in children as well as adults, screening for impaired awareness of hypoglycemia is an impor-

tant component of routine diabetes care and can help identify patients at increased risk of having a severe hypoglycemic event.

Our rates of impaired awareness of hypoglycemia are consistent with those in a previous study reported by Barkai et al. (13). In this prospective study of 130 children and adolescents with type 1 diabetes, impaired awareness was reported by 37% of patients. Patients with impaired awareness had a much greater frequency of hypoglycemia-related coma or seizure (14.6 vs. 1.2 episodes per 100 patient-years), and their overall incidence of hypoglycemia-related coma or seizure was 6.2 per 100 patient-years (13). Clearly, despite changes in insulin therapy in the last decade, hypoglycemia unawareness remains common.

Our results are also consistent with several recent studies in adults with type 1 diabetes. The prevalence of impaired

awareness is similar to that in adults despite a shorter duration of diabetes in children. There are also differences in treatment regimens and counterregulatory hormone and symptom responses to hypoglycemia (14–16). Geddes et al. (17) reported the prevalence of impaired awareness of hypoglycemia in ~20% of a large, unselected adult population with type 1 diabetes. These patients also had a 6-fold increase in the frequency of severe hypoglycemia in the preceding year. Similar rates of prevalence of impaired awareness and the association with severe hypoglycemia in adults have been reported by others (18).

Hypoglycemia unawareness has been extensively studied in adult patients. In both adults and adolescents, it is associated with defective counterregulatory hormone response, also known as hypoglycemia-associated autonomic failure (19). In this present study, we found that more children with recurrent hypoglycemia reported impaired awareness of hypoglycemia. This finding is not surprising given that even short, prior exposure to hypoglycemia can reduce the magnitude of epinephrine and other counterregulatory hormone responses as well as the autonomic symptom responses to a subsequent hypoglycemic episode (20). This shifts the glycemic threshold for these responses to a lower level of plasma glucose, which further increases the risk of subsequent severe hypoglycemic episodes. Hypoglycemia is more frequent in the young (21), which may explain the higher frequency of impaired awareness in children and adolescents. In adults, hypoglycemia unawareness is often associated with older age and longer duration of diabetes

Table 2—*Characteristics of children and adolescents with type 1 diabetes with recurrent and nonrecurrent hypoglycemia in the previous year*

	Recurrent hypoglycemia	Nonrecurrent hypoglycemia	P
n (%)	38 (6)	618 (94)	
Sex (male/female)	26/12	291/327	NS
Age at diagnosis (years)	6.6 ± 3.6	7.4 ± 4.1	NS
Age at questionnaire (years)	12.8 ± 4.1	12.8 ± 4.0	NS
Duration of diabetes (years)	6.2 ± 3.6	5.4 ± 3.9	NS
A1C (%) since diagnosis	8.5 ± 0.9	8.5 ± 1.0	NS
Severe hypoglycemia: episodes in preceding year	96	65	
Rate of severe hypoglycemia (episodes/100 patient-years)	252.6	10.5	<0.01
Impaired awareness of hypoglycemia (%)	47	28	0.031

Data are means ± SD unless indicated otherwise.

Table 3—*Characteristics of children and adolescents with duration of diabetes of >5 and <5 years*

	Duration <5 years	Duration >5 years	P
n (%)	359/656 (55)	297/656 (45)	
Sex (male/female)	182/177	135/162	NS
Age at diagnosis (years)	9.1 ± 4.2	5.4 ± 3.1	<0.001
Age at questionnaire (years)	11.7 ± 4.2	15.0 ± 3.0	<0.001
Duration of diabetes (years)	2.5 ± 1.4	8.4 ± 2.9	<0.001
A1C (%) since diagnosis	8.20 ± 1.0	8.8 ± 1.0	<0.001
Severe hypoglycemia: episodes in preceding year	64	97	
Rate of severe hypoglycemia (episodes/ 100 patient-years)	17.8	32.6	<0.001
Impaired awareness of hypoglycemia (%)	31	27	NS

Results expressed in mean ± SD unless otherwise indicated.

(17,22). In our study, however, patients with a duration of diabetes >5 years did not have higher rates of impaired hypoglycemia awareness compared with patients with a duration of <5 years.

Impaired hypoglycemia awareness is clearly a significant problem for children and adolescents with type 1 diabetes, and these children have a greater risk of having a hypoglycemia-related coma or seizure. This risk adds to the considerable burden of disease for families. There is evidence, however, that in adults with hypoglycemia unawareness, this phenomenon can be reversed by meticulously avoiding hypoglycemia for 2–3 weeks (23,24), although this is difficult to accomplish in young children. It is likely that the pathophysiology of the genesis of hypoglycemia unawareness and its associated counterregulatory hormone deficit is similar in the young to that in adults because attempts to restore responses by strictly avoiding hypoglycemia, at least in preliminary studies, appear to be successful (25).

Acknowledgments— This work was supported by a Juvenile Diabetes Research Foundation/National Health and Medical Research Council Special Program Grant.

No potential conflicts of interest relevant to this article were reported.

We thank the families and children of Princess Margaret Hospital Diabetes Clinic for participating in this study.

References

1. Cryer PE. Hypoglycaemia: the limiting factor in the glycaemic management of type I and type II diabetes. Diabetologia 2002;45:937–948
2. Diabetes Control and Complications Trial Research Group. The effect of intensive treatment of diabetes on the development and progression of long-term complications in insulin-dependent diabetes mellitus. N Engl J Med 1993;329:977–986
3. Rovet JF, Ehrlich RM, Czuchta D. Intellectual characteristics of diabetic children at diagnosis and one year later. J Pediatr Psychol 1990;15:775–788
4. Ryan C, Vega A, Drash A. Cognitive deficits in adolescents who developed diabetes early in life. Pediatrics 1985;75:921–927
5. Northam EA, Anderson PJ, Jacobs R, et al. Neuropsychological profiles of children with type 1 diabetes 6 years after disease onset. Diabetes Care 2001;24:1541–1546
6. Ho MS, Weller NJ, Ives FJ, et al. Prevalence of structural central nervous system abnormalities in early-onset type 1 diabetes mellitus. J Pediatr 2008;153:385–390
7. Tupola S, Rajantie J, Akerblom HK. Experience of severe hypoglycaemia may influence both patient's and physician's subsequent treatment policy of insulin-dependent diabetes mellitus. Eur J Pediatr 1998;157:625–627
8. Bulsara MK, Holman CD, van Bockxmeer FM, et al. The relationship between ACE genotype and risk of severe hypoglycaemia in a large population-based cohort of children and adolescents with type 1 diabetes. Diabetologia 2007;50:965–971
9. Davis EA, Keating B, Byrne GC, et al. Hypoglycemia: incidence and clinical predictors in a large population-based sample of children and adolescents with IDDM. Diabetes Care 1997;20:22–25
10. Clarke WL, Cox DJ, Gonder-Frederick LA, et al. Reduced awareness of hypoglycemia in adults with IDDM: a prospective study of hypoglycemic frequency and as-sociated symptoms. Diabetes Care 1995; 18:517–522
11. Geddes J, Wright RJ, Zammitt NN, et al. An evaluation of methods of assessing impaired awareness of hypoglycemia in type 1 diabetes. Diabetes Care 2007;30:1868–1870
12. Bulsara MK, Holman CD, Davis EA, et al. The impact of a decade of changing treatment on rates of severe hypoglycemia in a population-based cohort of children with type 1 diabetes. Diabetes Care 2004;27:2293–2298
13. Barkai L, Vamosi I, Lukacs K. Prospective assessment of severe hypoglycaemia in diabetic children and adolescents with impaired and normal awareness of hypoglycaemia. Diabetologia 1998;41:898–903
14. McCrimmon RJ, Gold AE, Deary IJ, et al. Symptoms of hypoglycemia in children with IDDM. Diabetes Care 1995;18:858–861
15. Amiel SA, Simonson DC, Sherwin RS, et al. Exaggerated epinephrine responses to hypoglycemia in normal and insulin-dependent diabetic children. J Pediatr 1987;110:832–837
16. Jones TW, Boulware SD, Kraemer DT, et al. Independent effects of youth and poor diabetes control on responses to hypoglycemia in children. Diabetes 1991;40:358–363
17. Geddes J, Schopman JE, Zammitt NN, et al. Prevalence of impaired awareness of hypoglycaemia in adults with type 1 diabetes. Diabet Med 2008;25:501–504
18. ter Braak EWMT, Appelman AMMF, van de Laak MF, et al. Clinical characteristics of type 1 diabetic patients with and without severe hypoglycemia. Diabetes Care 2000;23:1467–1471
19. Cryer PE. Mechanisms of hypoglycemia-associated autonomic failure and its component syndromes in diabetes. Diabetes 2005;54:3592–3601
20. Ovalle F, Fanelli CG, Paramore DS, et al. Brief twice-weekly episodes of hypoglycemia reduce detection of clinical hypoglycemia in type 1 diabetes mellitus. Diabetes 1998;47:1472–1479
21. Diabetes Control and Complications Trial Research Group. Effect of intensive diabetes treatment on the development and progression of long-term complications in adolescents with insulin-dependent diabetes mellitus: Diabetes Control and Complications Trial. J Pediatr 1994;125:177–188
22. Hepburn DA, Patrick AW, Eadington DW, et al. Unawareness of hypoglycaemia in insulin-treated diabetic patients: prevalence and relationship to autonomic neuropathy. Diabet Med 1990;7:711–717
23. Cranston I, Lomas J, Maran A, et al. Restoration of hypoglycaemia awareness in patients with long-duration insulin-de-

pendent diabetes. Lancet 1994;344:283–287

24. Fanelli C, Pampanelli S, Epifano L, et al. Long-term recovery from unawareness, deficient counterregulation and lack of cognitive dysfunction during hypoglycae-mia, following institution of rational, intensive insulin therapy in IDDM. Diabetologia 1994;37:1265–1276

25. Ly T, Hewitt J, Kendall J, et al. The use of real-time continuous glucose monitoring to correct hypoglycaemia unawareness in adolescents: initial data from a random-ised trial (Abstract). In *Proceedings of the APEG Annual Scientific Meeting, Canberra, Australia,* 2008. Morisset, NSW, Austra-lia, Australasian Paediatric Endocrine Group

Glucose Sensing During Hypoglycemia: Lessons From the Lab

Shortly after the introduction of insulin in the management of type 1 diabetes, clinicians became aware of the potential for insulin therapy to induce iatrogenic hypoglycemia. Hypoglycemia remains the major adverse effect of insulin therapy and has emerged as a significant limitation to achieving near-normal glucose control, which is required to reduce the risk of microvascular complications. The average individual with type 1 diabetes experiences around two episodes of symptomatic hypoglycemia per week. In the recent U.K. Hypoglycemia Study (1), the incidence of severe hypoglycemia (requiring external assistance) was 110 episodes per 100 patient-years in subjects with duration of diabetes <5 years and 320 episodes per 100 patient-years in subjects with duration of diabetes >15 years. Thus, despite the introduction of insulin analogues and improved delivery systems, hypoglycemia remains a major concern for individuals with type 1 and long-duration type 2 diabetes as well as their caregivers.

When glucose levels fall, a sequence of counterregulatory responses is triggered, which mainly involves the suppression of endogenous insulin secretion and the release of counterregulatory hormones that act rapidly to promote endogenous glucose production and limit peripheral glucose utilization. As glucose levels fall further, subjective awareness of hypoglycemia results in behavioral changes that ordinarily lead an individual to seek food. In healthy individuals, this homeostatic mechanism works well and hypoglycemia is rare, but for individuals with type 1 diabetes, these compensatory systems are disrupted at every level. First, for most individuals insulin delivery to the systemic circulation following a subcutaneous injection will continue despite the development of hypoglycemia. Second, almost all individuals with type 1 diabetes will over time develop defects in the hormonal counterregulatory defense against hypoglycemia. Within 5 years of diagnosis of type 1 diabetes, hypoglycemia fails to stimulate release of the major counterregulatory hormone glucagon (2). As a result, individuals with type 1 diabetes are particularly dependent on the sympathoadrenal (primarily epinephrine and norepinephrine) response to low blood glucose. However, within 10 years of diagnosis, the majority of patients develop additional impairments in sympathoadrenal and other neurohormonal responses against hypoglycemia (2). In addition, symptom awareness becomes impaired in individuals with type 1 diabetes. This combination of disrupted physiological and behavioral responses to hypoglycemia markedly increases the risk of suffering severe hypoglycemia in patients with type 1 diabetes.

To understand why glucose counterregulation is impaired in diabetes requires a greater knowledge of where and how hypoglycemia is sensed, how hypoglycemia-sensitive cells trigger a counterregulatory response, and how the presence of diabetes influences these mechanisms. Research in this area has in recent years focused on animal and more basic models, although the groundwork for this was laid by a series of elegant human studies in the 1980s and 1990s. In this review, I will examine the literature, largely based on rodent studies, that is beginning to shed some light on the mechanisms that underpin hypoglycemia detection. This review will focus on the role of the ventromedial hypothalamus (VMH) (Fig. 1), a key central glucose-sensing region involved in the detection of hypoglycemia, to illustrate the advances that have been made in this field of research.

The hypoglycemia sensors

Under most physiological conditions glucose is the primary fuel for the brain. The brain accounts for more than half the body's glucose use and because fuel stores such as glycogen are limited, it is very dependent on a continuous supply from the circulation. This probably explains why the glucose sensors thought to be dominant during hypoglycemia are found in the brain. Neurons shown to be regulated by glucose have been found in a number of brain areas that share certain common features (3). Within the brain they localize to regions adjacent to the III or IV ventricle or to the circumventricular organs (these are regions of the brain where the blood-brain barrier is leaky or absent). This potentially allows glucose sensing neurons direct sampling and, hence, monitoring of glucose levels in the blood, brain, and cerebrospinal flid. This is important because the presence of the blood-brain barrier ensures that brain glucose levels are only ~10–30% of the levels seen in the blood (4). Thus, glucose-sensing neurons are able to integrate changes in glucose within each of these different regions.

The VMH was shown to play a significant role in the detection of insulin-induced hypoglycemia in a series of in vivo rodent studies in the 1990s. Borg et al. (5) were able to demonstrate that chemical destruction of the VMH in a rodent model with ibotenic acid caused ~75% reduction in the hormonal counterregulatory response to acute hypoglycemia. Subsequently, they showed that the local perfusion, using microdialysis in awake unrestrained rats, of the VMH with 2-deoxyglucose (a nonmetabolizable form of glucose that effectively causes local hypoglycemia) stimulated a classic systemic counterregulatory response (6). Finally, and perhaps most convincingly, they demonstrated again with microdialysis that local perfusion of the VMH with glucose, maintaining glucose levels in this select brain region during systemic insulin-induced hypoglycemia, markedly suppressed the hormonal counterregulatory response (7). The addition of tracer to the perfusate (6), as well as the lesion studies (5), confirmed that the intervention in these studies was local to the VMH. In addition, a number of electrophysiological studies from hypothalamic slice preparations have shown that the VMH contains neurons that respond directly to low glucose (8), as do dissociated VMH neurons (9). Finally, transgenic mice that lack the vesicular glutamate transporter VGLuT2 selectively in steroidogenic factor-1 (SF1) neurons, which in rodents are only expressed in the VMH, show markedly impaired counterregulatory hormonal responses to acute insulin-induced hypoglycemia (10). Taken together these studies all point toward the VMH playing

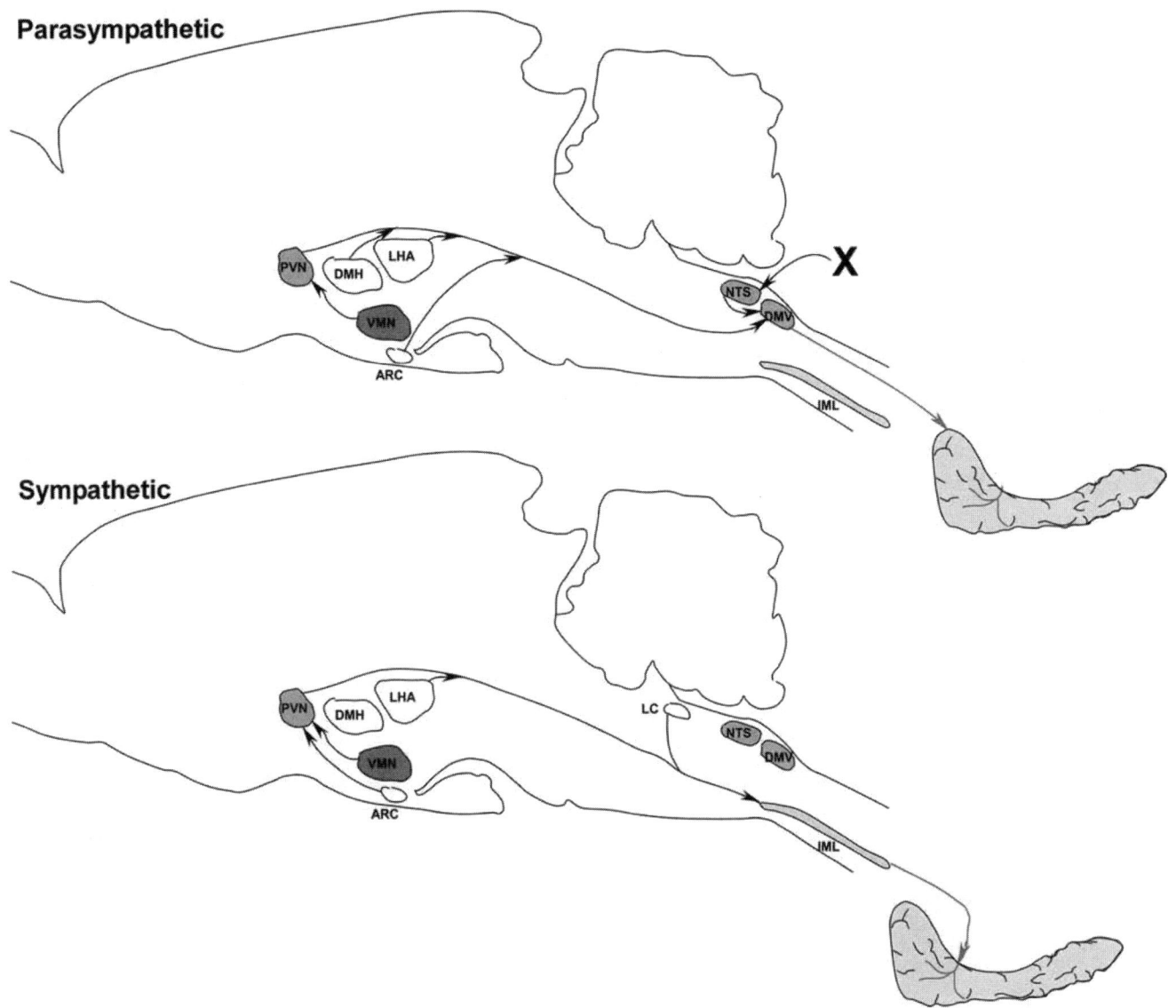

Figure 1—*Neural pathways linking the VMH via sympathetic and parasympathetic neurons to the pancreas. Retrograde neuronal tracer studies using pseudorabies virus microinjected into the pancreas of the rats established the VMH as a third-order neuron reaching the parasympathetic and sympathetic innervation of the pancreas via the paraventricular hypothalamic nucleus (PVN) and interomediolateral (IML) nucleus as well as the dorsal motor nucleus of the vagus (DMV), respectively. The dorsomedial hypothalamus (DMH) and lateral hypothalamus (LHA) also feed into this pathway as well as the nucleus tractus solitarius (NTS) in the hindbrain, each of which plays a role on glucose sensing. The nucleus tractus solitarius also is the likely point of integration of inputs from peripheral sensors via vagal afferents (X). Reprinted with permission from Buijs et al. (11).*

an important role in the mechanism by which the brain detects a falling glucose and triggers a counterregulatory hormone response.

For normal glucagon and epinephrine counterregulation to occur, neural pathways must exist between the glucose-sensing regions of the brain such as the VMH and the pancreatic α-cell and adrenal medulla, respectively. These pathways have not yet been fully elucidated. However, using pseudorabies virus as a retrograde tracer, Buijs et al. (11) were able to characterize sympathetic and parasympathetic inputs to the pancreas.

In this neuroanatomical study, the VMH was identified as a third-order neuron (the last of three neurons in a pathway that ultimately leads to the discharge of a neurotransmitter into the synaptic cleft) innervating the pancreas by way of other nuclei in the hypothalamus and thalamus and, subsequently, the dorsal motor nucleus of the vagus (parasympathetic) and intermediolateral cell column (sympathetic) (Fig. 1). These studies provide a potential neural pathway through which VMH glucose-sensing neurons could initiate glucose counterregulation during hypoglycemia, although why, given the

major role that the VMH appears to play in coordinating the counterregulatory response in vivo, this should be an indirect one is not clear. It should also be pointed out that if the VMH is not a primary sensing region but rather an important relay station for other brain regions, then this pathway may be even more indirect.

Glucose-sensing neurons are not unique to the brain and have also been identified in the intestine, hepatoportal vein, and carotid body as well as the classic glucose sensor the pancreatic β-cell (3). The hepato-portal glucose sensor in particular appears to play a significant role when glucose levels fall slowly (12) and links to central glucose sensors via capsaicin-sensitive sensory neurons (13). It is interesting to speculate whether both central and peripheral sensors may form a neural network of glucose-sensing cells designed to monitor and maintain glucose homeostasis. Certainly, evidence of presynaptic regulation of VMH glucose-sensing neurons by glucose-sensing neurons in other brain regions has been demonstrated (14). Moreover, and particularly in the brain, glucose-sensing neurons are generally located in areas involved in the control of the autonomic nervous system, neuroendocrine function, nutrient metabolism, and energy homeostasis. What this effectively means is that brain glucose-sensing neurons are able to receive inputs from blood nutrient levels, a variety of endocrine hormones, as well as from numerous peripheral and central sensory systems.

Mechanisms of glucose sensing

The defining feature of a glucose-sensing neuron is that it can use glucose not simply as a fuel but as a signaling molecule that regulates its activity. Such specialized neurons were first demonstrated by Oomura et al. (15) in 1969. These neurons are glucose sensing in so far as glucose is the major metabolic substrate for the brain, but the fact that these neurons can use other fuels such as lactate produced either by astrocytes (16) or delivered locally (17) to alter their function suggests that it is more likely glucose oxidation–derived intracellular ATP that determines the activity of these neurons. This is intriguing because neuronal levels of ATP are generally thought to be well maintained, which means that there would need to be subcellular compartmentalization of the glucose-sensing apparatus to provide sensing capability. Such compartmentalization has been shown within pancreatic β-cells (18).

The VMH, like other central glucose-sensing regions, has been shown to contain neurons whose activity is altered in response to changes of glucose within the physiological range. Two predominant subtypes of glucose-sensing neurons have been identified: namely, glucose-excited (GE) neurons whose activity increases as glucose levels rise and glucose-inhibited (GI) neurons whose activity decreases as glucose levels rise (8). The prevailing theory in the field at the moment is that these neurons use sensing mechanisms very similar to those found in the pancreatic β-

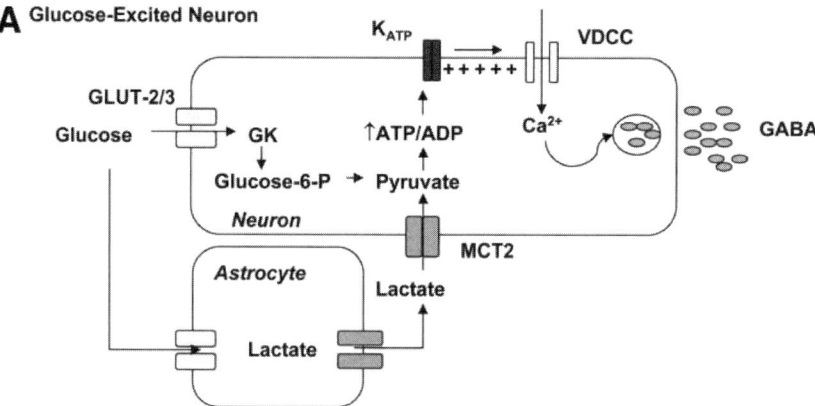

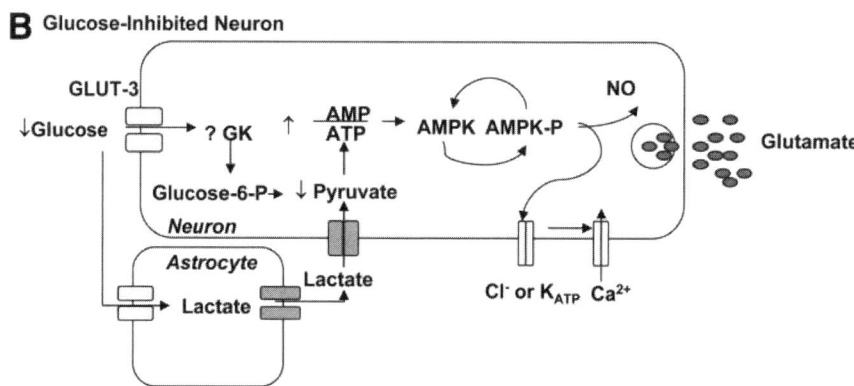

Figure 2—*Hypothetical sensing mechanism of GE (A) and GI (B) neurons. Glucose enters the GE neuron through GLUT2 or GLUT3 and is phosphorylated by glucokinase, acting as the gatekeeper and regulating the production of cytosolic ATP in a subcellular compartment. The ATP closes K_{ATP} channels in the plasma membrane causing depolarization. In turn, this leads to Ca^{2+} influx through voltage-dependent calcium channels (VDCC), stimulating neurotransmitter release and/or increased action potential frequency. Lactate, produced locally by astrocytes or arriving systemically, enters the neuron via monocarboxylate transporter-2 (MCT2) and can then be metabolized to form ATP. In GI neurons, glucokinase may once again act as the gatekeeper. A falling glucose results in an increase in the AMP:ATP ratio activating AMPK and stimulates the formation of NO, which may diffuse out to adjacent glial cells or act as a neurotransmitter. In addition, AMPK may act on chloride (Cl) channels leading to neuronal depolarization and neurotransmitter release and/or increased action potential frequency.*

and α-cells (19). In this paradigm, the GE neuron is analogous to the pancreatic β-cell whereas the GI neuron behaves like the α-cell (Fig. 2).

The VMH β-cell

Insulin secretion from the pancreatic β-cell follows membrane depolarization, which in turn is a response to a rise in glucose within the islet. Key steps in this process are though to be *1*) entry of glucose into the β-cell via the high-capacity GLUT (GLUT2) to allow rapid equilibration of extracellular and cytosolic glucose; *2*) phosphorylation of glucose by the low-affinity hexokinase, glucokinase, linking changes in extracellular glucose with proportional changes in the cytosolic ATP:ADP ratio; and *3*) closure of ATP-sensitive K^+ channel (K_{ATP}) in the plasma membrane of metabolism that leads to depolarization and increased electrical activity. There is some support for this mechanism being resent in VMH GE neurons. GLUT2, glucokinase, and the Kir6.2 subunit of the K_{ATP} channel are expressed in some but not all VMH GE neurons (9). Electrophysiological studies suggest glucokinase plays a regulatory role in VMH GE neuron sensing ability (20), whereas selective downregulation of glucokinase in primary VMH neuronal cultures led to the loss of all demonstrable glucose-sensing activity (21). In addition, in vivo microinjection of glucokinase activators or selective downregulation of VMH glucokinase modifies the counterregulatory response to acute hypoglycemia (22).

Similarly, K_{ATP} channels have been demonstrated throughout the brain, including hypothalamic regions thought to be involved in glucose sensing (23). Using single-cell RT-PCR to analyze glucose-sensing neurons (identified electrophysiologically in a hypothalamic slice preparation), investigators have shown they express mRNA for Kir6.2 and sulfonurea receptor-1 (SUR1), the two subunits that comprise the K_{ATP} channel in the pancreatic β-cell (9). In addition, electrophysiological studies in rat (20,24) and mouse (25) VMH have demonstrated that sulfonylureas (agents that block the K_{ATP} channel) can alter the response of GE neurons to changes in ambient glucose, and Kir6.2 knockout mice show impaired glucose counterregulation to systemic hypoglycemia (25). Finally, in vivo perfusion of VMH of rodents with glibenclamide (a K_{ATP} channel blocker) suppresses (26) whereas diazoxide (a K_{ATP} channel opener) amplifies (27) hormonal counterregulatory responses to acute hypoglycemia.

These studies provide support for the β-cell model, but inconsistencies in the literature are apparent that mean this hypothesis is not yet established. For instance, extracellular levels of glucose in the brain are only about 10–30% of the levels found in blood. Microdialysis studies in rats (4,28) and human subjects (29) have shown that the extracelullar fluid (ECF) glucose levels to which neurons are exposed are in the range of 1–2 mmol/l under basal conditions and fall markedly during acute hypoglycemia (~0.5 mmol/l) (30). This means that during hypoglycemia, brain ECF glucose levels are well beneath the range in which glucokinase or GLUT2 usually act in a regulatory manner. In addition, using genetically targeted luciferases to monitor cytosolic ATP, Ainscow et al. (31) were unable to detect a rise in ATP during exposure of hypothalamic neurons to a high glucose, although they were able to see increased cytosolic ATP in β-cells, hypothalamic astroglia, and cerebeller neurons. Interestingly, transgenic mice that express GLUT2 only in astroglial cells in the central nervous system are rescued from the defect in counterregulation seen in whole body GLUT2$^{-/-}$ mice (32), raising the intriguing possibility that astroglial cells might function as detectors of extracellular glucose change. Tanycytes, which are specialized glial cells that line the dorsal lateral, ventral lateral, and floor of the third ventricle express GLUT2; glucokinase; and the K_{ATP} channel send long processes that terminate in the VMH (33).

Burdakov et al. (34) have proposed two further possibilities through which glucose might activate glucose-sensing neurons that do not involve the metabolism of glucose. In the first, glucose transport is coupled directly with the transmembrane movement of ions, such as those used by sodium-glucose cotransporters (SGLTs). In this way, an inward current is generated while glucose is transported into the neuron, and this leads to depolarization and increased excitability. Phloridizin, a nonselective inhibitor of SGLTs, inhibits glucose-induced excitation of VMH neurons (20). Alternatively, glucose might bind to an extracellular receptor that could alter electrical activity without transporting the glucose into the neuron (34). Recently, such a mechanism has been demonstrated in GI orexigenic neurons in the lateral hypothalamus (35).

Once a change in glucose is sensed by the GE neuron, it needs to then communicate that signal to a downstream neuron in the pathway that leads eventually to glucose counterregulation. In general, neural communication relies on the release of classic neurotransmitters such as GABA, neuropeptides, or unconventional transmitters such as nitric oxide (NO). No definitive transmitter has been identified for GE neurons; it is very possible that a number of transmitters and peptides are important, but most current data support a role for the inhibitory neurotransmitter GABA. GAD, the rate-limiting enzyme in GABA synthesis, is expressed in 56% of GE and 36% of GI neurons (9). In vivo antagonism of the VMH GABA receptor amplifies the counterregulatory hormone response to acute hypoglycemia (36), and VMH GABA release is regulated by K_{ATP} channel modulation (37). Finally, GABA tone in the VMH is increased following recurrent hypoglycemia (38).

The VMH α-cell
GI neurons show a decrease in activity as glucose levels rise (8). It is perhaps easier to think of GI neurons as those glucose-sensing neurons that become more active when glucose levels fall, and as such they may use signaling mechanisms more relevant to the pancreatic α-cell. Unfortunately, like the α-cell, the signaling pathways used by the GI neuron are not well understood. This may reflect the fact that they appear to be few in number, comprising only 3–14% of neurons in the VMH nucleus (14,39). Although recent evidence suggests GI neurons may be more prev-

alent, when improved slice techniques are used in conjunction with novel methods for identifying GI neurons (e.g., membrane potential dyes) as many as ~30–40% of all neurons in the VMH are reported to be GI neurons (40).

Current evidence favors a role for AMP-activated protein kinase (AMPK) in the sensing pathway used by GI neurons. AMPK has been described as an intracellular fuel gauge in that it is activated in response to a rise in the intracellular ratio of AMP:ATP and acts to switch off energy-consuming anabolic processes and switch on energy-producing catabolic processes (41). Canabal et al. (40) demonstrated that in VMH GI neurons exposed to 2.5 mmol/l glucose, AICAR (an activator of AMPK) mimicked the excitatory effect of low glucose (0.5 mmol/l) on action potential frequency. Both low glucose and AICAR were shown to mediate their effects, in part, through an increase in NO production in GI neurons. Conversely, increased NO production in response to low glucose was blocked by compound C, an inhibitor of AMPK (40). In a related series of studies, Mountjoy et al. (42) reported that activation of AMPK with AICAR or inhibition with compound C altered neuronal activity in GI but not GE neurons in an ex vivo hypothalamic cell culture system obtained from the medio-basal (including VMH and Arc) hypothalamus. In this study, AMPK had no effect on the K_{ATP} channel (42), but others have suggested AMPK may instead act on a chloride channel to depolarize the plasma membrane (43). In rodent studies, in vivo pharmacological activation of AMPK in the VMH during acute hypoglycemia amplifies the glucose counterregulatory response in normal Sprague-Dawley rats (44) and restores the hormonal counterregulatory response to hypoglycemia in rats with defective counterregulation (45). Conversely, downregulation of AMPK in the VMH using specific RNA interference suppresses the counterregulatory response to acute hypoglycemia (46). In addition, mice that selectively lack the α-catalytic subunit of AMPK in proopiomelanocortin or agouti gene–related protein neurons (both neuronal types are located in the medio-basal hypothalamus and are involved in feeding behavior and energy homeostasis) lose the responsiveness of these neurons to changes in extracellular glucose (47).

As in the GE neuron, the mode of neurotransmission in GI neurons has yet to be established. Local administration of norepinephrine to the hypothalamus increases circulating glucose and counterregulatory hormones, whereas norepinephrine receptor antagonists block the counterregulatory response to 2-deoxyglucose (DG) (48). Glucoprivation induced through 2-DG (49) or insulin (50) increases VMH norepinephrine levels, whereas local perfusion of the VMH with glucose during systemic hypoglycemia prevents the local increase in norepinephrine (51). Intriguingly, terminals from noradrenergic neurons form a shell around the VMH, implying that the detection of hypoglycemia by these neurons takes place at a site distant from the VMH. Brainstem norepinephrine cell groups, for instance, which respond to glucoprivation, project to the VMH and may ultimately form a neural circuit through which peripheral and hypothalamic glucose sensors integrate (52).

Additionally, a potential role for the excitatory transmitter glutamate recently has been revealed. Neurons in the VMH are largely glutaminergic and express high levels of the vesicular glutamate transporter VGLuT2. Mice lacking VGLuT2 selectively in steroidogenic factor-1 (a transcription factor unique to a population of VMH neurons) neurons show a markedly suppressed counterregulatory response to hyperinsulinemic hypoglycemia (10). These findings support a potential role for excitatory glutaminergic transmission in the output signal from VMH GI neurons. Finally, the unconventional transmitter NO may also play a role in GI neuron signaling (40).

Recurrent hypoglycemia and glucose sensing

Studies in rodent models suggest that recurrent hypoglycemia results in altered glucose sensing within the brain. Recurrent hypoglycemia lowers the glucose level at which activation of glucose-inhibited neurons in the VMH is initiated (53). Moreover, in vivo activation of AMPK in the VMH of rats that have experienced prior recurrent hypoglycemia can restore hormonal counterregulatory responses to a subsequent hypoglycemic challenge (45). Similarly, opening of K_{ATP} channels in the VMH of recurrently hypoglycemic rats leads to the restoration of normal counterregulatory responses to subsequent hypoglycemia (27).

There are a number of potential explanations for altered glucose sensing in the VMH following recurrent hypoglycemia. One possibility is that glucose sensing neurons are seeing higher glucose and/or ATP levels during a subsequent hypoglycemic challenge caused by an increased supply of fuel through altered glucose or alternate fuel transport. However, whereas these changes suggest an increased capacity to transport fuels across the blood-brain barrier and into glucose-sensing neurons, the data from human studies have been mixed with some indicating increased whole brain glucose, or acetate, uptake after chronic hypoglycemia and others showing no change (3). Alternatively, the VMH might obtain additional metabolic substrates from more local sources. Brain glycogen can act as a fuel reserve during acute hypoglycemia (54), and brain glycogen levels may actually increase in response to an acute episode of hypoglycemia (54). Glycogen supercompensation could provide an additional fuel reserve that leads to defective glucose sensing during a subsequent episode of hypoglycemia. However, brain glycogen levels appear to be very low and in rodents return to baseline levels within 24 h of a hypoglycemic episode (55).

It has also emerged that within the brain there exist mechanisms for regulating the magnitude of the neuroendocrine response to acute hypoglycemia. The corticotrophin-releasing hormone (CRH) family of ligands and receptors form an ancient and highly conserved means of regulating the neuroendocrine stress response. At key sites involved with autonomic activation within the brain, CRH acting through the CRH receptor (CRHr)-1 appears to lead to an amplification of the autonomic response to stress, whereas urocortin (part of the CRH family of peptides) acting through the CRHr2 receptor suppresses the autonomic response to stress (56). We recently were able to show that such a mechanism operated in the VMH with urocortin locally delivered to the VMH markedly suppressing the counterregulatory response to acute hypoglycemia (57), whereas CRH amplified the response (58). Thus, an alteration in the balance between those mechanisms that regulate the hypoglycemia stress response might contribute to the development of defective counterregulation.

If our model is correct, these studies suggest that the balance between GE and GI neuronal activity is altered by recurrent hypoglycemia. The important point here is that both the GE and GI neurons operate over a range of glucose values and therefore are not either on or off but rather the balance tips in favor of one or other population as the glucose levels fluctuate. We would anticipate that GE neurons (acting to suppress counterregulation) are more likely to be active and/or GI neurons (acting to amplify counterregulation) less likely to be active following recurrent hypoglycemia. Consistent with this hypothesis, there is increased GABAergic inhibitory tone (38) (hypothetically GE mediated) and reduced AMPK activity (59) (hypothetically GI mediated) in the VMH following recurrent hypoglycemia, the net effect being that full glucose counterregulation is initiated at a lower glucose level. This gives individuals less time to react to, and seek treatment for, hypoglycemia.

SUMMARY — Within the body a number of highly specialized regions sense alterations in glucose levels and, in the case of hypoglycemia, this leads to the generation of a glucose counterregulatory defense response. The VMH, discussed in detail in this article, reflects only one of a number of brain regions thought to be important in the detection of hypoglycemia, and together these brain regions may form an integrated neural network coordinating physiological and behavioral responses to a hypoglycemic challenge. Glucose-sensing neurons, by virtue of specific sensing systems, directly or indirectly translate the rate or quantity of glucose oxidation into a neural signal that alters neuronal firing rates. These neurons appear to use signaling mechanisms that parallel those used by pancreatic β- and α-cells. The GE neuron, more likely to operate under conditions of euglycemia or hyperglycemia, may use glucokinase as its key regulatory step and the K_{ATP} channel to then translate that signal into altered neuronal firing rates. In contrast, the GI neuron, active under hypoglycemic conditions, may be dependent on alterations in intracellular AMPK activity that, in turn, may act via NO to alter neuronal firing rates. Potentially, the counterbalance between GI and GE neuronal activity forms the most sensitive means of regulating and maintaining blood glucose within a narrow physiological range as well as ensuring an adequate supply of glucose to the brain. Recurrent exposure to hypoglycemia disturbs this relationship in a number of ways, which may include an increased capacity of glucose-sensing regions of the brain to use glucose and/or alternate fuels, as well as changes in both the mechanisms that sense glucose and those that fine-tune the hypoglycemic stress response, the net effect being to reduce the glucose level at which counterregulation is initiated.

RORY MCCRIMMON

From the Department of Internal Medicine, Yale University School of Medicine, New Haven, Connecticut.
Corresponding author: Rory J. McCrimmon, rory.mccrimmon@yale.edu.

Received 21 January 2009 and accepted 16 March 2009.
DOI: 10.2337/dc09-0123

Acknowledgments— This research was supported by a research grant from the National Institute of Diabetes and Digestive and Kidney Diseases (NIDDK) (69831) and the Juvenile Diabetes Research Foundation.

No potential conflicts of interest relevant to this article were reported.

The author acknowledges the postdoctoral fellows and technical staff who contributed greatly to the research that underpins this article.

● ●

References

1. UK Hypoglycaemia Study Group. Risk of hypoglycaemia in types 1 and 2 diabetes: effects of treatment modalities and their duration. Diabetologia 2007;50:1140-1147
2. Mokan M, Mitrakou A, Veneman T, Ryan C, Korytkowski M, Cryer P, Gerich J. Hypoglycemia unawareness in IDDM. Diabetes Care 1994;17:1397–1403
3. McCrimmon R. The mechanisms that underlie glucose sensing during hypoglycaemia in diabetes. Diabet Med 2008;25:513–522
4. McNay EC, Gold PE. Extracellular glucose concentrations in the rat hippocampus measured by zero-net-flux: effects of microdialysis flow rate, strain, and age (Letter). Journal of Neurochemistry 1999;72:785–790
5. Borg WP, During MJ, Sherwin RS, Borg MA, Brines ML, Shulman GI. Ventromedial hypothalamic lesions in rats suppress counterregulatory responses to hypoglycemia. J Clin Invest 1994;93:1677–1682
6. Borg WP, Sherwin RS, During MJ, Borg MA, Shulman GI. Local ventromedial hypothalamus glucopenia triggers counterregulatory hormone release. Diabetes 1995;44:180–184
7. Borg MA, Sherwin RS, Borg WP, Tamborlane WV, Shulman GI. Local ventromedial hypothalamus glucose perfusion blocks counterregulation during systemic hypoglycemia in awake rats. J Clin Invest 1997;99:361–365
8. Routh VH. Glucose-sensing neurons: are they physiologically relevant? Physiol Behav 2002;76:403–413
9. Kang L, Routh VH, Kuzhikandathil EV, Gaspers LD, Levin BE. Physiological and molecular characteristics of rat hypothalamic ventromedial nucleus glucosensing neurons. Diabetes 2004;53:549–559
10. Tong Q, Ye C, McCrimmon RJ, Dhillon H, Choi B, Kramer MD, Yu J, Yang Z, Christiansen LM, Lee CE, Choi CS, Zigman JM, Shulman GI, Sherwin RS, Elmquist JK, Lowell BB. Synaptic glutamate release by ventromedial hypothalamic neurons is part of the neurocircuitry that prevents hypoglycemia. Cell Metab 2007;5:383-393
11. Buijs RM, Chun SJ, Niijima A, Romijn HJ, Nagai K. Parasympathetic and sympathetic control of the pancreas: a role for the suprachiasmatic nucleus and other hypothalamic centers that are involved in the regulation of food intake. J Comp Neurol 2001;431:405–423
12. Saberi M, Bohland M, Donovan CM. The locus for hypoglycemic detection shifts with the rate of fall in glycemia: the role of portal-superior mesenteric vein glucose sensing. Diabetes 2008;57:1380–1386
13. Fujita S, Bohland M, Sanchez-Watts G, Watts AG, Donovan CM. Hypoglycemic detection at the portal vein is mediated by capsaicin-sensitive primary sensory neurons. Am J Physiol Endocrinol Metab 2007;293:E96–E101
14. Song Z, Levin BE, McArdle JJ, Bakhos N, Routh VH. Convergence of pre- and postsynaptic influences on glucosensing neurons in the ventromedial hypothalamic nucleus. Diabetes 2001;50:2673-2681
15. Oomura Y, Ono T, Ooyama H, Wayner MJ. Glucose and osmosensitive neurones of the rat hypothalamus. Nature 1969;222:282–284
16. Magistretti PJ, Sorg O, Naichen Y, Pellerin L, de Rham S, Martin JL. Regulation of astrocyte energy metabolism by neurotransmitters. Ren Physiol Biochem 1994;17:168–171
17. Borg MA, Tamborlane WV, Shulman GI, Sherwin RS. Local lactate perfusion of the ventromedial hypothalamus suppresses hypoglycemic counterregulation. Diabetes 2003;52:663–666
18. Kennedy HJ, Pouli AE, Ainscow EK, Jouaville LS, Rizzuto R, Rutter GA. Glucose generates sub-plasma membrane ATP microdomains in single islet beta-cells: potential role for strategically located mitochondria. J Biol Chem 1999;274:13281–13291
19. Sherwin RS. Bringing light to the dark side of insulin: a journey across the blood-brain barrier. Diabetes 2008;57:2259–2268
20. Yang XJ, Kow LM, Funabashi T, Mobbs CV. Hypothalamic glucose sensor: similarities to and differences from pancreatic β-cell mechanisms. Diabetes 1999;48:1763–1772
21. Kang L, Dunn-Meynell AA, Routh VH, Gaspers LD, Nagata Y, Nishimura T, Eiki J, Zhang BB, Levin BE. Glucokinase is a critical regulator of ventromedial hypothalamic neuronal glucosensing. Diabetes 2006;55:412–420 [erratum appears in Diabetes 2006;55:862]
22. Levin BE, Becker TC, Eiki J, Zhang BB, Dunn-Meynell AA. Ventromedial hypothalamic glucokinase is an important mediator of the counterregulatory response to insulin-induced hypoglycemia. Diabetes 2008;57:1371–1379
23. Ashford ML, Boden PR, Treherne JM. Glucose-induced excitation of hypothalamic neurones is mediated by ATP-sensitive K+ channels. Pflugers Arch 1990;415:479–483
24. Ashford ML, Boden PR, Treherne JM. Tolbutamide excites rat glucoreceptive ventromedial hypothalamic neurones by indirect inhibition of ATP-K+ channels. Br J Pharmacol 1990;101:531–540
25. Miki T, Liss B, Minami K, Shiuchi T, Saraya A, Kashima Y, Horiuchi M, Ashcroft F, Minokoshi Y, Roeper J, Seino S. ATP-sensitive K+ channels in the hypothalamus are essential for the maintenance of glucose homeostasis (Letter). Nat Neurosci 2001;4:507–512
26. Evans ML, McCrimmon RJ, Flanagan DE, Keshavarz T, Fan X, McNay EC, Jacob RJ, Sherwin RS. Hypothalamic ATP-sensitive K^+ channels play a key role in sensing hypoglycemia and triggering counterregulatory epinephrine and glucagon responses. Diabetes 2004;53:2542–2551
27. McCrimmon RJ, Evans ML, Fan X, McNay EC, Chan O, Ding Y, Zhu W, Gram DX, Sherwin RS. Activation of ATP-sensitive K^+ channels in the ventromedial hypothalamus amplifies counterregulatory hormone responses to hypoglycemia in normal and recurrently hypoglycemic rats. Diabetes 2005;54:3169–3174
28. McNay EC, Gold PE. Age-related differences in hippocampal extracellular fluid glucose concentration during behavioral testing and following systemic glucose administration. J Gerontol Series A Biol Sci Med Sci 2001;56:B66–B71
29. Abi-Saab WM, Maggs DG, Jones T, Jacob R, Srihari V, Thompson J, Kerr D, Leone P, Krystal JH, Spencer DD, During MJ, Sherwin RS. Striking differences in glucose and lactate levels between brain extracellular fluid and plasma in conscious human subjects: effects of hyperglycemia and hypoglycemia. J Cereb Blood Flow Metab 2002;22:271–279
30. de Vries MG, Arseneau LM, Lawson ME, Beverly JL. Extracellular glucose in rat ventromedial hypothalamus during acute and recurrent hypoglycemia. Diabetes 2003;52:2767–2773

31. Ainscow EK, Mirshamsi S, Tang T, Ashford ML, Rutter GA. Dynamic imaging of free cytosolic ATP concentration during fuel sensing by rat hypothalamic neurones: evidence for ATP-independent control of ATP-sensitive K(+) channels. J Physiol 2002;544:429–445

32. Marty N, Dallaporta M, Foretz M, Emery M, Tarussio D, Bady I, Binnert C, Beermann F, Thorens B. Regulation of glucagon secretion by glucose transporter type 2 (glut2) and astrocyte-dependent glucose sensors (Letter). J Clin Invest 2005; 115:3545–3553

33. Garcia MA, Millan C, Balmaceda-Aguilera C, Castro T, Pastor P, Montecinos H, Reinicke K, Zuniga F, Vera JC, Onate SA, Nualart F. Hypothalamic ependymal-glial cells express the glucose transporter GLUT2, a protein involved in glucose sensing. J Neurochem 2003;86:709–724

34. Burdakov D, Luckman SM, Verkhratsky A. Glucose-sensing neurons of the hypothalamus. Philos Trans R Soc Lond B Biol Sci 2005;360:2227–2235

35. Gonzalez JA, Jensen LT, Fugger L, Burdakov D. Metabolism-independent sugar sensing in central orexin neurons. Diabetes 2008;57:2569–2576

36. Chan O, Zhu W, Ding Y, McCrimmon RJ, Sherwin RS. Blockade of GABA$_A$ receptors in the ventromedial hypothalamus further stimulates glucagon and sympathoadrenal but not the hypothalamo-pituitary-adrenal response to hypoglycemia. Diabetes 2006; 55:1080–1087

37. Chan O, Lawson M, Zhu W, Beverly JL, Sherwin RS. ATP-sensitive K$^+$ channels regulate the release of GABA in the ventromedial hypothalamus during hypoglycemia. Diabetes 2007;56:1120–1126

38. Chan O, Cheng H, Herzog R, Czyzyk D, Zhu W, Wang A, McCrimmon RJ, Seashore MR, Sherwin RS. Increased GABAergic tone in the ventromedial hypothalamus contributes to suppression of counterregulatory responses after antecedent hypoglycemia. Diabetes 2008;57: 1363–1370

39. Dunn-Meynell AA, Routh VH, Kang L, Gaspers L, Levin BE. Glucokinase is the likely mediator of glucosensing in both glucose-excited and glucose-inhibited central neurons. Diabetes 2002;51:2056-2065

40. Canabal DD, Song Z, Potian JG, Beuve A, McArdle JJ, Routh VH. Glucose, insulin, and leptin signaling pathways modulate nitric oxide synthesis in glucose-inhibited neurons in the ventromedial hypothalamus. Am J Physiol Regul Integr Comp Physiol 2007;292:R1418–R1428

41. Hardie DG, Carling D. The AMP-activated protein kinase: fuel gauge of the mammalian cell? Eur J Biochem 1997;246:259–273

42. Mountjoy PD, Bailey SJ, Rutter GA. Inhibition by glucose or leptin of hypothalamic neurons expressing neuropeptide Y requires changes in AMP-activated protein kinase activity. Diabetologia 2007;50: 168–177

43. Fioramonti X, Contie S, Song Z, Routh VH, Lorsignol A, Penicaud L. Characterization of glucosensing neuron subpopulations in the arcuate nucleus: integration in neuropeptide Y and pro-opio melanocortin networks? Diabetes 2007;56:1219-1227

44. McCrimmon RJ, Fan X, Ding Y, Zhu W, Jacob RJ, Sherwin RS. Potential role for AMP-activated protein kinase in hypoglycemia sensing in the ventromedial hypothalamus. Diabetes 2004;53:1953-1958

45. McCrimmon RJ, Fan X, Cheng H, McNay E, Chan O, Shaw M, Ding Y, Zhu W, Sherwin RS. Activation of AMP-activated protein kinase within the ventromedial hypothalamus amplifies counterregulatory hormone responses in rats with defective counterregulation. Diabetes 2006; 55:1755–1760

46. McCrimmon RJ, Shaw M, Fan X, Cheng H, Ding Y, Wang A, Sherwin RS. AMP-activated protein kinase (AMPK): a key mediator of hypoglycemia-sensing in the ventromedial hypothalamus (VMH). Diabetes 2006;55(Suppl.1):A15

47. Claret M, Smith MA, Batterham RL, Selman C, Choudhury AI, Fryer LG, Clements M, Al-Qassab H, Heffron H, Xu AW, Speakman JR, Barsh GS, Viollet B, Vaulont S, Ashford ML, Carling D, Withers DJ. AMPK is essential for energy homeostasis regulation and glucose sensing by POMC and AgRP neurons (Letter). J Clin Invest 2007;117:2325–2336

48. Smythe GA, Edwards SR. A role for central postsynaptic alpha 2-adrenoceptors in glucoregulation. Brain Res 1991;562: 225–229

49. Beverly JL, de Vries MG, Beverly MF, Arseneau LM. Norepinephrine mediates glucoprivic-induced increase in GABA in the ventromedial hypothalamus of rats. Am J Physiol Regul Integr Comp Physiol 2000;279:R990–R996

50. Beverly JL, De Vries MG, Bouman SD, Arseneau LM. Noradrenergic and GABAergic systems in the medial hypothalamus are activated during hypoglycemia. Am J Physiol Regul Integr Comp Physiol 2001;280: R563–R569

51. de Vries MG, Lawson MA, Beverly JL. Hypoglycemia-induced noradrenergic activation in the VMH is a result of decreased ambient glucose. Am J Physiol Regul Integr Comp Physiol 2005;289:R977–R981

52. Ritter S, Dinh TT, Zhang Y. Localization of hindbrain glucoreceptive sites controlling food intake and blood glucose. Brain Res 2000;856:37–47

53. Song Z, Routh VH. Recurrent hypoglycemia reduces the glucose sensitivity of glucose-inhibited neurons in the ventromedial hypothalamus nucleus. Am J Physiol Regul Integr Comp Physiol 2006;291:R1283–R1287

54. Choi IY, Seaquist ER, Gruetter R. Effect of hypoglycemia on brain glycogen metabolism in vivo. J Neurosci Res 2003;72: 25–32

55. Herzog RI, Chan O, Yu S, Dziura J, McNay EC, Sherwin RS. Effect of acute and recurrent hypoglycemia on changes in brain glycogen concentration. Endocrinology 2008;149:1499–1504

56. Bale TL, Vale WW. CRF and CRF receptors: role in stress responsivity and other behaviors. Annu Rev Pharmacol Toxicol 2004;44:525–527

57. McCrimmon RJ, Song Z, Cheng H, McNay EC, Weikart-Yeckel C, Fan X, Routh VH, Sherwin RS. Corticotrophin-releasing factor receptors within the ventromedial hypothalamus regulate hypoglycemia-induced hormonal counterregulation. J Clin Invest 2006;116:1723–1730

58. Cheng H, Zhou L, Zhu W, Wang A, Tang C, Chan O, Sherwin RS, McCrimmon RJ. Type 1 corticotrophin-releasing factor receptors in the ventromedial hypothalamus promote hypoglycemia-induced hormonal counterregulation. Am J Physiol 2007

59. Alquier T, Kawashima J, Tsuji Y, Kahn BB. Role of hypothalamic adenosine 5'-monophosphate-activated protein kinase in the impaired counterregulatory response induced by repetitive neuroglucopenia. Endocrinology 2007;148:1367–1375

Mechanisms of Insulin Resistance After Insulin-Induced Hypoglycemia in Humans: The Role of Lipolysis

Paola Lucidi, Paolo Rossetti, Francesca Porcellati, Simone Pampanelli, Paola Candeloro,
Anna Marinelli Andreoli, Gabriele Perriello, Geremia B. Bolli, and Carmine G. Fanelli

OBJECTIVE—Changes in glucose metabolism occurring during counterregulation are, in part, mediated by increased plasma free fatty acids (FFAs), as a result of hypoglycemia-activated lipolysis. However, it is not known whether FFA plays a role in the development of posthypoglycemic insulin resistance as well.

RESEARCH DESIGN AND METHODS—We conducted a series of studies in eight healthy volunteers using acipimox, an inhibitor of lipolysis. Insulin action was measured during a 2-h hyperinsulinemic-euglycemic clamp (plasma glucose [PG] 5.1 mmol/l) from 5:00 P.M. to 7:00 P.M. or after a 3-h morning hyperinsulinemic-glucose clamp (from 10 A.M. to 1:00 P.M.), either euglycemic (study 1) or hypoglycemic (PG 3.2 mmol/l, studies 2–4), during which FFA levels were allowed to increase (study 2), were suppressed by acipimox (study 3), or were replaced by infusing lipids (study 4). [6,6-^{2}H$_2$]-Glucose was infused to measure glucose fluxes.

RESULTS—Plasma adrenaline, norepinephrine, growth hormone, and cortisol levels were unchanged ($P > 0.2$). Glucose infusion rates (GIRs) during the euglycemic clamp were reduced by morning hypoglycemia in study 2 versus study 1 (16.8 ± 2.3 vs. 34.1 ± 2.2 µmol/kg/min, respectively, $P < 0.001$). The effect was largely removed by blockade of lipolysis during hypoglycemia in study 3 (28.9 ± 2.6 µmol/kg/min, $P > 0.2$ vs. study 1) and largely reproduced by replacement of FFA in study 4 (22.3 ± 2.8 µmol/kg/min, $P < 0.03$ vs. study 1). Compared with study 2, blockade of lipolysis in study 3 decreased endogenous glucose production (2 ± 0.3 vs. 0.85 ± 0.1 µmol/kg/min, $P < 0.05$) and increased glucose utilization (16.9 ± 1.85 vs. 28.5 ± 2.7 µmol/kg/min, $P < 0.05$). In study 4, GIR fell by ~23% (22.3 ± 2.8 µmol/kg/min, vs. study 3, $P = 0.058$), indicating a role of acipimox per se on insulin action.

CONCLUSION—Lipolysis induced by hypoglycemia counterregulation largely mediates posthypoglycemic insulin resistance in healthy subjects, with an estimated overall contribution of ~39%. *Diabetes* **59:1349–1357, 2010**

P hysiological responses to insulin-induced hypoglycemia in humans are well established (1,2). Timely increments in secretion of counterregulatory hormones and specific symptom appearance prevent further fall in plasma glucose concentration (3). Counterregulatory hormones are all similarly critical in defense against hypoglycemia (3). These "anti-insulin" responses last several hours after a hypoglycemic episode ends (4). This condition of posthypoglycemic insulin resistance translating into postmeal hyperglycemia was described first by Somogyi (5) after his observation that overtreatment with evening regular insulin can result in hyperglycemia the following morning (6). In the clinical setting, this process can contribute to the instability of the metabolic control in patients with diabetes (7). With intermediate- and long-acting insulin as well as continuous subcutaneous insulin infusion currently available, fasting hyperglycemia after nocturnal hypoglycemia is either infrequent (7) or modest (8). Posthypoglycemic insulin resistance nevertheless results in significant postmeal hyperglycemia (9).

Mintz et al. (10) and Oakley et al. (11) described reduced rebound hyperglycemia after hypoglycemia in hypophysectomized patients, proposing a role for growth hormone and cortisol in the pathogenesis of posthypoglycemic insulin resistance, whereas Popp et al. (12) documented impaired glucose recovery from acute hypoglycemia induced by an intravenous insulin bolus after β-adrenergic blockade, suggesting an involvement of catecholamines, at least in the acute phase. In the mid-1980s, Bolli et al. (13) provided evidence that posthypoglycemic hyperglycemia in patients with type 1 diabetes is the result of counterregulatory hormonal response to hypoglycemia in concert with prevalent plasma insulin concentration, and that all of the hormones but glucagon may play a role. Long-lasting posthypoglycemic insulin resistance (up to 7–8 h) is induced in its early phase primarily by epinephrine response and in its late phase by growth hormone and cortisol (14–19). The mechanisms by which the counterregulatory hormones adrenaline, growth hormone, and cortisol induce posthypoglycemic insulin resistance are attributed to increased endogenous glucose production (liver and kidney) and suppressed glucose utilization (peripheral tissues, mainly muscles). However, it is possible that other mechanisms, i.e., indirect mechanisms, may also contribute. Indeed, earlier observations (20,21) indicate that activation of lipolysis, i.e., an increase in plasma free fatty acids (FFAs) and glycerol, plays a critical role in mediating the effects of catecholamines and other lipolytic, counterregulatory hormones in the defense against acute, insulin-induced hypoglycemia. It is conceivable that the same mechanisms continue to operate immediately after hypoglycemia and contribute to insulin resistance in subsequent hours.

The present series of studies was undertaken *1*) to establish whether increased availability of FFA substrate after lipolysis and/or lipid oxidation in response to acute, insulin-induced hypoglycemia plays a role in the pathogenesis of posthypoglycemic insulin resistance, and if so, *2*) to quantitate its contribution, and *3*) to determine whether its

From the Department of Internal Medicine, Section of Internal Medicine, Endocrinology and Metabolism, University of Perugia, Perugia, Italy.
Corresponding author: Geremia B. Bolli, gbolli@unipg.it.
Submitted 25 May 2009 and accepted 26 February 2010. Published ahead of print at http://diabetes.diabetesjournals.org on 18 March 2010. DOI: 10.2337/db09-0745.

effects are mediated by the liver or peripheral tissues, or both.

RESEARCH DESIGN AND METHODS

Subjects. The study was carried out according to the Declaration of Helsinki after obtaining written informed consent from all subjects. Eight healthy volunteers (three women and five men) with no family history of diabetes or other endocrine diseases and who were not taking any medications participated in the study, which had been approved by the local ethics committee. Their mean ($\pm$ SE) age was 28 $\pm$ 1.8 years and their mean BMI (kg/m^2) was 22.8 $\pm$ 0.7. All subjects were studied on four different occasions, in random order, with an interval between studies of at least 2 weeks.

Protocol. On all occasions, subjects presented to the Clinical Research Center of the Department of Internal Medicine, Endocrinology and Metabolism, University of Perugia at 6:00 A.M. after an overnight fast of 10 h. They were placed on bed rest and maintained a supine position until the end of the experiments at 7:00 P.M. To obtain arterialized-venous blood samples, a dorsal vein of a hand was cannulated retrogradely with a 18-gauge catheter needle, and the hand was maintained at 65°C in a thermoregulated Plexiglas box (22). An antecubital vein of the contralateral arm was cannulated with an 18-gauge catheter needle for infusions. Insulin, stable isotope–labeled tracers, and variable glucose (20% solution) were infused in all studies, whereas a heparin and lipid solution was infused only in study 4. Potassium chloride at the rate of 5 mEq/h was also infused along with saline in all clamp studies to prevent hypokalemia. All infusions were performed with separate syringe pumps (Harvard Apparatus, Inc., The Ealing Co., South Natick, MA). Both forearm venous lines were kept patent by saline solution infused at a rate of 30 ml/h. At 7:00 A.M., a primed 16-μmol/kg sterile, pyrogen-free constant infusion (0.22 μmol/kg/min) of [6,6-^{2}H$_2$]-glucose (Cambridge Isotopes Laboratories, Cambridge, MA) was started and maintained throughout to determine glucose kinetics as previously described (23,24). Three hours were allowed for isotopic equilibration, after which baseline blood samples were taken. Euglycemic and hypoglycemic clamps were achieved by a variable rate of infusion of 20% glucose enriched to 2.5% with [6,6-^{2}H$_2$]-glucose, to avoid non–steady-state errors in measurement of glucose turnover (25) and to maintain a blood glucose concentration at euglycemia (5.5 mmol/l) and hypoglycemia (3.2 mmol/l), respectively.

Lipid and carbohydrate oxidation expenditure were measured in all subjects by indirect calorimetry (26) for a 30-min period at baseline (-30 to 0 min) and during the last 30 min of each hour throughout. At 45 min before beginning experiments, a transparent plastic ventilated hood was placed over the subject's head and made airtight around the neck. Air flow and O$_2$ and CO$_2$ concentrations in the expired and inspired air were measured by a computerized continuous open-circuit system (Deltatrac; Datex Instruments, Helsinki, Finland) (27) that has a precision of 2.5% for oxygen consumption and 1.0% for carbon dioxide production. Protein oxidation was estimated from urinary excretion of urea.

Subjects underwent either a 3-h hyperinsulinemic-euglycemic (study 1), or hypoglycemic clamp (studies 2–4) in the morning between 10:00 A.M. and 1:00 P.M., (time segment 0–180 min [t_1]). In studies 3–4, acipimox, an inhibitor of lipolysis, was given to suppress lipolysis. In study 4, to quantify the effects of acipimox per se on glucose metabolism, a lipid emulsion and heparin were infused to reproduce plasma FFA and glycerol concentrations similar to those of study 2 with spontaneous hypoglycemic activation of lipolysis. In t_1, regular insulin (Eli Lilly Italia SpA), diluted to 1 unit/ml in 100 ml of saline solution containing 2 ml of the subject's blood, was infused at the rate of 1 mU/kg/min. Glucose was infused at variable rate to maintain euglycemia in study 1, whereas hypoglycemia (3.2 $\pm$ 0.1 mmol/l) was allowed to occur in studies 2–4. Acipimox 250 mg (5-methyl-pyrazene-carboxylic acid 4-oxide, Olbetam; Pfizer Italia srl, Latina, Italy) was given orally at 0 and 180 min to inhibit lipolysis in studies 3–4. To establish whether acipimox had effects other than antilipolysis, a triglyceride emulsion of 10% Intralipid (Fresenius Kabi, Verona, Italy; 10% soybean oil, 1.2% egg yolk phospholipids, and 2.25% glycerol) and heparin (Normoparin, heparin sodium; Farmaceutici Caber SpA, Ferrara, Italy) was infused at a variable rate (up to 1 ml/min and 0.2 units/kg/min for Intralipid and heparin, respectively) in study 4 to reproduce the increase in FFAs and glycerol observed in study 2. At 420 min, lipid/heparin infusion was halved (lipids 0.5 ml/kg/min and heparin 0.1 unit/kg/min), and at 480 min the heparin infusion was further reduced to 0.05 units/kg/min. Intralipid and heparin infusion rates were chosen based on pilot experiments as well as experience from previous studies in our laboratory (20).

At 1:00 P.M. (180 min) insulin infusion was stopped and euglycemia was recovered with variable glucose infusion in the time segment 180–420 min (t_2) in all studies. At 4:00 P.M. (360 min), another capsule of acipimox 250 mg was given to maintain suppression of lipolysis in studies 3–4. Between 5:00 and 7:00 P.M. (time segment 420–540 min [t_3]) subjects underwent a 2-h hyperin-

sulinemic-euglycemic clamp to measure insulin sensitivity. Insulin infusion was started again at 420 min in t_3 at the constant rate of 1 mU/kg/min together with glucose infused at a variable rate to maintain euglycemia throughout. After collection of the final samples at 540 min, the subjects were fed. Finally, when plasma glucose was stable, intravenous lines were removed and the subjects discharged.

Analyses. Arterialized blood samples were taken before beginning the isotope infusion to determine background glucose enrichments. To determine glucose concentrations and kinetics, arterialized blood samples were taken every 10 min during the last 30 min of the basal period and every 20 min during the insulin clamps. All blood samples were drawn into tubes containing EDTA and centrifuged. Plasma was stored at -80°C. Glucose enrichment was determined on its penta-acetate (penta-O-acetyl-β-D-glucopyranose) derivative by gas chromatography–mass spectrometry (gas chromatography HP 5890 II, mass spectrometry HP 5972A; Hewlett-Packard, Palo Alto, CA) in electron impact ionization mode monitoring the ions 200 and 202 for the unlabeled and D-[6,6-^{2}H$_2$]glucose, respectively (24). To maintain euglycemia and hypoglycemia, arterialized blood glucose was measured every 3–7 min (Beckman Glucose Analyzer II; Beckman Instruments, Fullerton, CA). Blood samples were collected at 30-min intervals and assayed for alanine (28), insulin (20), glucagon (20), cortisol (20), growth hormone (20), adrenaline and norepinephrine (20), FFA (Wako NEFA C test kit; Wako Chemicas, Neuss, Germany), 3-β-OH-butyrate (28), and glycerol (28). For FFA determination, blood (2 ml) was collected in tubes containing 50 μl of the lipoproteinlipase inhibitor diethyl-p-nitrophenyl-phosphate (Paraoxon; Sigma Chemical, St. Louis, MO) diluted to 0.04% in diethyl ether (29). Urine was collected from the onset to the end of each study period to determine nitrogen excretion using the Kjeldahl method (30).

Calculations. Oxidation rates for carbohydrate and fat were calculated from indirect calorimetric measurements by averaging the data over the 30 min of measurements during each hour (31). Nonoxidative glucose utilization was calculated by subtracting the rate of glucose oxidation from the total rate of glucose uptake (31). Protein oxidation rate was measured from urinary nitrogen excretion before and during insulin infusion adjusted for changes in serum urea during insulin infusion (32).

Tracer-to-tracee ratio for glucose was calculated as the ratio between the master peak (M) and the enriched peak (M+2) after subtracting the background enrichment. The calculations were based on a steady-state assumption. For glucose, the total rate of appearance (R_a) and disappearance (R_d) was calculated as follows (μmol/kg/min): $R_a = (F_{total}/E_{glucose}) - \text{GIR}$ and $R_d = (F_{total}/E_{glucose})$. F_{total} is the total infusion rate of glucose tracer (μmol/kg/min). $E_{glucose}$ is the enrichment of glucose in plasma (tracer-to-tracee ratio). Glucose infusion rate (GIR) is the exogenous glucose administered during the clamp.

Statistics. Data in text are given as means $\pm$ SE. Statistical analysis was performed by using mixed-model repeated-measures ANOVA, with Huynh-Feldt adjustment for nonsphericity. Post hoc comparisons (Newman-Keuls test) were carried out to pinpoint specific differences on significant interaction terms. $P < 0.05$ was considered to indicate statistically significant difference. A sample size of eight was chosen based on the calculation that it achieves 88% power to detect a difference of 6.6 μmol/kg/min between study 3 (lipolysis blocked by acipimox) and study 4 (lipolysis blocked by acipimox and plasma FFAs replaced) with an SD of 6.0 μmol/kg/min and a significance level (alpha) of 0.05 using a two-sided one-sample t test. We conducted the statistical analyses using NCSS/PASS 2007 software (Kaysville, UT).

RESULTS

Plasma glucose and insulin concentrations and rates of glucose infusion. In t_1, plasma glucose was maintained at baseline euglycemia in study 1 (hyperinsulinemic-euglycemic clamp; Fig. 1). In studies 2–4, plasma glucose was allowed to decrease to a nadir of 3.2 $\pm$ 0.1 mmol/l between 30 and 180 min ($P > 0.2$ between studies 2 and 4). Thereafter, plasma glucose increased to euglycemic levels of study 1 by 300 min and remained euglycemic until the end of the study (540 min).

Plasma insulin was not different in the four studies. Hypoglycemia in study 2 resulted in lower glucose infusion rates required to maintain euglycemia between 300 and 420 min of t_2 compared with euglycemic study 1 (3.1 $\pm$ 1.3 vs. 6.1 $\pm$ 1.5 μmol/kg/min, $P = 0.037$). However, when lipolysis was blocked by acipimox in study 3, the rate of glucose infusion increased to values similar to those of

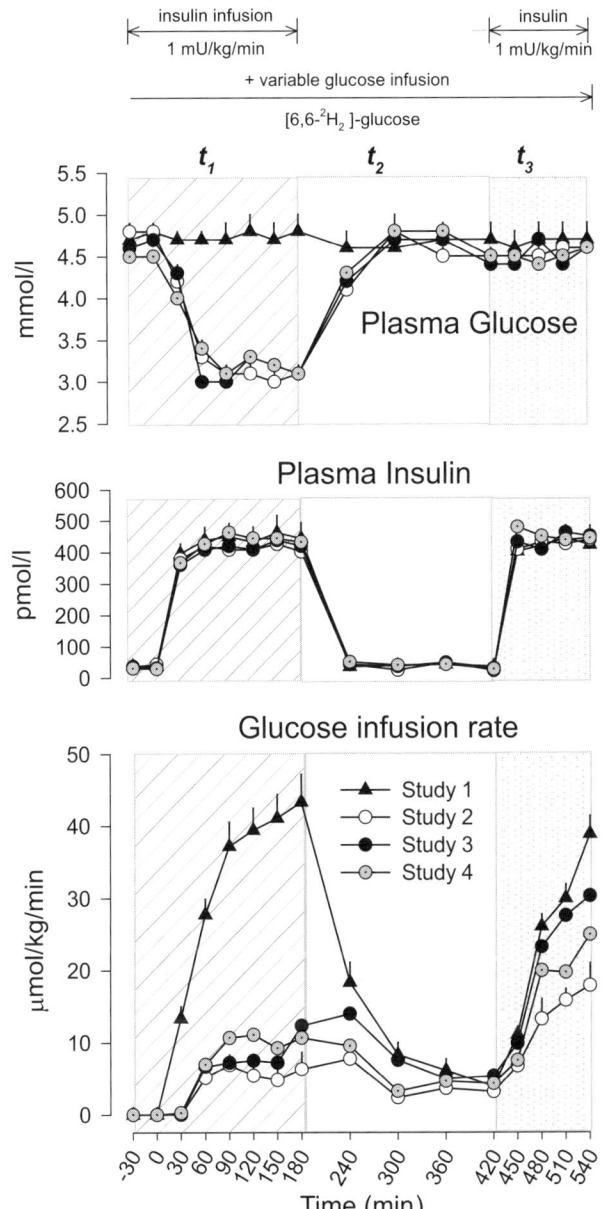

FIG. 1. Plasma glucose, insulin concentrations, and rates of glucose infusion in study 1 (euglycemia), study 2 (hypoglycemia), study 3 (hypoglycemia + acipimox), and study 4 (hypoglycemia + acipimox + heparin + intralipid). The diagonal area depicts t_1 (0–180 min, euglycemia or hypoglycemia), the white area depicts t_2 (180–420 min, euglycemia or recovery to hypoglycemia), and the dotted area depicts t_3 (420–540 min, euglycemic clamp) of each study.

study 1 (5.9 ± 6.1 vs. 12 ± 2.2 μmol/kg/min, $P > 0.2$). Finally, when FFAs and glycerol were replaced in study 4, the rate of glucose infusion was again reduced to values similar to those of study 2 (4.1 ± 1.9 vs. 3.1 ± 1.3 μmol/kg/min, $P = 0.124$). In the hyperinsulinemic-euglycemic clamp of t_3 (420–540 min), the rate of glucose infusion required to maintain euglycemia was reduced by morning hypoglycemia in study 2 (510–540 min, 16.8 ± 2.3 vs. 34.1 ± 2.2 μmol/kg/min, study 2 vs. study 1, respectively, $P < 0.001$), but the effect was largely removed by blockade of lipolysis during hypoglycemia in study 3 (28.9 ± 2.6 μmol/kg/min, $P > 0.2$ vs. study 1), and largely reproduced

by replacement of FFAs and glycerol in study 4 (22.3 ± 2.8 μmol/kg/min, $P < 0.03$ vs. study 1) (Fig. 1).

Rates of endogenous glucose production, glucose utilization, and glucose and lipid oxidation. Hypoglycemia in study 2 compared with study 1 euglycemia resulted in increase in endogenous glucose production, suppression of utilization and oxidation of glucose, and stimulation of lipid oxidation in t_2 (Fig. 2). In particular, endogenous glucose production and lipid oxidation were significantly greater (9.0 ± 0.9 vs. 5.9 ± 0.3 μmol/kg/min, $P = 0.01$, 5.5 ± 0.5 vs. 4.0 ± 0.4 μmol/kg/min, $P = 0.07$, study 2 vs. 1, respectively). Blockade of lipolysis (study 3) largely reversed these effects, which were reproduced by replacement of FFAs and glycerol (study 4). In addition, in t_3, the morning hypoglycemia of study 2 compared with the euglycemic study 1, respectively resulted in lower suppression of endogenous glucose production (2 ± 0.3 vs. 0.1 ± 0.1 μmol/kg/min), lower oxidation (4.2 + 0.45 vs. 6.95 + 0.7 μmol/kg/min, $P < 0.01$) and utilization (16.9 ± 1.85 vs. 31.9 ± 3.15 μmol/kg/min, $P = 0.001$) of glucose, and less suppression of lipid oxidation (5 ± 0.45 vs. 3.1 ± 0.3 μmol/kg/min, $P = 0.01$). However, blockade of lipolysis (study 3) largely reversed all these changes (endogenous glucose production 0.85 ± 0.1 μmol/kg/min, glucose oxidation 8.8 ± 1.05 μmol/kg/min, glucose utilization 28.5 ± 2.7 μmol/kg/min, lipid oxidation 2.9 ± 0.25 μmol/kg/min). Finally, replacement of FFAs and glycerol largely reproduced the effect observed in study 2 (Fig. 2).

In t_3, nonoxidative rates of glucose utilization (total glucose utilization rates minus glucose oxidation rates from indirect calorimetry) were 78, 75, 69, and 86% in studies 1, 2, 3, and 4, respectively, of the overall glucose utilization. The replacement of FFA levels in study 4 with concomitant administration of acipimox significantly increased nonoxidative rates of glucose utilization compared with study 3 ($P = 0.02$).

Plasma counterregulatory hormones concentrations. Baseline plasma concentrations of all counterregulatory hormones were not different in studies 1–4 (Fig. 3). Plasma glucagon decreased slightly in the euglycemic time segment t_1 of study 1. In contrast, in the hypoglycemia studies 2–4, plasma glucagon increased at 180 min and then returned to baseline values. Plasma adrenaline did not change in study 1, whereas it increased similarly in studies 2–4 by 180 min and, subsequently, returned to baseline values by 240 min. Plasma norepinephrine concentrations increased slightly between 30 and 180 min and were not different in all four studies. Plasma growth hormone did not change (baseline 2.0 ± 0.3 μg/dl) in the euglycemic study 1. In studies 2–4, plasma growth hormone peaked at 180 min (12 ± 0.3, 17 ± 2, 9.4 ± 1.8 μg/dl, respectively, $P < 0.01$ vs. study 1). There was a trend of a greater response of plasma growth hormone in study 3 compared with study 2 ($P = 0.07$) and study 4 ($P = 0.08$). Plasma cortisol decreased slightly in the euglycemic study 1, whereas it increased similarly in studies 2–4 ($P < 0.05$ vs. study 1) at 180 min. Afterward, plasma cortisol decreased to baseline values by 300 min.

In t_3, plasma concentrations of counterregulatory hormones glucagon, adrenaline, norepinephrine, growth hormone, and cortisol were not different among the four studies.

Plasma FFA, glycerol, β-hydroxybutyrate, lactate, and alanine concentrations. In t_1, plasma FFAs decreased after initiation of insulin infusion from an averaged baseline of 0.40 ± 0.03 to a nadir of 0.09 ± 0.02

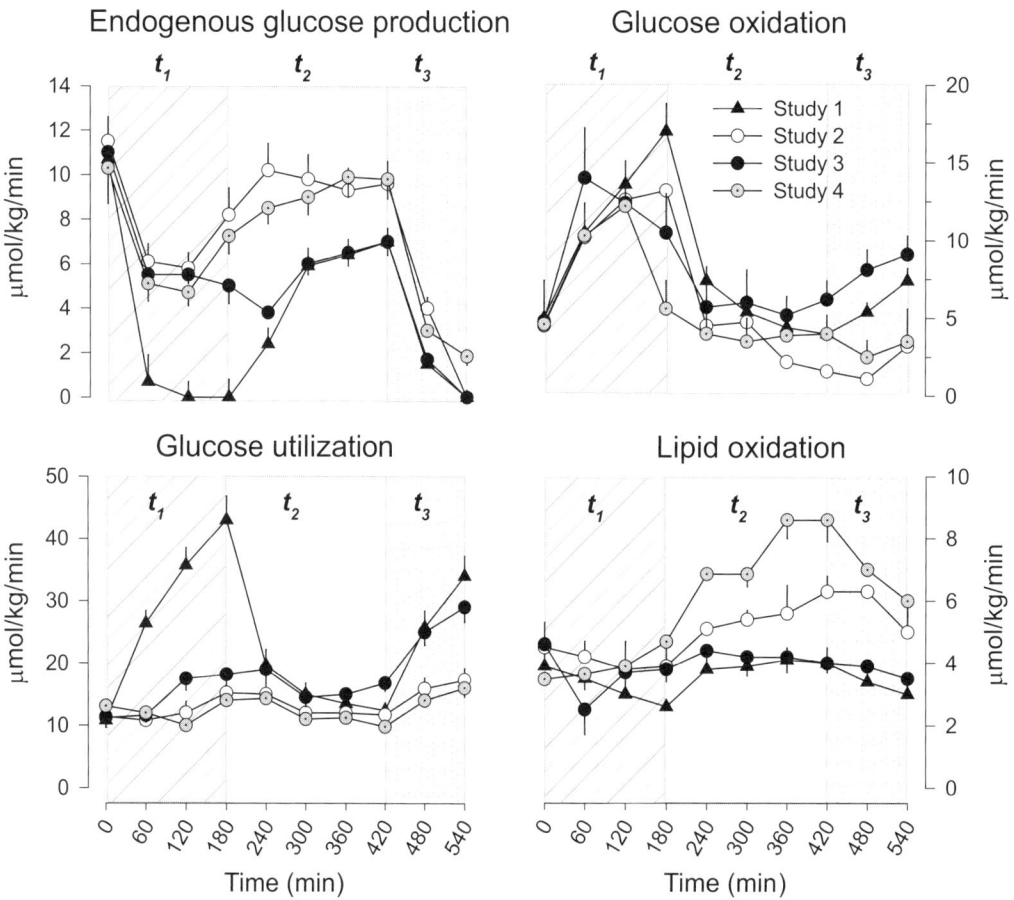

FIG. 2. Glucose utilization, endogenous glucose production, glucose oxidation, and lipid oxidation in study 1 (euglycemia), study 2 (hypoglycemia), study 3 (hypoglycemia + acipimox), and study 4 (hypoglycemia + acipimox + heparin + intralipid). The diagonal area depicts t_1 (0–180 min, euglycemia or hypoglycemia), the white area depicts t_2 (180–420 min, euglycemia or recovery to hypoglycemia), and the dotted area depicts t_3 (420–540 min, euglycemic clamp) of each study.

mmol/l at 180 min with no differences in studies 1–3 (Fig. 4). After discontinuing insulin infusion (180 min), plasma FFAs returned to values similar to those of baseline by 420 min of t_2. In the same segment of t_2, plasma FFA levels were at all times less suppressed in study 2 compared with studies 1 and 3 ($P < 0.05$). Finally, replacement of FFAs and glycerol in study 4 reproduced plasma FFA concentrations similar to those of study 2 and greater than those of studies 1 and 3 ($P < 0.05$).

After an initial suppression, plasma glycerol concentrations increased by 240 min (150 ± 23 mmol/l) in study 2. In studies 1 and 3, plasma glycerol concentrations were suppressed throughout, whereas in study 4 exogenous lipid emulsion produced plasma concentrations in the range of those of study 2. Plasma β-hydroxybutyrate followed a pattern similar to that of plasma FFA in all studies, although it was higher in study 2 compared with study 4.

In the euglycemic study 1, plasma lactate (baseline 1.0 ± 0.2 mmol/l) did not change. In studies 2–4, plasma lactate baseline values were similar to those of study 1, however plasma concentrations increased and peaked at 180 min (1.5 ± 0.24, 1.6 ± 0.17, and 1.5 ± 0.16 mmol/l, studies 2, 3, and 4, respectively); afterward, they decreased to baseline values by 240 min.

Plasma alanine concentrations did not change signifi-

cantly from baseline in all studies. In t_3, baseline (420 min) plasma FFA, glycerol, and β-hydroxybutyrate concentrations were significantly higher in studies 2 and 4 than studies 1 and 3. However, after insulin infusion, plasma FFA, glycerol, and β-hydroxybutyrate concentrations decreased in study 2 to concentrations similar to those of studies 1 and 3. In study 4, these metabolites followed the same pattern observed in studies 1–3. Plasma lactate concentrations increased slightly and similarly in all studies. Plasma alanine did not change, although levels tended to be higher in studies 3–4 ($P = 0.081$) (Fig. 4).

Effect of acipimox per se on insulin action. Mean values of GIR and rates of endogenous glucose production and glucose utilization calculated during the last 30 min of the euglycemic clamp in t_3 allow estimation of the likely contribution of acipimox per se, independent of the decrease in circulating FFA levels, on insulin action. In study 3, inhibition of lipolysis by acipimox determined an increase in GIR, paralleled by a similar increment of glucose disappearance, of ~72% compared with study 2 (28.9 ± 2.6 vs. 16.8 ± 2.3 μmol/kg/min, respectively, $P = 0.009$). When plasma FFA and glycerol levels were replaced by infusing lipids and lipolysis was still blocked by acipimox in study 4, GIR was still higher by ~ 33% compared with study 2 (22.3 ± 2.8 μmol/kg/min, vs. study 2, $P = 0.026$). This indicates a role of acipimox per se on insulin action and

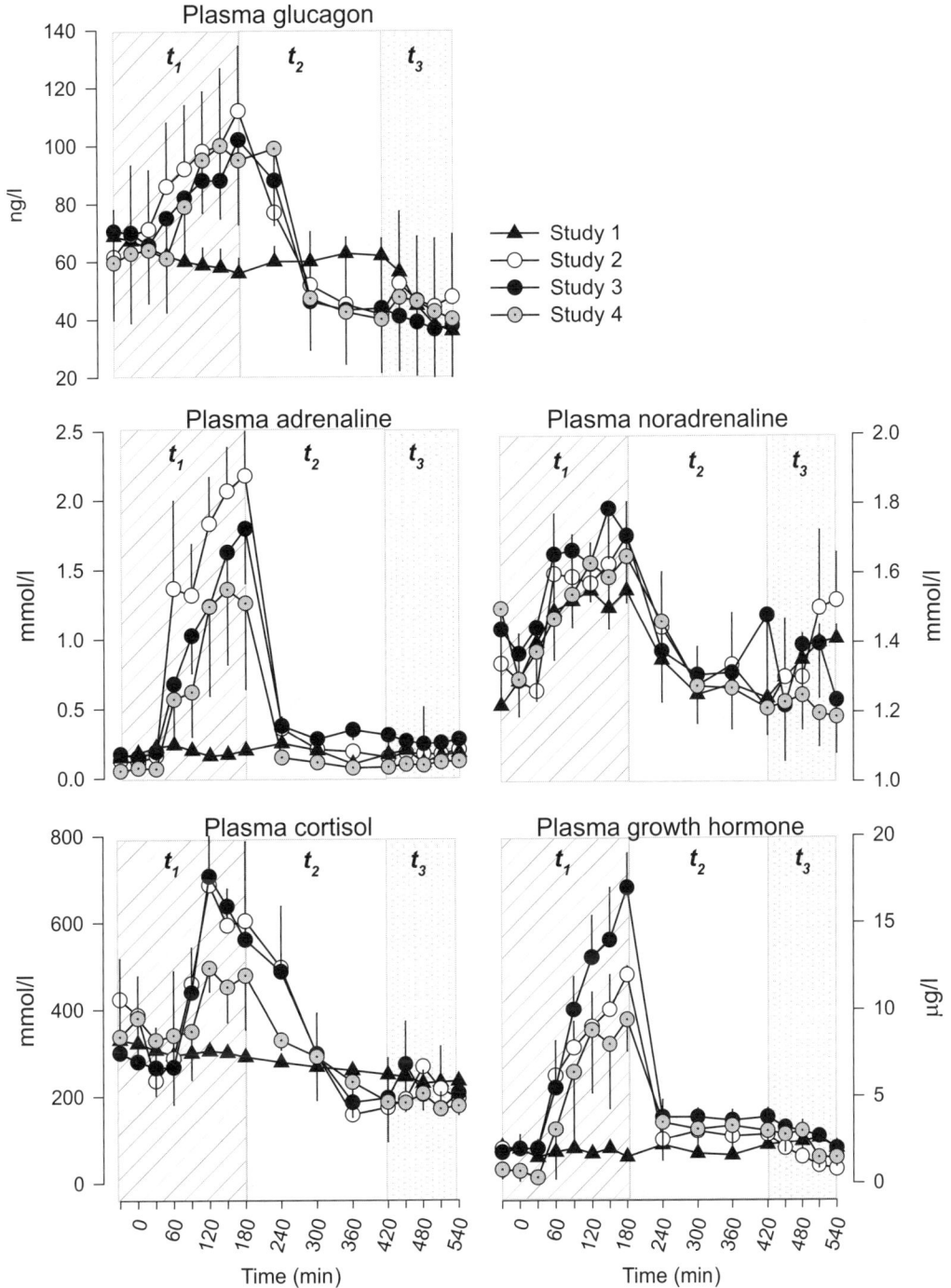

FIG. 3. Plasma counterregulatory hormones glucagon, adrenaline, norepinephrine, cortisol, and growth hormone in study 1 (euglycemia), study 2 (hypoglycemia), study 3 (hypoglycemia + acipimox), and study 4 (hypoglycemia + acipimox + heparin + intralipid). The diagonal area depicts t_1 (0–180 min, euglycemia or hypoglycemia), the white area depicts t_2 (180–420 min, euglycemia or recovery to hypoglycemia), and the dotted area depicts t_3 (420–540 min, euglycemic clamp) of each study.

quantifies its relative contribution to the effects observed in study 3. Accordingly, the overall contribution of lipolysis to posthypoglycemic insulin resistance was estimated to be ~39%.

DISCUSSION

The results indicate the following: First, the counterregulatory hormonal response to hypoglycemia contributes to reduced insulin action up to 9 h after an acute hypoglycemic episode. Second, this posthypoglycemic insulin resistance is generated by the counterregulatory hormones that act in part indirectly by activating lipolysis (contribution of 39%), and in part directly, i.e., by lipolysis-independent mechanisms (contribution of ~60%). Third, the mechanisms of posthypoglycemic insulin resistance induced by lipolysis include increase in endogenous

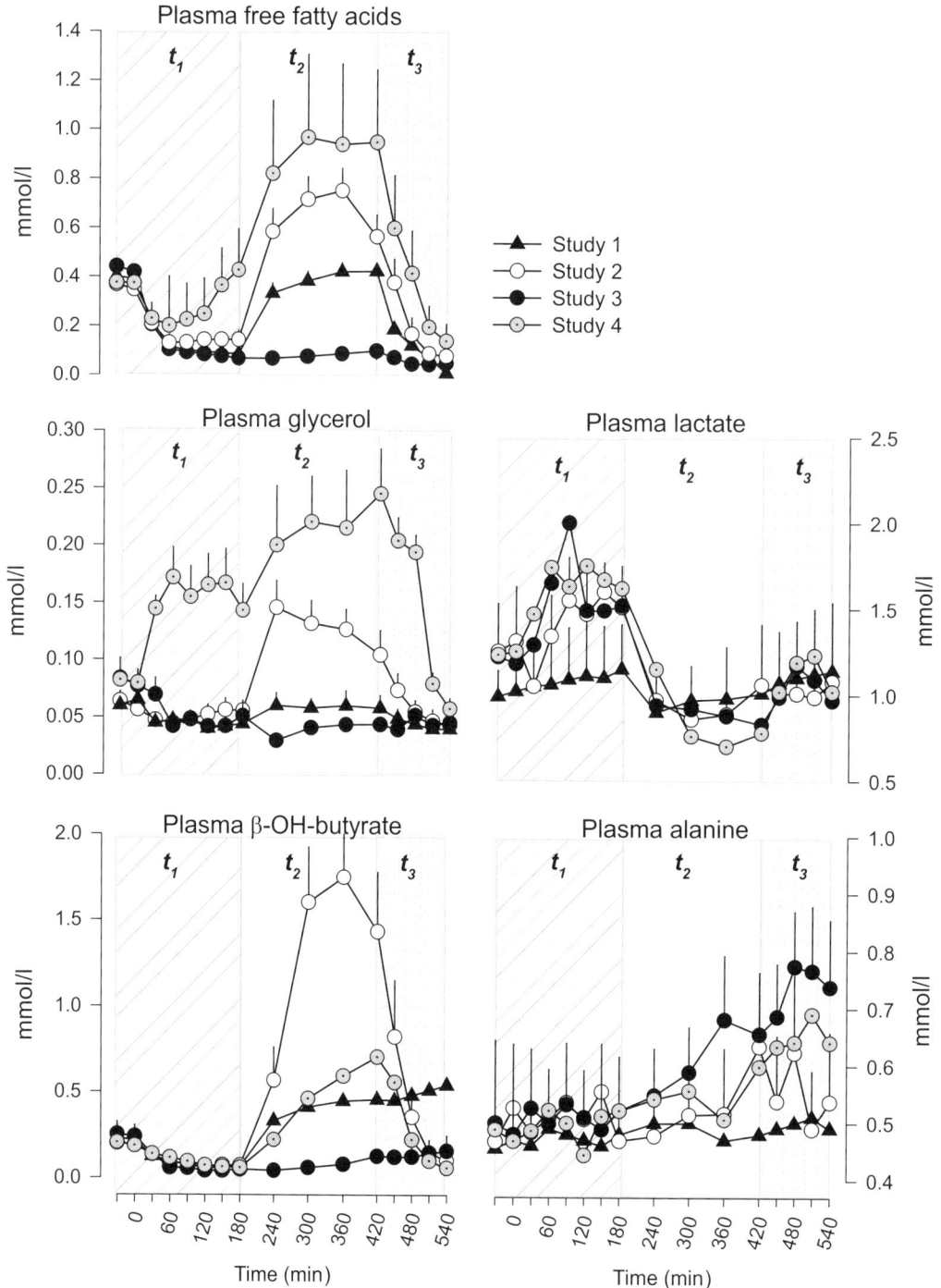

FIG. 4. Plasma nonglucose substrates free fatty acids, glycerol, β-OH-butyrate, lactate, and alanine in study 1 (euglycemia), study 2 (hypoglycemia), study 3 (hypoglycemia + acipimox), and study 4 (hypoglycemia + acipimox + heparin + intralipid). The diagonal area depicts t_1 (0–180 min, euglycemia or hypoglycemia), the white area depicts t_2 (180–420 min, euglycemia or recovery to hypoglycemia), and the dotted area depicts t_3 (420–540 min, euglycemic clamp) of each study.

glucose production, suppression of peripheral utilization and oxidation of glucose, and increase lipid oxidation. Thus, the adipose tissue plays a pivotal role in determining and sustaining posthypoglycemic insulin resistance in humans.

In a late phase of hypoglycemia, a large part of the anti-insulin effects of counterregulatory hormones, mainly catecholamines, on production and utilization of glucose is not direct but is mediated by stimulation of lipolysis (20,21).

The novel finding of the present study is that hypoglycemia-induced lipolysis also exerts long-lasting effects by blunting insulin action after restoration of euglycemia.

Administration of acipimox (study 3) suppressed lipolysis (as reflected by plasma FFA and glycerol concentrations) and markedly reduced lipid oxidation. This was associated with suppression of endogenous glucose production by 42%, increased glucose utilization by 64%, and increased glucose oxidation by 100%.

The mechanisms of regulation of glucose metabolism by fatty acids is not completely understood. The initial hypothesis of competition between FFAs and glucose for oxidation has been proposed by Randle et al. based on studies in vitro (33). Increased availability and oxidation of free fatty acids would increase levels of acetyl-CoA and citrate. The former inhibits pyruvate dehydrogenase, which in turn decreases glucose oxidation. The latter inhibits phosphofructokinase, which in turn decreases glycolysis and glucose utilization. Other studies in humans have demonstrated that the overall effect of elevation of levels of free fatty acids is increased lipid oxidation and suppressed oxidation and utilization of glucose (34), thus creating a condition of free fatty acid–induced insulin resistance (35). However, in addition to the hypothesis of Randle et al., it is likely FFAs interfere with insulin-stimulated glucose transport activity in muscles and induce insulin resistance by altering insulin signaling through insulin receptor substrate-1–associated phosphatidylinositol 3-kinase, resulting in decreased insulin-stimulated glucose transport activity (36).

It is likely that both glycerol and FFA contributed to the increase in the rate of hepatic glucose production observed in study 4 compared with study 3 (20). However, the design of the present experiments does not allow us to distinguish between the relative contribution of glycerol and FFAs to the increased hepatic glucose production.

All counterregulatory hormones increased in response to hypoglycemia (studies 1–3). However, with the exception of growth hormone (GH), which tended to be greater when lipolysis was blocked (study 3) compared with when lipolysis was allowed to occur (study 2) or FFA levels and glycerol were replaced (study 4), their levels were similar in studies 1–3. This effect on GH can be related to the lack of suppressive action of lower FFA levels on growth hormone secretion in study 3 (37).

From our study it is not possible to define the relative role of the individual counterregulatory hormones in the posthypoglycemic insulin resistance. However, because counterregulatory hormones were not affected by blockade of lipolysis, with the exception of GH, one might be tempted to speculate that, in addition to catecholamines (12), GH might direct, to some extent, the phenomenon of free fatty acid–induced posthypoglycemic insulin resistance. Indeed, earlier evidence points toward a critical role of GH and cortisol in insulin resistance after insulin-induced hypoglycemia (17,35). The elevation of norepinephrine in study 1 in which there was no hypoglycemia has to be considered as a response to insulin per se during the hyperinsulinemic-euglycemic clamp in t_1 and t_3. In fact, hyperinsulinemia per se stimulates sympathetic neural activity including norepinephrine elevation (38).

It is interesting to note that in one study the suppressive effect of acipimox on FFA and glycerol levels did inhibit recovery from hypoglycemia in a model of acute hypoglycemia induced by a 30-min insulin infusion in healthy subjects (39). However, the study did not examine the same effect in a model of more clinical prolonged hypoglycemia. It is possible that increased FFA and glycerol levels to hypoglycemia decrease insulin response during subsequent hypoglycemia. In fact, whereas antecedent hypoglycemia blunts neuroendocrine (and symptomatic) responses to subsequent hypoglycemia (4), Davis and Tate have shown that FFA levels and glucose infusion rates during subsequent afternoon hypoglycemia were higher and lower, respectively, after antecedent morning hypo-

glycemia compared with antecedent morning euglycemia, resulting in greater insulin resistance compensating for diminished neuroendocrine responses (40). More recently, it has been shown that insulin resistance can last up to 18 h after two brief episodes of antecedent hypoglycemia (4). In contrast, posthypoglycemic insulin resistance after antecedent hypoglycemia has not been studied in type 1 diabetic subjects. However, in those individuals, antecedent hypoglycemia is the major cause of hypoglycemia-associated autonomic failure syndrome, which, by reducing both symptoms of and physiological defense against developing hypoglycemia, favors severe hypoglycemia (41).

Hypoglycemia can be common also in people with type 2 diabetes, particularly under intensive glucose treatment (42,43). Whether the phenomenon of posthypoglycemic insulin resistance, demonstrated in healthy subjects in our present study, operates in people with type 2 diabetes who are already insulin resistant to some degree, thus contributing to worsened posthypoglycemia (hyper)glycemia, is not known.

Acipimox, a nicotinic acid analog and a potent inhibitor of lipolysis (44), is an established therapy for dyslipidemia. The antilipolytic action of acipimox is mediated through suppression of intracellular cAMP levels, with the subsequent decrease in cAMP-dependent protein kinase activity, leading to the reduced activity of hormone-sensitive lipase (45). Compared with nicotinic acid, acipimox has fewer side effects (light flushing) and a longer duration of action (46). In addition, by lowering circulating FFAs, acute administration of acipimox has been shown to improve insulin sensitivity in lean (47) and obese subjects and people with type 2 diabetes (48,49). The results of the present study are in line with earlier reports (50) indicating that acipimox improves insulin sensitivity by decreasing circulating FFA levels. In addition, our data show that acipimox also directly enhances insulin sensitivity. In fact, in study 3, GIR required to maintain euglycemia during the clamp (t_3) was greater than in study 4, in which acipimox was given as in study 3 and plasma FFA levels were replaced by infusion of lipids, but higher than in study 2. If acipimox had no effects on insulin sensitivity, GIR would have approximately matched rates observed in study 2. In addition, glucose oxidation was not affected by acipimox, suggesting that the increase in GIR stimulated by acipimox (~33%) must be accounted for by glucose storage as glycogen (nonoxidative glucose utilization).

Although our study reports the new finding that lipolysis induced by hypoglycemia counterregulation mediates in part posthypoglycemic insulin resistance, it has limitations. First, the study sample size was limited. It was, however, adequately powered to examine the issue and conducted under carefully controlled conditions. Second, although acipimox has been extensively adopted in metabolic studies (21,37,49,50), its use to investigate the role of lipolysis in posthypoglycemic insulin resistance may have exerted enhancing effects on in vivo insulin action independent of lipolysis and plasma FFA levels. We attempted to overcome this problem by planning study 4 to correct for the direct effects of acipimox on insulin action. Third, the results of our study have been obtained in healthy subjects and may not be immediately extrapolated to subjects with diabetes until specific studies are performed. Despite these limitations, the present study speaks to a major role of lipolysis in the pathogenesis of posthypoglycemic insulin resistance.

In conclusion, the present study demonstrates that the

activation of lipolysis by counterregulatory hormones in response to hypoglycemia (indirect effects) accounts for ~39% of the total effect on late posthypoglycemic insulin resistance. It is tempting to speculate that the late posthypoglycemic insulin resistance originates as a defensive mechanism to protect against recurrence of hypoglycemia after recent, antecedent hypoglycemia episode by limiting peripheral utilization and oxidation of glucose, thus increasing its availability for the brain. However, in subjects with type 1 diabetes, and long-term type 2 diabetes (in which pancreatic B-cell function is either totally or largely lost), posthypoglycemic insulin resistance may result in significant hyperglycemia especially after a meal, and interfere with day-long blood glucose control (7). In addition, in insulin-resistant type 2 diabetic patients, the reduced insulin action after hypoglycemia may exaggerate the preexisting insulin resistance and aggravate the cardiovascular risk.

ACKNOWLEDGMENT

No potential conflicts of interest relevant to this article were reported.

REFERENCES

1. Mitrakou A, Ryan C, Veneman T, Mokan M, Jenssen T, Kiss I, Durrant J, Cryer P, Gerich J. Hierarchy of glycemic thresholds for counterregulatory hormone secretion, symptoms, and cerebral dysfunction. Am J Physiol 1991;260:E67–E74
2. Fanelli C, Pampanelli S, Epifano L, Rambotti AM, Ciofetta M, Modarelli F, Di Vincenzo A, Annibale B, Lepore M, Lalli C. Relative roles of insulin and hypoglycaemia on induction of neuroendocrine responses to, symptoms of, and deterioration of cognitive function in hypoglycaemia in male and female humans. Diabetologia 1994;37:797–807
3. Bolli GB, Fanelli CG. Physiology of glucose counterregulation to hypoglycemia. Endocrinol Metab Clin North Am 1999;28:467–493, v
4. Heller SR, Cryer PE. Reduced neuroendocrine and symptomatic responses to subsequent hypoglycemia after 1 episode of hypoglycemia in nondiabetic humans. Diabetes 1991;40:223–226
5. Somogyi M. Effect of insulin hypoglycemia on alimentary hyperglycemia. J Biol Chem 1951;193:859–871
6. Somogyi M. Exacerbation of diabetes by excess insulin action. Am J Med 1959;169–191
7. Perriello G, De Feo P, Torlone E, Calcinaro F, Ventura MM, Basta G, Santeusanio F, Brunetti P, Gerich JE, Bolli GB. The effect of asymptomatic nocturnal hypoglycemia on glycemic control in diabetes mellitus. N Engl J Med 1988;319:1233–1239
8. Havlin CE, Cryer PE. Nocturnal hypoglycemia does not commonly result in major morning hyperglycemia in patients with diabetes mellitus. Diabetes Care 1987;10:141–147
9. Frier BM, Corrall RJ, Ashby JP, Baird JD. Attenuation of the pancreatic beta cell response to a meal following hypoglycaemia in man. Diabetologia 1980;18:297–300
10. Mintz DH, Finster JL, Taylor AL, Fefer A. Hormonal genesis of glucose intolerance following hypoglycemia. Am J Med 1968;45:187–197
11. Oakley NW, Jacobs HS, Turner RC, Williams J, Aquino Cdos S, Nabarro JD. The effect of hypoglycaemia on oral glucose tolerance in normal subjects and patients with pituitary and adrenal disorders. Clin Sci 1970;39:663–674
12. Popp DA, Shah SD, Cryer PE. Role of epinephrine-mediated β-adrenergic mechanisms in hypoglycemic glucose counterregulation and posthypoglycemic hyperglycemia in insulin-dependent diabetes mellitus. J Clin Invest 1982;69:316–326
13. Bolli GB, Gottesman IS, Campbell PJ, Haymond MW, Cryer PE, Gerich JE. Glucose counterregulation and waning of insulin in the Somogyi phenomenon (posthypoglycemic hyperglycemia). N Engl J Med 1984;311:1214–1219
14. Attvall S, Eriksson BM, Fowelin J, von Schenck H, Lager I, Smith U. Early posthypoglycemic insulin resistance in man is mainly an effect of beta-adrenergic stimulation. J Clin Invest 1987;80:437–442
15. Attvall S, Fowelin J, von Schenck H, Lager I, Smith U. Insulin resistance in type 1 (insulin-dependent) diabetes following hypoglycaemia–evidence for the importance of beta-adrenergic stimulation. Diabetologia 1987;30:691–697
16. Fowelin J, Attvall S, von Schenck H, Smith U, Lager I. Characterization of the late posthypoglycemic insulin resistance in insulin-dependent diabetes mellitus. Metabolism 1990;39:823–826
17. Fowelin J, Attvall S, Von Schenck H, Smith U, Lager I. Combined effect of growth hormone and cortisol on late posthypoglycemic insulin resistance in humans. Diabetes 1989;38:1357–1364
18. Kollind M, Adamson U, Lins PE. Studies of insulin resistance following hypoglycemia in insulin-dependent diabetes mellitus. Acta Med Scand 1988;223:153–157
19. Kollind M, Adamson U, Lins PE, Curstedt T. Importance of growth hormone for blood glucose regulation following insulin-induced nocturnal hypoglycemia in insulin-dependent diabetes mellitus. Acta Med Scand 1988;223:159–164
20. Fanelli CG, De Feo P, Porcellati F, Perriello G, Torlone E, Santeusanio F, Brunetti P, Bolli GB. Adrenergic mechanisms contribute to the late phase of hypoglycemic glucose counterregulation in humans by stimulating lipolysis. J Clin Invest 1992;89:2005–2013
21. Fanelli C, Calderone S, Epifano L, De Vincenzo A, Modarelli F, Pampanelli S, Perriello G, De Feo P, Brunetti P, Gerich JE. Demonstration of a critical role for free fatty acids in mediating counterregulatory stimulation of gluconeogenesis and suppression of glucose utilization in humans. J Clin Invest 1993;92:1617–1622
22. McGuire EA, Helderman JH, Tobin JD, Andres R, Berman M. Effects of arterial versus venous sampling on analysis of glucose kinetics in man. J Appl Physiol 1976;41:565–573
23. Tserng KY, Kalhan SC. Calculation of substrate turnover rate in stable isotope tracer studies. Am J Physiol 1983;245:E308–E311
24. Wolfe RR. Radioactive and Stable Isotope Tracers in Biomedicine: principles and practice of kinetic analysis. New York, Wiley-Liss, 1992, p. 425–426
25. Gastaldelli A, Coggan AR, Wolfe RR. Assessment of methods for improving tracer estimation of non-steady-state rate of appearance. J Appl Physiol 1999;87:1813–1822
26. Jequier E. Direct and indirect calorimetry in man. In *Substrate and Energy Metabolism*. Garrow JS, Halliday D, Eds. London, Wiley & Son, Ltd., 1985, p. 82–92
27. Meriläinen PT. Metabolic monitor. Int J Clin Monit Comput 1987;4:167–177
28. Lowry O, Passoneau J. Typical fluorometric procedures for metabolite assays. In A Flexible System for Enzimatic Analysis. Lowry O, Passoneau J, Eds. New York, Academic Press, Inc., 1972, p. 89–92
29. Hawk PB. Kjedal method. In Practical Physiology Chemistry. Hawk P, Oser B, Summerson W, Eds. Philadelphia, Blakiston. 1947, p. 814–822
30. Miles J, Glasscock R, Aikens J, Gerich J, Haymond M. A microfluorometric method for the determination of free fatty acids in plasma. J Lipid Res 1983;24:96–99
31. Ferrannini E. The theoretical bases of indirect calorimetry: a review. Metabolism 1988;37:287–301
32. Tappy L, Owen OE, Boden G. Effect of hyperinsulinemia on urea pool size and substrate oxidation rates. Diabetes 1988;37:1212–1216
33. Randle PJ, Garland PB, Hales CN, Newsholme EA. The glucose-fatty acid cycle: its role in insulin sensitivity and the metabolic disturbances of diabetes mellitus. *Lancet*. 1963;1:785–789
34. Bonadonna RC, Zych K, Boni C, Ferrannini E, DeFronzo RA. Time dependence of the interaction between lipid and glucose in humans. Am J Physiol 1989;257(Pt. 1):E49–E56
35. Clore JN, Brennan JR, Gebhart SP, Newsome HH, Nestler JE, Blackard WG. Prolonged insulin resistance following insulin-induced hypoglycaemia. Diabetologia 1987;30:851–858
36. Dresner A, Laurent D, Marcucci M, Griffin ME, Dufour S, Cline GW, Slezak LA, Andersen DK, Hundal RS, Rothman DL, Petersen KF, Shulman GI. Effects of free fatty acids on glucose transport and IRS-1-associated phosphatidylinositol 3-kinase activity. J Clin Invest 1999;103:253–259
37. Peino R, Cordido F, Peñalva A, Alvarez CV, Dieguez C, Casanueva FF. Acipimox-mediated plasma free fatty acid depression per se stimulates growth hormone (GH) secretion in normal subjects and potentiates the response to other GH-releasing stimuli. J Clin Endocrinol Metab 1996;81:909–913
38. Paramore DS, Fanelli CG, Shah SD, Cryer PE. Forearm norepinephrine spillover during standing, hyperinsulinemia, and hypoglycemia. Am J Physiol 1998;275:E872–E881
39. Newrick PG, Braatvedt G, Stansbie D, Corrall RJ. Suppression of lipolysis in normal man does not inhibit recovery from insulin-induced hypoglycaemia. Eur J Clin Invest 1993;23:53–56
40. Davis SN, Tate D. Effects of morning hypoglycemia on neuroendocrine and metabolic responses to subsequent afternoon hypoglycemia in normal man. J Clin Endocrinol Metab 2001;86:2043–2050

41. Cryer PE. Mechanisms of hypoglycemia-associated autonomic failure and its component syndromes in diabetes. Diabetes 2005;54:3592–3601

42. U.K. prospective diabetes study 16: overview of 6 years' therapy of type II diabetes: a progressive disease: U.K. Prospective Diabetes Study Group. Diabetes 1995;44:1249–1258

43. Action to Control Cardiovascular Risk in Diabetes Study Group, Gerstein HC, Miller ME, Byington RP, Goff DC Jr, Bigger JT, Buse JB, Cushman WC, Genuth S, Ismail-Beigi F, Grimm RH Jr, Probstfield JL, Simons-Morton DG, Friedewald WT. Effects of intensive glucose lowering in type 2 diabetes. N Engl J Med 2008;358:2545–2559

44. Christie AW, McCormick DK, Emmison N, Kraemer FB, Alberti KG, Yeaman SJ. Mechanism of anti-lipolytic action of acipimox in isolated rat adipocytes. Diabetologia 1996;39:45–53

45. Aktories K, Schultz G, Jakobs KH. Inhibition of adenylate cyclase and stimulation of a high affinity GTPase by the antilipolytic agents, nicotinic acid, acipimox and various related compounds. Arzneimittelforschung 1983;33:1525–1527

46. Fuccella LM, Goldaniga G, Lovisolo P, Maggi E, Musatti L, Mandelli V, Sirtori CR. Inhibition of lipolysis by nicotinic acid and by acipimox. Clin Pharmacol Ther 1980;28:790–795

47. Fulcher GR, Walker M, Catalano C, Farrer M, Alberti KG. Acute metabolic and hormonal responses to the inhibition of lipolysis in non-obese patients with non-insulin-dependent (type 2) diabetes mellitus: effects of acipimox. Clin Sci (Lond) 1992;82:565–571

48. Fulcher GR, Walker M, Catalano C, Agius L, Alberti KG. Metabolic effects of suppression of nonesterified fatty acid levels with acipimox in obese NIDDM subjects. Diabetes 1992;41:1400–1408

49. Vaag A, Skött P, Damsbo P, Gall MA, Richter EA, Beck-Nielsen H. Effect of the antilipolytic nicotinic acid analogue acipimox on whole-body and skeletal muscle glucose metabolism in patients with non-insulin-dependent diabetes mellitus. J Clin Invest 1991;88:1282–1290

50. Walker M, Agius L, Orskov H, Alberti KG. Peripheral and hepatic insulin sensitivity in non-insulin-dependent diabetes mellitus: effect of nonesterified fatty acids. Metabolism 1993;42:601–608

Ventromedial Hypothalamic Nitric Oxide Production Is Necessary for Hypoglycemia Detection and Counterregulation

Xavier Fioramonti,[1] Nicolas Marsollier,[2] Zhentao Song,[1] Kurt A. Fakira,[1] Reema M. Patel,[1] Stacey Brown,[3] Thibaut Duparc,[4] Arnaldo Pica-Mendez,[1] Nicole M. Sanders,[5] Claude Knauf,[4] Philippe Valet,[4] Rory J. McCrimmon,[4] Annie Beuve,[1] Christophe Magnan,[2] and Vanessa H. Routh[1]

OBJECTIVE—The response of ventromedial hypothalamic (VMH) glucose-inhibited neurons to decreased glucose is impaired under conditions where the counterregulatory response (CRR) to hypoglycemia is impaired (e.g., recurrent hypoglycemia). This suggests a role for glucose-inhibited neurons in the CRR. We recently showed that decreased glucose increases nitric oxide (NO) production in cultured VMH glucose-inhibited neurons. These in vitro data led us to hypothesize that NO release from VMH glucose-inhibited neurons is critical for the CRR.

RESEARCH DESIGN AND METHODS—The CRR was evaluated in rats and mice in response to acute insulin-induced hypoglycemia and hypoglycemic clamps after modulation of brain NO signaling. The glucose sensitivity of ventromedial nucleus glucose-inhibited neurons was also assessed.

RESULTS—Hypoglycemia increased hypothalamic constitutive NO synthase (NOS) activity and neuronal NOS (nNOS) but not endothelial NOS (eNOS) phosphorylation in rats. Intracerebroventricular and VMH injection of the nonselective NOS inhibitor N^G-monomethyl-L-arginine (L-NMMA) slowed the recovery to euglycemia after hypoglycemia. VMH L-NMMA injection also increased the glucose infusion rate (GIR) and decreased epinephrine secretion during hyperinsulinemic/hypoglycemic clamp in rats. The GIR required to maintain the hypoglycemic plateau was higher in nNOS knockout than wild-type or eNOS knockout mice. Finally, VMH glucose-inhibited neurons were virtually absent in nNOS knockout mice.

CONCLUSIONS—We conclude that VMH NO production is necessary for glucose sensing in glucose-inhibited neurons and full generation of the CRR to hypoglycemia. These data suggest that potentiating NO signaling may improve the defective CRR resulting from recurrent hypoglycemia in patients using intensive insulin therapy. *Diabetes* **59:519–528, 2010**

From the [1]Department of Pharmacology and Physiology, New Jersey Medical School, Newark, New Jersey; the [2]National Center for Scientific Research, University Paris Diderot, Paris, France; the [3]Department of Internal Medicine, Yale University School of Medicine, New Haven, Connecticut; the [4]INSERM U858, Institut de Medecine Moleculaire de Rangueil, IFR150, Université Paul Sabatier, Toulouse, France; and the [5]Division of Endocrinology/Metabolism, Veterans Affairs Puget Sound Health Care System, Seattle, Washington.

Corresponding author: Vanessa H. Routh, routhvh@umdnj.edu.

Received 20 March 2009 and accepted 8 November 2009. Published ahead of print at http://diabetes.diabetesjournals.org on 23 November 2009. DOI: 10.2337/db09-0421.

Intensive insulin therapy significantly reduces the onset and progression of hyperglycemia-related complications in patients with type 1 and advanced type 2 diabetes. However, intensive insulin therapy also causes a clinically adverse effect: hypoglycemia (1). Powerful neuroendocrine and autonomic counterregulatory mechanisms protect the brain from hypoglycemia (2,3). These protective mechanisms, known as the counterregulatory response (CRR) to hypoglycemia, involve the release of hormones (e.g., glucagon, epinephrine) that restore euglycemia by stimulating hepatic glucose production and inhibiting peripheral glucose uptake (3). Although the physiology of the CRR is well understood, the underlying cellular mechanisms by which the brain senses hypoglycemia and initiates the CRR remain elusive.

During hypoglycemia, central and peripheral glucose sensors detect declining glucose levels (4). In the brain, the ventromedial hypothalamus, which includes the arcuate nucleus and the ventromedial nucleus (VMN), is important in the initiation of the CRR (5–7). This region contains specialized glucose-sensing neurons (GSNs). Ventromedial hypothalamic (VMH) GSN electrical activity is regulated by physiologically relevant changes in extracellular glucose levels (8–11). Glucose-excited neurons decrease, whereas glucose-inhibited neurons increase, their input resistance, membrane potential, and action potential frequency when extracellular glucose is reduced (10). Many studies suggest that VMH glucose-inhibited neurons play a critical role in the control of the CRR (4). For example, the response of VMH glucose-inhibited neurons to decreased glucose is impaired under conditions where the CRR is impaired (e.g., recurrent hypoglycemia) (12,13).

Nitric oxide (NO) is a gaseous messenger produced by NO synthase (NOS). Two classes of NOS have been identified in the brain: the inducible NOS (iNOS) and the constitutive NOS, which includes the neuronal NOS (nNOS) and endothelial NOS (eNOS) isoforms (14). Hypothalamic NO is involved in the regulation of food intake and glucose homeostasis (15–18). In support of this, we have recently shown that VMH glucose-inhibited neurons produce NO via nNOS in response to decreased extracellular glucose levels (19,20). Therefore, in this study, we test the hypothesis that NO production by VMH glucose-inhibited neurons is necessary for the CRR to hypoglycemia. We tested this hypothesis using a combination of in vivo and in vitro techniques in wild-type rats and mice as well as in transgenic nNOS and eNOS knockout mice.

RESEARCH DESIGN AND METHODS

All procedures were approved by the Institutional Animal Care and Use Committee at the University of Medicine and Dentistry of New Jersey. Adult male Sprague-Dawley rats were purchased from Charles River. Adult 5- to 8-week-old C57BL/6J wild-type, nNOS knockout (B6.129S4-Nos1^{tm1Plh}/J), and eNOS knockout (B6.129P2-Nos3^{tm1Unc}/J) mice were purchased from The Jackson Laboratory (Bar Harbor, ME). Animals were housed individually and maintained on a 12-h light/12-h dark schedule at 22–23°C with ad libitum access to food and water.

In vivo experiments

Surgical procedures. Rats were anesthetized with sodium pentobarbital (50 mg/kg i.p.; Ovation) and mice, with ketamine/xylazine (80/8 mg/kg i.p.; Bioniche-Pharma/Lloyd Laboratories). Vascular catheters were surgically implanted in the left carotid and/or the right jugular vein in rats, and a vascular catheter was implanted in the right jugular vein in mice. The catheters were filled with heparin (10 units/ml) and flushed every other day. Additionally, rats received a stereotaxic implantation of microinjection cannula guide positioned 1-mm dorsal to the ventromedial hypothalamus or in the right lateral ventricle according to stereotaxic coordinates (VMH cannulation; from bregma: −2.5 mm anterior-posterior, −2.8 mm medial-lateral, and −8.5 mm dorsal-ventral, at an angle of 20°; intracerebroventricular [ICV] cannulation; from bregma: −1.0 mm anterior-posterior, −1.4 mm medial-lateral, and −4.0 mm dorsal-ventral). Animals were allowed 5–7 days to recover from surgery and were handled every day. Animals that did not recover to their presurgery body weights were excluded from the study. For probe placement, at the end of each experiment, cannula placement was verified by methyl-blue (Sigma) injection.

Experimental procedures. Animals undergoing hyperinsulinemic/hypoglycemic clamps were either fasted overnight (rats) or for 5 h (9:00 A.M. to 2:00 P.M.; mice). Two hours before the start of the study, catheters were externalized outside the cage to minimize investigator interaction and were connected to infusion pumps. Starting 30 min before insulin injection (see below), one group of rats was infused intracerebroventricularly (0.4 μl/min, 2 h), whereas another group was injected in the ventromedial hypothalamus (0.1 μl/min, 10 min) with one of the following compounds in artificial cerebrospinal fluid (aCSF; containing in mM: 135 NaCl, 5 KCl, 1 CaCl$_2$, 1 MgCl$_2$, 10 HEPES, pH = 7.4): N^G-monomethyl-L-arginine (L-NMMA; 50 mmol/l in aCSF), 1H-[1,2,4]-oxadiazolo-[4,3-a]quinoxalin-1–1 (ODQ; 0.1 mmol/l in aCSF containing 0.1% DMSO). The control for L-NMMA was injected with aCSF, whereas the control for ODQ was injected with DMSO (0.1% in aCSF).

Acute insulin infusion. Rats (100–150 g) were injected with an insulin bolus (1 unit/kg; regular human insulin; Eli-Lilly) through the jugular catheter 30 min after ICV or VMH infusion. Blood glucose was monitored every 15 min from −30 to 120 min after insulin infusion via tail prick.

Hyperinsulinemic/hypoglycemic clamp. Starting 30 min after VMH or ICV infusion, rats (300–350 g) or mice (7–8 weeks old) were injected through the jugular catheter with an insulin bolus (rats: 0.4 units/kg; mice: 1 unit/kg) to decrease glycemia to ~50 mg/dl within 30–40 min. This time course was used based on the results of Saberi et al. (21), suggesting that brain versus peripheral glucose sensors predominate in CRR initiation when blood glucose decreases rapidly. After this bolus, animals were perfused with insulin at 1.2 units · kg^{-1} · h^{-1} for 90 (rats) or 120 (mice) min. Glucose (20%) was co-perfused with insulin to maintain plasma glucose level of ~50 mg/dl. The concentration of blood glucose was measured every 10 min via tail prick. For clamps carried out in rats, arterial blood samples (500 μl) taken from the carotid catheter were collected at 0, 30, 60, and 90 min for subsequent measurement of plasma glucagon, epinephrine, and norepinephrine. Glucocorticoid levels were not measured because they are not an essential aspect of the recovery from an acute hypoglycemic challenge (for review, see [22]). For glucagon, 250 μl of blood was collected in chilled tubes containing EGTA (1.6 mg/ml; Sigma) and aprotinin (250 KIU/ml; Sigma). For catecholamines, blood was collected in chilled tubes containing reduced glutathione (1.2 mg/ml; Sigma) and EDTA (1.8 mg/ml; Sigma). After removal of plasma, erythrocytes from experimental rats were resuspended in an equivalent volume of sterile NaCl 0.9% and reinfused after each blood sampling to prevent volume depletion. For mice clamp, trunk blood was collected at the end of the clamp in chilled tubes containing reduced glutathione (1.2 mg/ml; Sigma) and EDTA (1.8 mg/ml; Sigma) for plasma epinephrine and norepinephrine measurement.

Plasma glucagon and catecholamine determination. Plasma glucagon concentrations were determined using commercially available radioimmunoassay kits (Linco Research). Plasma epinephrine and norepinephrine concentrations were analyzed by high-performance liquid chromatography using electrochemical detection (ESA Biosciences, Acton, MA).

Phosphorylated-NOS Western blot. Rats (100–150 g) were injected with saline or insulin (2 units/kg, s.c.) and killed 60 min after by an overdose of sodium pentobarbital (Euthasol, Virbac, Fort Worth, TX). The ventral hypo-

thalamus was quickly harvested, snap frozen, and stored at −80°C. Brain samples were lysed over ice in lysis buffer (150 mmol/l NaCl, 0.02% sodium azide, 10 mmol/l HEPES, 50 mmol/l NaF, 0.1% SDS, 0.5% deoxycholic acid, 1% Nonidet P-40, 0.2 mmol/l phenylmethylsulfonyl fluoride, 2 μg/ml pepstatin-A, 2 μg/ml leupeptin, and 2 μg/ml aprotinin). Cytosolic lysate supernatants were collected by centrifugation at 14,000g for 10 min at 4°C. Protein (15 μg) was electrophoresed and transferred to nitrocellulose membranes. Immunodetection with primary antibodies was performed for 12 h at 4°C: phosphorylated-NOS (P-nNOS; nNOS-Ser 1717) 1:5,000 (Millipore), phosphorylated eNOS (eNOS-Ser 1177) 1:5,000, and nNOS and eNOS 1:2,500 (Cell Signaling). After washing, secondary antibody (donkey anti-rabbit; Jackson ImmunoResearch) was added at 1:1,000 for 1 h at room temperature. Signals are visualized using ECL kit (Thermo) and quantified using Scion Image. Results are presented as percentage of control after normalization to total nNOS/eNOS.

NOS activity. NOS activity was quantified using the radiodetection kit (Calbiochem) based on the biochemical conversion of [^{3}H-]L-arginine to [^{3}H-]L-citrulline by NOS. To distinguish Ca^{2+}-dependent constitutive NOS activity (nNOS + eNOS), from Ca^{2+}-independent iNOS activity, hypothalamic homogenates were prepared as above and divided into two sets of samples, one of which omitted calcium in the assay medium for measurement of iNOS activity.

In vitro experiments

Electrophysiology. Coronal brain slices (250 μm) from wild-type and nNOS knockout mice (5–7 weeks old) were prepared as previously described (8,23). Briefly, viable neurons were visualized under infrared differential-interference contrast microscopy (DM LFS microscope; Leica Microsystems). Current clamp recordings (standard whole-cell configuration) from VMN neurons were performed using a MultiClamp 700A (Axon Instruments) and analyzed using pCLAMP9 software. During recording, brain slices were perfused at 10 ml/min with normal oxygenated artificial cerebrospinal fluid containing (in mM): 126 NaCl, 1.9 KCl, 1.2 KH$_2$PO$_4$, 26 NaHCO$_3$, 2.4 CaCl$_2$, 1.3 MgCl$_2$, 2.5 glucose; 300–310 mOsM, pH 7.4). Borosilicate pipettes (3–5 MΩ; Sutter Instrument) were filled with an intracellular solution containing (in mM): 128 K-gluconate, 10 KCl, 4 KOH, 10 HEPES, 4 MgCl$_2$, 0.5 CaCl$_2$, 5 EGTA, and 2 Na$_2$ATP (pH 7.2; 290–300 mOsM). Membrane potential, action potential frequency, and input resistance in response to constant hyperpolarizing pulse (20 pA) were monitored as extracellular glucose level was changed from 2.5 to 0.1 mmol/l as described in figures.

Cellular imaging. VMH neurons were prepared using a protocol modified from Murphy et al. (24,25) (see supplementary data for detailed protocol, available in an online appendix at http://diabetes.diabetesjournals.org/cgi/content/full/db09hyphen]0421/DC1). VMH neurons were perfused in a closed chamber at 0.6 ml/min with oxygenated extracellular solution containing (in mM): 132 NaCl, 5 KCl, 0.45 KH$_2$PO$_4$, 0.45 NaH$_2$PO$_4$, 1.2 CaCl$_2$, 0.5 MgCl$_2$, 0.4 MgSO$_4$, 5 HEPES, 2.5 glucose (pH 7.3; osmolarity adjusted to 300–310 mOsM) in the presence of 0.5% membrane potential dye (FLIPR-MPD; Molecular Devices, Sunnyvale, CA). After 10 min of equilibration, VMH neurons were perfused with the same extracellular solution containing 0.1 mmol/l glucose for 15 min followed by 15 min at 2.5 mmol/l glucose. Image acquisition and analysis were performed as previously described (24,25). Neurons were considered as glucose-inhibited neurons when their fluorescence intensity reversibly increased more than 25% in response to 0.1 mmol/l glucose. Data are expressed in percentage of glucose-inhibited neurons detected per dish.

Hypothalamic NO real-time measurement. Wild-type mice were killed by decapitation without anesthesia. The hypothalamus was quickly harvested and maintained in 200 μl Krebs-Ringer oxygenated solution containing 2.5 mmol/l glucose at 37°C. A NO-specific amperometric probe (ISO-NOPF100; World Precision Instruments [WPI], Sarasota, FL) was implanted directly in the tissue and NO release was monitored. The hypothalamus was exposed to the following sequence of glucose concentrations (15 min each): 2.5, 0.1, and 2.5 mmol/l. The concentration of NO gas in the tissue was measured in real time with the data acquisition system LabTrax (WPI) connected to the free radical analyzer Apollo1000 (WPI). Data acquisition and analysis were performed with DataTrax2 software (WPI). The NO-specific amperometric probe was calibrated as previously described (26).

Data analysis. All data are presented as mean ± SEM. Statistical analysis was performed using Graphpad Prism 4.0 by two-way ANOVA followed by Bonferroni post hoc test, one-way ANOVA followed by Dunnett post hoc test, or unpaired *t* test as described in the figure legends. $P < 0.05$ indicates statistical significance.

RESULTS

Hypoglycemia activates ventral hypothalamic nNOS.

We have previously shown that decreased glucose concentration increases NO production in cultured VMH glucose-

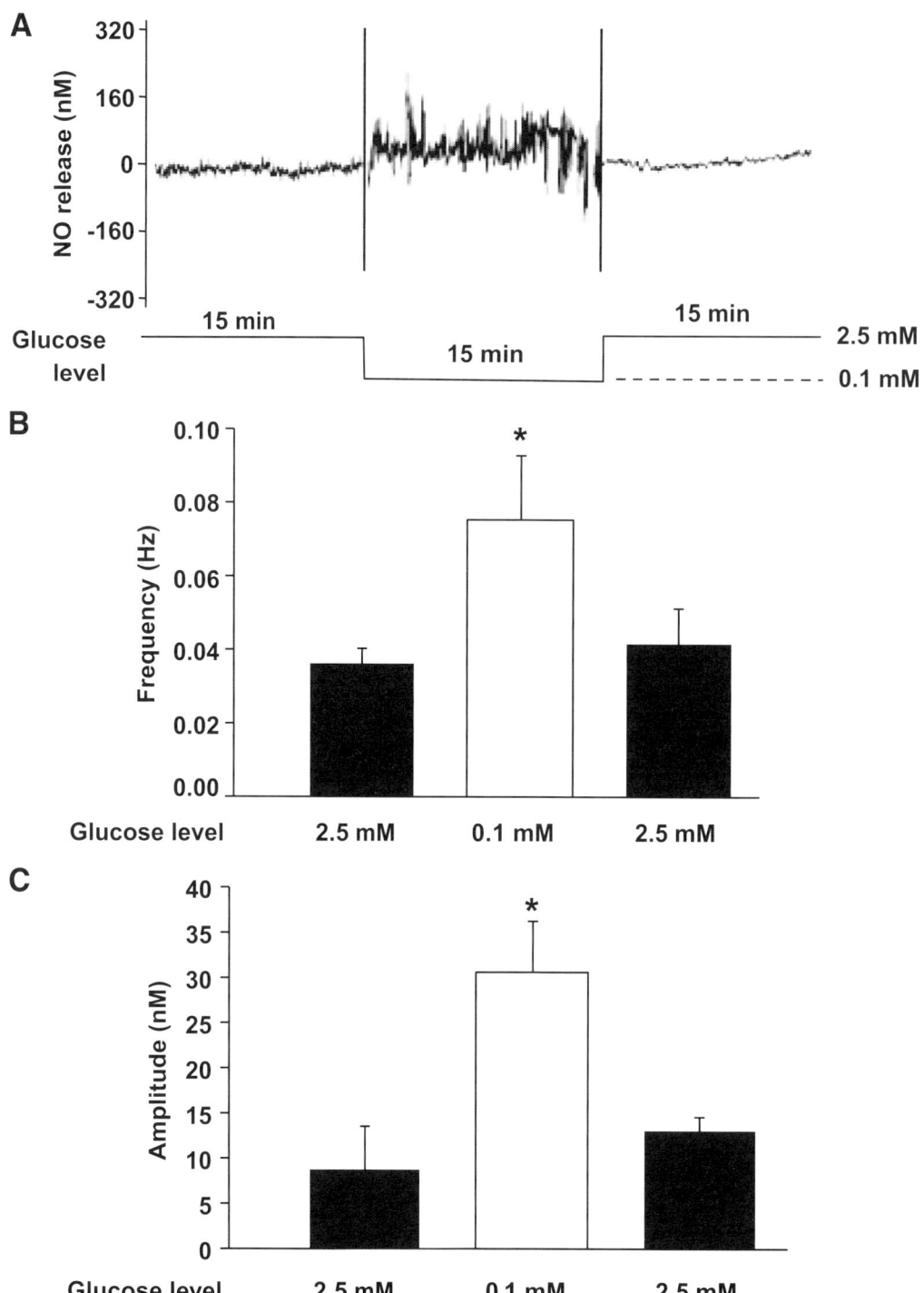

FIG. 1. Decreased glucose increases VMH NO release. *A*: Representative trace of ex vivo amperometric measurements of NO release from mouse hypothalamus in response to an extracellular glucose decrease from 2.5 to 0.1 mmol/l. *B*: Mean frequency and (*C*) mean amplitude of NO release calculated during the last 10-min recording for each glucose level (*n* = 4). *$P < 0.05$ vs. 2.5 mmol/l glucose (one-way ANOVA).

inhibited neurons in vitro using a membrane sensitive dye (20). To confirm that decreased glucose increases hypothalamic NO production, we performed amperometric measurement of NO release in hypothalamic chunks ex vivo using an NO-sensitive electrode. As shown in Figure 1, decreased glucose from 2.5 to 0.1 mmol/l significantly increases the amplitude (3.5-fold; $P < 0.05$) and frequency (2.1-fold; $P < 0.05$) of NO release. NO release returned to

baseline when extracellular solution was subsequently raised to 2.5 mmol/l glucose (Fig. 1).

To provide in vivo evidence that hypoglycemia increases hypothalamic NO production, constitutive (nNOS and eNOS) and inducible (iNOS) activity was determined in ventral hypothalamus from rats 60 min after insulin injection. Insulin-hypoglycemia significantly increased constitutive NOS activity by 1.45 ± 0.11-fold. iNOS activity was

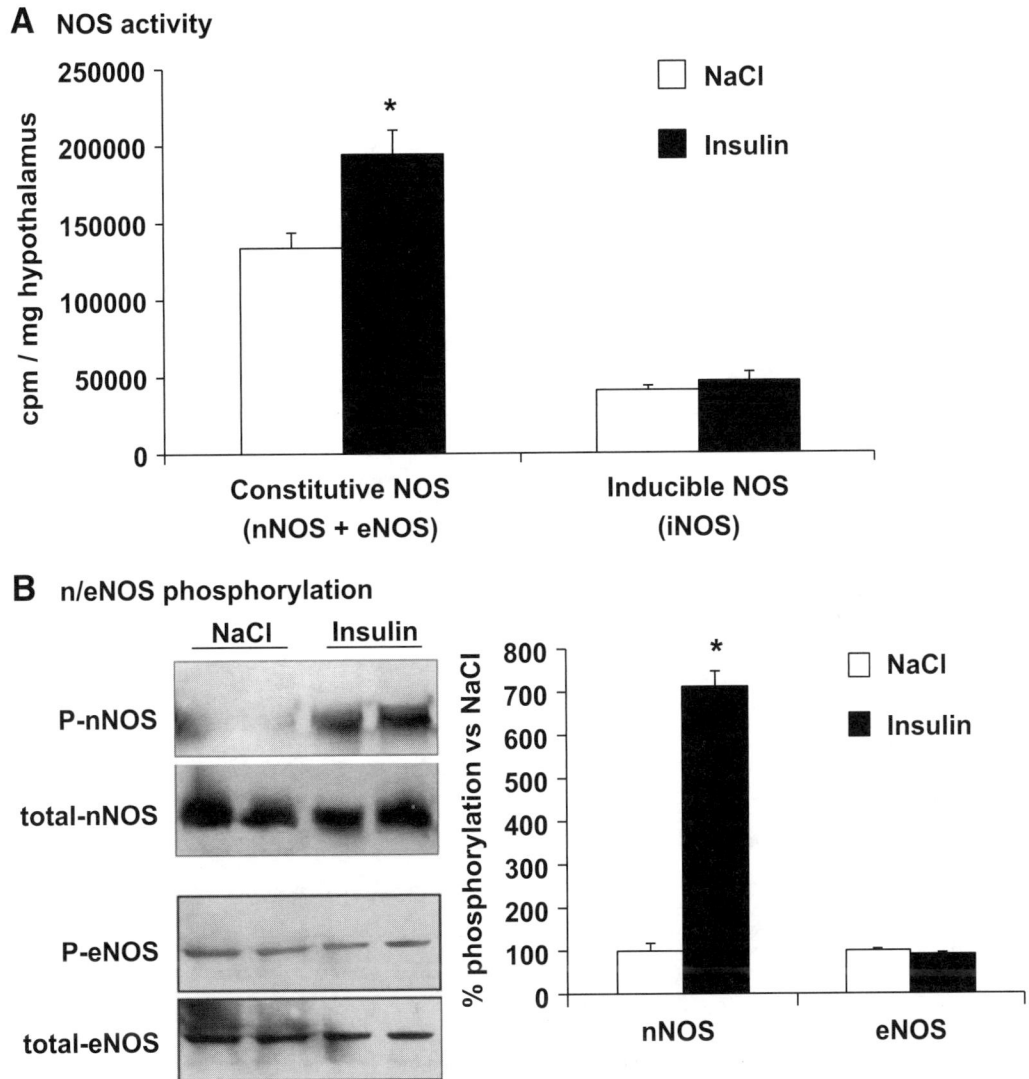

FIG. 2. Hypoglycemia increases ventral hypothalamic nNOS activity. *A*: Ventral hypothalamic constitutive (e/nNOS) or inducible (iNOS) NOS activity from rats injected subcutaneously with saline (control, $n = 6$) or insulin (2 units/kg; $n = 6$) 60 min after injection. *B*: Representative Western blot (*left panel*) of ventral hypothalamic total nNOS, phosphorylated nNOS (P-nNOS), total eNOS, and P-eNOS from control or insulin-treated rats injected subcutaneously with saline ($n = 5$) or insulin ($n = 5$) 60 min after injection. The *right panel* shows the quantification of the ratio between P-nNOS or P-eNOS and total nNOS or eNOS, respectively. Data are means ± SEM and represented as percentage of saline where the control group was considered to be 100%. *$P < 0.05$ vs. control (unpaired t test).

not changed (Fig. 2*A*). Cortical constitutive NOS activity was not changed in insulin-induced hypoglycemia treated rats versus control (data not shown). To determine whether nNOS or eNOS is primarily responsible for hypoglycemia-induced hypothalamic NO production, Western blots against the phosphorylated nNOS and eNOS forms were performed. nNOS phosphorylation was significantly increased by 7.26 ± 0.36-fold, whereas eNOS phosphorylation was not changed (Fig. 2*B*), suggesting that nNOS activation was responsible for increased VMH constitutive NOS activity during insulin-induced hypoglycemia. These data strongly suggest that insulin-induced hypoglycemia stimulates nNOS-derived VMH NO production.

Inhibition of VMH NO signaling impairs the CRR to hypoglycemia. We first evaluated the effect of brain NO on the counterregulatory response to acute insulin-induced hypoglycemia. As shown in Fig. 3, rats infused with the nonselective NOS inhibitor L-NMMA either intracere-

broventricularly or into the ventromedial hypothalamus showed significantly lower glycemia at 60 and 90 min after insulin injection compared with control. Many of the effects of NO are mediated by its receptor, soluble guanylyl cyclase (sGC) (14). Inhibition of VMH sGC with ODQ decreased the glycemia at 45, 60, 90, and 120 min after insulin injection (Fig. 3*B*).

To confirm that VMH NO production is involved in the CRR, we performed hyperinsulinemic/hypoglycemic clamps (5,6,21,27). During the hypoglycemic clamp, blood glucose was decreased to similar levels in control (52 ± 1.1 mg/dl) and treated (54 ± 1.0 mg/dl) animals (Fig. 4). Administration of the nonselective NOS inhibitor L-NMMA in the ventromedial hypothalamus significantly increased the glucose infusion rate (GIR) necessary to maintain the hypoglycemia plateau (Fig. 4). Changes in GIR were associated with significant decreases in epinephrine levels at 60 and 90 min in L-NMMA–treated animals (Fig. 4). Glucagon (Fig. 4) and norepinephrine (data not shown)

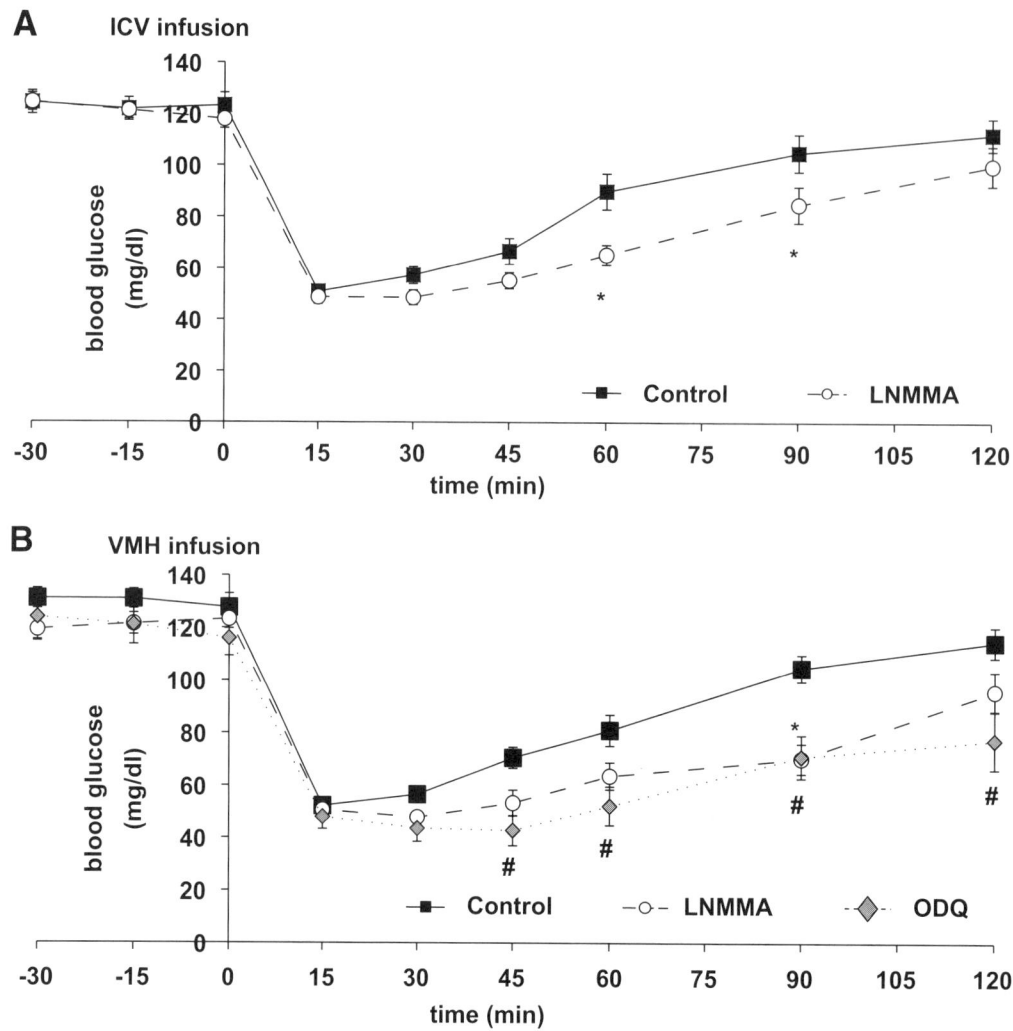

FIG. 3. VMH NO signaling is necessary for recovery to euglycemia after insulin-induced hypoglycemia. Blood glucose levels in response to insulin-induced hypoglycemia (1 unit/kg, i.v.) in rats receiving (A) ICV perfusion of aCSF (controls; n = 14) or L-NMMA (50 mmol/l; n = 14), or (B) unilateral VMH injection of aCSF (n = 7), L-NMMA (50 mmol/l, n = 7), or ODQ (0.1 mmol/l, n = 5). *, #P < 0.05 vs. control (two-way ANOVA).

levels were not significantly reduced. Taken together, these data show that the VMH NO-sGC signaling pathway is necessary for the full generation of the sympathoadrenal response to hypoglycemia.

VMH nNOS is involved in the CRR to hypoglycemia. To confirm that VMH nNOS derived-NO is involved in the CRR, we performed hyperinsulinemic/hypoglycemic clamps in wild-type, nNOS, and eNOS knockout mice. The GIR required to maintain the hypoglycemic plateau over the last 30 min was significantly higher in nNOS knockout and lower in eNOS knockout mice compared with wild type (wild type: 17.4 ± 1.6 mg $\cdot$ kg$^{-1} \cdot$ min^{-1}; nNOS: 31.1 ± 1.7 mg $\cdot$ kg$^{-1} \cdot$ min^{-1}; eNOS: 12.8 ± 1.1 mg $\cdot$ kg$^{-1} \cdot$ min^{-1}; $P < 0.05$; Fig. 5B). At the end of the clamp, epinephrine levels were significantly reduced in the nNOS knockout compared with wild-type or eNOS knockout mice (Fig. 5C). There was no difference in plasma norepinephrine levels between groups (data not shown). Because the initial blood glucose level was lower in nNOS knockout than wild-type mice (nNOS knockout: 136 ± 6.4 mg/dl versus wild type: 179 ± 7.5 mg/dl; $P < 0.05$), we measured plasma insulin and liver glycogen content in another group of mice after 5-h fast. Neither plasma insulin nor liver

glycogen concentration was different between nNOS knockout and wild-type mice (insulin: wild type: 0.58 ± 0.2 versus nNOS: 0.52 ± 0.1 ng/ml; glycogen: wild type: 23.5 ± 2.8 versus nNOS: 24.7 ± 5.3 mg/g of liver; $n = 4$; $P > 0.05$). These data show that NO produced specifically by the nNOS isoform is necessary for the full generation of the CRR.

nNOS is necessary for glucose sensing by VMH glucose-inhibited neurons. Data from our laboratory and others suggest that VMN GSNs play a role in sensing hypoglycemia and initiating the CRR (9,13,27–32). Because we showed above that the CRR is impaired in nNOS knockout mice, we wanted to determine whether the glucose sensitivity of GSNs is also impaired. We used whole-cell current clamp recording techniques to measure the membrane potential, action potential frequency (APF), and input resistance of VMN neurons in response to decreased glucose levels from 2.5 to 0.1 mmol/l in wild-type and nNOS knockout mice. In wild-type mice, three neurons (3 of 36, 8%) were identified as glucose-excited neurons by a decrease in their membrane potential, APF, and input resistance in response to 2.5–0.1 mmol/l glucose decrease, whereas 11 neurons (11 of 36, 30%) increased

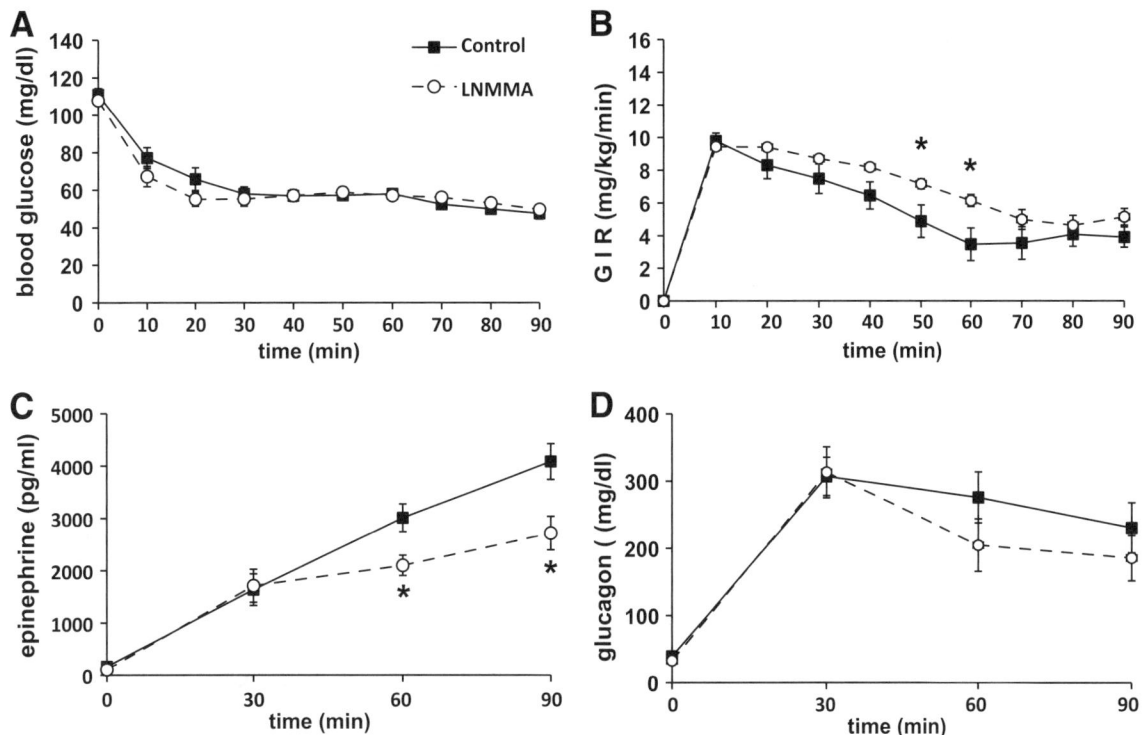

FIG. 4. VMH NOS inhibition impairs the CRR to hypoglycemia. Blood glucose level (*A*); GIR (*B*); plasma epinephrine (*C*), and glucagon levels (*D*) during hyperinsulinemic/hypoglycemic clamp (1.2 units · kg⁻¹ · h⁻¹) of animals injected bilaterally in the ventromedial hypothalamus with aCSF (controls; $n = 8$) or L-NMMA (50 mmol/l; $n = 6$). *$P < 0.05$ vs. controls (two-way ANOVA).

membrane potential, APF, and input resistance in response to decreased glucose and were identified as glucose-inhibited neurons (Fig. 6*A*). In nNOS knockout mice, four neurons (4 of 25, 16%) were identified as glucose-excited neurons (Fig. 6*B*). In contrast, no glucose-inhibited neurons (0 of 25) were found in nNOS knockout mice VMN. Results are summarized in Fig. 6*C*. We confirmed these electrophysiology data using a membrane potential sensitive dye in cultured VMH neurons. Whereas 13.0 ± 1.2% of VMH neurons were glucose-inhibited neurons in wild-type mice (14 dishes; 1,352 neurons; 7 mice), only 2.4 ± 0.6% were glucose-inhibited neurons in nNOS knockout mice (12 dishes; 961 neurons; 3 mice; $P < 0.05$). These data suggest that VMH glucose-inhibited neuron glucose sensing is impaired in nNOS knockout mice.

DISCUSSION

This study confirms that decreased glucose increases VMH NO production in vivo. Moreover, this study supports our novel hypothesis that NO production is necessary for the full generation of the CRR and glucose sensing in VMH glucose-inhibited neurons. Pharmacological inhibition of VMH NO signaling decreases blood glucose recovery and impairs the CRR after hypoglycemia. Interestingly, the impaired CRR in mice lacking nNOS is associated with an almost complete loss of VMH glucose-inhibited neurons, consistent with our recently published data showing that NO production is required for glucose-inhibited neurons to sense glucose (24). We have previously shown that VMH glucose-inhibited neurons are less sensitive to decreased glucose under conditions where the CRR is also impaired. These data suggested a role for VMH glucose-inhibited neurons in the CRR (12,13,28,31,33). Our current data

strengthen the hypothesis that detection of hypoglycemia by VMH glucose-inhibited neurons is a necessary step in the full generation of the CRR.

We found previously, using in vitro cellular imaging, that among cultured VMH neurons only glucose-inhibited neurons produce NO in response to decreased glucose. nNOS, but not eNOS, mediates NO production in VMH glucose-inhibited neurons (20). In the present study, we confirm this finding by showing that decreased glucose increases VMH NO release using an NO-sensitive electrode. Moreover, insulin-induced hypoglycemia in vivo increases VMH NOS activity and nNOS phosphorylation. Because insulin increases nNOS-derived NO production in cultured VMH neurons (20), insulin injection may contribute to the increased VMH NO production during this clinically relevant form of hypoglycemia. These data strongly support our hypothesis that nNOS activation during insulin-induced hypoglycemia induces VMH NO production in vivo. Cabou et al. (16) recently suggested that cerebral insulin injection during euglycemia increases hypothalamic NO production through eNOS. Insulin-induced hypoglycemia did not increase eNOS activity in our study. Moreover, because Cabou et al. did not evaluate nNOS activity, they did not rule out a role for this NOS isoform in response to cerebral insulin injection. It is possible that prolonged hyperinsulinemia and/or recurrent episodes of insulin-induced hypoglycemia further increase VMH NO production through a combined increase in nNOS and eNOS activity.

What is the role of VMH NO production in energetic homeostasis during energy deficit? One putative function for VMH NO production is to increase cerebral blood flow, leading to increased local nutrient availability. Human and

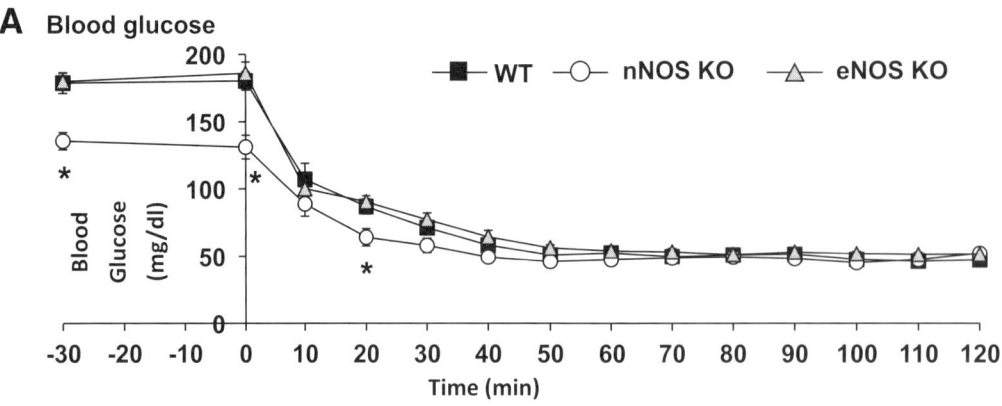

A Blood glucose

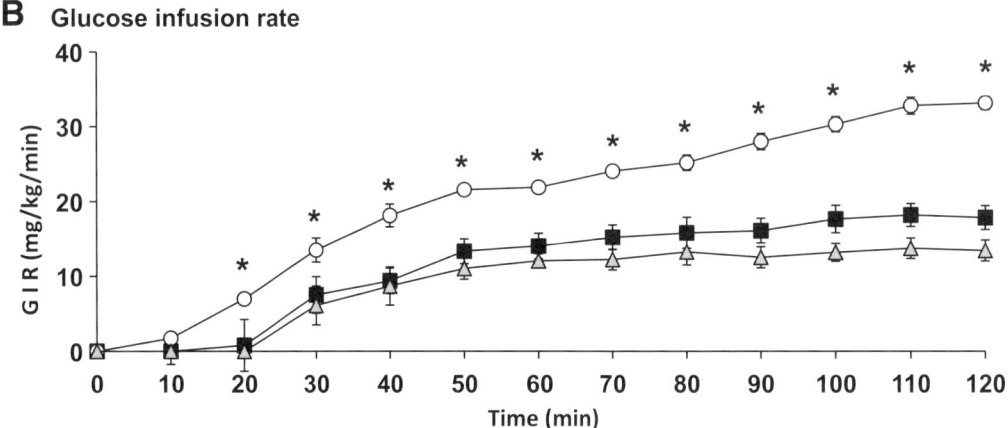

B Glucose infusion rate

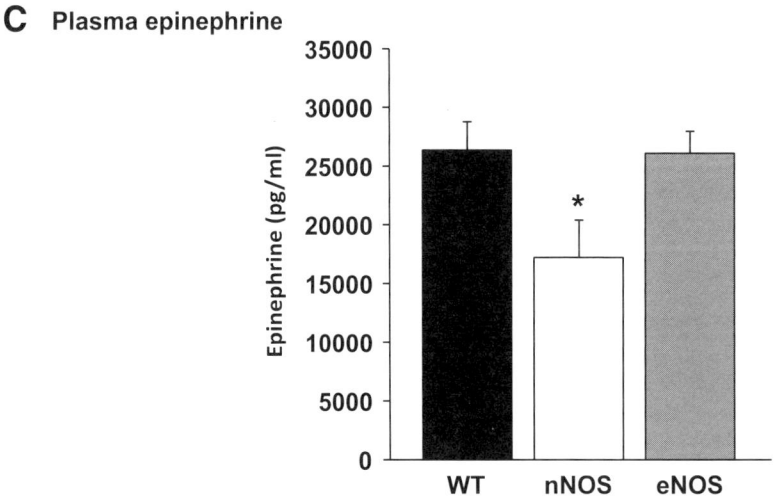

C Plasma epinephrine

FIG. 5. nNOS is necessary for full initiation of the CRR. Blood glucose concentration (*A*), glucose infusion rate (*B*), and plasma epinephrine taken at the end of the clamp (*C*) of wild-type (WT) (*n* = 14), eNOS (*n* = 6), and nNOS (*n* = 7) knockout mice during hyperinsulinemic/hypoglycemic clamp (1.2 units · kg^{-1} · h^{-1}). *$P < 0.05$ vs. wild type (two-way ANOVA).

animal studies show that insulin-induced hypoglycemia is associated with increased cerebral blood flow in many brain areas including the hypothalamus (34–36). For example, Page et al. (37) recently showed that decreased blood glucose increased hypothalamic blood flow prior to the release of CRR hormones. One of the main physiological functions of NO is related to the vascular system. The role of eNOS-mediated NO production in peripheral vasorelaxation is well established (38). One of the unique features of NO as a neurotransmitter is the ability to diffuse across cell membranes (14). Thus, although we did not see an increase in eNOS activity in our studies, NO produced in VMH glucose-inhibited neurons may diffuse to adjacent vascular smooth muscle cells lining cerebral vasculature and cause vasodilatation. However, we think that this is unlikely because Horinaka et al. (39) and Paulson (40) showed that increased cerebral blood flow in response to hypoglycemia was NO independent. These

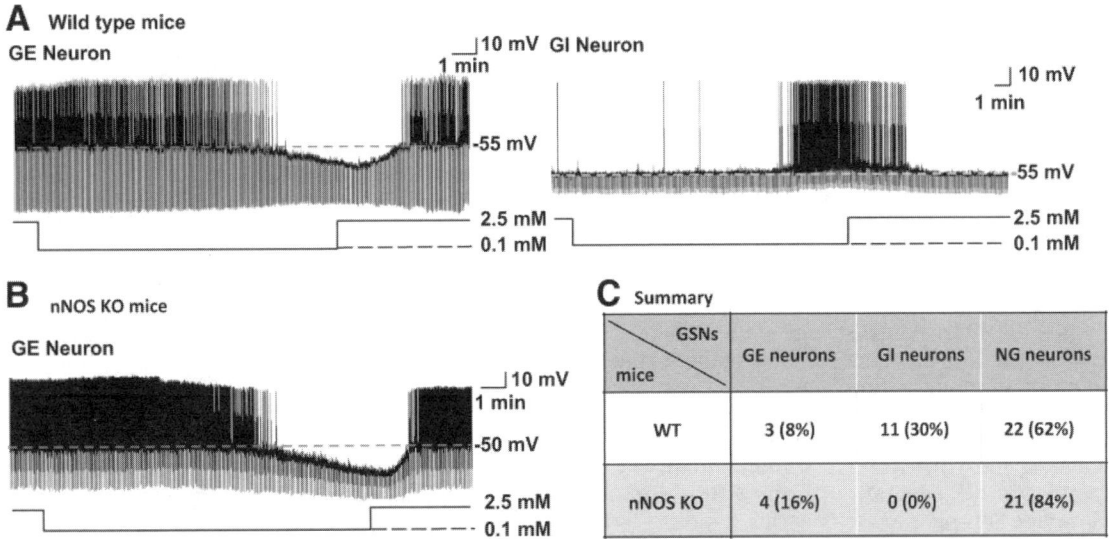

FIG. 6. nNOS is necessary for glucose sensing by VMN glucose-inhibited neurons. Representative whole-cell current-clamp recordings of VMN glucose-excited and glucose-inhibited neurons in brain slices from wild-type (WT) mice (*A*) or nNOS knockout mice (*B*). The dotted lines represent the resting membrane potential. Glucose concentration changes are schematically displayed below each recording. Downward deflections in whole-cell current-clamp recordings represent the membrane voltage responses to constant hyperpolarizing currents. (*C*) Table summarizing the number (and %) of VMN glucose-excited (GE), glucose-inhibited (GI), or nonglucose-sensitive (NG) neurons in wild-type or nNOS knockout mice.

data suggest that VMH nNOS-mediated NO production does not play a role in blood flow regulation. This is consistent with other studies that suggest a role for the β-adrenergic receptor and/or the ATP-sensitive K^+ channel (K_{ATP}) in hypoglycemia-induced increases in cerebral blood flow (41,42).

Another function of VMH NO production is through the CRR. We used two complementary approaches to show that VMH NO production is a physiologically required step in the full generation of the CRR. First, inhibition of VMH NO production slows down the recovery to euglycemia in response to acute insulin-induced hypoglycemia. Although this is the most physiological evaluation of the CRR, it is difficult to reliably compare the levels of counterregulatory hormones between treatments due to variation in the actual degree of hypoglycemia. Thus, we also used the "gold standard" technique for studying the CRR: hyperinsulinemic/hypoglycemic clamps. Here we found that VMH NOS inhibition increases the GIR and decreases epinephrine production during hypoglycemic clamps. Moreover, the GIR is significantly greater and epinephrine production lower in nNOS knockout versus wild-type mice. These data confirm our hypothesis that VMH NO plays an important role in the control of the CRR. However, it is also clear that the CRR was not completely abolished by either L-NMMA injection or in the nNOS knockout mice. These findings are consistent with parallel regulation of the CRR by other central or peripheral glucose sensors. Finally, both eNOS and nNOS knockout mice exhibit insulin resistance (18,43). In eNOS knockout mice, there was a decrease in the GIR to maintain the hypoglycemic plateau that may reflect insulin resistance (18,43). The milder insulin resistance in nNOS knockout mice probably did not affect the GIR due to the high insulin concentration used for the hypoglycemic clamp.

The next step was to explore the molecular and cellular mechanisms by which VMH NO production contributes to the CRR. Our previous studies suggested a role for VMN glucose-inhibited neurons in the generation of the CRR

because their response to decreased glucose is impaired when the CRR is impaired (12,13,28,31,33). We have recently shown that NO production via nNOS is necessary for VMN glucose-inhibited neurons to depolarize in response to decreased glucose (24). In the present study, VMH glucose-inhibited neurons were not detected in nNOS knockout mice in response to decreased extracellular glucose from 2.5 to 0.1 mmol/l. This glucose concentration decrease, although supraphysiologic, was necessary because we have previously shown that recurrent episodes of hypoglycemia decrease the response of VMH glucose-inhibited neurons to decreased glucose. In fact, after recurrent hypoglycemia the response of VMH glucose-inhibited neurons to a glucose decrease from 2.5 to 0.5 mmol/l was almost undetectable; however their response to a glucose decrease from 2.5 to 0.1 mmol/l was intact (13). Thus, using a glucose decrease to 0.1 mmol/l suggests that functional VMH glucose-inhibited neurons are almost absent in nNOS knockout mice. The CRR was also impaired in nNOS knockout mice. These data reinforce our hypothesis that activation of VMH glucose-inhibited neurons in response to decreased glucose is critical for the full generation of the CRR. Restoration of VMH NO expression in nNOS knockout mice would lend further strength to this conclusion. However, the effects of NO are highly dependent on the localization of intracellular NO production, which, in turn, is highly dependent on intracellular NOS localization (14). Overexpressing nNOS or injecting NO donors into the ventromedial hypothalamus of nNOS knockout mice would not mimic physiological NO production and could lead to difficulties in data interpretation. Our data suggest also that the NO receptor sGC mediates the effect of VMH NO on the CRR. sGC is expressed in all VMH neurons including glucose-inhibited neurons (20). Cyclic guanosine monophosphate produced by sGC has been shown to modulate neuronal activity (17,44). Taken together, these data suggest that decreased glucose depolarizes VMH glucose-inhibited neurons through NO-sGC signaling and leads to full generation of the CRR.

On the other hand, our data suggest that VMH glucose-inhibited neurons are not the only mediator of the CRR because the CRR is still present, albeit impaired, in the absence of NO signaling. VMH glucose-excited neurons are normal in nNOS knockout mice. Moreover, Miki et al. (30) showed that the CRR was impaired and VMH glucose-excited neurons were absent in K_{ATP}-deficient mice. Therefore, it is likely that VMH glucose-inhibited and glucose-excited neurons as well as extrahypothalamic glucose sensors are needed for the full generation of the CRR. Interestingly, glucagon but not epinephrine secretion in response to hypoglycemia was impaired in the K_{ATP}-deficient mice (30). In contrast our data indicate that inhibition of VMH NO signaling impairs epinephrine but not glucagon or norepinephrine secretion in response to hypoglycemia. This suggests that different glucose sensors may control unique elements of the CRR.

In conclusion, the VMH NO-sGC signaling pathway is a key component in the generation of the CRR. Moreover, our data provide strong support for our hypothesis that VMH glucose-inhibited neurons play a crucial role in the central detection of hypoglycemia and generation of the CRR. These data also suggest that potentiating NO signaling may enhance epinephrine secretion and glucose recovery in diabetic patients exposed to recurrent hypoglycemia. The role of NO signaling in epinephrine secretion in response to hypoglycemia is extremely relevant for patients with type 1 diabetes who lack a glucagon response. Thus, the NO-sGC signaling pathway may offer new therapeutic targets to improve the treatment of patients with type 1 and advanced type 2 diabetes using intensive insulin therapy.

ACKNOWLEDGMENTS

This work was supported in part by the Juvenile Diabetes Research Foundation (X.F. and V.H.R.) and the National Institutes of Health (2RO1-DK-55619 and 1RO1-DK-64566) (V.H.R.). X.F. was also supported in part by the Philippe Foundation.

No potential conflicts of interest relevant to this article were reported.

REFERENCES

1. The Diabetes Control and Complications Trial Research Group. The effect of intensive treatment of diabetes on the development and progression of long-term complications in insulin-dependent diabetes mellitus. N Engl J Med 1993;329:977–986
2. Amiel SA, Tamborlane WV, Simonson DC, Sherwin RS. Defective glucose counterregulation after strict glycemic control of insulin-dependent diabetes mellitus. N Engl J Med 1987;316:1376–1383
3. Cryer PE. Glucose counterregulation in man. Diabetes 1981;30:261–264
4. Routh VH, Song Z, Liu X. The role of glucosensing neurons in the detection of hypoglycemia. Diabetes Technol Ther 2004;6:413–421
5. Borg MA, Sherwin RS, Borg WP, Tamborlane WV, Shulman GI. Local ventromedial hypothalamus glucose perfusion blocks counterregulation during systemic hypoglycemia in awake rats. J Clin Invest 1997;99:361–365
6. Borg WP, During MJ, Sherwin RS, Borg MA, Brines ML, Shulman GI. Ventromedial hypothalamic lesions in rats suppress counterregulatory responses to hypoglycemia. J Clin Invest 1994;93:1677–1682
7. Borg WP, Sherwin RS, During MJ, Borg MA, Shulman GI. Local ventromedial hypothalamus glucopenia triggers counterregulatory hormone release. Diabetes 1995;44:180–184
8. Fioramonti X, Contié S, Song Z, Routh VH, Lorsignol A, Pénicaud L. Characterization of glucosensing neuron subpopulations in the arcuate nucleus: integration in neuropeptide Y and pro-opio melanocortin networks? Diabetes 2007;56:1219–1227
9. Kang L, Routh VH, Kuzhikandathil EV, Gaspers LD, Levin BE. Physiological and molecular characteristics of rat hypothalamic ventromedial nucleus glucosensing neurons. Diabetes 2004;53:549–559
10. Song Z, Levin BE, McArdle JJ, Bakhos N, Routh VH. Convergence of pre- and postsynaptic influences on glucosensing neurons in the ventromedial hypothalamic nucleus. Diabetes 2001;50:2673–2681
11. Wang R, Liu X, Hentges ST, Dunn-Meyhell AA, Levin BE, Wang W, Routh VH. The regulation of glucose-excited neurons in the hypothalamic arcuate nucleus by glucose and feeding relevant peptides. Diabetes 2004;53:1959–1965
12. Powell AM, Sherwin RS, Shulman GI. Impaired hormonal responses to hypoglycemia in spontaneously diabetic and recurrently hypoglycemic rats: reversibility and stimulus specificity of the deficits. J Clin Invest 1993;92:2667–2674
13. Song Z, Routh VH. Recurrent hypoglycemia reduces the glucose sensitivity of glucose-inhibited neurons in the ventromedial hypothalamus nucleus. Am J Physiol Regul Integr Comp Physiol 2006;291:R1283-R1287
14. Guix FX, Uribesalgo I, Coma M, Muñoz FJ. The physiology and pathophysiology of nitric oxide in the brain. Prog Neurobiol 2005;76:126–152
15. Cabou C, Campistron G, Marsollier N, Leloup C, Cruciani-Guglielmacci C, Pénicaud L, Drucker DJ, Magnan C, Burcelin R. Brain glucagon-like peptide-1 regulates arterial blood flow, heart rate, and insulin sensitivity. Diabetes 2008;57:2577–2587
16. Cabou C, Cani PD, Campistron G, Knauf C, Mathieu C, Sartori C, Amar J, Scherrer U, Burcelin R. Central insulin regulates heart rate and arterial blood flow: an endothelial nitric oxide synthase-dependent mechanism altered during diabetes. Diabetes 2007;56:2872–2877
17. Riediger T, Giannini P, Erguven E, Lutz T. Nitric oxide directly inhibits ghrelin-activated neurons of the arcuate nucleus. Brain Res 2006;1125:37–45
18. Shankar RR, Wu Y, Shen HQ, Zhu JS, Baron AD. Mice with gene disruption of both endothelial and neuronal nitric oxide synthase exhibit insulin resistance. Diabetes 2000;49:684–687
19. Canabal DD, Potian JG, Duran RG, McArdle JJ, Routh VH. Hyperglycemia impairs glucose and insulin regulation of nitric oxide production in glucose-inhibited neurons in the ventromedial hypothalamus. Am J Physiol Regul Integr Comp Physiol 2007;293:R592-R600
20. Canabal DD, Song Z, Potian JG, Beuve A, McArdle JJ, Routh VH. Glucose, insulin, and leptin signaling pathways modulate nitric oxide synthesis in glucose-inhibited neurons in the ventromedial hypothalamus. Am J Physiol Regul Integr Comp Physiol 2007;292:R1418-R1428
21. Saberi M, Bohland M, Donovan CM. The locus for hypoglycemic detection shifts with the rate of fall in glycemia: the role of portal-superior mesenteric vein glucose sensing. Diabetes 2008;57:1380–1386
22. Cryer PE. Role of growth hormone in glucose counterregulation. Horm Res 1996;46:192–194
23. Fioramonti X, Lorsignol A, Taupignon A, Pénicaud L. A new ATP-sensitive K+ channel-independent mechanism is involved in glucose-excited neurons of mouse arcuate nucleus. Diabetes 2004;53:2767–2775
24. Murphy BA, Fakira KA, Song Z, Beuve A, Routh VH. AMP-activated protein kinase and nitric oxide regulate the glucose sensitivity of ventromedial hypothalamic glucose-inhibited neurons. Am J Physiol Cell Physiol 2009;297:C750-C758.
25. Murphy BA, Fioramonti X, Jochnowitz N, Fakira K, Gagen K, Contie S, Lorsignol A, Penicaud L, Martin WJ, Routh VH. Fasting enhances the response of arcuate neuropeptide Y-glucose-inhibited neurons to decreased extracellular glucose. Am J Physiol Cell Physiol 2009;296:C746-C756
26. Knauf C, Prevot V, Stefano GB, Mortreux G, Beauvillain JC, Croix D. Evidence for a spontaneous nitric oxide release from the rat median eminence: influence on gonadotropin-releasing hormone release. Endocrinology 2001;142:2343–2350
27. McCrimmon RJ, Fan X, Cheng H, McNay E, Chan O, Shaw M, Ding Y, Zhu W, Sherwin RS. Activation of AMP-activated protein kinase within the ventromedial hypothalamus amplifies counterregulatory hormone responses in rats with defective counterregulation. Diabetes 2006;55:1755–1760
28. Borg MA, Tamborlane WV, Shulman GI, Sherwin RS. Local lactate perfusion of the ventromedial hypothalamus suppresses hypoglycemic counterregulation. Diabetes 2003;52:663–666
29. Kang L, Dunn-Meynell AA, Routh VH, Gaspers LD, Nagata Y, Nishimura T, Eiki J, Zhang BB, Levin BE. Glucokinase is a critical regulator of ventromedial hypothalamic neuronal glucosensing. Diabetes 2006;55:412–420
30. Miki T, Liss B, Minami K, Shiuchi T, Saraya A, Kashima Y, Horiuchi M, Ashcroft F, Minokoshi Y, Roeper J, Seino S. ATP-sensitive K+ channels in the hypothalamus are essential for the maintenance of glucose homeostasis. Nat Neurosci 2001;4:507–512
31. Song Z, Routh VH. Differential effects of glucose and lactate on glucosens-

ing neurons in the ventromedial hypothalamic nucleus. Diabetes 2005;54: 15–22

32. Levin BE, Becker TC, Eiki J, Zhang BB, Dunn-Meynell AA. Ventromedial hypothalamic glucokinase is an important mediator of the counterregulatory response to insulin-induced hypoglycemia. Diabetes 2008;57:1371–1379

33. McCrimmon RJ, Song Z, Cheng H, McNay EC, Weikart-Yeckel C, Fan X, Routh VH, Sherwin RS. Corticotrophin-releasing factor receptors within the ventromedial hypothalamus regulate hypoglycemia-induced hormonal counterregulation. J Clin Invest 2006;116:1723–1730

34. Bryan RM, Jr, Eichler MY, Johnson TD, Woodward WT, Williams JL. Cerebral blood flow, plasma catecholamines, and electroencephalogram during hypoglycemia and recovery after glucose infusion. J Neurosurg Anesthesiol 1994;6:24–34

35. Bryan RM, Jr, Hollinger BR, Keefer KA, Page RB. Regional cerebral and neural lobe blood flow during insulin-induced hypoglycemia in unanesthetized rats. J Cereb Blood Flow Metab 1987;7:96–102

36. Kennan RP, Takahashi K, Pan C, Shamoon H, Pan JW. Human cerebral blood flow and metabolism in acute insulin-induced hypoglycemia. J Cereb Blood Flow Metab 2005;25:527–534

37. Page KA, Arora J, Qiu M, Relwani R, Constable RT, Sherwin RS. Small decrements in systemic glucose provoke increases in hypothalamic blood flow prior to the release of counterregulatory hormones. Diabetes 2009; 58:448–452

38. Moncada S, Palmer RM, Higgs EA. Nitric oxide: physiology, pathophysiology, and pharmacology. Pharmacol Rev 1991;43:109–142

39. Horinaka N, Artz N, Jehle J, Takahashi S, Kennedy C, Sokoloff L. Examination of potential mechanisms in the enhancement of cerebral blood flow by hypoglycemia and pharmacological doses of deoxyglucose. J Cereb Blood Flow Metab 1997;17:54–63

40. Paulson OB. Blood-brain barrier, brain metabolism and cerebral blood flow. Eur Neuropsychopharmacol 2002;12:495–501

41. Hollinger BR, Bryan RM. Beta-receptor-mediated increase in cerebral blood flow during hypoglycemia. Am J Physiol 1987;253:H949-H955

42. Horinaka N, Kuang TY, Pak H, Wang R, Jehle J, Kennedy C, Sokoloff L. Blockade of cerebral blood flow response to insulin-induced hypoglycemia by caffeine and glibenclamide in conscious rats. J Cereb Blood Flow Metab 1997;17:1309–1318

43. Duplain H, Burcelin R, Sartori C, Cook S, Egli M, Lepori M, Vollenweider P, Pedrazzini T, Nicod P, Thorens B, Scherrer U. Insulin resistance, hyperlipidemia, and hypertension in mice lacking endothelial nitric oxide synthase. Circulation 2001;104:342–345

44. Ahern GP, Klyachko VA, Jackson MB. cGMP and S-nitrosylation: two routes for modulation of neuronal excitability by NO. Trends Neurosci 2002;25:510–517

Effects of Acute Insulin-Induced Hypoglycemia on Spatial Abilities in Adults With Type 1 Diabetes

Rohana J. Wright, mrcp[1]
Brian M. Frier, md[1,2]
Ian J. Deary, phd[2,3]

OBJECTIVE — To examine the effects of acute insulin-induced hypoglycemia on spatial cognitive abilities in adult humans with type 1 diabetes.

RESEARCH DESIGN AND METHODS — Sixteen adults with type 1 diabetes underwent two counterbalanced experimental sessions: euglycemia (blood glucose 4.5 mmol/l [81 mg/dl]) and hypoglycemia (2.5 mmol/l [45 mg/dl]). Arterialized blood glucose levels were maintained using a hyperinsulinemic glucose clamp technique. During each session, subjects underwent detailed assessment of spatial abilities from the Kit of Factor-Referenced Cognitive Tests and two tests of general cognitive function.

RESULTS — Spatial ability performance deteriorated significantly during hypoglycemia. Results for the Hidden Patterns, Card Rotations, Paper Folding, and Maze Tracing tests were all impaired significantly ($P \leq 0.001$) during hypoglycemia, as were results for the Cube Comparisons Test ($P = 0.03$). The Map Memory Test was not significantly affected by hypoglycemia.

CONCLUSIONS — Hypoglycemia is a common side effect of insulin therapy in individuals with type 1 diabetes, and spatial abilities are of critical importance in day-to-day functioning. The deterioration in spatial abilities observed during modest experimental hypoglycemia provides novel information on the cerebral hazards of hypoglycemia that has potential relevance to everyday activities.

Diabetes Care 32:1503–1506, 2009

H ypoglycemia is a common effect of insulin treatment of diabetes. Strict glycemic control limits the development and severity of vascular complications of diabetes, but hypoglycemia is a frequent consequence. Strict glycemic control can increase the incidence of severe hypoglycemia by threefold (1). Hypoglycemia has an adverse effect on cognitive functions, as the human brain relies solely on glucose as its source of energy (2). It has a pronounced effect on complex cognitive tasks both in diabetic and nondiabetic individuals, whereas simple mental tasks are relatively unaffected (2). Cognitive function deteriorates when arterialized blood glucose concentrations decline to <3.0 mmol/l (3–6). Simple and choice reaction times, speed of mathematical calculation, verbal fluency, attention, memory, and psychomotor function have all been demonstrated to be affected during hypoglycemia (7–10). The recovery of different aspects of cognitive function may vary from between 40 and 90 min after restoration of blood glucose to normal (2,11).

Whereas hypoglycemia impairs many domains of cognitive function, the effect of hypoglycemia on spatial cognitive abilities has not been investigated in detail, although spatial ability is undoubtedly a component of some of the tests used to assess other aspects of cognition (12).

Spatial abilities may be defined as the ability to generate, retain, retrieve, and transform or manipulate structured visual images to orientate and interpret the surrounding environment. In real-life terms, spatial ability is concerned with how human beings deal with issues concerning two- and three-dimensional objects, space, navigation, and pathfinding. Practical daily cognition often involves inferring how shapes and objects will appear and function when they are rotated or otherwise oriented or viewed differently. In everyday interactions with the environment, this process is very important, with particular relevance for complex tasks such as driving and map reading. A large variety of mental tests are available for the assessment of spatial abilities. Largely, these tests can be separated into tests of spatial perception, namely the ability to determine spatial relations despite distracting information; spatial visualization, which is the ability to manipulate complex, multistep spatial information; and mental rotation, which is the ability to rotate two- or three-dimensional figures in one's mind (13). The present study was designed to investigate the effects of acute insulin-induced hypoglycemia on spatial abilities in adults with type 1 diabetes, using a well-characterized battery of spatial tests that incorporate all of these components of spatial cognition.

RESEARCH DESIGN AND
METHODS — Sixteen adults with type 1 diabetes (seven male and nine female) participated in the study. Subjects were recruited from the diabetes clinic at the Royal Infirmary of Edinburgh. Baseline demographic characteristics were a median age of 28 years (interquartile range 25–37.5 years), median duration of diabetes 10 years (4.2–19 years), BMI (means ± SD) 26.4 ± 4.01 kg/m², and A1C 7.91 ± 0.92%. A1C was measured by high-performance liquid chromatography (nondiabetic reference range 5.0–6.05%; Bio-Rad Laboratories, Munich, Germany) and was Diabetes Control and Complications Trial–aligned. The subjects had no history of hypertension or macrovascular disease, and microvascu-

From the [1]Department of Diabetes, Royal Infirmary of Edinburgh, Edinburgh, U.K.; the [2]Centre for Cognitive Ageing and Cognitive Epidemiology, University of Edinburgh, Edinburgh, U.K.; and the [3]Department of Psychology, University of Edinburgh, Edinburgh, U.K.
Corresponding author: Ian J. Deary, i.j.deary@ed.ac.uk.
Received 4 February 2009 and accepted 30 April 2009.
Published ahead of print at http://care.diabetesjournals.org on 1 June 2009. DOI: 10.2337/dc09-0212.

lar disease was excluded before recruitment. The presence of retinopathy was sought using digital retinal photography, neuropathy was assessed by clinical examination, and nephropathy was identified by the presence of microalbuminuria. Subjects were excluded if they had a history of impaired awareness of hypoglycemia or a history of a previous severe reaction to hypoglycemia. None of the participants had a history of head injury, seizure, blackouts, alcohol or drug abuse, or psychiatric illness. Subjects were not taking any medications other than insulin or the oral contraceptive pill. All subjects gave written informed consent before participating in the study, which had been approved by the local research ethics committee.

Each subject underwent two laboratory sessions, separated by at least 2 weeks. The study was conducted at the Clinical Research Facility at the Royal Infirmary of Edinburgh. A modified hyperinsulinemic glucose clamp (14) was used to maintain blood glucose at a predetermined level: euglycemia at 4.5 mmol/l (81 mg/dl) and hypoglycemia at 2.5 mmol/l (45 mg/dl). Each subject underwent a euglycemia study and a hypoglycemia study in a randomized, counterbalanced fashion. The subjects were blinded to the experimental condition.

Study procedure
The experimental session began at 0830 h. All subjects monitored their blood glucose with care for the preceding 48 h, including bedtime testing, and the study was postponed if they had any blood glucose value <3.5 mmol/l or any symptoms suggestive of hypoglycemia. After an overnight fast the subjects omitted their morning insulin dose. A retrograde intravenous cannula for regular blood glucose sampling was inserted into the nondominant hand and was placed in a heated blanket to arterialize the venous blood (15). A further cannula in the nondominant antecubital fossa was used to infuse soluble insulin (Human Actrapid; Novo Nordisk Pharmaceuticals, Crawley, U.K.) and 20% dextrose. Insulin was infused at a constant rate of 1.5 mU · kg^{-1} · min^{-1} using a Gemini PCI pump (Alaris Medical Systems, San Diego, CA). Dextrose (20%) was infused at a rate that varied according to the arterialized blood glucose concentration, which was measured at 5-min intervals using the glucose oxidase method (2300 Stat; YSI, Yellow Springs, OH).

On each study day, the arterialized blood glucose was initially stabilized at 4.5 mmol/l for a period of 30 min. It was then either maintained at that level throughout the study (euglycemia condition) or it was lowered over 20 min to 2.5 mmol/l and maintained at that level for the duration of the study (hypoglycemia condition). The experimental period lasted for 60 min, after which time the blood glucose concentration was restored to 4.5 mmol/l. Subjects were given a meal after completion of each study.

Cognitive function tests
Tests of spatial ability were drawn from the French and Ekstrom Kit of Factor-Referenced Cognitive Tests (16,17). In addition, the Digit Symbol Substitution Test and Trail Making B Test were administered to confirm the recognized effect of hypoglycemia on cognitive function, as described previously (7–10).

Spatial ability tests
Hidden patterns test. The Hidden Patterns Test requires subjects to identify a figure that is hidden among other lines. The figure is the same throughout, with the same orientation, and subjects have 3 min to correctly identify as many of the patterns in which the figure is concealed as possible.

Card rotations test. The Card Rotations Test requires the subject to look closely at a shape on the left-hand side of a page and then assess whether the eight shapes on the right-hand side are the same shape rotated through a variable number of degrees or whether the shapes are different and have in fact been reversed or are a mirror image of the initial shape. Three minutes are allowed to complete as many items as possible.

Cube comparisons test. This test involves pairs of cubes, such as the wooden building blocks played with by children, with a letter or shape on each facet of the cube. Subjects have 3 min to analyze as many pairs of cubes as possible and must determine whether the two cubes could be the same cube viewed from different sides or whether they must be different cubes if the letters on the sides did not correspond with each other had the cube been turned over.

Paper folding test. The Paper Folding Test involves showing participants a sequence of folds in a piece of paper, through which a set of holes is then punched. The participants must choose which of a set of punched and unfolded

papers corresponds to the one they have just seen.

Map memory test. This is a test of the subject's ability to remember the position of buildings on a street map. Four minutes are permitted to memorize the map and then a further 4 min to place the buildings correctly on a blank version of the map.

Maze tracing test. This is a test of the subject's ability to find a path through a maze quickly. A pencil line must be drawn through the maze without crossing any of the "walls." The maze is broken down into blocks, and the score is the number of blocks that are successfully navigated in 3 min.

Other cognitive function tests
Digit symbol substitution test. This test is from the Wechsler Adult Intelligence Scale-III and assesses the ability of the subject to perform coding as quickly as possible. The subject is given a key of numbers 1–9, which each have a corresponding symbol. They must then fill in as many symbols as possible for a list of numbers in 120 s.

Trail making B test. The Trail Making B Test is a computerized version of the test and similar in principle to the classic test from the Halstead Reitan battery. It is used to assess complex visual processing and also assesses motor function with regard to visual motor tracking. It is performed on a handheld computer. The subject is presented with a grid containing letters and numbers in a random order and must connect the numbers and letters in numerical and alphabetical order, alternating the number with the letter in fashion "1-A-2-B-3-C . . ." etc.

Hypoglycemia symptom score. The Edinburgh Hypoglycemia Scale was used to assess the symptoms experienced by subjects during each experimental session. It is a validated self-rating questionnaire comprising a list of common symptoms of hypoglycemia that can be classified into autonomic, neuroglycopenic, and nonspecific symptoms. Each symptom is scored on a Likert scale from 1 (not present) to 7 (intensely present) (18).

Statistical analysis
Results were analyzed using SPSS (version 15.0 for Windows; SPSS, Chicago, IL). A general linear model (repeated-measures ANOVA) was used, with order of session (euglycemia-hypoglycemia or hypoglycemia-euglycemia) as a between-subjects factor and condition (euglycemia

Table 1—*Spatial ability test scores*

Spatial test	Euglycemia score	Hypoglycemia score	P	Cohen's d	η_p^2
Hidden Patterns	94.5 ± 21.8	73.7 ± 21.0	<0.001	0.97	0.627
Card Rotations	51.9 ± 15.5	40.4 ± 18.7	0.001	0.67	0.580
Cube Comparison	11.7 ± 4.1	9.4 ± 5.7	0.03	0.46	0.298
Paper Folding	6.0 ± 1.9	4.7 ± 2.0	0.001	0.67	0.604
Map Memory	8.6 ± 3.1	7.8 ± 2.1	0.3	0.30	0.081
Maze Tracing	11.1 ± 3.0	9.4 ± 2.5	<0.001	0.62	0.621

Data are means ± SD. Significance level was $P < 0.05$; effect sizes were computed as Cohen's d and η_p^2.

or hypoglycemia) as a within-subjects factor. $P < 0.05$ was considered to be significant. Effect sizes were calculated using η_p^2 to assess the degree to which hypoglycemia accounts for the variance in results, and Cohen's d was used to establish the extent of any effects of hypoglycemia on spatial abilities. Results are expressed as means ± SD unless stated otherwise.

RESULTS

Blood glucose
The target blood glucose levels were achieved for each experimental condition. The blood glucose concentration achieved during the hypoglycemia condition was 2.46 ± 0.22 mmol/l and during the euglycemia condition was 4.53 ± 0.24 mmol/l.

Symptom scores
Significant increments occurred in total autonomic ($P < 0.001$), total neuroglycopenic ($P < 0.001$), and malaise symptom scores (<0.001) during hypoglycemia.

General cognitive function
In the present study, scores achieved for the Digit Symbol Substitution Test were significantly lower during the hypoglycemia study period (72.4 ± 20.2) compared with those during euglycemia (84.6 ± 20.7) ($P < 0.001$), confirming that a standard measure of speed of information processing was significantly impaired at blood glucose concentrations of 2.5 mmol/l. Performance on the Trail Making B Test was statistically not impaired by hypoglycemia, with a score of 50.4 ± 20.9 s during hypoglycemia and a score of 38.9 ± 11.5 s during euglycemia ($P = 0.07$).

Spatial ability
Hypoglycemia resulted in a significantly lower score on all of the spatial ability tests except the Map Memory Test (Table 1). Cohen's d results have shown that the impact of hypoglycemia on these spatial abilities was medium to large. Moreover, the η_p^2 values indicate that the hypoglycemia condition accounted for a large proportion of the variance in the results (Table 1). No significant effects were observed of order of exposure to glycemic condition or test battery.

CONCLUSIONS — Acute, insulin-induced hypoglycemia causes significant decrements in most spatial cognitive abilities examined here in a group of adults with uncomplicated type 1 diabetes. This impairment of function was accompanied by a deterioration in speed of mental processing as demonstrated by the decrement in score for the Digit Symbol Substitution Test. The effect sizes obtained indicate the development of medium to large decrements in spatial abilities during hypoglycemia in adults with type 1 diabetes.

The present study examined a group of subjects with type 1 diabetes and did not include a control group of nondiabetic subjects. Although this is a limitation of the present study, in reality it is the everyday effect of hypoglycemia on this group of individuals that is of clinical importance.

Other studies assessing the effects of hypoglycemia on aspects of cognitive function have used tests that require a spatial ability component (12), but to our knowledge no previous study has used a test battery specifically examining spatial abilities, although it has clear importance in the safe conduct of tasks such as driving, which rely heavily upon the interpretation of the surrounding environment.

The Map Memory Test was not affected significantly by the glycemic condition. This test assesses both spatial ability and visual memory. This finding is consistent with previous studies that examined memory function using visual memory tests from the Wechsler Adult Intelligence Scale, which also showed that visual memory is preserved during acute hypoglycemia (19). It is also notable that the Map Memory Test, unlike the other tests used here, does not have multiple items, and so its scores may be more idiosyncratic.

Spatial ability relies on cerebral pathways that predominantly involve the right cerebral hemisphere, particularly the parietal lobe. The frontal cortex, thalamus, and, to some extent, the cerebellum are also involved in the coordination of spatial cognition (20,21). Neuroimaging studies during hypoglycemia have shown attenuation of functional response, e.g., blood oxygenation level–dependent activation, in the premotor and supplementary motor cortex, consistent with recognized areas of importance in spatial functioning (22). In addition, it has been shown previously that general fluid intelligence is impaired during hypoglycemia, and it is fluid intelligence rather than crystallized intelligence that is responsible for spatial cognition (10).

In summary, the present study has shown that acute hypoglycemia has an adverse effect on spatial abilities. These novel data are important for two reasons. First, with regard to our understanding of the domains of cognitive function that experience decrements during hypoglycemia, spatial abilities were a lacuna that has now been partly filled. Second, spatial abilities are relevant to the everyday activities of individuals with type 1 diabetes, and there are now data to show that part of the inability to manage complex tasks during hypoglycemia is the inability to efficiently carry out spatial cognitive operations.

Acknowledgments— This work was supported by the Biotechnology and Biological Sciences Research Council, the Engineering and Physical Sciences Research Council, the Economic and Social Research Council, and the Medical Research Council. B.M.F. and I.J.D. are members of The University of Edinburgh Centre for Cognitive Ageing and Cognitive Epidemiology, part of the cross-council Lifelong Health and Wellbeing Initiative.

No potential conflicts of interest relevant to this article were reported.

References
1. The Diabetes Control and Complications Trial Research Group. The effect of intensive insulin treatment of diabetes on the

development and progression of long term complications. N Engl J Med 1993; 329:977–986

2. Deary IJ. Symptoms of hypoglycaemia and effects on mental performance and emotions. In *Hypoglycaemia in Clinical Diabetes*. 2nd ed. Frier BM, Fisher M, Eds. Chichester, U.K., John Wiley & Sons, 2007, p. 25–48

3. Hoffman RG, Speelman DJ, Hinnen DA, Conley KL, Guthrie RA, Knapp RK. Changes in cortical functioning with acute hypoglycemia and hyperglycemia in type 1 diabetes. Diabetes Care 1989;12: 193–197

4. Mitrakou A, Ryan C, Veneman T, Mokan M, Jenssen T, Kiss I, Durrant J, Cryer P, Gerich J. Hierarchy of glycemic thresholds for counterregulatory hormone secretion, symptoms, and cerebral dysfunction. Am J Physiol 1991;260:E67–E74

5. Widom B, Simonson DJ. Glycemic control and neuropsychologic function during hypoglycemia in patients with insulin-dependent diabetes. Ann Intern Med 1990;112:904–912

6. Wirsen A, Tallroth G, Lindgren M, Agardh C. Neuropsychological performance differs between type 1 diabetic and normal men during insulin-induced hypoglycaemia. Diabet Med 1992;9:156–165

7. McAulay V, Ferguson SC, Deary IJ, Frier BM. Acute hypoglycemia in humans causes attentional dysfunction while nonverbal intelligence is preserved. Diabetes Care 2001;24:1745–1750

8. Sommerfield AJ, Deary IJ, McAulay V, Frier BM. Moderate hypoglycemia impairs multiple memory functions in healthy adults. Neuropsychology 2003; 17:125–132

9. Sommerfield AJ, Deary IJ, McAulay V, Frier BM. Short-term, delayed, and working memory are impaired during hypoglycemia in individuals with type 1 diabetes. Diabetes Care 2003;26:390–396

10. Warren RE, Allen KA, Sommerfield AJ, Deary IJ, Frier BM. Acute hypoglycemia impairs non-verbal intelligence. Diabetes Care 2004;27:1447–1448

11. Zammitt NN, Warren RE, Deary IJ, Frier BM. Delayed recovery of cognitive function following hypoglycemia in adults with type 1 diabetes: effect of impaired awareness of hypoglycemia. Diabetes 2008;57:732–736

12. Geddes J, Deary IJ, Frier BM. Effects of acute insulin-induced hypoglycaemia on psychomotor function: people with type 1 diabetes are less affected than nondiabetic adults. Diabetologia 2008;51: 1814–1821

13. Linn MC, Petersen AC. Emergence and characterisation of gender differences in spatial abilities: a meta-analysis. Child Dev 1985;56:1479–1498

14. De Fronzo R, Tobin JD, Andres R. Glucose clamp technique: a method for quantifying insulin secretion and resistance. Am J Physiol 1979;273:E214–E223

15. Abumrad NN, Rabin D, Diamond MP, Lacy WW. Use of a heated superficial hand vein as an alternative site for the measurement of amino acid concentrations and for the study of glucose and ala-nine kinetics in man. Metabolism 1981; 30:936–940

16. Ekstrom RB, French JW, Harman HH, Dermen D. *Kit of Factor-Referenced Cognitive Tests.* Princeton, NJ: Educational Testing Service, 1976

17. Ekstrom RB, French JW, Harman HH. Cognitive factors: their identification and replication. Multivariate Behav Res Monogr 1979;79:3–84.

18. Gold AE, MacLeod KM, Frier BM. Frequency of severe hypoglycemia in patients with type 1 diabetes with impaired awareness of hypoglycemia. Diabetes Care 1994;17:697–703

19. Warren RE, Zammitt NN, Deary IJ, Frier BM. The effects of acute hypoglycaemia on memory acquisition and recall and prospective memory in type 1 diabetes. Diabetologia 2007;50:178–185

20. Harris IM, Egan GF, Sonkkila C, Tochon-Danguy HJ, Paxinos G, Watson JDG. Selective right parietal lobe activation during mental rotation. Brain 2000;123: 65–73

21. Vogel JJ, Bowers CA, Vogel DS. Cerebral lateralization of spatial abilities: a meta-analysis. Brain Cogn 2003;52:197–204

22. Rosenthal JM, Amiel SA, Yaguez L, Bullmore E, Hopkins D, Evans M, Pernet A, Reid H, Giampetro V, Andrew CM, Suckling J, Simmons A, Williams SCR. The effect of acute hypoglycemia on brain function and activation: a functional magnetic resonance imaging study. Diabetes 2001;50:1618–1626

Attenuated Sympathoadrenal Responses, but Not Severe Hypoglycemia, During Aggressive Glycemic Therapy of Early Type 2 Diabetes

Stephanie A. Amiel[1] and Philip E. Cryer[2]

Iatrogenic hypoglycemia is a major limiting factor in the strict glycemic management of diabetes (1,2). Hypoglycemia can cause recurrent morbidity in many people with type 1 diabetes and also in some with advanced type 2 diabetes (2,3). Rarely fatal, fear of hypoglycemia precludes maintenance of euglycemia over a lifetime with diabetes and full realization of the vascular benefits of glycemic control. Hypoglycemic events compromise defenses against subsequent falling plasma glucose concentrations and thus cause a vicious cycle of recurrent hypoglycemia.

Hypoglycemia in diabetes is fundamentally the result of episodes of therapeutic hyperinsulinemia caused by treatment with an insulin secretagogue or insulin. In general, the incidence of iatrogenic hypoglycemia is a function of the degree of β-cell failure (1,2,4), and risk is predicted by the absence of evidence of endogenous insulin secretion (C-peptide) (5). Incidence of hypoglycemia is lower in people with type 2 diabetes, who are not usually completely insulin deficient, than in those with type 1 diabetes, and this is especially true early in the course of type 2 diabetes. However, the incidence of hypoglycemia increases progressively over time (6), ultimately approximating that in those with type 1 diabetes (7,8), as type 2 diabetic individuals approach the insulin-deficient end of the spectrum. Because type 2 diabetes is ~20-fold more prevalent than type 1 diabetes and many people with type 2 diabetes ultimately require treatment with insulin, most episodes of iatrogenic hypoglycemia, including severe hypoglycemia, occur in those with type 2 diabetes (1–3,9).

The key physiological defenses against falling plasma glucose concentrations are *1*) a decrease in insulin secretion; *2*) an increase in glucagon secretion; and, in the absence of the latter, *3*) an increase in epinephrine secretion (1,2). The behavioral defense is carbohydrate ingestion prompted by perception of the largely sympathetic neural neurogenic symptoms that cause the individual to become aware of hypoglycemia (10,11). Although these mechanisms are intact early in the course of type 2 diabetes when endogenous insulin deficiency is only relative, the insulin and glucagon responses are typically compromised in people with absolute endogenous insulin deficiency in type 1 diabetes (1,2,12) and in those with advanced type 2 diabetes (13). Epinephrine, sympathetic nervous system, and symptomatic responses are further compromised in a subset of patients, causing, in large part, the clinical syndrome of hypoglycemia unawareness with a greatly increased risk of severe hypoglycemic episodes (14). Because experimentally induced recent antecedent hypoglycemia (as well as exercise and the state of deep sleep) produces defective epinephrine, sympathetic neural, and symptom responses to subsequent hypoglycemia (15,16) and to underscore the key role of the attenuated sympathoadrenal responses in defense against severe hypoglycemia, this pathophysiology has been termed hypoglycemia-associated autonomic failure (HAAF) in diabetes (1,2,13). The attenuated epinephrine secretory response causes defective glucose counterregulation in the setting of absolute β-cell failure. The concept of HAAF was developed in the context of type 1 diabetes (1,2), and its role in the pathogenesis of hypoglycemia in type 2 diabetes (1,2,9) remains to be clarified.

As reported in this issue of *Diabetes*, Davis et al. (17) address this issue, studying 15 patients with relatively early type 2 diabetes. Mean duration of known diabetes was only 6 years. At baseline patients had no evidence of compromised physiological or behavioral defenses against hypoglycemia. Even after overnight insulin infusions to maintain near euglycemia, mean fasting plasma C-peptide concentrations were higher than those of patients with type 1 diabetes (18,19). Importantly, insulin secretion as assessed by C-peptide levels fell appropriately, by ~75%, when plasma glucose concentrations were lowered to 3.3 mmol/l (60 mg/dl), just below the postabsorptive physiological range of ~3.9–6.1 mmol/l (70–110 mg/dl). At a plasma glucose concentration of 3.3 mmol/l (60 mg/dl), increments in plasma glucagon and epinephrine were similar to those of nondiabetic control patients, and muscle sympathetic nerve activity (MSNA) and symptomatic responses were enhanced. Perhaps this reflects the experience of hyperglycemia, as the mean A1C was just over 10%, indicating very poor glycemic control. Exaggerated counterregulatory response to hypoglycemia in those with type 2 diabetes has been described previously (20).

In the patients with poor glycemic control in Davis et al.'s study, two episodes of subphysiological plasma glucose concentrations reduced an array of responses (including glucagon and epinephrine, MSNA, and symptoms) to hypoglycemia the following day (17). This has been well documented in nondiabetic subjects and those with type 1 and type 2 diabetes (1,2,12). However, it is of interest that

From the [1]Department of Medicine, King's College London School of Medicine, London, U.K.; and the [2]Division of Endocrinology, Metabolism and Lipid Research, Washington University School of Medicine, St. Louis, Missouri.

Corresponding author: Stephanie A. Amiel, stephanie.amiel@kcl.ac.uk.

DOI: 10.2337/db08-1647

See accompanying original article, p. 701.

this was demonstrated following low plasma glucose levels as high as 3.3 mmol/l (60 mg/dl) (17).

The novelty of the Davis et al. study is that, following the first hypoglycemia investigation, patients were brought into strict glycemic control with intensification of lifestyle and oral agent therapy, reducing mean A1C levels to 6.7% in 6 months with, remarkably, no overall weight gain. Treatment was associated with an increase in self-reported glucose levels <3.9 mmol/l (70 mg/dl) from 1.1 to 3.2 per patient per month on intensive home monitoring, although only four patients reported glucose levels <2.8 mmol/l (50 mg/dl). Unfortunately, the extent to which any of these were symptomatic was not reported, and it is not clear that the self-monitoring was as intensive before the intensification of therapy. There were no episodes of major hypoglycemia. This change in glycemic experience was associated with a substantial reduction in the plasma epinephrine, MSNA, and symptomatic responses to plasma glucose concentrations of 3.3 mmol/l (60 mg/dl) (~50, 66, and 40%, respectively), a novel finding in early type 2 diabetes, although it has been shown in advanced type 2 diabetes that required insulin to improve control (21). Notably, in the Davis et al. study, decrements in insulin secretion and increments in glucagon secretion were not reduced, and only the epinephrine responses were reduced significantly compared with those of healthy control subjects.

Coupled with reports of other investigators cited by Davis et al. (17), these data provide further insight into the pathophysiology of glucose counterregulation in diabetes by the application of state-of-the-art assessment methods in a clinically relevant setting. The data provide both further documentation that sympathoadrenal and symptomatic responses to hypoglycemia are exaggerated in early type 2 diabetic patients with poor glycemic control and new evidence that aggressive glycemic therapy in these patients results in attenuation of responses to subsequent low plasma glucose concentrations (17). This effect is most plausibly attributed to reduced exposure to hyperglycemia and an increased frequency of subphysiological glucose levels during intensive therapy. Further, immediately antecedent iatrogenic hypoglycemia causes a further reduction in the vigor of the counterregulatory responses.

Are there clinical implications from these data? Hypoglycemia sufficient to cause cognitive impairment (not measured by Davis et al.) can diminish quality of life. Functional sympathoadrenal failure might be relevant to the pathogenesis of rare, but potentially fatal, ventricular arrhythmias (22). Concern has arisen about the possible involvement of hypoglycemia in the adverse effects of rapid intensification of diabetes therapies in late and complicated type 2 diabetes (23,24). In the present study, it is noteworthy that in patients with relatively early type 2 diabetes the changes seen in the responses to experimentally induced hypoglycemia were not associated with an increased frequency of major clinical hypoglycemia, perhaps because β-cell failure was not sufficient to cause loss of the insulin and glucagon responses (1,2). Data from follow-up studies show the prolonged benefit of early intensive glucose management in preventing vascular complications of diabetes (25,26). These data, taken in context with other published work showing possible problems of taking action much later in the course of the disease, would seem to be a further encouragement to implementing good control of diabetes as early as possible.

ACKNOWLEDGMENTS

The original cited work of P.E.C. has been supported, in part, by U.S. Public Health Service National Institutes of Health grants R37 DK27085, MO1 RR00036 (now UL1 RR24992), and P60 DK20579 and by a fellowship award from the American Diabetes Association.

P.E.C. has served as a consultant to MannKind, Marcadia Biotech, Medtronic MiniMed, and Merck in the past year. S.A.A. has served on advisory boards for Medtronic Minimed, Amylin Europe, Eli Lilly U.K., NovoNordisk, Novartis, and Merck Sharp and Dohme. No other potential conflicts of interest relevant to this article were reported.

REFERENCES

1. Cryer PE: The barrier of hypoglycemia in diabetes. *Diabetes* 57:3169–3167, 2008
2. Cryer PE: *Hypoglycemia in Diabetes: Pathophysiology Prevalence and Prevention*. Alexandria, VA, American Diabetes Association, 2009
3. Zammitt NN, Frier BM: Hypoglycemia in type 2 diabetes: pathophysiology, frequency, and effects of different treatment modalities. *Diabetes Care* 28:2948–2961, 2005
4. Donnelly LA, Morris AD, Frier BM, Ellis JD, Donnan PT, Durrant R, Band MM, Reekie G, Leese GP, The DARTS/MEMO Collaboration: Frequency and predictors of hypoglycaemia in type 1 and insulin-treated type 2 diabetes: a population-based study. *Diabet Med* 22:749–755, 2005
5. Mühlhauser I, Overmann H, Bender R, Bott U, Berger M: Risk factors for severe hypoglycaemia in adult patients with type 1 diabetes: a prospective population-based study. *Diabetologia* 41:1274–1282, 1998
6. UK Prospective Diabetes Study (UKPDS) Group: Intensive blood-glucose control with sulphonylureas or insulin compared with conventional treatment and risk of complications in patients with type 2 diabetes (UKPDS 33). *Lancet* 352:837–853, 1998
7. Leese GP, Wang J, Broomhall J, Kelly P, Marsden A, Morrison W, Frier BM, Morris AD, DARTS/MEMO Collaboration: Frequency of severe hypoglycemia requiring emergency treatment in type 1 and type 2 diabetes: a population-based study of health service resource use. *Diabetes Care* 26:1176–1180, 2003
8. U.K. Hypoglycaemia Study Group: Risk of hypoglycaemia in type 1 and 2 diabetes: effects of treatment modalities and their duration. *Diabetologia* 50:1140–1147, 2007
9. Amiel SA, Dixon TD, Mann R, Jameson K: Hypoglycaemia in type 2 diabetes. *Diabet Med* 25:245–254, 2008
10. Towler DA, Havlin CE, Craft S, Cryer PE: Mechanism of awareness of hypoglycemia: perception of neurogenic (predominantly cholinergic) rather than neuroglycopenic symptoms. *Diabetes* 42:1791–1798, 1993
11. DeRosa MA, Cryer PE: Hypoglycemia and the sympathoadrenal system: neurogenic symptoms are largely the result of sympathetic neural, rather than adrenomedullary, activation. *Am J Physiol Endocrinol Metab* 287:E32–E41, 2004
12. Dagogo-Jack SE, Craft S, Cryer PE: Hypoglycemia-associated autonomic failure in insulin-dependent diabetes mellitus. *J Clin Invest* 91:819–828, 1993
13. Segel SA, Paramore DS, Cryer PE: Hypoglycemia-associated autonomic failure in advanced type 2 diabetes. *Diabetes* 51:724–733, 2002
14. Ryder RE, Owens DR, Hayes TM, Ghatei MA, Bloom SR: Unawareness of hypoglycaemia and inadequate hypoglycaemic counterregulation: no causal relation with diabetic autonomic neuropathy. *BMJ* 301:783–787, 1990
15. Heller S, Cryer PE: Reduced neuroendocrine and symptomatic responses to subsequent hypoglycemia after 1 episode of hypoglycemia in nondiabetic humans. *Diabetes* 40:223–226, 1991
16. Davis SN, Shavers C, Mosqueda-Garcia R, Costa F: Effects of differing antecedent hypoglycemia on subsequent counterregulation in normal humans. *Diabetes* 46:1328–1335, 1997
17. Davis SN, Mann S, Briscoe VJ, Ertl AC, Tate DB: Effects of intensive therapy and antecedent hypoglycemia on counterregulatory responses to hypoglycemia in type 2 diabetes. *Diabetes* 58:701–709, 2009
18. Gjessing HJ, Matzen LE, Faber OK, Frølund A: Fasting plasma C-peptide, glucagon stimulated plasma C-peptide, and urinary C-peptide in relation to clinical type of diabetes. *Diabetologia* 32:305–311, 1989

19. Service FJ, Rizza RA, Zimmerman BR, Dyck PJ, O'Brien PC, Melton LJ III: The classification of diabetes by clinical and C-peptide criteria: a prospective population-based study. *Diabetes Care* 20:198–201, 1997

20. Spyer G, Hattersely AT, Macdonald IA, Amiel SA, MacLeod KM: Hypoglycaemic counterregulation at "normal" blood glucose concentrations in patients with well-controlled type 2 diabetes. *Lancet* 356:1970–1974, 2000

21. Korzon-Burakowska A, Hopkins D, Matyka K, Lomas J, Pernet A, Macdonald IA, Amiel SA: Effects of glycemic control on protective responses against hypoglycemia in type 2 diabetes. *Diabetes Care* 21:282–290, 1998

22. Adler GK, Bonyhay I, Failing H, Waring E, Dotson S, Freeman R: Antecedent hypoglycemia impairs autonomic cardiovascular function: implications for rigorous glycemic control. *Diabetes* 58:360–366, 2009

23. Robinson RT, Harris ND, Ireland RH, Macdonald IA, Heller SR: Changes in cardiac repolarization during clinical episodes of nocturnal hypoglycaemia in adults with type 1 diabetes. *Diabetologia* 47:312–315, 2004

24. Dluhy RG, McMahon GT: Intensive glycemic control in the ACCORD and ADVANCE trials. *N Engl J Med* 358:2630–2633, 2008

25. Diabetes Control and Complications Trial/Epidemiology of Diabetes Interventions and Complications (DCCT/EDIC) Study Research Group: Intensive diabetes treatment and cardiovascular disease in patients with type 1 diabetes. *N Engl J Med* 353:2643–2653, 2005

26. Holman RR, Paul SK, Ethel MA, Matthews DR, Neil HAW: 10-year follow-up of intensive glucose control in type 2 diabetes. *N Engl J Med* 359:1577–1589, 2008

Effects of Antecedent GABA$_A$ Activation With Alprazolam on Counterregulatory Responses to Hypoglycemia in Healthy Humans

Maka S. Hedrington,[1] Stephnie Farmerie,[1] Andrew C. Ertl,[1] Zhihui Wang,[1] Donna B. Tate,[1] and Stephen N. Davis[1,2]

OBJECTIVE—To date, there are no data investigating the effects of GABA$_A$ activation on counterregulatory responses during repeated hypoglycemia in humans. The aim of this study was to determine the effects of prior GABA$_A$ activation using the benzodiazepine alprazolam on the neuroendocrine and autonomic nervous system (ANS) and metabolic counterregulatory responses during next-day hypoglycemia in healthy humans.

RESEARCH DESIGN AND METHODS—Twenty-eight healthy individuals (14 male and 14 female, age 27 ± 6 years, BMI 24 ± 3 kg/m^2, and A1C $5.2 \pm 0.1\%$) participated in four randomized, double-blind, 2-day studies. Day 1 consisted of either morning and afternoon 2-h hyperinsulinemic euglycemia or 2-h hyperinsulinemic hypoglycemia (2.9 mmol/l) with either 1 mg alprazolam or placebo administered 30 min before the start of each clamp. Day 2 consisted of a single-step hyperinsulinemic-hypoglycemic clamp of 2.9 mmol/l.

RESULTS—Despite similar hypoglycemia (2.9 ± 1 mmol/l) and insulinemia (672 ± 108 pmol/l) during day 2 studies, GABA$_A$ activation with alprazolam during day 1 euglycemia resulted in significant blunting ($P < 0.05$) of ANS (epinephrine, norepinephrine, muscle sympathetic nerve activity, and pancreatic polypeptide), neuroendocrine (glucagon and growth hormone), and metabolic (glucose kinetics, lipolysis, and glycogenolysis) counterregulatory responses. GABA$_A$ activation with alprazolam during prior hypoglycemia caused further significant ($P < 0.05$) decrements in subsequent glucagon, growth hormone, pancreatic polypeptide, and muscle sympathetic nerve activity counterregulatory responses.

CONCLUSIONS—Alprazolam activation of GABA$_A$ pathways during day 1 hypoglycemia can play an important role in regulating a spectrum of key physiologic responses during subsequent (day 2) hypoglycemia in healthy man. *Diabetes* **59: 1074–1081, 2010**

From the [1]Department of Medicine, Vanderbilt University, Nashville, Tennessee; and the [2]Department of Medicine, Veterans Affairs, Nashville, Tennessee.

Corresponding author: Stephen N. Davis, sdavis@medicine.umaryland.edu.

Received 13 October 2009 and accepted 6 January 2010. Published ahead of print at http://diabetes.diabetesjournals.org on 19 January 2010. DOI: 10.2337/db09-1520. Clinical trial reg. no. NCT00592332, clinicaltrials.gov.

Hypoglycemia continues to be the major limiting factor to good glycemic control in patients with diabetes. During the last two decades, there have been many studies demonstrating that antecedent hypoglycemia can blunt counterregulatory responses to subsequent hypoglycemia in healthy and type 1 and type 2 diabetic individuals (1). Despite the clinical importance and many elegant studies addressing this topic, there remain gaps in our knowledge regarding the mechanisms regulating neuroendocrine and autonomic nervous system (ANS) responses during episodes of repeated hypoglycemia in man.

The three major acute neuroendocrine/ANS counterregulatory defenses against a falling plasma glucose include release of glucagon and epinephrine combined with inhibition of endogenous insulin release. All of these mechanisms either fail (i.e., insulin modulation and glucagon release within ~5 years of type 1 diabetes duration) or become substantially reduced with disease duration (type 2 diabetes). Furthermore, repeated hypoglycemia has been demonstrated to reduce epinephrine and glucagon responses, which are important defenses against subsequent falling blood glucose levels in both type 1 (epinephrine) and type 2 (epinephrine and glucagon) diabetes (2).

For many years, the problem of severe or frequent hypoglycemia was thought to be confined almost exclusively to type 1 diabetes. Recent multicenter trials aimed at improving glycemic control both within hospitals and in the community have identified excess adverse events and death plausibly related to hypoglycemia in type 2 diabetes (3,4). The glucagon response to hypoglycemia is initially relatively preserved in type 2 diabetes (although there is decrease with disease duration) (5). However, as the prevalence of hypoglycemia is increasing in type 2 diabetes, it continues to be of importance to understand the mechanisms regulating release of both glucagon and epinephrine during repeated episodes of hypoglycemia.

γ-Aminobytyric acid (GABA) is a major inhibitory neurotransmitter. Previous studies have demonstrated increases in GABAergic tone within the ventromedial hypothalamus in rats with repeated hypoglycemia, which is associated with blunted glucagon and epinephrine responses (6). Chan et al. (7) have also demonstrated that blockade of GABA$_A$ receptors within the ventromedial hypothalamus in rats results in increased glucagon and epinephrine responses during hypoglycemia. Studies investigating the effects of GABA$_A$ modulation on counterregulatory responses during hypoglycemia in humans are scarce. In fact, previous studies have used activation of GABA$_A$ receptors rather than changes in GABA concen-

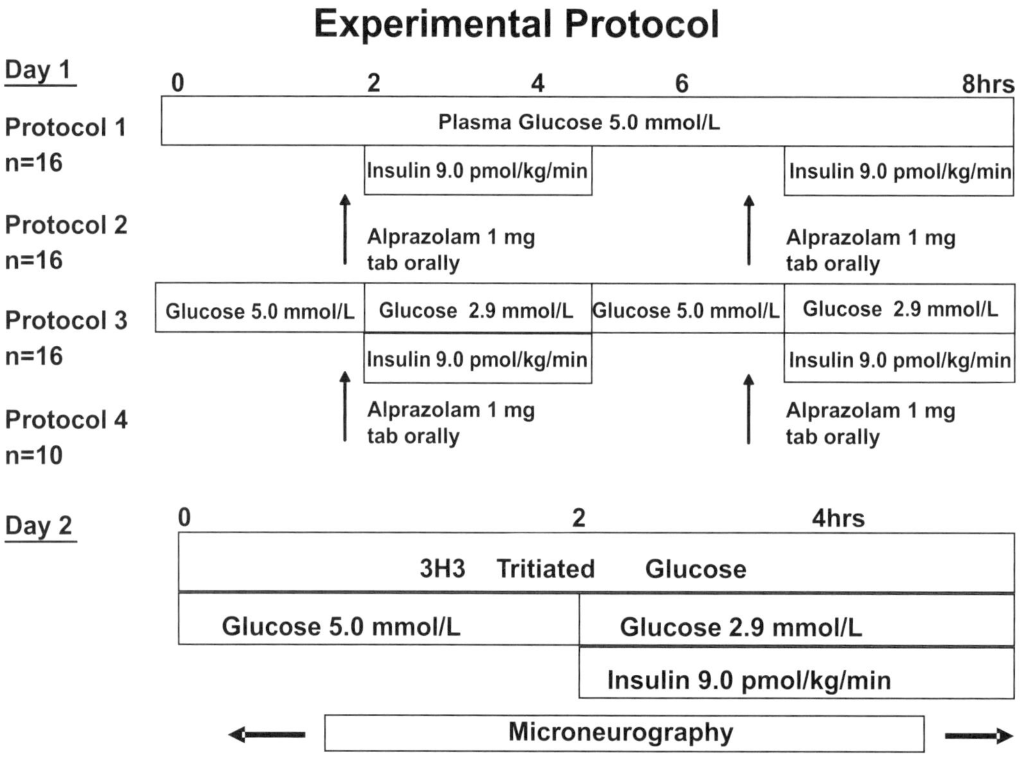

Experimental Protocol

FIG. 1. Study procedures.

trations to investigate the role of GABAergic pathways in ANS and neuroendocrine counterregulatory responses during hypoglycemia in humans and primates. van Vugt et al. (8) demonstrated that alprazolam (a potent pharmacologic activator of the benzodiazepine-GABA_A receptor) can inhibit anterior pituitary neuroendocrine responses during acute hypoglycemia in rhesus monkeys. Giordano et al. (9) reported that alprazolam also reduced neuroendocrine and epinephrine responses to acute intravenous insulin bolus–induced hypoglycemia in healthy humans. Breier et al. (10), using a model of 2-deoxyglucose–induced glucoprivic stress in humans, also demonstrated that alprazolam blunted ACTH and epinephrine responses during neuroglycopenia. Lastly, Smith et al. (11), using modafinil to acutely lower GABA levels during clamped hypoglycemia in healthy humans, reported increased heart rate and improved cognitive function with the drug. Thus, available data would indicate that GABA_A activation can acutely reduce, whereas GABA_A blockade can increase, neuroendocrine and sympathoadrenal responses to hypoglycemia. However, it is unknown whether GABA_A activation can play a mechanistic role in causing neuroendocrine and ANS failure during repeated hypoglycemia in healthy humans. Therefore, in the present study, we have tested the hypothesis that antecedent pharmacologic activation of benzodiazepine-GABA_A receptors with alprazolam can result in counterregulatory failure during next-day hypoglycemia in healthy humans.

RESEARCH DESIGN AND METHODS

Twenty-eight healthy individuals (14 male and 14 female, aged 27 ± 6 years, BMI 24 ± 3 kg/m^2, and A1C $5.2 \pm 0.1\%$) were studied. Subjects were nonsmokers, had no family history of diabetes, and were not taking any medications. All subjects had normal liver, renal, and hematological parameters. Studies were approved by the Vanderbilt University Human Subjects

Institutional Review Board, and all subjects gave informed written and verbal consent.

Experimental design. The volunteers participated in four separate, randomized, double-blind 2-day experiments, with differing day 1 protocols, separated by at least 2 months (Fig. 1). Women were studied at the same point in their menstrual cycle for each arm of the study so as to reduce variability associated with phase of menstrual cycle. All subjects were instructed to avoid intense exercise and alcohol and to consume their usual weight-maintaining diet for 3 days before each study. Each subject was admitted to the Vanderbilt University Clinical Research Center the evening before an experiment. The next morning, after an overnight 10-h fast, subjects had intravenous cannulae placed into each arm under local 1% lidocaine anesthesia. One cannula was placed in a retrograde fashion into a vein in the back of the hand. This hand was placed in a heated box (55–60°C) so that arterialized blood could be obtained (12). The other cannula was placed in the contralateral arm for infusions of dextrose, insulin, potassium chloride, and labeled glucose.

Day 1 consisted of different antecedent challenges (morning and afternoon hypoglycemia or euglycemia with or without prior [30 min before each clamp] administration of 1 mg alprazolam or placebo in a randomized double-blind manner) (Fig. 1). Day 1 studies consisted of a baseline period (0–120 min) and a 2-h hyperinsulinemic experimental clamp period (120–240 min). An insulin-infusion solution was prepared with normal saline containing 3% (vol/vol) of the subject's own plasma. At the onset of the experimental period, a primed continuous infusion of insulin (Eli Lilly, Indianapolis, IN) was administered at a rate of 9 pmol $\cdot$ kg^{-1} $\cdot$ min^{-1} for 120 min (Medfusion 3010; Medex-A Furon Healthcare Company, Deluth, GA). Potassium chloride (5 mmol/h; Imed pump) was also infused during the clamp period to reduce insulin-induced hypokalemia. Plasma glucose levels were measured every 5 min, and a variable infusion of 20% dextrose was adjusted so that plasma glucose levels were held constant (13) in the prior euglycemia studies. During hypoglycemia, the rate of fall of glucose was controlled (0.08 mmol/min) and the hypoglycemic nadir (3.0 mmol/l) was achieved and held constant using a modification of the glucose clamp technique (14). After completion of the initial 2-h test period, plasma glucose was maintained at euglycemia for 2 h. At that point, insulin was restarted, and a second hyperinsulinemic-euglycemic clamp, or hyperinsulinemic-hypoglycemic clamp, identical to that of the morning's study was performed (i.e., 1 mg alprazolam or placebo administered 30 min before the start of glucose clamp). At completion of the second glucose clamp, subjects consumed a standardized meal and a bedtime snack prior to 10 P.M. and remained in the Clinical Research Center.

Day 2 hypoglycemia. Day 2 was identical for all four protocols and was started after an overnight 10-h fast. Each study consisted of a tracer equilibration period (0–90 min), a basal period (90–120 min), and a 2-h experimental period (120–240 min). A primed (18 μCi) continuous infusion (0.18 μCi/min) of high-pressure liquid chromatography–purified [3-3H] glucose (11.5 mCi/mmol/l; Perkin Elmer Life Sciences, Boston, MA) was administered starting at 0 min and continued throughout the study for measurement of glucose kinetics. Also during the equilibration period, isolation of the peroneal nerve for microneurography (technique described below) was started. At the onset of the experimental period, a primed constant (9 pmol · kg^{-1} · min^{-1}) infusion of insulin was started and continued for the next 2 h. The rate of fall of glucose was controlled (~0.08 mmol/min), and the hypoglycemic nadir (2.9–3.0 mmol/l) was achieved and then held constant for the remainder of the study.

Tracer calculations. Glucose R_a, endogenous glucose production (EGP), and glucose utilization (R_d) were calculated according to the methodology of Wall et al. (15). EGP was calculated by determining the total R_a (which comprises both EGP and any exogenous glucose infused to maintain the desired hypoglycemia) and subtracting from it the amount of exogenous glucose infused. It is now recognized that this approach is not fully quantitative because it underestimates the total R_a and R_d that can be obtained. The use of a highly purified tracer and taking measurements under steady-state conditions (i.e., constant specific activity) in the presence of low glucose flux eliminates most, if not all, of the problems. To minimize changes in specific activity, isotope delivery was increased commensurate with increases in exogenous glucose infusion. For this study, only glucose flux results from the basal and the final 30-min periods of the hypoglycemic clamps are reported.

Direct measurement of muscle sympathetic nerve activity via microneurography. Muscle sympathetic nerve activity (MSNA) was recorded because it provides a measurement of direct sympathetic nervous system activity during insulin-induced hypoglycemia (16). MSNA was measured in the peroneal nerve at the level of the fibular head or popliteal fossa. A recording of MSNA was considered adequate when there was 1) spontaneous appearance of pulse-linked bursts, 2) increased nerve activity during phase II (hypotensive phase) and suppressed activity during phase IV (blood pressure overshoot) of the Valsalva maneuver, 3) increased nerve activity in response to held expiration (apnea), or 4) proprioceptive afferent signals in response to stretching the tendons in the foot or tapping the muscle belly but not cutaneous stimulation by stroking the skin.

Sympathetic nerve activity was expressed as bursts per minute. Measurements of MSNA were made from original tracings or online recordings (DI-220; Dataq Instruments, Akron, OH) by an operator blinded to the sequence of experiments. Bursts were selected if the signal:noise ratio was >2:1.

Analytical methods. The collection and processing of blood samples have previously been described (17). Plasma glucose concentrations were measured in triplicate using the glucose oxidase method with a glucose analyzer (Beckman, Fullerton, CA). Blood for hormones and intermediary metabolites were drawn twice during the basal period and every 15 min during the experimental period. Glucagon was measured according to the method of Aguilar-Parada et al. (18), with an interassay coefficient of variation (CV) of 15%. Insulin was measured as previously described (19), with an interassay CV of 11%. Catecholamines were determined by high-pressure liquid chromatography (20), with an interassay CV of 12% for both epinephrine and norepinephrine. We made two modifications to the procedure for catecholamine determination: 1) we used a five-point rather than one-point standard calibration curve, and 2) we spiked the initial and final samples of plasma with known amounts of epinephrine and norepinephrine so that accurate identification of the relevant catecholamine peaks could be made. Growth hormone (21) (interassay CV 8%), cortisol (Clinical Assays Gamma Coat Radioimmunoassay kit) (interassay CV 6%), pancreatic polypeptide (interassay CV 8%) (22), and glucagon (Linco Research, St. Louis, MO) (interassay CV 15%) were measured using radioimmunoassay techniques. Lactate and β-hydroxybutyrate were measured on deproteinized whole blood using the methodology of Lloyd et al. (23). Nonesterified fatty acids (NEFAs) were measured using a WAKO kit (24).

Cardiovascular parameters. Heart rate and systolic, diastolic, and mean arterial blood pressure were measured noninvasively by a Dinamap (Critikon, Tampa, FL) every 10 min throughout each 2-h insulin clamp. Hypoglycemic symptoms were quantified using a previously validated semiquantitative questionnaire (25). Each individual was asked to rate his or her experience of the symptoms twice during the control period and every 15 min during experimental periods. Symptoms measured included the following: sweaty, tremor/shaky, hot, thirsty/dry mouth, agitation/irritability, palpitations, tired/fatigued, confusion, dizzy, difficulty thinking, blurriness of vision, and sleepy.

The ratings of the first six symptoms were summed to get the autonomic score while the ratings from the last six symptoms provide a neuroglycopenic symptom score.

Statistical analysis. Data are expressed as means ± SE and were analyzed using standard parametric one- and two-way ANOVA with repeated measures where appropriate (SigmaStat; SPSS Science, Chicago, IL). Tukey's post hoc analysis was used to delineate statistical significance across time within each group and for each group compared with the prior euglycemia control group. A P value of <0.05 was accepted as statistically significant. The baseline and final 30 min of hypoglycemia on day 2 were compared for most parameters because steady-state glucose levels, insulin levels, and glucose infusion rates were achieved by this time. Baseline period data represent an average of two time points (110 and 120 min), and final 30-min data represent an average of three measurements taken during this time (210, 225, and 240 min).

RESULTS

Day 1 glucose and insulin levels. Plasma glucose levels were similar in the morning and afternoon during the prior euglycemic studies with and without alprazolam (5.2 ± 0.1 mmol/l). Plasma glucose during the day 1 morning and afternoon hypoglycemia studies were also similar with and without alprazolam (2.9 ± 0.1 mmol/l). Plasma insulin levels were similar among all groups during the morning and afternoon hyperinsulinemic-euglycemic and -hypoglycemic clamps (672 ± 108 pmol/l).

Day 2 glucose, insulin, and neuroendocrine counterregulatory hormones. Plasma glucose was equivalent (2.9 ± 0.1 mmol/l) during all of day 2 hypoglycemia. Plasma insulin was also similar (612 ± 58 pmol/l) during all of day 2 hypoglycemia studies (Fig. 2).

Plasma glucagon levels (Fig. 3) were significantly reduced (P < 0.01) during the final 30 min of day 2 hypoglycemia following day 1 euglycemia and alprazolam (131 ± 21 ng/l) and day 1 hypoglycemia (132 ± 18 ng/l) compared with day 1 euglycemia (241 ± 34 ng/l). Day 1 hypoglycemia and alprazolam resulted in a greater reduction (P < 0.05) in day 2 glucagon (76 ± 8 ng/l) than that in the other groups during day 2 hypoglycemia.

Day 2 growth hormone responses were also lower (P < 0.05) following day 1 euglycemia and alprazolam (20 ± 4 μg/l) than those of day 1 euglycemia (31 ± 5 μg/l) or day 1 hypoglycemia (28 ± 4 μg/l). Growth hormone responses were further reduced (P < 0.05) following day 1 hypoglycemia and alprazolam (13 ± 3 μg/l) compared with those of day 1 hypoglycemia and day 1 hypoglycemia and alprazolam (Fig. 3). Day 2 plasma cortisol responses were similar in all groups following the differing day 1 interventions.

ANS responses during day 2 hypoglycemia. Day 2 plasma epinephrine levels (Fig. 4) were significantly lower (P < 0.05) during the final 30 min of hypoglycemia following day 1 euglycemia and alprazolam (3,397 ± 339 pmol/l), day 1 hypoglycemia (2,230 ± 290 pmol/l), and day 1 hypoglycemia and alprazolam (2,943 ± 515 pmol/l) than those of day 1 euglycemia (4,209 ± 389 pmol/l).

Day 2 baseline and final 30 min of hypoglycemia norepinephrine values (Fig. 4) were also significantly lower (P < 0.05) following day 1 euglycemia and alprazolam (0.7 ± 0.1 and 1.2 ± 0.16 nmol/l, respectively) and day 1 hypoglycemia and alprazolam (0.6 ± 0.1 and 1.5 ± 0.15 nmol/l) than those of day 1 euglycemia (1.1 ± 0.1 and 1.9 ± 0.17 nmol/l). Pancreatic polypeptide levels during the final 30 min of day 2 hypoglycemia were also significantly lower (P < 0.05) after day 1 euglycemia and alprazolam (163 ± 27 pmol/l), day 1 hypoglycemia (197 ± 28 pmol/l), and (P < 0.01) day 1 hypoglycemia and alprazolam (128 ± 32 pmol/l) than those of day 1 euglycemia (263 ± 33 pmol/l).

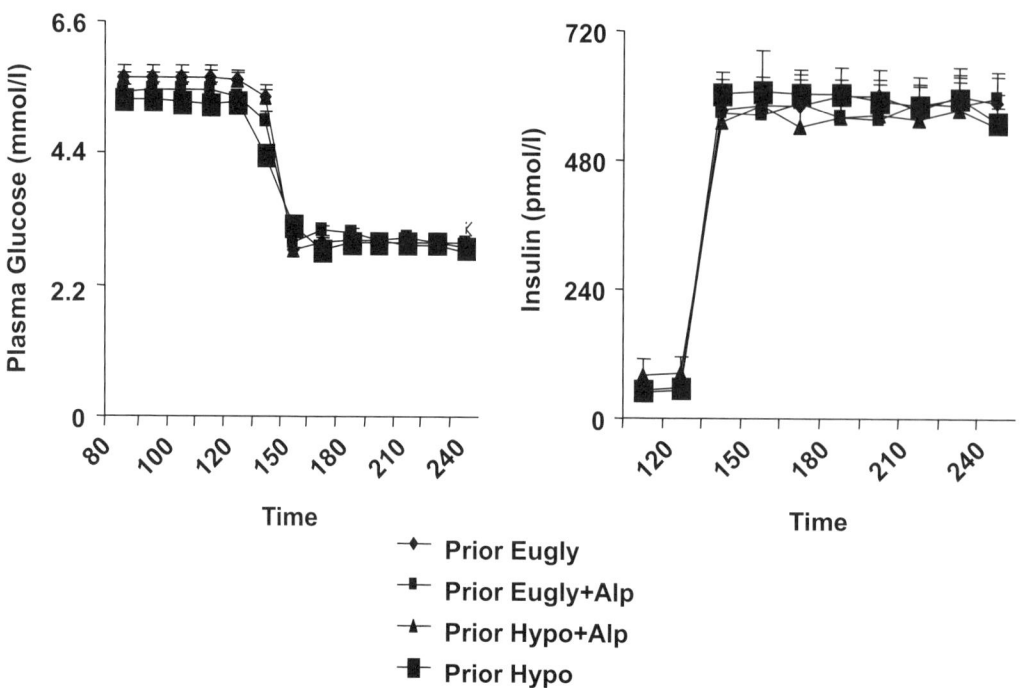

FIG. 2. Plasma glucose and insulin levels during day 2 hypoglycemia in healthy individuals fasted overnight following either day 1 euglycemia (Eugly), day 1 euglycemia and alprazolam (Eugly+Alp), day 1 hypoglycemia (Hypo), or day 1 hypoglycemia and alprazolam (Hypo+Alp).

Day 2 pancreatic polypeptide responses were blunted by a greater extent ($P < 0.05$) following day 1 alprazolam and hypoglycemia compared with day 1 hypoglycemia and day 1 euglycemia.

Basal MSNA (Fig. 5) was significantly reduced ($P < 0.05$) following day 1 alprazolam administration. MSNA responses during the final 30 min of day 2 hypoglycemia were also reduced following day 1 euglycemia and alprazolam ($\Delta3 \pm 1$ bursts/min) and day 1 hypoglycemia ($\Delta7 \pm 2$ bursts/min) compared with those ($\Delta12 \pm 2$) following day 1 euglycemia. MSNA responses were blunted by a greater extent ($P < 0.05$) following day 1 hypoglycemia and alprazolam ($\Delta-2 \pm 1$ bursts/min) than those of day 1 euglycemia and alprazolam, day 1 hypoglycemia, or day 1 euglycemia.

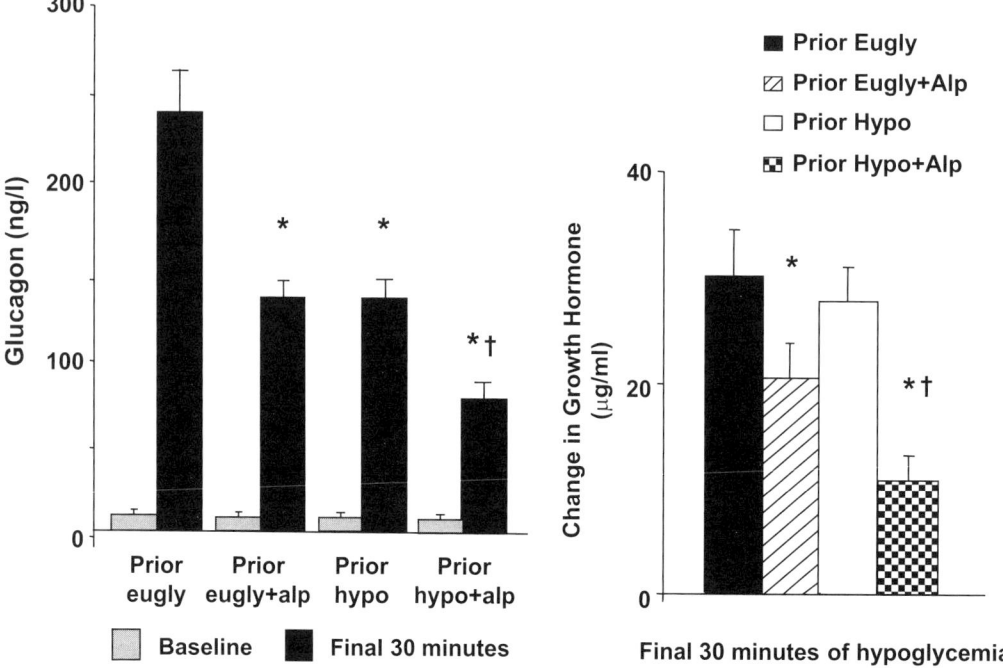

FIG. 3. Day 2 glucagon and growth hormone responses (baseline and final 30 min of hypoglycemia) in healthy individuals fasted overnight following either day 1 euglycemia (Eugly), day 1 euglycemia and alprazolam (Eugly+Alp), day 1 hypoglycemia (Hypo), or day 1 hypoglycemia and alprazolam (Hypo+Alp). *Final 30-min levels are significantly reduced ($P < 0.05$) compared with those of day 1 euglycemia. †Final 30-min levels are significantly reduced ($P < 0.05$) compared with day 1 euglycemia and alprazolam, day 1 hypoglycemia, and day 1 euglycemia.

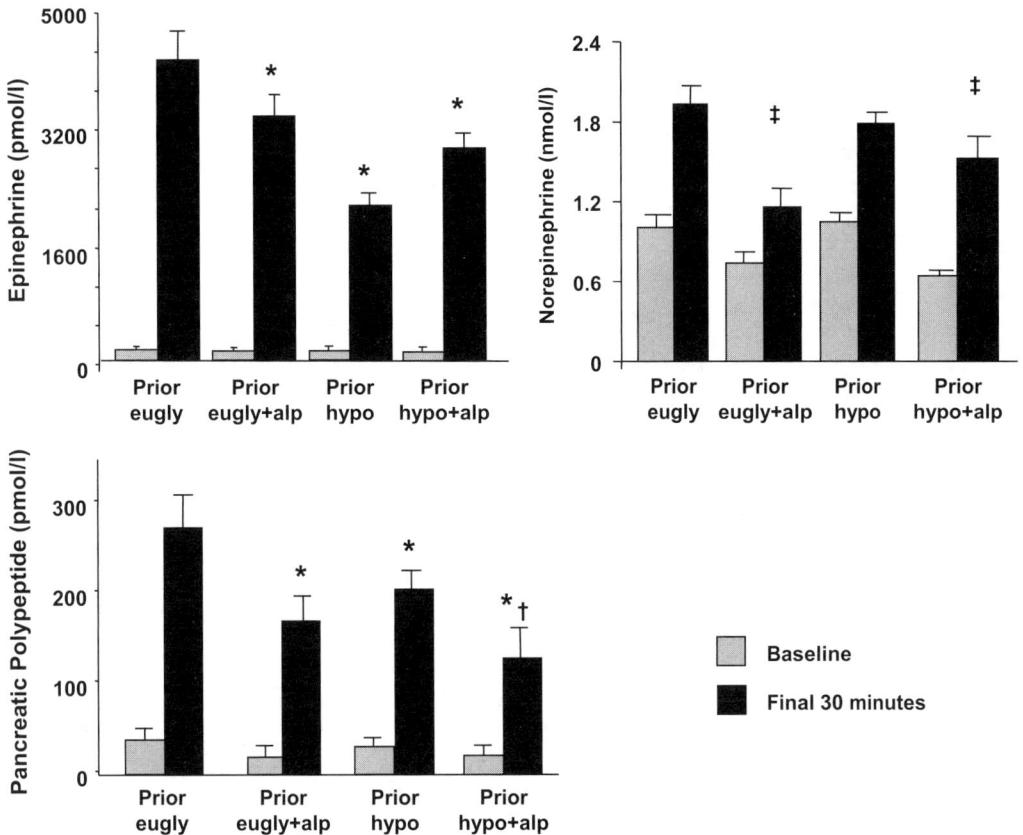

FIG. 4. Day 2 epinephrine, norepinephrine, and pancreatic polypeptide (baseline and final 30 min of hypoglycemia) in healthy individuals fasted overnight following either day 1 euglycemia (eugly), day 1 euglycemia and alprazolam (eugly+alp), day 1 hypoglycemia (hypo), or day 1 hypoglycemia and alprazolam (hypo+alp). *Final 30-min levels are significantly reduced ($P < 0.05$) compared with those of day 1 euglycemia. ‡Basal and final 30-min norepinephrine values are significantly reduced ($P < 0.05$) compared with those of day 1 euglycemia.

Day 2 glucose kinetics. Rates of EGP were significantly reduced ($P < 0.05$) during the final 30 min of day 2 hypoglycemia following day 1 euglycemia and alprazolam, day 1 hypoglycemia, and day 1 hypoglycemia and alprazolam (7.2 ± 1.7, 6.1 ± 1.6, and 8.8 ± 1.1 $\mu mol \cdot kg^{-1} \cdot min^{-1}$, respectively) with those of day 1 euglycemia (12.2 ± 1.7 $\mu mol \cdot kg^{-1} \cdot min^{-1}$) (Table 1). Glucose infusion rates were significantly increased ($P < 0.05$) during the final 30 min of day 2 hypoglycemia following day 1 euglycemia and alprazolam, day 1 hypoglycemia, and day 1 hypoglycemia and alprazolam (7.5 ± 1.1, 8.8 ± 3.3, and 8.3 ± 2.2 $\mu mol \cdot kg^{-1} \cdot min^{-1}$, respectively) compared with 2.5 ± 1.1 $\mu mol \cdot kg^{-1} \cdot min^{-1}$ following day 1 euglycemia.

Day 2 intermediary metabolism. Blood lactate levels were significantly reduced ($P < 0.05$) basally and during the final 30 min of day 2 hypoglycemia following day 1 euglycemia and alprazolam and day 1 hypoglycemia and alprazolam compared with day 1 euglycemia (Table 2). Plasma NEFA levels were also significantly reduced ($P < 0.05$) at baseline and during the final 30 min of hypoglycemia following both day 1 alprazolam groups. NEFA levels were also reduced ($P < 0.05$) during the final 30 min of day 2 hypoglycemia following day 1 hypoglycemia (Table 2).

Day 2 cardiovascular responses and symptom responses. There were similar changes in blood pressure (systolic, diastolic, and mean arterial pressure) and heart rate during the final 30 min of hypoglycemia in all groups (Table 3). Hypoglycemic symptoms were reduced in all groups during the final 30 min of day 2 hypoglycemia.

Following day 1 euglycemia and alprazolam, symptoms were reduced by ~25%, which did not reach statistical significance. Following day 1 hypoglycemia and alprazolam and day 1 hypoglycemia, there were significant reductions ($P < 0.05$) of 30 and 38%, respectively. Day 2 autonomic and neuroglycopenic symptom scores were similarly reduced following day 1 hypoglycemia or day 1 hypoglycemia and alprazolam.

DISCUSSION

This study tested the hypothesis that day 1 pharmacologic activation of $GABA_A$ receptors in healthy man with alprazolam can blunt neuroendocrine and ANS responses to day 2 hypoglycemia. Our results demonstrate that prior $GABA_A$ receptor activation with alprazolam has widespread effects to blunt anterior pituitary, sympathoadrenal, parasympathetic, and sympathetic neural counterregulatory responses to next-day hypoglycemia. $GABA_A$ activation resulted in significant blunting of a spectrum of key neuroendocrine, ANS, and metabolic counterregulatory responses/mechanisms (glucagon, epinephrine, endogenous glucose production, and lipolysis) during next-day hypoglycemia.

Numerous studies have investigated the mechanisms responsible for the acquired ANS and neuroendocrine counterregulatory failure occurring following hypoglycemia (1). To date, a unifying mechanism responsible for the syndrome of acquired hypoglycemia-associated counterregulatory failure

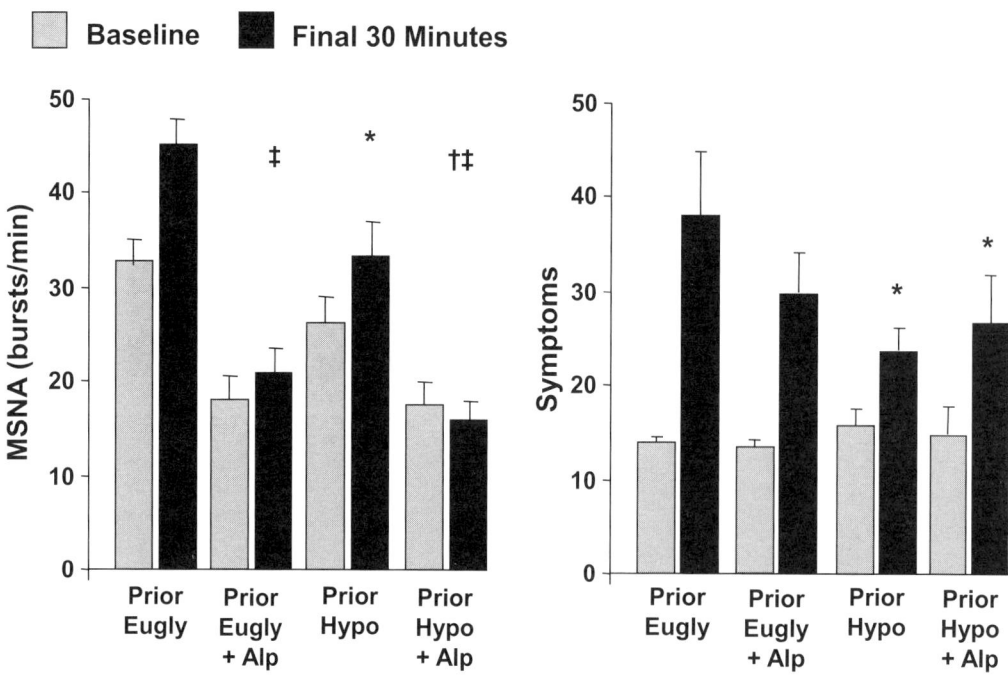

FIG. 5. MSNA and hypoglycemia symptoms at baseline (gray boxes) and during final 30 min (black boxes) of day 2 hypoglycemia in healthy individuals fasted overnight following either day 1 euglycemia (Eugly), day 1 euglycemia and alprazolam (Eugly+Alp), day 2 hypoglycemia (Hypo), or day 2 hypoglycemia and alprazolam (Hypo+Alp). *Final 30-min levels are significantly reduced ($P < 0.05$) compared with those of day 1 euglycemia. †Final 30-min responses are significantly reduced ($P < 0.05$) compared with those of day 1 euglycemia and alprazolam, day 1 hypoglycemia, and day 1 euglycemia. ‡Basal and final 30-min levels are significantly reduced ($P < 0.05$) compared with those of prior euglycemia.

has not been determined (26). GABA is a major inhibitory neurotransmitter and is known to regulate many physiologic responses (27–29). Previous work has demonstrated that increases of gabergic tone in the ventromedial nucleus in rats can downregulate counterregulatory responses to hypoglycemia and indeed subsequent hypoglycemia (6). Additionally, blockade of GABA$_A$ in the ventromedial nucleus of rats

increases neuroendocrine and sympathetic nervous system responses to hypoglycemia (7). Determination of the effects of activation of specific gabergic neurons in discrete areas of the human brain is not possible at this time. To overcome this limitation, previous studies have used alprazolam, a commonly used anxiolytic to specifically activate brain benzodiazepine-GABA$_A$ receptors (8,9). Two previous studies (one in primates and the other in healthy humans) have demon-

TABLE 1
Rates of endogenous glucose production, glucose disappearance, and glucose infusion during baseline and final 30 min of hypoglycemia in men fasted overnight following day 1 euglycemia, day 1 euglycemia and alprazolam, day 1 hypoglycemia, and day 1 hypoglycemia and alprazolam

	Baseline period	Final 30 min hypoglycemia
Endogenous glucose production ($\mu mol \cdot kg^{-1} \cdot min^{-1}$)		
Euglycemia	9.9 ± 0.6	$13.2 \pm 1.7*$
Euglycemia and alprazolam	9.9 ± 1.1	$7.2 \pm 1.7*†$
Hypoglycemia	11.6 ± 0.6	$6.1 \pm 1.7*†$
Hypoglycemia and alprazolam	11.0 ± 1.1	$8.8 \pm 1.1*†$
R_d ($\mu mol \cdot kg^{-1} \cdot min^{-1}$)		
Euglycemia	10.5 ± 2.2	$15.6 \pm 1.7*$
Euglycemia and alprazolam	9.9 ± 0.6	$14.8 \pm 1.7*$
Hypoglycemia	11.6 ± 1.7	$14.9 \pm 1.1*$
Hypoglycemia and alprazolam	10.5 ± 1.1	$17.1 \pm 1.7*$
Glucose infusion rate ($\mu mol \cdot kg^{-1} \cdot min^{-1}$)		
Euglycemia	0	2.5 ± 1.1
Euglycemia and alprazolam	0	$7.5 \pm 1.1†$
Hypoglycemia	0	$8.8 \pm 3.3†$
Hypoglycemia and alprazolam	0	$8.3 \pm 2.2†$

*$P < 0.05$: significantly different from baseline. †$P < 0.05$: significantly different from euglycemic controls.

TABLE 2
Intermediary metabolite levels during baseline and final 30 min of hyperinsulinemic hypoglycemia in healthy individuals fasted overnight following day 1 euglycemia, day 1 euglycemia and alprazolam, day 1 hypoglycemia, and day 1 hypoglycemia and alprazolam

	Baseline period	Final 30 min hypoglycemia
Blood lactate (mmol/l)		
Euglycemia	0.9 ± 0.1	$1.4 \pm 0.1*$
Euglycemia and alprazolam	$0.6 \pm 0.1†$	$1.1 \pm 0.1*‡$
Hypoglycemia	0.9 ± 0.1	$1.4 \pm 0.1*$
Hypoglycemia and alprazolam	$0.6 \pm 0.1†$	$0.9 \pm 0.1*‡$
Plasma NEFA ($\mu mol/l$)		
Euglycemia	329 ± 43	$147 \pm 22*$
Euglycemia and alprazolam	$174 \pm 27†$	$80 \pm 12*‡$
Hypoglycemia	346 ± 31	$98 \pm 23*†$
Hypoglycemia and alprazolam	$186 \pm 40†$	$73 \pm 21*‡$
Blood β-hydroxybutyrate ($\mu mol/l$)		
Euglycemia	40 ± 20	$10 \pm 4*$
Euglycemia and alprazolam	70 ± 10	$33 \pm 20*$
Hypoglycemia	30 ± 8	$9 \pm 2*$
Hypoglycemia and alprazolam	20 ± 10	$10 \pm 5*$

*$P < 0.05$ significantly different from baseline. †$P < 0.05$ significantly different from euglycemia and hypoglycemia. ‡$P < 0.05$ significantly different from euglycemia.

TABLE 3

Cardiovascular responses during baseline and final 30 min of hyperinsulinemic hypoglycemia in men fasted overnight following day 1 euglycemia, day 1 euglycemia and alprazolam, day 1 hypoglycemia, and day 1 hypoglycemia and alprazolam

	Baseline period	Final 30 min hypoglycemia
Monthly systolic blood pressure (mmHg)		
Euglycemia	111 ± 3	119 ± 4*
Euglycemia and alprazolam	116 ± 4	126 ± 5*
Hypoglycemia	114 ± 3	123 ± 4*
Hypoglycemia and alprazolam	120 ± 6	131 ± 9*
Monthly diastolic blood pressure (mmHg)		
Euglycemia	69 ± 3	62 ± 2*
Euglycemia and alprazolam	73 ± 3	68 ± 3*
Hypoglycemia	67 ± 3	68 ± 4*
Hypoglycemia and alprazolam	73 ± 3	66 ± 4*
Monthly mean arterial pressure (mmHg)		
Euglycemia	82 ± 4	78 ± 4
Euglycemia and alprazolam	82 ± 3	79 ± 4
Hypoglycemia	81 ± 2	79 ± 2
Hypoglycemia and alprazolam	85 ± 4	83 ± 5
Heart rate (bpm)		
Euglycemia	63 ± 3	76 ± 5*
Euglycemia and alprazolam	62 ± 3	72 ± 4*
Hypoglycemia	65 ± 4	75 ± 4*
Hypoglycemia and alprazolam	65 ± 3	74 ± 3*

*$P < 0.05$ significantly different from baseline.

strated that acute alprazolam administration blunts neuroendocrine and sympathetic nervous system responses during intravenouos insulin bolus–induced hypoglycemia (8,9). In the present study, prior GABA$_A$ activation with alprazolam during day 1 euglycemia resulted in significant reductions in ANS and neuroendocrine responses during next-day hypoglycemia. Multiple limbs of the ANS response to hypoglycemia were blunted by prior GABA$_A$ activation. Epinephrine, norepinephrine, MSNA, and hypoglycemic symptoms were reduced, indicating a diffuse blunting effect upon the sympathetic nervous system. Furthermore, basal sympathetic neural outflow was also reduced by prior GABA$_A$ activation. Additionally, pancreatic polypeptide, a marker of parasympathetic nervous system activity, was also significantly reduced. The site of GABA$_A$ sensing to downregulate the ANS responses cannot be precisely determined in this study. The down regulation of MSNA responses points to central nervous system sensing. However, there are GABA$_A$ receptors in islet cells that may be regulating the pancreatic polypeptide and glucagon responses. Additionally, previous work has demonstrated that GABA$_A$ receptors may also modulate catecholamine secretion directly from the adrenal medulla (30). Day 1 GABA$_A$ activation with alprazolam also reduced the response of growth hormone and glucagon during day 2 hypoglycemia. The regulation of glucagon release during hypoglycemia is still under study. Previous work has provided evidence for local control (i.e., within the pancreatic islets) of glucagon release secondary to inhibition of β-cell insulin release (31). Other studies have pointed to regulation via the ANS (32). In the present study, we cannot definitively state whether prior activation of GABA$_A$ inhibited glucagon release via a direct effect on pancreatic islets or via inhibition of neural (presumably ANS) pathways.

Similar to the findings of Giodano et al. (7) in humans and Chan et al. (8) in rats, we did not find significant reductions of cortisol during hypoglycemia following alprazolam. However, both Breir et al. (10), using 2-deoxyglycose glucose to create a glucoprivic state in humans, and Giodano et al. (9) reported that ACTH levels were blunted during hypoglycemia following acute GABA$_A$ activation with alprazolam. We did not measure ACTH in the current study, but our finding that growth hormone responses were blunted following alprazolam supports previous findings that GABA$_A$ activation can blunt hypothalamo-anterior pituitary responses during hypoglycemia in humans.

Important metabolic counterregulatory responses/mechanisms were also blunted by GABA$_A$ activation. Endogenous glucose production, lipolysis (as reflected by NEFA levels), and glycogenolysis (as reflected by lactate levels) were blunted during day 2 hypoglycemia following alprazolam. These reduced metabolic counterregulatory responses during day 2 hypoglycemia can be explained by the blunted ANS and neuroendocrine drive caused by the GABA$_A$ activation. The reduced day 2 basal NEFA and lactate levels following day 1 alprazolam may also be explained by the observed reduced sympathetic neural activity (i.e., reduced lipolysis and glycogenolysis) (27). Blood pressure and heart rate responses were not different during day 2 hypoglycemia in any of the groups despite the differences in ANS activity. The mechanism for this finding is not known but may be explained by offsetting effects of GABA$_A$ activation on the sympathetic and parasympathetic nervous system.

This present study also studied whether activation of GABA$_A$ receptors during prior hypoglycemia had any additional effects on subsequent counterregulatory responses. Our results do demonstrate that pharmacologic activation of GABA$_A$ receptors during prior hypoglycemia with alprazolam results in additional blunting of some counterregulatory responses. Epinephrine and norepinephrine responses were not further blunted during day 2 hypoglycemia by the addition of alprazolam during day 1 hypoglycemia. Additionally, important metabolic counterregulatory mechanisms such as glucose kinetics (EGP, glucose disappearance, and lipolysis) were not farther decreased by the combination of hypoglycemia and GABA$_A$ activation). However, MSNA, glucagon, pancreatic polypeptide, and growth hormone responses were further reduced following day 1 hypoglycemia and alprazolam. We believe that there may be two possible explanations for this finding: 1) the combination of hypoglycemia and alprazolam resulted in greater activation of GABA$_A$ receptors or 2) prior alprazolam and hypoglycemia operate through different mechanisms for which the combined effects are additive. Our results also suggest that blunted counterregulatory responses are not due to exhaustion of individual neuroendocrine hormones and that the ANS response to hypoglycemia is heterogeneous, with some elements more susceptible to downregulation following certain stimuli (i.e., GABA$_A$ activation) than others (in this study, MSNA and parasympathetic nervous system were more susceptible than adrenomedullary and symptom responses). Lastly, although this is a study investigating physiologic responses to hypoglycemia in healthy subjects, it may be useful to discuss the possible clinical implications of our study. Benzodiazepines are commonly used in the clinical management of patients with diabetes. The findings that alprazolam can significantly reduce key neuroendocrine and ANS counterregulatory responses during next-day hypoglycemia and that the combination of prior hypoglycemia with alprazolam can further blunt certain counterregulatory responses raise concerns about the possible effects of benzodiazepines on the prevalence of hypoglycemia in clinical practice.

The dose of alprazolam (1 mg before each of two glucose clamps) used in the present study was relatively modest. In the U.S., the drug is approved to be used up to a dose of 10 mg daily. The present study dose of alprazolam was typical of usual starting doses, which range from 0.5 to 1 mg three times a day. However, we do want to point out that the present study was not a clinical outcomes study. We were using alprazolam as a specific pharmacologic probe for GABA$_A$ activation. As a result of to the present study design, we cannot comment whether higher (or lower) doses of day 1 alprazolam would have had greater or lesser effects on day 2 counterregulatory responses. It should also be noted that although alprazolam has a quick onset of action reaching maximum levels within 1–2 h, the plasma half-life is longer with a typical duration of 9–11 h. Thus, as day 2 hypoglycemia was induced ~21 h after the last administration of alprazolam, it is possible that the day 1 administration of the drug still resulted in some acute effects during subsequent (day 2) hypoglycemia. However, what is clear from the present study is that submaximal activation of GABA$_A$ receptors can result in rapid and widespread downregulation of subsequent homeostatic responses to hypoglycemia in healthy man.

In summary, this study has demonstrated that prior activation of GABA$_A$ receptors by alprazolam can produce a spectrum of reduced ANS (adrenomedullary, direct sympathetic nerve activity, and parasympathetic nervous system), neuroendocrine (growth hormone and glucagon), and metabolic (endogenous glucose production, lipolysis, and glycogenolysis) counterregulatory responses during next-day hypoglycemia. We conclude that prior activation of GABA$_A$ pathways can play an important role in regulating a number of key physiologic responses to subsequent hypoglycemia in healthy man. Further studies are required to determine whether GABA$_A$ receptors exert similar effects in individuals with diabetes.

ACKNOWLEDGMENTS

This work was supported by National Institutes of Health grants R01 DK-069803, M01 RR-000095, P01 HL-056693, and P60 DK-020593.

No potential conflicts of interest relevant to this article were reported.

We are thankful for the expert technical assistance of Eric Allen and Wanda Snead. We also thank the nursing staff of the Vanderbilt General Clinical Research Center and Jan Botts Hicks for her expert secretarial skills.

REFERENCES

1. Cryer PE. Mechanisms of sympatho-adrenal failure and hypoglycemia in diabetes. J Clin Invest 2006;116:1470–1473
2. Cryer PE. Hypoglycemia: still the limiting factor in the glycemic management of diabetes. Endocr Pract 2008;14:750–756
3. Action to Control Cardiovascular Risk in Diabetes (ACCORD) Study Group. Effects of intensive glucose lowering in type 2 diabetes. N Engl J Med 2008;358:2545–2559
4. NICE–Sugar Study Investigators. Intensive versus conventional glucose control in critically ill patients. N Engl J Med 2009;360:1283–1297
5. Segel SA, Paramore DS, Cryer PE. Hypoglycemia-associated autonomic failure in advanced type 2 diabetes. Diabetes 2002;51:724–733
6. Chan O, Cheng H, Herzog R, Czyzyk D, Zhu W, Wang A, McCrimmon RJ, Seashore MR, Sherwin RS. Increased GABAergic tone in the ventromedial

hypothalamus contributes to suppression of counterregulatory responses after antecedent hypoglycemia. Diabetes 2008;57:1363–1370
7. Chan O, Zhu W, Ding Y, McCrimmon RJ, Sherwin RS. Blockade of GABA$_A$ receptors in the ventromedial hypothalamus further stimulates glucagon and sympathoadrenal but not the hypothalamo-pituitary-adrenal response to hypoglycemia. Diabetes 2006;55:1080–1087
8. Van Vugt DA, Washburn DL, Farley AE, Reid RL. Hypoglycemia-induced inhibition of LH and stimulation of ACTH secretion in the rhesus monkey is blocked by alprazolam. Neuroendocrinology 1997;65(5):344–352
9. Giordano R, Grottoli S, Brossa P, Pellegrino M, Destefanis S, Lanfranco F, Gianotti L, Ghigo E, Arvat E. Alprazolam (a benzodiazepine activating GABA receptor) reduces the neuroendocrine responses to insulin-induced hypoglycaemia in humans. Clin Endocrinol (Oxf) 2003;59:314–320
10. Breier A, Davis O, Buchanan R, Listwak SJ, Holmes C, Pickar D, Goldstein DS. Effects of alprazolam on pituitary-adrenal and catecholaminergic responses to metabolic stress in humans. Biol Psychiatry 1992;32:880–890
11. Smith D, Pernet A, Rosenthal JM, Bingham EM, Reid H, Macdonald IA, Amiel SA. The effect of modafinil on counter-regulatory and cognitive responses to hypoglycaemia. Diabetologia 2004;47:1704–1711
12. Abumrad NN, Rabin D, Diamond MC, Lacy WW. Use of a heated superficial hand vein as an alternative site for measurement of amino acid concentration and for the study of glucose and alanine kinetics in man. Metabolism 1981;30:936–940
13. DeFronzo RA, Tobin K, Andres R. Glucose clamp technique: a method for quantifying insulin secretion and resistance. Am J Physiol 1979;237:E216–E223
14. Amiel SA, Tamborlane W, Simonson D, Sherwin RS. Defective glucose counterregulation after strict glycemic control of insulin-dependent diabetes mellitus. N Engl J Med 1987;31:1376–1383
15. Wall JS, Steele R, Debodo RD, Altszuler N. Effect of insulin on utilization and production of circulating glucose. Am J Physiol 1957;189:43–50
16. Wallin BG, Sundlof G, Eriksson BM, Dominiak P, Grobecker H, Lindblad LE. Plasma noradrenaline correlates to sympathetic muscle nerve activity in normotensive man. Acta Physiol Scand 1981;111:69–73
17. Cherrington AD, Williams PE, Harris MS. Relationship between the plasma glucose level and glucose uptake in the conscious dog. Metabolism 1978;27:787–791
18. Aguilar-Parada E, Eisentraut AM, Unger RH. Pancreatic glucagon secretion in normal and diabetic subjects. Am J Med Sci 1969;257:415–419
19. Wide L, Porath J. Radioimmunoassay of proteins with the use of sephadex-coupled antibodies. Biochim Biophys Acta 1966;130:257–260
20. Causon R, Caruthers M, Rodnight R. Assay of plasma catecholamines by liquid chromatography with electrical detection. Anal Biochem 1981;116:223–226
21. Hunter W, Greenwood F. Preparation of [131I]-labeled human growth hormone of high specific activity. Nature 1962;194:495–496
22. Hagopian W, Lever E, Cen D, Emmounoud D, Polonsky K, Pugh W, Moosa A, Jaspan JB. Predominance of renal and absence of hepatic metabolism of pancreatic polypeptide in the dog. Am J Physiol 1983;245:171–177
23. Lloyd B, Burrin J, Smythe P, Alberti KGMM. Enzymatic fluorometric continuous-flow assays for blood glucose lactate, pyruvate, alanine, glycerol, and 3-hydroxybutyrate. Clin Chem 1978;24:1724–1729
24. Ho RJ. Radiochemical assay of long chain fatty acid using 63NI as tracer. Anal Biochem 1970;26:105–113
25. Dreary L, Hepburn D, Macleod K, Frier BM. Partitioning the symptoms of hypoglycemia using multi-sample confirmatory factor analysis. Diabetologia 1993;36:761–770
26. Cryer PE. Diverse causes of hypoglycemia-associated autonomic failure in diabetes. N Engl J Med 2004;350:2272–2279
27. McCann SM, Rettori V. Gamma amino bytyric acid (GABA) controls anterior pituitary hormone secretion. Adv Biochem Psychopharmacol 1986;42:173–189
28. Lang CH. Inhibition of central GABAA receptors enhances hepatic glucose production and peripheral glucose uptake. Brain Res Bull 1995;37:611–616
29. Beverly JL, DeVries M, Bouman S, Arseneau L. Noradrenergic and GABAergic systems in the medial hypothalamus are activated during hypoglycemia. Am J Physiol Reg Int Comp Physiol 2001;280:R563–R569
30. Castro E, Oset-Gasque M, Gonzalez M. GABAA and GABAB receptors are functionally active in the regulation of catecholamine secretion by bovine chromaffin cells. J Neurosci Res 1989;23:290–296
31. Raju B, Cryer PE. Loss of the decrement in intraislet insulin plausibly explains loss of the glucagons response to hypoglycemia in insulin-deficient diabetes: documentation of the intraislet insulin hypothesis in humans. Diabetes 2005;54:757–764
32. Havel PJ, Ahren B. Activation of autonomic nerves and the adrenal medulla contributes to increased glucagon secretion during moderate insulin–induced hypoglycemia in women. Diabetes 1997;46:801–807

Human Brain Glycogen Metabolism During and After Hypoglycemia

Gülin Öz,[1] Anjali Kumar,[2] Jyothi P. Rao,[2] Christopher T. Kodl,[2] Lisa Chow,[2] Lynn E. Eberly,[3] and Elizabeth R. Seaquist[2]

OBJECTIVE—We tested the hypotheses that human brain glycogen is mobilized during hypoglycemia and its content increases above normal levels ("supercompensates") after hypoglycemia.

RESEARCH DESIGN AND METHODS—We utilized in vivo ^{13}C nuclear magnetic resonance spectroscopy in conjunction with intravenous infusions of [^{13}C]glucose in healthy volunteers to measure brain glycogen metabolism during and after euglycemic and hypoglycemic clamps.

RESULTS—After an overnight intravenous infusion of 99% enriched [1-^{13}C]glucose to prelabel glycogen, the rate of label wash-out from [1-^{13}C]glycogen was higher (0.12 ± 0.05 vs. 0.03 ± 0.06 μmol $\cdot$ g^{-1} $\cdot$ h^{-1}, means $\pm$ SD, $P < 0.02$, $n = 5$) during a 2-h hyperinsulinemic-hypoglycemic clamp (glucose concentration 57.2 ± 9.7 mg/dl) than during a hyperinsulinemic-euglycemic clamp (95.3 ± 3.3 mg/dl), indicating mobilization of glucose units from glycogen during moderate hypoglycemia. Five additional healthy volunteers received intravenous 25–50% enriched [1-^{13}C]glucose over 22–54 h after undergoing hyperinsulinemic-euglycemic (glucose concentration 92.4 ± 2.3 mg/dl) and hyperinsulinemic-hypoglycemic (52.9 ± 4.8 mg/dl) clamps separated by at least 1 month. Levels of newly synthesized glycogen measured from 4 to 80 h were higher after hypoglycemia than after euglycemia ($P \leq 0.01$ for each subject), indicating increased brain glycogen synthesis after moderate hypoglycemia.

CONCLUSIONS—These data indicate that brain glycogen supports energy metabolism when glucose supply from the blood is inadequate and that its levels rebound to levels higher than normal after a single episode of moderate hypoglycemia in humans. *Diabetes* **58:1978–1985, 2009**

G lucose is the primary fuel for the adult brain. During euglycemia and hyperglycemia, the brain receives more glucose from the blood than it utilizes and normal metabolism can be maintained. However, how the energy needs of the brain are met during hypoglycemia has been a matter of debate. Mobilization of glucose stored in the form of glycogen is one potential mechanism that could support brain metab-

olism when blood glucose is low. Glycogen content of the brain has been measured at 3–10 μmol/g (1–4), an amount much higher than brain glucose at euglycemia (1–1.5 μmol/g) (5). Although brain glycogen content is much lower than liver (200–400 μmol/g) (6) and muscle (80 μmol/g) (7), we have previously estimated that it can augment cerebral energy needs during short periods of glucose deficit in humans (4). In the current study, we addressed this question in normal human volunteers using nuclear magnetic resonance (NMR) methodology first developed in rats (8) and then translated to humans (9,10). With this technique, [^{13}C]glucose is administered intravenously and its incorporation into and wash-out from brain glycogen is tracked (9,10). [1-^{13}C]glucose has been the substrate of choice since the NMR signal of [1-^{13}C]glucose in glycogen is well resolved from those of free [1-^{13}C]glucose and other glucosyl positions. The ^{13}C NMR measurement of brain glycogen was recently validated by comparing glycogen concentrations obtained in vivo in rats to those measured in extracted tissue by a standard biochemical assay (11).

Using ^{13}C NMR, we recently estimated that 3–4 μmol/g glucose is stored in the form of glycogen in the awake human brain (4). This is in agreement with a measurement of 5–6 μmol/g in normal gray and white matter obtained by biopsies during surgery of patients with epilepsy (12) because anesthesia is known to trigger glycogen accumulation (13). Based on these studies, the glycogen content of the brain represents a significant glucose reservoir relative to free glucose. We found that human brain glycogen turns over very slowly relative to the cerebral rate of glucose utilization (CMR_{glc}) under normal physiology (4), similar to what has been observed in the rodent brain (1,8,14). Namely, at euglycemia and hyperglycemia, bulk brain glycogen turns over at a rate that is ~1–2% of CMR_{glc} (15–18) in both humans and rodents. Importantly, glycogen synthesis and breakdown rates can be altered by many factors, such as nutrients, neurotransmitters, and hormones, including glucose and insulin (19–22). The low metabolic rate of glycogen under normal physiology, together with the capacity to acutely regulate glycogen synthase and phosphorylase in response to nutritional and hormonal state, indicate that glycogen may serve as an emergency reservoir when glucose supply from the blood is inadequate. Indeed, brain glycogen is mobilized during hypoglycemia in the rodent brain (23–26), but whether a similar event occurs in humans during hypoglycemia is unknown.

In rodents, brain glycogen was observed to rebound to levels higher than normal, a phenomenon termed "supercompensation," after a single hypoglycemic episode (23). This led to the hypothesis that glycogen may be involved in the pathogenesis of hypoglycemia unawareness by supplying extra fuel to the brain during episodes experienced

From the [1]Center for MR Research, Department of Radiology, Medical School, University of Minnesota, Minneapolis, Minnesota; the [2]Department of Medicine, Medical School, University of Minnesota, Minneapolis, Minnesota; and the [3]Division of Biostatistics, School of Public Health, University of Minnesota, Minneapolis, Minnesota.

Corresponding author: Gülin Öz, gulin@cmrr.umn.edu.

Received 16 February 2009 and accepted 1 June 2009.

Published ahead of print at http://diabetes.diabetesjournals.org on 5 June 2009. DOI: 10.2337/db09-0226.

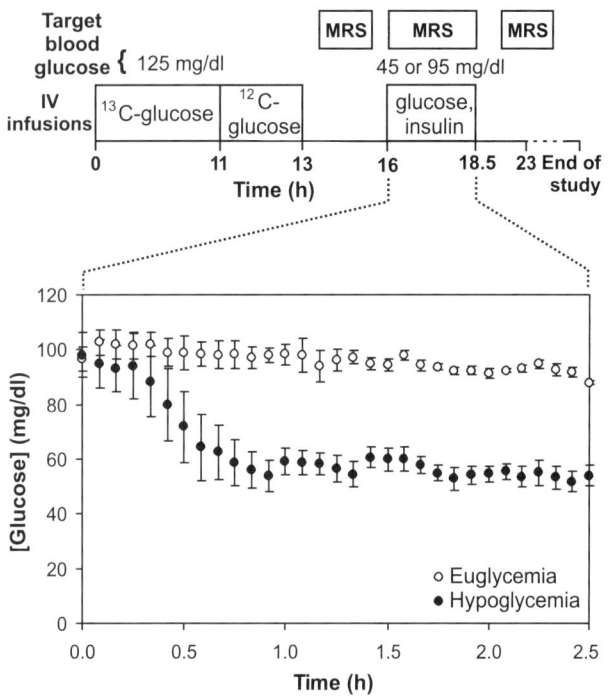

FIG. 1. Experimental protocol of the glycogen utilization study. Average (±SEM) blood glucose levels during the hyperinsulinemic-hypoglycemic and hyperinsulinemic-euglycemic clamps are also shown.

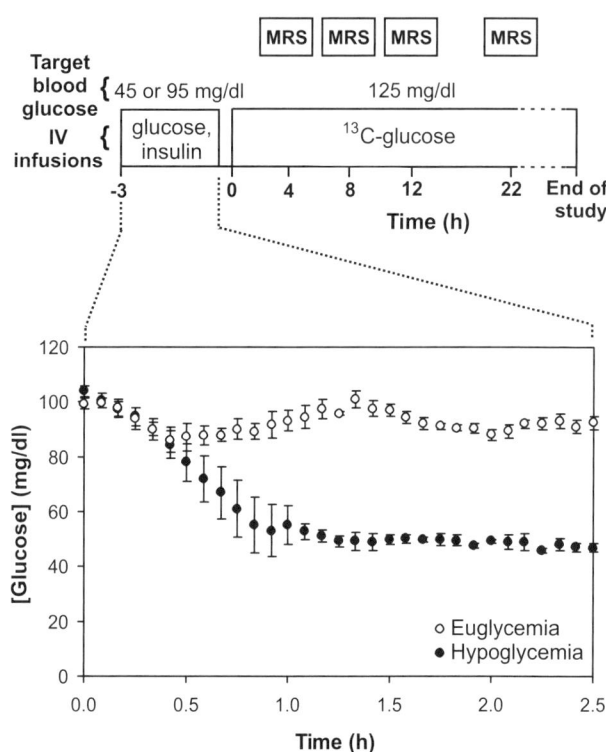

FIG. 2. Experimental protocol of the glycogen supercompensation study. Average (±SEM) blood glucose levels during the hyperinsulinemic-hypoglycemic and hyperinsulinemic-euglycemic clamps are also shown.

soon after the initial hypoglycemia (23,27). Glycogen supercompensation has not yet been studied in the human brain.

The aims of the current study were *1*) to assess glycogen mobilization in the human brain during moderate hypoglycemia and *2*) to determine if the glycogen synthesis rate is increased after a hypoglycemic episode indicating supercompensation in the human brain.

RESEARCH DESIGN AND METHODS

Glycogen utilization study. Five healthy volunteers (four men and one woman age 43 ± 13 years, BMI 25 ± 3 kg/m², means ± SD) on no medications participated in a paired experiment after giving informed consent using procedures (Fig. 1) approved by the University of Minnesota Institutional Review Board. Subjects were studied on two separate occasions separated by at least 1 week, with each subject serving as their own control. Subjects reported to the General Clinical Research Center (GCRC) at 6:00 P.M. after starting a fast at 2:00 P.M. Intravenous catheters were placed antegrade in contralateral arms for [¹³C]glucose infusion and blood sampling. At 7:00 P.M., a bolus of [1-¹³C]glucose was given to rapidly raise blood glucose enrichment. A continuous infusion was then given at a variable rate to maintain blood glucose 25% above basal levels to minimize endogenous hepatic glucose production and achieve stable glucose enrichments, because postprandial insulin levels are known to suppress hepatic glucose output (28). Blood glucose was measured on an automatic glucose meter (OneTouch SureStep; Lifescan, Milpitas, CA). Additional samples were collected hourly and immediately frozen for the later determination of isotopic enrichment of plasma glucose by gas chromatography–mass spectroscopy (GC-MS) as described previously (15). A total of 186 g of [1-¹³C]glucose (Isotec, Miamisburg, OH, and Cambridge Isotope Laboratories, Andover, MA; prepared as 20% weight/volume D-glucose in water with 99% isotopic enrichment) was administered for 11.1 ± 1.2 h to prelabel glycogen. Subjects were then given an unlabeled glucose infusion for 1.6 ± 0.6 h to wash-out [¹³C]glucose from blood so that [1-¹³C]glucose removed from glycogen would not be replenished by plasma [1-¹³C]glucose.

After the wash-out period, subjects were transferred to the Center for Magnetic Resonance Research (CMRR) for a baseline scan, which was omitted in one subject. They were prepared for a 2-h hyperinsulinemic clamp study by retrograde placement of a third intravenous catheter into a foot to provide venous access for arterialized blood sampling (29) while the subject

was in the magnet. The two-arm intravenous catheters were used for administration of glucose, insulin (2 mU · kg⁻¹ · min⁻¹) and potassium phosphate (4 mEq/h). Glucose (20% dextrose in water) was titrated to achieve target blood glucose of 45 mg/dl (2.5 mmol/l) on one occasion and 95 mg/dl (5.3 mmol/l) on the other occasion, in random order. Blood was obtained every 5 min for immediate measurement of glucose using an autoanalyzer (Analox Instruments, Lunenburg, MA). During the hypoglycemic clamps, blood was also sampled every 30 min for the later determination of glucagon, catecholamines, growth hormone, and cortisol. Four [1-¹³C]glycogen NMR spectra were acquired using methods described below while blood glucose levels were clamped at the target levels, starting 4.9 ± 1.3 h after the end of the [1-¹³C]glucose infusion. Subjects were then removed from the magnet, the insulin and potassium infusions were stopped, glucose was administered to bring the blood glucose to 95 mg/dl, and subjects were fed a regular meal. Additional spectroscopic measurements of [¹³C]glycogen were obtained at ~23, 28, 38, and 46 h after the start of the [¹³C]glucose infusion.

Glycogen supercompensation study. Five healthy volunteers (four men and one woman, age 43 ± 14 years, BMI 26 ± 4 kg/m², means ± SD) on no medications participated in a paired experiment after giving informed consent using procedures (Fig. 2) approved by the University of Minnesota Institutional Review Board. Subjects were studied on two occasions separated by at least 1 month. Subjects reported at 7:00 A.M. to the GCRC in the fasting state. Two intravenous catheters were placed antegrade in contralateral arms for administration of glucose, insulin, and KPhos. Each volunteer underwent a 2-h hyperinsulinemic-euglycemic clamp on one occasion and a hyperinsulinemic-hypoglycemic clamp on the other, in random order, as described above. After the clamp, the insulin and potassium infusions were stopped and glucose was administered to bring the blood glucose to 95 mg/dl. Thirty minutes after the end of the clamp, [1-¹³C]glucose infusion was started with an initial bolus to rapidly raise blood glucose enrichment. The two-arm intravenous lines were used for [¹³C]glucose infusion and blood sampling. The infusion rate was adjusted to maintain blood glucose 25% above basal levels. A total of 820–1,420 g of [1-¹³C]glucose (25–50% isotopic enrichment) was administered over 22–54 h. During the infusion, additional blood samples were collected and frozen for the later determination of isotopic enrichment of plasma glucose by GC-MS. Subjects were transferred to the CMRR to acquire [1-¹³C]glycogen NMR spectra at ~4, 8, 12, 22, 29, 35, 46, 53, 60, 70, and 80 h after the start of the [1-¹³C]glucose infusion. During the infusion, subjects

TABLE 1
Comparison of glucose and glycogen measurements before clamps in the utilization study (means ± SD between subjects)

	Euglycemia study	Hypoglycemia study	P (paired t test)
[Mean plasma glucose] during overnight infusion (mg/dl)	129 ± 13	129 ± 22	0.97
Mean isotopic enrichment of plasma glucose during overnight infusion (%)	83 ± 9	78 ± 11	0.22
[^{13}C-glycogen] at baseline (μmol/g)	1.2 ± 0.2	1.3 ± 0.2	0.86
[Newly synthesized glycogen] at baseline (μmol/g)*	1.4 ± 0.3	1.5 ± 0.2	0.36
[^{13}C-glycogen] at the beginning of clamp (μmol/g)†	1.4 ± 0.1	1.2 ± 0.3	0.12
[Newly synthesized glycogen] at the beginning of clamp (μmol/g)†	1.7 ± 0.3	1.5 ± 0.2	0.24

*Newly synthesized: corrected for plasma glucose isotopic enrichment during infusions. †These are the glycogen levels obtained in the first 30 min of the 2-h clamps.

were fed isocaloric, low-carbohydrate meals designed to minimize the impact of dietary carbohydrate on [^{13}C]glucose enrichment.

NMR spectroscopy. All measurements were performed on a 4-tesla, 90-cm bore magnet (Oxford Magnet Technology, Oxford, U.K.) with an INOVA console (Varian, Palo Alto, CA). Subjects were positioned supine on the patient bed with the occipital lobe just above the ^{1}H/^{13}C surface coil (30). Subjects wore earplugs to minimize exposure to gradient noise and were positioned in the coil holder using cushions to minimize head movement.

The [1-^{13}C]glycogen NMR signal localized in a $7 \times 5 \times 6$ cm^3 voxel in the occipital lobe was acquired as described previously (4,9,10). Each spectrum/data point presented here was acquired over 30 min. The amount of ^{13}C label in the C1 position of glycogen was quantified by the external reference method (9,10). The [1-^{13}C]glycogen concentrations were divided by the plasma glucose isotopic enrichment to correct for differences in isotopic enrichment between subjects and to determine the newly synthesized glycogen concentrations.

Modeling glycogen turnover. A model of glycogen metabolism (4) was fitted to the time courses of [^{13}C]glycogen using the software SAAM II (The SAAM Institute, Seattle, WA). Data from the euglycemic clamp studies of each subject were used for modeling, together with their blood glucose isotopic enrichment time courses as input function. Glycogen synthase (V_{syn}) and phosphorylase (V_{phos}) rates were set to be equal and brain glycogen concentration was set to be constant. Thus, the fitted variables were total glycogen concentration (Glyc) and turnover rate $V_{syn} = V_{phos}$. The cerebral metabolic rate of glucose (CMR$_{glc}$) in the human brain was assumed to be 0.4 μmol · g^{-1} · min^{-1} = 24 μmol · g^{-1} · h^{-1} (15) and the glucose-6-phosphate concentration 0.1 μmol/g (14). Sensitivity analysis indicated that the results were not affected over large ranges of both of these variables (18–30 μmol · g^{-1} · h^{-1} for CMR$_{glc}$ and up to 1 μmol/g for glucose-6-phosphate concentration). Concentration and rate estimates are reported as means ± SD.

Statistical analysis. In the utilization study, summary statistics and paired t tests were used to compare within-subject differences in plasma glucose, glucose enrichment, and glycogen on hypoglycemic versus euglycemic study days, at each baseline and during clamps. Repeated measures ANOVA was used to compare euglycemic measures to hypoglycemic measures of glycogen, for both within-clamp measures and after-clamp measures. In the supercompensation study, summary statistics and paired t tests were used to compare within-subject differences in plasma glucose, plasma insulin, and the 4-h glycogen measurement on hypoglycemic versus euglycemic study days.

RESULTS

Glycogen utilization study. Brain glycogen of five healthy volunteers was prelabeled via an overnight intravenous infusion of [1-^{13}C]glucose before a euglycemic or hypoglycemic clamp study in the scanner (Fig. 1). Average plasma glucose levels and isotopic enrichments during the overnight infusion were not significantly different for the euglycemia versus hypoglycemia study days, leading to equal glycogen prelabeling before both clamp studies (Table 1). Target levels for blood glucose during the clamps were reached in ~30 min after starting the insulin infusion (Fig. 1). Average blood glucose concentration during the hypoglycemic clamps was 57.2 ± 9.7 mg/dl and during the euglycemic clamps 95.1 ± 3.3 mg/dl. The hypoglycemic glucose concentration was slightly above our target level mainly because of one subject who did not require glucose infusion and stayed above 60 mg/dl during the clamp period. Average blood glucose during the hypo-

glycemic clamps of the other four subjects was 53.3 ± 4.7 mg/dl. Counterregulation during hypoglycemia was demonstrated by measurement of serum glucagon, growth hormone, cortisol, and catecholamines (Fig. 3). The residual plasma glucose enrichment after the chase with [^{12}C]glucose (Fig. 1) during the hypoglycemic clamps tended to be higher than that during the euglycemic clamps (22 ± 14 vs. 11 ± 4%, $P = 0.13$, paired t test) likely because of mobilization of [^{13}C]-labeled hepatic glycogen during hypoglycemia. However, considering the approximately twofold higher glucose concentrations during the euglycemic clamps, the level of cerebral [^{13}C]glucose available for incorporation into glycogen was equal between the hypoglycemic and euglycemic clamps, which was also apparent from the residual glucose peaks in the spectra (Fig. 4A).

The glycogen signal was stable during the euglycemic clamps, while it decreased during the hypoglycemic clamps (Fig. 4A), indicating mobilization of glucose units from glycogen during moderate hypoglycemia. Average glycogen integrals, each normalized to first clamp measure, during euglycemia were higher than during hypoglycemia (0.98 ± 0.05 vs. 0.87 ± 0.08, $P < 0.0001$, repeated measures ANOVA) (Fig. 4B). Glycogen utilization was confirmed by a higher rate at which newly synthesized glycogen levels decreased during hypoglycemia (0.12 ± 0.05 μmol · g^{-1} · h^{-1}) than during euglycemia (0.03 ± 0.06 μmol · g^{-1} · h^{-1}, $P < 0.02$, paired t test). This label wash-out rate during euglycemia was the same as we previously observed after an 11-h prelabeling period (4). To further analyze the consistency between our previous observations during euglycemia and slight hyperglycemia and this study, we fitted a model of glycogen turnover to the time courses of [^{13}C]glycogen obtained during the euglycemia studies of the five volunteers. This resulted in estimates of glycogen content of 4.3 ± 0.2 μmol/g and turnover rate ($V_{syn} = V_{phos}$) of 0.18 ± 0.01 μmol · g^{-1} · h^{-1}, indicating a turnover time constant of 24 h, in excellent agreement with prior results (4).

Newly synthesized glycogen levels after the clamp (at 23, 28, 38, and 46 h time points) were not different for euglycemia versus hypoglycemia studies ($P = 0.64$, repeated measures ANOVA). Note that the "newly synthesized glycogen" levels refer to measured [^{13}C]glycogen levels divided by the isotopic enrichment of plasma glucose during the preclamp infusions; therefore, they do not necessarily reflect new glycogen synthesized after the clamps. Based on the lower [^{13}C]glycogen levels at the end of the hypoglycemic clamps, one might expect the glycogen measurements after hypoglycemia to also be lower than those after euglycemia. However, the average plasma

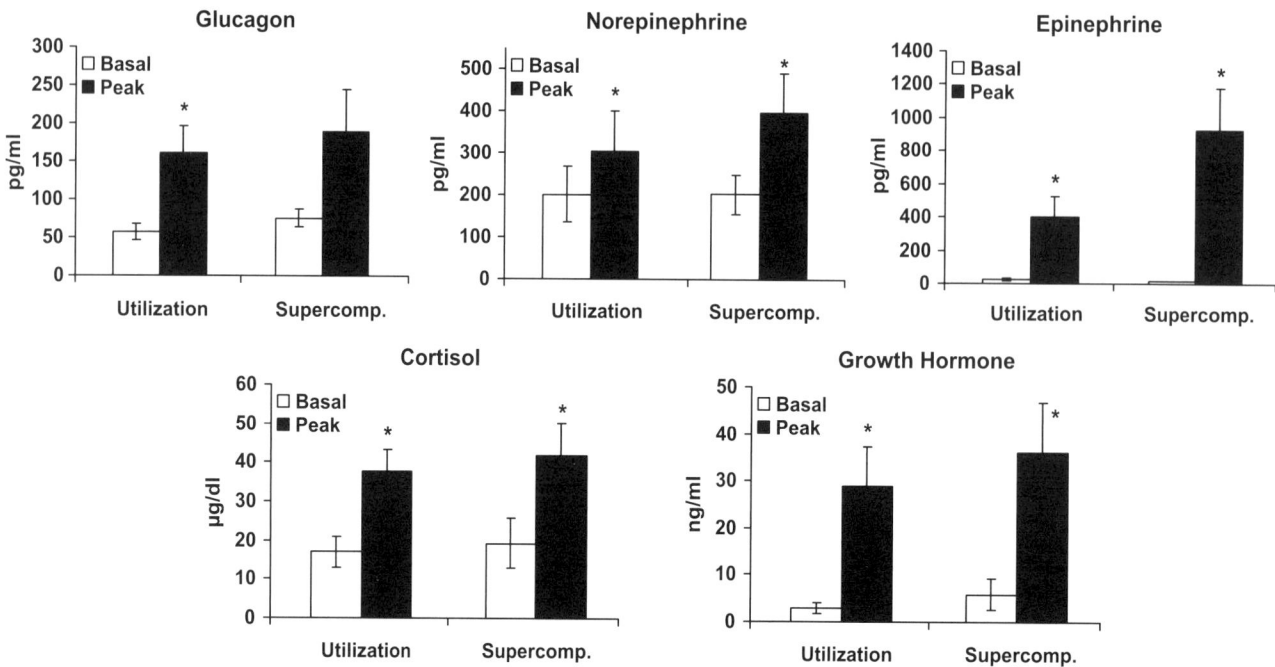

FIG. 3. Counterregulatory hormone response during the hypoglycemic clamps in the glycogen utilization and supercompensation (Supercomp) studies. Basal (5 min and immediately before the clamp) versus peak (maximum observed over the 2-h clamp period) values (average ± SEM) are shown. * $P < 0.05$, paired t test.

glucose isotopic enrichment at the end of the hypoglycemic clamps was $13 \pm 11\%$ (as opposed to $2 \pm 1\%$ at the end of the euglycemic clamps) and this enriched glucose could have been incorporated into glycogen once blood glucose levels were rescued, thereby equalizing [^{13}C]glycogen levels in the following scans. This effect would have been augmented by glycogen supercompensation after hypoglycemia. Therefore, we investigated if glycogen synthesis was increased after hypoglycemia in the next set of experiments.

Glycogen supercompensation study. In this experiment, label incorporation from intravenous [1-^{13}C]glucose into brain glycogen was measured after a euglycemic or hypoglycemic clamp (Fig. 2). Target levels for blood glucose during the clamps were reached in 40–60 min after starting the insulin infusion (Fig. 2). Average blood glucose concentration was 52.9 ± 4.8 mg/dl (means ± SD between subjects) during the hypoglycemic clamps and 92.4 ± 2.3 mg/dl during the euglycemic clamps. Counterregulation during hypoglycemia was demonstrated by measurement of serum glucagon, growth hormone, cortisol, and catecholamines (Fig. 3). Average plasma glucose levels during the [1-^{13}C]glucose infusion were 115 ± 8 mg/dl and average insulin levels 40 ± 12 mU/l, with no difference between the euglycemia and hypoglycemia studies ($P = 0.38$ for glucose levels and 0.51 for insulin, paired t test) (Fig. 5A and B). Steady ^{13}C isotopic enrichment levels in blood glucose were achieved during the long infusions as demonstrated by data obtained in one subject in Fig. 5C. We fitted a model of glycogen turnover to the time courses of [^{13}C]glycogen obtained during the euglycemia studies of the five volunteers. This resulted in estimates of glycogen content of 3.5 ± 0.1 μmol/g and turnover rate ($V_{syn} = V_{phos}$) of 0.20 ± 0.01 μmol · g^{-1} · h^{-1}, in agreement with the results of the glycogen utilization study and our prior published results for euglycemia and slight hyperglycemia (4). The newly synthesized glycogen

levels were higher after hypoglycemia than after euglycemia across all time points during and after the ^{13}C-glucose infusions (Fig. 6, $P \leq 0.01$ paired t test for each subject separately), indicating increased glycogen synthesis after hypoglycemia. The glycogen synthesis rate can be estimated from the initial rate of label incorporation when ^{13}C enrichment of glycogen is negligible and the labeling kinetics primarily represents synthesis. The first glycogen data point obtained from each volunteer at 4 h was used for this purpose. The synthesis rate of glycogen was 0.25 ± 0.03 μmol · g^{-1} · h^{-1} after euglycemia and 0.32 ± 0.05 μmol · g^{-1} · h^{-1} after hypoglycemia ($P < 0.02$, paired t test). The difference between newly synthesized glycogen levels increased steadily over time during the [^{13}C]glucose infusion (Fig. 6) reaching ~ 1 μmol/g at 34 h, indicating a net synthesis of ~ 1 μmol/g glycogen occurred over this time period.

DISCUSSION

Here we present the first evidence for glycogen utilization during, and supercompensation after, moderate hypoglycemia in the healthy human brain. Using ^{13}C NMR, we found that brain glycogen content decreased by $\sim 15\%$ during modest hypoglycemia, whereas it was unchanged under isoinsulinemic euglycemia. Our data also indicate that brain glycogen content increased after a period of modest hypoglycemia but did not change after isoinsulinemic euglycemia in a second group of healthy volunteers.

In the utilization experiment, we detected glycogen mobilization by an increased ^{13}C label wash-out from prelabeled glycogen during hypoglycemia relative to euglycemia. The ^{13}C label was incorporated into glycogen mainly via turnover, as net synthesis does not occur at the euglycemia and slight hyperglycemia we utilized during prelabeling (4). Hence, the total and labeled glycogen

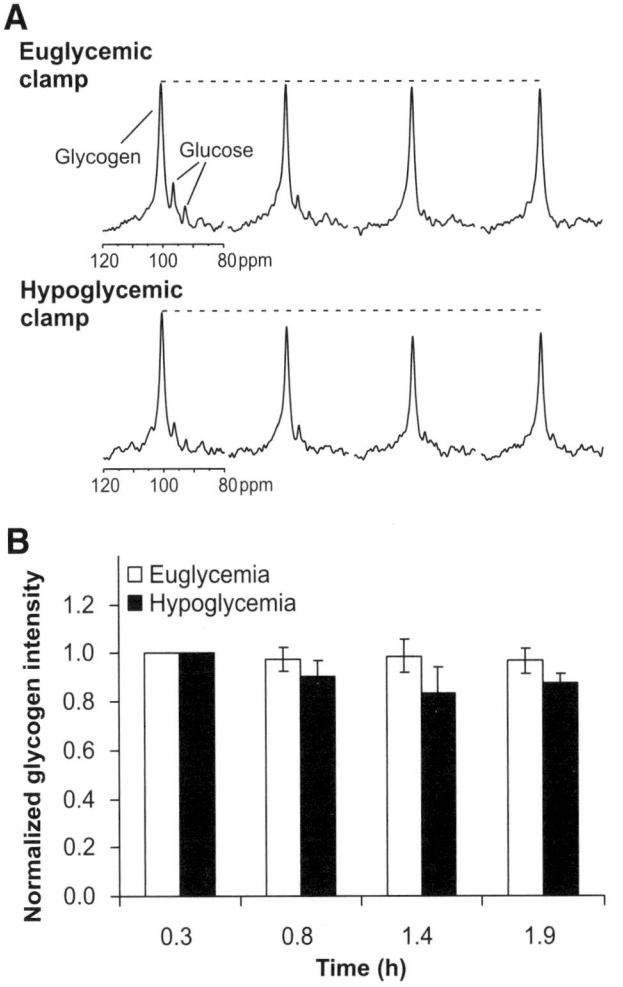

FIG. 4. Glycogen utilization during moderate hypoglycemia in the human brain. *A*: Proton-decoupled ¹³C NMR spectra acquired over four consecutive 30-min periods during the hypoglycemic and euglycemic clamps of the utilization study. The C1 peak of glycogen at 100.5 ppm and the two C1 glucose peaks originating from α- and β-glucose are marked. Spectra were averaged over the five subjects (4,096 transients per spectrum per subject with a repetition time of 0.45 s) and normalized with respect to the first half-hour spectrum. The volume-of-interest was 210 ml (7 × 5 × 6 cm³) in the occipital lobe. *B*: Glycogen integrals over four consecutive 30-min periods normalized to the spectrum acquired during the first 30 min of the clamp. Error bars indicate SD between subjects.

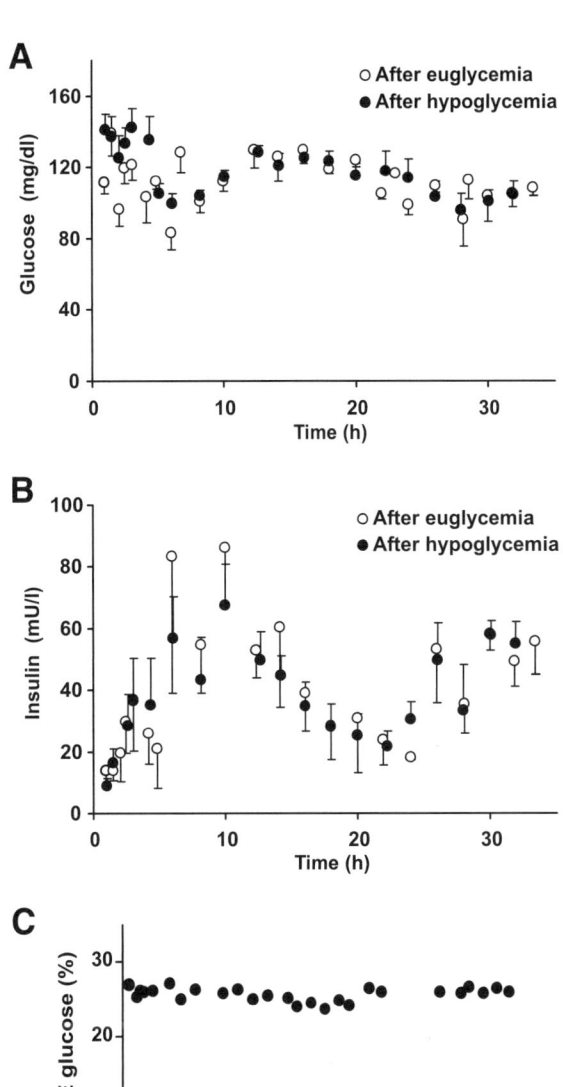

FIG. 5. Glucose, insulin and ¹³C isotopic enrichment (IE) in the blood of volunteers after the euglycemic and hypoglycemic clamps in the supercompensation study. *A* and *B*: Plasma glucose and insulin levels (average ± SEM) during the [1-¹³C]glucose infusion are shown for those time points where data are available from two or more subjects. Only one volunteer was infused with glucose longer than 34 h. *C*: Stability of ¹³C enrichment of plasma glucose in one volunteer. [1-¹³C]glucose (29% enriched) was administered intravenously for 54 h as also apparent from the rapid drop in isotopic enrichment after this time point.

levels were equal before the hypoglycemic and euglycemic clamps. We designed the study with an ~1- to 2-h [¹²C]glucose infusion after the ¹³C to chase the [¹³C]glucose from blood, such that any [¹³C]glucose removed from glycogen during the clamps would not be replenished by [¹³C]glucose from the blood, increasing our chances to detect glycogen mobilization. Ideally, one would turn over all glycogen molecules before the clamp and keep the isotopic enrichment of the blood constant and equal to that of glycogen (31) during the clamps such that the glycogenolysis rate would equal the rate of label wash-out from glycogen. However, it takes 3–5 days to turn over the total human brain glycogen pool (4) and it is very difficult to keep blood isotopic enrichments constant during hypoglycemia based on our prior experience, making this experimental design unfeasible in humans. The isotopic enrichment of glucose during hypoglycemia in our studies tended to be higher than during euglycemia (22 vs. 11%),

which might have even reduced the difference in [¹³C]glycogen levels between the hypoglycemic and euglycemic clamps. We do not expect this to be a factor because the [¹³C]glucose levels available for incorporation into glycogen were comparable during the two clamps considering the higher glucose levels during euglycemia. In theory, the increased label wash-out from glycogen during hypoglycemia may have been because of increased turnover; however, this possibility is highly unlikely considering the known reciprocal regulation of glycogen synthase and phosphorylase (22).

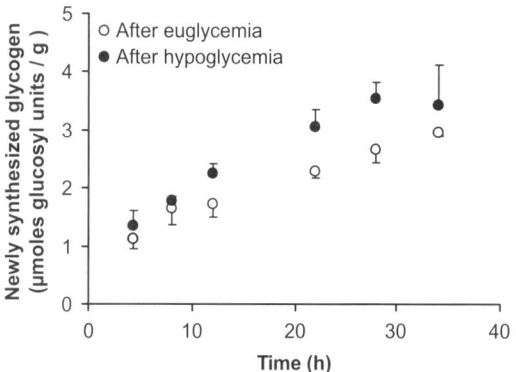

FIG. 6. Glycogen supercompensation after moderate hypoglycemia in the human brain. Newly synthesized glycogen concentrations (average ± SD) during ^{13}C glucose infusions after euglycemic and hypoglycemic clamps are shown for those time points where data are available from two or more subjects.

Our observations demonstrate that the human brain employs mechanisms of hypoglycemia response that are similar to those in the rodent brain (23–26). The [^{13}C]glycogen signal decreases with a rate of ~64%/h in the rat brain at ~1.5 mmol/l blood glucose (23) and ~10%/h in the human brain at ~3 mmol/l blood glucose, indicating a mobilization rate commensurate with the severity of hypoglycemia. The rat study implied that glycogen was not mobilized until brain glucose levels were zero (23); however, in the current study brain glucose was 0.6–0.8 μmol/g based on reported glucose transport parameters for the human brain (5,32). At these glucose levels, hexokinase is 92–94% saturated ($K_M = 50$ μmol/l), whereas it is 95–97% saturated at euglycemia (1–1.5 μmol/g brain glucose). This slight desaturation of hexokinase may have been enough to trigger glycogen mobilization to supplement the glucose-6-phospate deficit. Alternatively, a more general brain stress response may have been operative, involving the activation of brainstem catecholaminergic neurons, shown to occur with hypoglycemia (33–35). In particular norepinephrine is very effective in increasing glycogen breakdown (22) and may do so in the absence of a significant glucose deficit. Interestingly, after treatment with a glycogen phosphorylase inhibitor to increase brain glycogen content, neuronal function is prolonged during severe hypoglycemia in rats (36), providing further evidence that the brain may rely on glycogen stores to augment reduced energy delivery during hypoglycemia.

We only utilized the data from the euglycemia studies to fit a glycogen metabolic model because the model assumes the data were collected under steady-state conditions, which was not true during hypoglycemia. With the euglycemia data, we obtained glycogen content and turnover values in agreement with our previous findings (4). To roughly estimate the glycogenolysis rate during hypoglycemia we used the formula d[^{13}C-glycogen]/dt = IE_{glc} × V_{syn} − IE_{glyc} × V_{phos}, using the average blood IE_{glc} (isotopic enrichment of free glucose) and assuming constant IE_{glyc} (isotopic enrichment of glycogen) during the 2-h clamps. IE_{glyc} was ~40% based on the measured [^{13}C]glycogen level relative to total glycogen (4). Because brain glucose isotopic enrichment closely follows the blood glucose isotopic enrichment, IE_{glc} was set equal to the average isotopic enrichment measured in the blood during the hypoglycemic clamps, 22%. The net glycogenolysis rate (V_{phos} − V_{syn}) could then be estimated by

investigating two limiting conditions, with V_{syn} set to 0 or to the turnover rate of glycogen, 0.18 μmol · g^{-1} · h^{-1}. This way we estimated a glycogenolysis rate of 0.22–0.30 μmol · g^{-1} · h^{-1}, that is, that 0.4–0.6 μmol/g glycogen was mobilized during the 2-h hypoglycemic clamp. This glycogenolysis rate still constitutes a very small fraction (~1%) of CMR_{glc} (if CMR_{glc} does not change under hypoglycemia) and shows that the blood supplies the majority of glucose utilized by the brain during moderate hypoglycemia. This was the case even during severe hypoglycemia in rats where glycogen was shown to supplement a small glucose deficit (23).

In the supercompensation experiment, we observed a higher synthesis rate for human brain glycogen after hypoglycemia versus euglycemia. This higher rate could not be because of any differences in insulin levels (23,31) as these were the same in the paired studies (Fig. 5B). Clearly, some of this synthesis had to replenish the glycogen mobilized during the 2-h hypoglycemia. However, because a net synthesis of ~1 μmol/g glycogen occurred during 34 h of [^{13}C]glucose infusion and only 0.4–0.6 μmol/g glycogen was mobilized during the prior hypoglycemic clamp, our data indicate that glycogen content was higher after moderate hypoglycemia. It would be ideal to observe [^{13}C]glycogen levels higher than the normal glycogen levels (3–4 μmol/g) to confirm supercompensation; however, this would require even longer experimental periods in humans than the 4 days in this study.

It is unlikely that the glycogen content of the brain can increase many-fold because of the restriction of brain volume within the skull and water retention by glycogen. However, up to fourfold increases above basal brain glycogen content have been observed (37) and can likely be accommodated because of the low glycogen content of the brain. Glycogen supercompensation has been observed after multiple metabolic stressors in the rodent brain, such as hypoxia (38), hypoglycemia (37), ischemia (37), brain injury (39), and sleep deprivation (3), and in other tissues, such as the muscle after exercise (40). Furthermore, supercompensation of muscle glycogen after its depletion with exercise is augmented with repeated bouts of exercise, that is, in exercise-trained rodents and humans (40). Therefore, glycogen supercompensation may be a protective measure taken by the affected tissue in preparation for the next bout of metabolic stress (38).

Our data that indicate supercompensation of human brain glycogen are in agreement with similar NMR studies in rats (23). Furthermore, glycogen supercompensation in the hypothalamus and cortex after recurrent glucopenia was demonstrated recently in a rat model of hypoglycemia-associated autonomic failure (HAAF) (41). Although these observations suggest that glycogen supercompensation may be involved in the development of hypoglycemia unawareness, recent experiments by Herzog et al. (24) failed to demonstrate glycogen supercompensation in the cortex, cerebellum and hypothalamus in awake rats 6 and 24 h after hypoglycemia. They attributed this failure to confirm the prior rat NMR study (23) to anesthesia and severe hyperglycemia levels used for the NMR experiments. However, our current data, that also indicate supercompensation, were acquired with awake humans maintained at mild hyperglycemia (115 mg/dl) during the [^{13}C]glucose infusion after the clamps (Fig. 5A). We suggest that the variability among measurements in animals studied at different time points might be the reason that Herzog et al. did not observe supercompensation after hypoglycemia in the rat model. In NMR experiments, time courses are monitored in individual subjects, thereby facilitating the observation of treatment effects relative to extraction studies where all data points are obtained from different animals. Indeed, in the Herzog et al. study, even though the cortical glycogen levels were almost doubled in cortex after recurrent versus acute hypoglycemia (~7 vs. 4 μmol/g), this difference was not statistically significant, likely because of the large variance between animals.

Taken together, our observations demonstrate that brain glycogen is a dynamic source of energy and provide the first support for the hypothesis that brain glycogen may be used to offset the loss of substrate that occurs in humans during hypoglycemia. They further demonstrate increased brain glycogen synthesis after moderate hypoglycemia in humans and indicate glycogen supercompensation. The potential involvement of glycogen in the development of HAAF in humans, and specifically if supercompensated glycogen provides additional substrate to the brain during subsequent hypoglycemic episodes, need to be investigated in future studies.

ACKNOWLEDGMENTS

This work was supported by the National Institutes of Health Grant R01 NS035192 (to E.R.S.). The CMRR is supported by National Center for Research Resources (NCRR) Biotechnology Research Resource Grant P41RR008079 and Neuroscience Center Core Blueprint Award P30NS057091. The GCRC is supported by NCRR Grant M01RR00400.

Parts of this study were presented in abstract form at the Scientific Meeting of the International Society for Magnetic Resonance in Medicine, Berlin, Germany, 19–25 May 2007; at the 67th Scientific Sessions of the American Diabetes Association, Chicago, Illinois, 22–26 June 2007; at the Perugia 2007 Hypoglycemia Symposium, Perugia, Italy, 12–15 May 2007; and at the 69th Scientific Sessions of the American Diabetes Association, New Orleans, Louisiana, 5–9 June 2009.

We thank the nurses and medical assistants of the GCRC for their enthusiastic support of the glucose infusion studies, the staff of the CMRR for maintaining and supporting the NMR system, Gregor Adriany for invaluable help with the NMR coil, and Alexander Shestov, Felipe Barros, and Gerry Dienel for discussions and comments on our work.

REFERENCES

1. Choi IY, Gruetter R. In vivo ^{13}C NMR assessment of brain glycogen concentration and turnover in the awake rat. Neurochem Int 2003;43:317–322
2. Cruz NF, Dienel GA. High glycogen levels in brains of rats with minimal environmental stimuli: implications for metabolic contributions of working astrocytes. J Cereb Blood Flow Metab 2002;22:1476–1489
3. Kong J, Shepel PN, Holden CP, Mackiewicz M, Pack AI, Geiger JD. Brain glycogen decreases with increased periods of wakefulness: implications for homeostatic drive to sleep. J Neurosci 2002;22:5581–5587
4. Öz G, Seaquist ER, Kumar A, Criego AB, Benedict LE, Rao JP, Henry PG, Van De Moortele PF, Gruetter R. Human brain glycogen content and metabolism: implications on its role in brain energy metabolism. Am J Physiol Endocrinol Metab 2007;292:E946–E951
5. Gruetter R, Ugurbil K, Seaquist ER. Steady-state cerebral glucose concentrations and transport in the human brain. J Neurochem 1998;70:397–408
6. Roden M, Petersen KF, Shulman GI. Nuclear magnetic resonance studies of hepatic glucose metabolism in humans. Recent Prog Horm Res 2001;56:219–237
7. Krssak M, Petersen KF, Bergeron R, Price T, Laurent D, Rothman DL, Roden M, Shulman GI. Intramuscular glycogen and intramyocellular lipid

8. Choi IY, Tkáč I, Ugurbil K, Gruetter R. Noninvasive measurements of [1-^{13}C]glycogen concentrations and metabolism in rat brain in vivo. J Neurochem 1999;73:1300–1308
9. Öz G, Henry PG, Seaquist ER, Gruetter R. Direct, noninvasive measurement of brain glycogen metabolism in humans. Neurochem Int 2003;43:323–329
10. Öz G, Henry PG, Tkáč I, Gruetter R. A localization method for the measurement of fast relaxing ^{13}C NMR signals in humans at high magnetic fields. Appl Magn Reson 2005;29:159–169
11. Lei H, Morgenthaler F, Yue T, Gruetter R. Direct validation of in vivo localized ^{13}C MRS measurements of brain glycogen. Magn Reson Med 2007;57:243–248
12. Dalsgaard MK, Madsen FF, Secher NH, Laursen H, Quistorff B. High glycogen levels in the hippocampus of patients with epilepsy. J Cereb Blood Flow Metab 2007;27:1137–1141
13. Brunner EA, Passonneau JV, Molstad C. The effect of volatile anaesthetics on levels of metabolites and on metabolic rate in brain. J Neurochem 1971;18:2301–2316
14. Watanabe H, Passonneau JV. Factors affecting the turnover of cerebral glycogen and limit dextrin in vivo. J Neurochem 1973;20:1543–1554
15. Gruetter R, Seaquist ER, Ugurbil K. A mathematical model of compartmentalized neurotransmitter metabolism in the human brain. Am J Physiol Endocrinol Metab 2001;281:E100–E112
16. Toyama H, Ichise M, Liow JS, Modell KJ, Vines DC, Esaki T, Cook M, Seidel J, Sokoloff L, Green MV, Innis RB. Absolute quantification of regional cerebral glucose utilization in mice by ^{18}F-FDG small animal PET scanning and 2-^{14}C-DG autoradiography. J Nucl Med 2004;45:1398–1405
17. Henry PG, Lebon V, Vaufrey F, Brouillet E, Hantraye P, Bloch G. Decreased TCA cycle rate in the rat brain after acute 3-NP treatment measured by in vivo ^{1}H-[^{13}C] NMR spectroscopy. J Neurochem 2002;82:857–866
18. Öz G, Berkich DA, Henry PG, Xu Y, LaNoue K, Hutson SM, Gruetter R. Neuroglial metabolism in the awake rat brain: CO_2 fixation increases with brain activity. J Neurosci 2004;24:11273–11279
19. Dringen R, Hamprecht B. Glucose, insulin, and insulin-like growth factor I regulate the glycogen content of astroglia-rich primary cultures. J Neurochem 1992;58:511–517
20. Hamai M, Minokoshi Y, Shimazu T. L-Glutamate and insulin enhance glycogen synthesis in cultured astrocytes from the rat brain through different intracellular mechanisms. J Neurochem 1999;73:400–407
21. Magistretti PJ, Morrison JH, Shoemaker WJ, Sapin V, Bloom FE. Vasoactive intestinal polypeptide induces glycogenolysis in mouse cortical slices: a possible regulatory mechanism for the local control of energy metabolism. Proc Natl Acad Sci U S A 1981;78:6535–6539
22. Magistretti PJ, Sorg O, Martin J. Regulation of glycogen metabolism in astrocytes: physiological, pharmacological, and pathological aspects. In Astrocytes: Pharmacology and Function. Murphy S, Ed. San Diego, CA, Academic Press, 1993, pp. 243–265
23. Choi IY, Seaquist ER, Gruetter R. Effect of hypoglycemia on brain glycogen metabolism in vivo. J Neurosci Res 2003;72:25–32
24. Herzog RI, Chan O, Yu S, Dziura J, McNay EC, Sherwin RS. Effect of acute and recurrent hypoglycemia on changes in brain glycogen concentration. Endocrinology 2008;149:1499–1504
25. Ratcheson RA, Blank AC, Ferrendelli JA. Regionally selective metabolic effects of hypoglycemia in brain. J Neurochem 1981;36:1952–1958
26. Agardh CD, Folbergrova J, Siesjo BK. Cerebral metabolic changes in profound, insulin-induced hypoglycemia, and in the recovery period following glucose administration. J Neurochem 1978;31:1135–1142
27. Gruetter R. Glycogen: the forgotten cerebral energy store. J Neurosci Res 2003;74:179–183
28. Alzaid AA, Dinneen SF, Turk DJ, Caumo A, Cobelli C, Rizza RA. Assessment of insulin action and glucose effectiveness in diabetic and nondiabetic humans. J Clin Invest 1994;94:2341–2348
29. Seaquist ER. Comparison of arterialized venous sampling from the hand and foot in the assessment of in vivo glucose metabolism. Metabolism 1997;46:1364–1366
30. Adriany G, Gruetter R. A half-volume coil for efficient proton decoupling in humans at 4 Tesla. J Magn Reson 1997;125:178–184
31. Morgenthaler FD, van Heeswijk RB, Xin L, Laus S, Frenkel H, Lei H, Gruetter R. Non-invasive quantification of brain glycogen absolute concentration. J Neurochem 2008;107:1414–1423
32. de Graaf RA, Pan JW, Telang F, Lee JH, Brown P, Novotny EJ, Hetherington HP, Rothman DL. Differentiation of glucose transport in human brain gray and white matter. J Cereb Blood Flow Metab 2001;21:483–492
33. Morilak DA, Fornal CA, Jacobs BL. Effects of physiological manipulations

on locus coeruleus neuronal activity in freely moving cats. III. Glucoregulatory challenge. Brain Res 1987;422:32–39

34. Lachuer J, Gaillet S, Barbagli B, Buda M, Tappaz M. Differential early time course activation of the brainstem catecholaminergic groups in response to various stresses. Neuroendocrinology 1991;53:589–596

35. Yuan PQ, Yang H. Neuronal activation of brain vagal-regulatory pathways and upper gut enteric plexuses by insulin hypoglycemia. Am J Physiol Endocrinol Metab 2002;283:E436–E448

36. Suh SW, Bergher JP, Anderson CM, Treadway JL, Fosgerau K, Swanson RA. Astrocyte glycogen sustains neuronal activity during hypoglycemia: studies with the glycogen phosphorylase inhibitor CP-316,819 ([R-R*,S*]-5-chloro-N-[2-hydroxy-3-(methoxymethylamino)-3-oxo-1-(phenylmet hyl)-propyl]-1H-indole-2-carboxamide). J Pharmacol Exp Ther 2007;321: 45–50

37. Folbergrova J, Katsura KI, Siesjo BK. Glycogen accumulated in the brain following insults is not degraded during a subsequent period of ischemia. J Neurol Sci 1996;137:7–13

38. Brucklacher RM, Vannucci RC, Vannucci SJ. Hypoxic preconditioning increases brain glycogen and delays energy depletion from hypoxia-ischemia in the immature rat. Dev Neurosci 2002;24:411–417

39. Shimizu N, Hamuro Y. Deposition of glycogen and changes in some enzymes in brain wounds. Nature 1958;181:781–782

40. Holloszy JO, Kohrt WM, Hansen PA. The regulation of carbohydrate and fat metabolism during and after exercise. Front Biosci 1998;3:D1011–D1027

41. Alquier T, Kawashima J, Tsuji Y, Kahn BB. Role of hypothalamic adenosine 5'-monophosphate-activated protein kinase in the impaired counterregulatory response induced by repetitive neuroglucopenia. Endocrinology 2007;148:1367–1375

Brain Insulin Action Regulates Hypothalamic Glucose Sensing and the Counterregulatory Response to Hypoglycemia

Kelly A. Diggs-Andrews,[1] Xuezhao Zhang,[1] Zhentao Song,[2] Dorit Daphna-Iken,[1] Vanessa H. Routh,[2] and Simon J. Fisher[1,3]

OBJECTIVE—An impaired ability to sense and appropriately respond to insulin-induced hypoglycemia is a common and serious complication faced by insulin-treated diabetic patients. This study tests the hypothesis that insulin acts directly in the brain to regulate critical glucose-sensing neurons in the hypothalamus to mediate the counterregulatory response to hypoglycemia.

RESEARCH DESIGN AND METHODS—To delineate insulin actions in the brain, neuron-specific insulin receptor knockout (NIRKO) mice and littermate controls were subjected to graded hypoglycemic (100, 70, 50, and 30 mg/dl) hyperinsulinemic (20 mU/kg/min) clamps and nonhypoglycemic stressors (e.g., restraint, heat). Subsequently, counterregulatory responses, hypothalamic neuronal activation (with transcriptional marker *c-fos*), and regional brain glucose uptake (via ^{14}C-2deoxyglucose autoradiography) were measured. Additionally, electrophysiological activity of individual glucose-inhibited neurons and hypothalamic glucose sensing protein expression (GLUTs, glucokinase) were measured.

RESULTS—NIRKO mice revealed a glycemia-dependent impairment in the sympathoadrenal response to hypoglycemia and demonstrated markedly reduced (3-fold) hypothalamic *c-fos* activation in response to hypoglycemia but not other stressors. Glucose-inhibited neurons in the ventromedial hypothalamus of NIRKO mice displayed significantly blunted glucose responsiveness (membrane potential and input resistance responses were blunted 66 and 80%, respectively). Further, hypothalamic expression of the insulin-responsive GLUT 4, but not glucokinase, was reduced by 30% in NIRKO mice while regional brain glucose uptake remained unaltered.

CONCLUSIONS—Chronically, insulin acts in the brain to regulate the counterregulatory response to hypoglycemia by directly altering glucose sensing in hypothalamic neurons and shifting the glycemic levels necessary to elicit a normal sympathoadrenal response. *Diabetes* 59:2271–2280, 2010

From the [1]Division of Endocrinology, Metabolism and Lipid Research, Department of Internal Medicine, Washington University School of Medicine, Saint Louis, Missouri; the [2]Department of Pharmacology and Physiology, New Jersey Medical School (UMDNJ), Newark, New Jersey; and the [3]Department of Cell Biology and Physiology, Washington University School of Medicine, Saint Louis, Missouri.

Corresponding author: Simon J. Fisher, sfisher@dom.wustl.edu.

Received 22 March 2010 and accepted 4 June 2010. Published ahead of print at http://diabetes.diabetesjournals.org on 14 June 2010. DOI: 10.2337/db10-0401.

Intensive insulin therapy markedly increases the risk of severe hypoglycemia in people with type 1 (1) and type 2 (2) diabetes. Thus, hypoglycemia is the rate-limiting step for tight glycemic management in diabetic patients. In response to hypoglycemia, glucose sensors in the central and peripheral nervous system coordinate efferent autonomic responses resulting in the release of key counterregulatory hormones—glucagon, norepinephrine, epinephrine, and cortisol. This coordinated response stimulates hepatic glucose output and restricts glucose utilization to increase blood glucose levels. Patients with diabetes often have an impaired ability to sense and respond to hypoglycemia (3–5) because several components of the counterregulatory response have been shown to be either absent (i.e., fall in insulin, rise in glucagon) or markedly blunted (i.e., the sympathoadrenal response) (6,7).

While hypoglycemia is caused by absolute or relative insulin excess, the role of insulin in regulating the counterregulatory response is unclear. Studies have demonstrated that increased insulin levels may augment (8–11), diminish (12), or not change (13–16) the sympathoadrenal response to hypoglycemia. Given recent evidence indicating that insulin acts in the brain (17), some studies have investigated whether insulin's putative actions in regulating the counterregulatory response might be mediated via actions in the central nervous system. Again, conflicting reports suggest that insulin may act centrally to enhance (18–20), reduce (21), or not alter (22) the sympathoadrenal response to hypoglycemia. If insulin acts in the brain, its likely site of action is glucose-sensing neurons located in the ventromedial hypothalamus (VMH) (21,23–26). These glucose-sensing neurons share metabolic similarities to other well-characterized glucose-sensing cells (i.e., pancreatic β-cells), especially with regard to glucose transport and metabolism (27–29). On the basis of the expression of insulin receptors in the majority of glucosensing neurons in the VMH (30), it is postulated that brain insulin action may mediate its effects on central glucose sensing by regulating expression of GLUTs and/or glucokinase.

In this study, the neuronal specific insulin-receptor knockout (NIRKO) mouse model, which chronically lacks central nervous system (CNS) insulin signaling (17,31), was used to investigate the role and mechanism by which brain insulin action regulates central glucose sensing and the counterregulatory response to hypoglycemia.

RESEARCH DESIGN AND METHODS

Mice homozygous for the floxed insulin receptor allele ($IR^{lox-lox}$) were bred with transgenic mice that express Cre recombinase cDNA from the rat nestin promoter to generate ($IR^{lox-lox}$:nestin-Cre$^{+/-}$) NIRKO mice (17). Genotypes were determined by PCR of tail DNA. Unless otherwise indicated, 2–4-month-old NIRKO ($IR^{lox-lox}$:nestin-Cre$^{+/-}$) and littermate control (control, $IR^{lox-lox}$: nestin-Cre$^{-/-}$) mice were used for these experiments. All mice were housed on a 12-h light/dark cycle and fed a standard rodent chow (Mouse Diet 9F, PMI Nutrition International, St. Louis, MO) ad libitum. All procedures were in accordance with the Guide for the Care and Use of Laboratory Animals of the National Institutes of Health and were approved by the Animal Studies Committee of Washington University.

Hypoglycemic-hyperinsulinemic glucose clamps. Mice anesthetized with ketamine/xylazine (87 and 13.4 mg/kg i.p.) were implanted with catheters (MRE 025, Braintree Scientific Inc., Braintree, MA) into both the right internal jugular and the left carotid or femoral artery. After a 5–7-day recovery period, hyperinsulinemic (20 mU/kg/min) hypoglycemic clamps were performed in 5-h fasted, awake, unrestrained, NIRKO and control mice (n = 6–9 per group). To create different degrees of hypoglycemic stress, arterial blood glucose was measured at 10-min intervals and the rate of intravenous 50% dextrose infusion was carefully adjusted to create equivalent levels of mild (70 mg/dl), moderate (50 mg/dl), and severe hypoglycemia (30 mg/dl) as well as a euglycemic (110 mg/dl) control. High-performance liquid chromatography–purified [3-^{3}H]-glucose tracer (NEN Life Science Products Inc., Boston, MA) was infused (10 µCi bolus and 0.1 µCi/min) for the assessment of hepatic glucose production (32). Three blood samples for hepatic glucose production determination were taken during the basal period and again during the last 0.5 h of the clamp. An additional blood sample was obtained for hormonal measurements during the basal period and at the end of the clamp.

Brain glucose uptake. Briefly, awake, unrestrained, cannulated NIRKO and littermate control mice (n = 6–9 per group) underwent a 2-h hyperinsulinemic (40 mU/kg/min) hypoglycemic (30 mg/dl) clamp protocol. At 45 min before the end of the clamp, a 5 µCi bolus of ^{14}C 2-deoxyglucose was rapidly infused intravenously and 10 timed arterial blood samples were collected for analysis of arterial plasma glucose and ^{14}C levels. Isotope concentrations in regions of interest were measured from 20 µm thick coronal serial sections after exposure to autoradiograph film via optical densitometry. Regional glucose uptake was calculated according to Sokoloff's equation using rat rate constants, as mice rate constants have not been established (33).

Hypoglycemia-induced c-fos expression. Awake, 5-h fasted NIRKO (n = 4) and littermate controls (n = 6) were given a single intraperitoneal injection of high-dose insulin (3.0–3.5 units/kg) to achieve a consistent and stable hypoglycemic insult (~30 mg/dl) for 2 h. Euglycemic controls (~110 mg/dl, n = 4 per group) were given an i.p. injection of saline. After a 2-h duration of hypoglycemia (or euglycemia), each cryoprotected brain was analyzed for c-fos expression.

Electrophysiological studies. Male 14–28-day-old NIRKO and littermate control mice were anesthetized and transcardially perfused with ice-cold oxygenated perfusion. Sections (350 µm) through the hypothalamus were made on a vibratome (Vibroslice; Camden Instruments). The brain slices were maintained at 34°C in oxygenated high-Mg^{2+} low-Ca^{2+} artificial cerebrospinal fluid (ACSF) for 30 min and then transferred to normal oxygenated ACSF for the remainder of the day. Viable neurons were visualized and studied under infrared differential-interference contrast microscopy using a Leica DMLS microscope equipped with a 40× long working-distance water-immersion objective. Current-clamp recordings (standard whole-cell recording configuration) from neurons in the VMH were made using an Axopatch 1D amplifier (Axon Instruments, Foster City, CA) as previously described (34,35). During recording, brain slices were perfused at 10 ml/min with normal oxygenated ACSF. Input resistance was calculated from the change in membrane potential in response to small 500-ms hyperpolarizing pulses (−10 to −20 pA) given every 3 s. The membrane potential response was measured only after the membrane response to altered extracellular glucose had stabilized, and this value was compared with controls that were measured immediately before changing extracellular glucose. Individual glucose-inhibited neurons were identified as those neurons that increased their action potential frequency, membrane potential, and input resistance with decreases in extracellular glucose from 2.5 to 0.1 mmol/l.

Restraint stress. Awake, 5-h fasted control and NIRKO mice (n = 6 per group) were placed in a mouse restrainer (Braintree Scientific, Braintree, MA) for 45 min to induce restraint stress. Cardiovascular parameters were obtained during the basal period and during the last 20 min of restraint stress using a tail-cuff system (Kent Scientific Corporation, Torrington, CT). Blood samples were taken by previously implanted arterial cannula at the beginning and end of the restraint period to measure plasma epinephrine levels.

Heat stress. Awake control and NIRKO mice (n = 6 per group) were exposed to an ambient temperature of 42°C for 90 min to induce heat stress. Blood samples were taken at the end of the heat stress period to measure catecholamines. Subsequently, cryoprotected brains were analyzed for heat stress–induced c-fos immunostaining.

Western blots. The medial basal hypothalamus, defined anatomically as posterior to the optic chiasm, anterior to the mammillary body, inferior to the thalamus, and ±1 mm lateral to the midline, was dissected and frozen for analysis. Homogenized hypothalamic protein extracts (20 µg for GLUT1 and GLUT3; 100 µg for GLUT4 and glucokinase) were fractionated by electrophoresis on a 10% Bis-Tris Criterion XT (Biorad, Hercules, CA) gel and subjected to transfer. The following primary antibodies were used: GLUT1 (1:5,000, Chemicon), GLUT3 (1:1,000, Chemicon), GLUT4 (1:1,000, kindly supplied by Dr. M. Mueckler), glucokinase (1:1,000, Calbiochem). The blots were developed using a horseradish peroxidase-conjugated secondary antibody (1:8,000). Primary antibody binding was detected by enhanced chemiluminescence reagents (Perkin Elmer, Wellesley, MA) on ISO-MAX films and quantified by ImageQuant software analysis (Amersham Pharmacia, Piscataway, NJ). An antibody against β-actin (1:2,000, Sigma, St. Louis, MO) served as a loading control.

Immunohistochemistry. Cryoprotected brains were processed for DAB 3,3′-diaminobenzidine peroxidose substrate immunohistochemistry or immunofluorescence. Briefly, free-floating hypothalamic sections (20–30 µm) throughout the VMH/arcuate nucleus (ARC) were taken from 1.46 to 1.82 mm caudal to bregma, blocked, and incubated overnight at 4°C in primary antibodies. The following antibody dilutions were used: GLUT4 (1:1,000), c-fos (1:2000, Ab-5, Calbiochem). For immunofluorescence, goat anti-rabbit Texas Red (1:200, Molecular Probes) was used as the secondary antibody. Subsequently, the sections were mounted on slides using Vectashield Mounting Medium (Vector Laboratories, Burlingame, CA). For DAB immunohistochemistry, immunoreactivity was performed with biotinylated goat anti-rabbit immunoglobulin G (1:200) using the Elite ABC kit (Vector Laboratories). As a negative control, alternative sections were incubated without primary antibodies. Regions of interest were identified using anatomical landmarks (36), and positively stained cells were counted by a blinded investigator. Four to six brain sections per mouse were quantified for statistical purposes.

RT-PCR. Sections (400 µm) were taken from brain sections 1.46–1.86 mm caudal to bregma. Bilateral punch biopsy samples (0.5 mm) from the VMH and ARC (0.75 mm from the piriform cortex) were collected from NIRKO mice and littermate controls (n = 7–8 per group). The mRNA extracted with Trizol (Invitrogen Corporation, Carlsbad, CA) was subject to quantitative two-step RT-PCR performed in triplicate in a fluorescent temperature cycler (GeneAmp 7,700 Sequence Detector, Applied Biosystems) with glucokinase primers (glucokinase probe 5′-/56-FAM/ACC GCC AAT GTG AGG TCG GCA/3BHQ_1/-3′; glucokinase reverse 5′-AGC CGG TGC CCA CAA TC-3′; and glucokinase forward 5′-CCA CAA TGA TCT CCT GCT ACT ATG A-3′). The results were quantified after normalizing to rRNA L32mRNA.

Plasma assays. Blood glucose was measured by a glucometer (Becton, Dickinson and Company, Franklin Lakes, NJ), while plasma glucose was assayed by the glucose oxidase method and a spectrophotometer (BioTek Instruments, Inc., Winooski, VT). Radioimmunoassays were performed for glucagon (LINCO Research, Inc., St. Charles, MO) and corticosterone (ICN Biomedicals, Inc., Costa Mesa, CA). Insulin was assayed by ELISA (Chrystal Chem. Inc., Downers Grove, IL). Plasma epinephrine and norepinephrine were measured with a single isotope derivative (radioenzymatic) method (37).

Statistics. All values are presented as the mean ± SEM. Statistical significance was set at $P < 0.05$, as determined by Student t test.

RESULTS

Brain insulin action is necessary for full sympathoadrenal response to hypoglycemia. To characterize the counterregulatory response to hypoglycemia, a series of hyperinsulinemic glucose clamps were performed. Blood glucose was clamped at 110, 70, 50, and 30 mg/dl in control and NIRKO mice to induce different degrees of hypoglycemia (mild = 70 mg/dl, moderate = 50 mg/dl, and severe hypoglycemia = 30 mg/dl) or no hypoglycemia (euglycemic clamp = 110 mg/dl) (Fig. 1). In response to insulin infusion, plasma insulin levels were similarly elevated in NIRKO and control mice (Fig. 2A). Severe hypoglycemia (30 mg/dl) resulted in a sixfold increase in glucagon levels and ~60% increase in corticosterone levels, but these increases were similar in both groups (Fig. 2B and C).

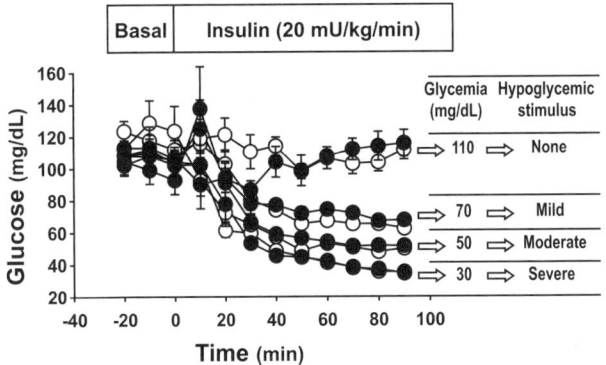

FIG. 1. Hyperinsulinemic, graded hypoglycemic clamps. Blood glucose levels are shown for NIRKO (filled circles) and control (open circles) mice (n = 6–8 mice per group). After basal sampling, insulin was infused (20 mU/kg/min) and blood glucose levels were measured at 10-min intervals via arterial sampling. By adjusting the rate of intravenous glucose infusion, glucose levels were carefully lowered, then clamped at matched, predetermined glycemic levels (110, 70, 50, and 30 mg/dl) to create different degrees of hypoglycemic stress (none, mild, moderate, and severe, respectively).

The epinephrine response was significantly impaired in NIRKO mice during moderate (50 mg/dl) and severe (30 mg/dl) hypoglycemia (Fig. 3A). The epinephrine responses

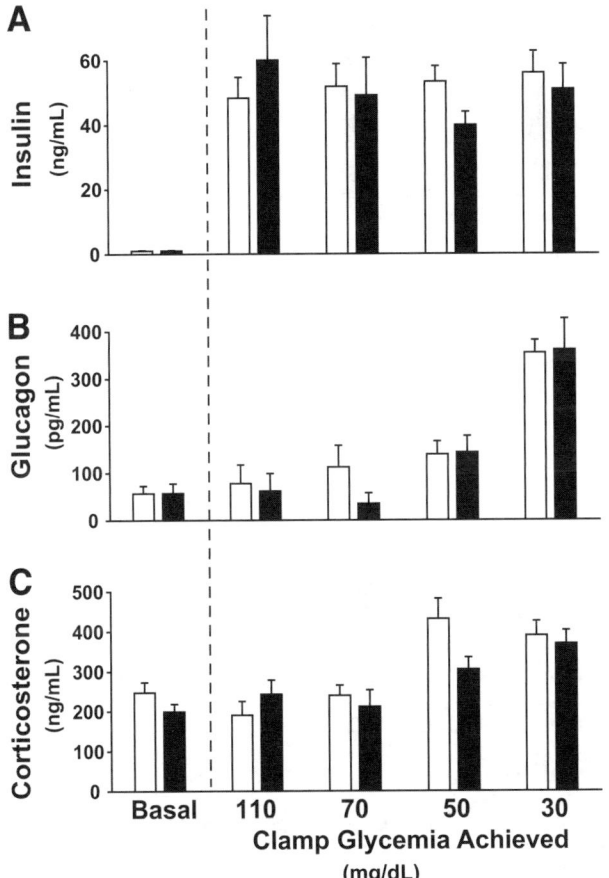

FIG. 2. Hormone levels during graded hyperinsulinemic glucose clamps. Results are shown for NIRKO (closed bars) and control (open bars) mice (n = 6–8 mice per group). A: By experimental design, insulin levels rose markedly and similarly between groups during the hyperinsulinemic clamps. B and C: Glucagon (B) and corticosterone (C) levels in both treatment groups rose significantly above basal levels ($P < 0.05$) during moderate and severe hypoglycemia but similarly between treatment groups.

were highly correlated to glycemia levels in both control ($R^2 = 0.76$) and NIRKO ($R^2 = 0.75$) mice but were different between groups as indicated by a shift in the hypoglyce-mia–epinephrine response curve (Fig. 3A, inset). Norepi-nephrine levels trended lower in NIRKO mice during moderate (50 mg/dl) and severe (30 mg/dl) hypoglycemia, but the difference did not reach significance (Fig. 3B). In response to the high dose of insulin (20 mU/kg/min), hepatic glucose production was completely inhibited dur-ing the hyperinsulinemic clamp at glycemic levels of 100, 70, and 50 mg/dl. During severe hypoglycemia (30 mg/dl), hepatic glucose production rose significantly; however, the rise in hepatic glucose production was significantly blunted in NIRKO mice (Fig. 3C).

Absent CNS insulin action impairs hypothalamic neu-ronal activation to hypoglycemia. To assess the brain's response to hypoglycemia, c-fos-based functional mapping was used to demonstrate activated neurons and functional circuits that respond to hypoglycemic stress (38). Eugly-cemic (~110 mg/dl) controls displayed low c-fos expres-sion in the hypothalamus (Fig. 4B). In response to insulin-induced hypoglycemia (31.5 ± 3.1 mg/dl), both NIRKO and control mice markedly increased c-fos expression within the paraventricular nucleus (PVN) of the hypothalamus (Fig. 4A). However, NIRKO animals showed a threefold impairment in c-fos activation as compared with controls (control: 99 ± 16 vs. NIRKO: 31 ± 5, $P < 0.01$) (Fig. 4B).

Impaired glucose sensing in individual glucose-inhib-ited neurons. Whole-cell current-clamp recordings were performed to evaluate the glucose sensitivity of individual glucose-inhibited neurons in the VMH. As expected for VMH glucose-inhibited neurons bathed in sufficient 2.5 mmol/l glucose, action potentials in this basal state were absent in recordings from both control and NIRKO mice. There were also no group differences in membrane poten-tial (MP) or input resistance (IR) in 2.5 mmol/l glucose (control: MP = −57 ± 4 mV, IR = 1,209 ± 272 MΩ; NIRKO: MP = −59 ± 3 mV, IR = 1,016 ± 162 MΩ). Further, no group differences were observed in glucose-inhibited neu-rons in response to a maximal glucose decrease from 2.5 to 0.1 mmol/l (not shown). In contrast, glucose-inhibited neurons in NIRKO mice had a significantly impaired change in membrane potential and input resistance (66 and 80% impairment, respectively) in response to a glu-cose decrease from 2.5 to 0.5 mmol/l (Fig. 4C and D).

Absent CNS insulin signaling does not influence re-sponse to restraint or heat stress. NIRKO and control mice were subjected to a mild stressor (restraint stress) and a more profound stressor (heat stress) to evaluate sympathoadrenal activation in response to glycemia-inde-pendent stress. In response to milder restraint stress, plasma epinephrine levels rose similarly twofold in both littermate controls and NIRKO mice (Fig. 5A). The physi-ological increased heart rate to restraint stress was also similar in control and NIRKO mice (Fig. 5B). Heat stress induced a more pronounced catecholamine elevation than restraint stress (to levels observed with hypoglycemia), but the rise in both epinephrine and norepinephrine in response to heat stress was again not significantly different between groups (Fig. 6C and D). To determine whether this defect in neuronal activation was unique to hypogly-cemia, c-fos expression was also assessed in response to heat stress. Increased c-fos expression was again noted in the PVN in response to heat stress (Fig. 6A), to levels observed with hypoglycemia; however, in response to heat stress, there was no difference in c-fos expression between

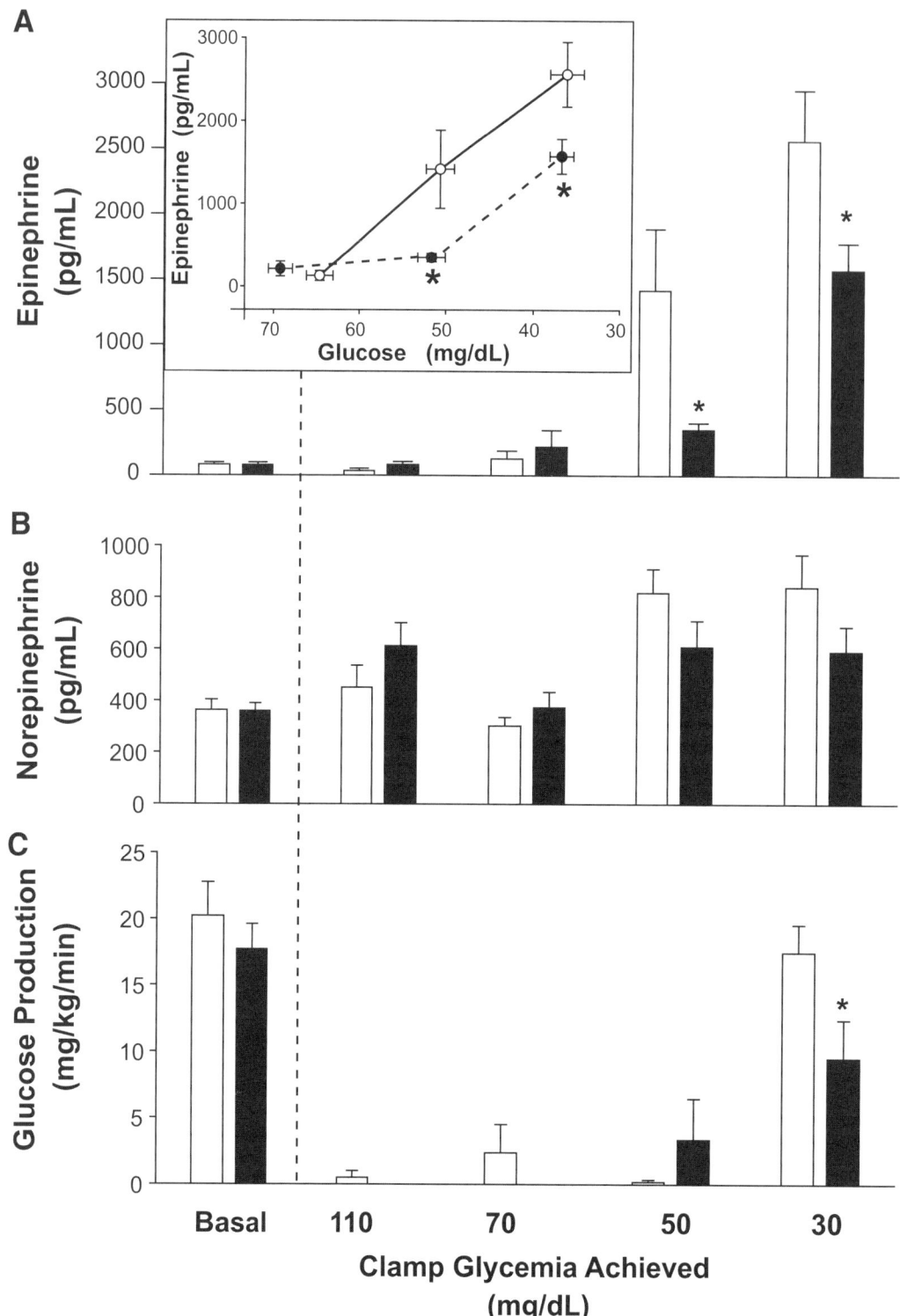

FIG. 3. Catecholamine and hepatic glucose production levels in a series of hyperinsulinemic glucose clamps. Results are shown for NIRKO (closed bars) and control (open bars) mice ($n = 6$–8 mice per group). A: The epinephrine response was significantly impaired in NIRKO mice ($P < 0.05$) during moderate (50 mg/dl) and severe (30 mg/dl) hypoglycemia. The inset picture demonstrates a shift in the hypoglycemia dose–response curve by the solid (controls) versus dashed (NIRKO) lines. B: Norepinephrine levels in both treatment groups rose significantly higher from the basal period during moderate and severe hypoglycemia, but there was no difference between NIRKO and control responses. C: Hepatic glucose production, in the basal period prior to insulin infusion, was the same in control and NIRKO mice. During the hyperinsulinemic glucose clamps at mild and moderate hypoglycemia, HGP was suppressed. Despite the hyperinsulinemia, during severe hypoglycemia (30 mg/dl), hepatic glucose production rose significantly but remained lower in NIRKO as compared with control mice. *$P < 0.05$.

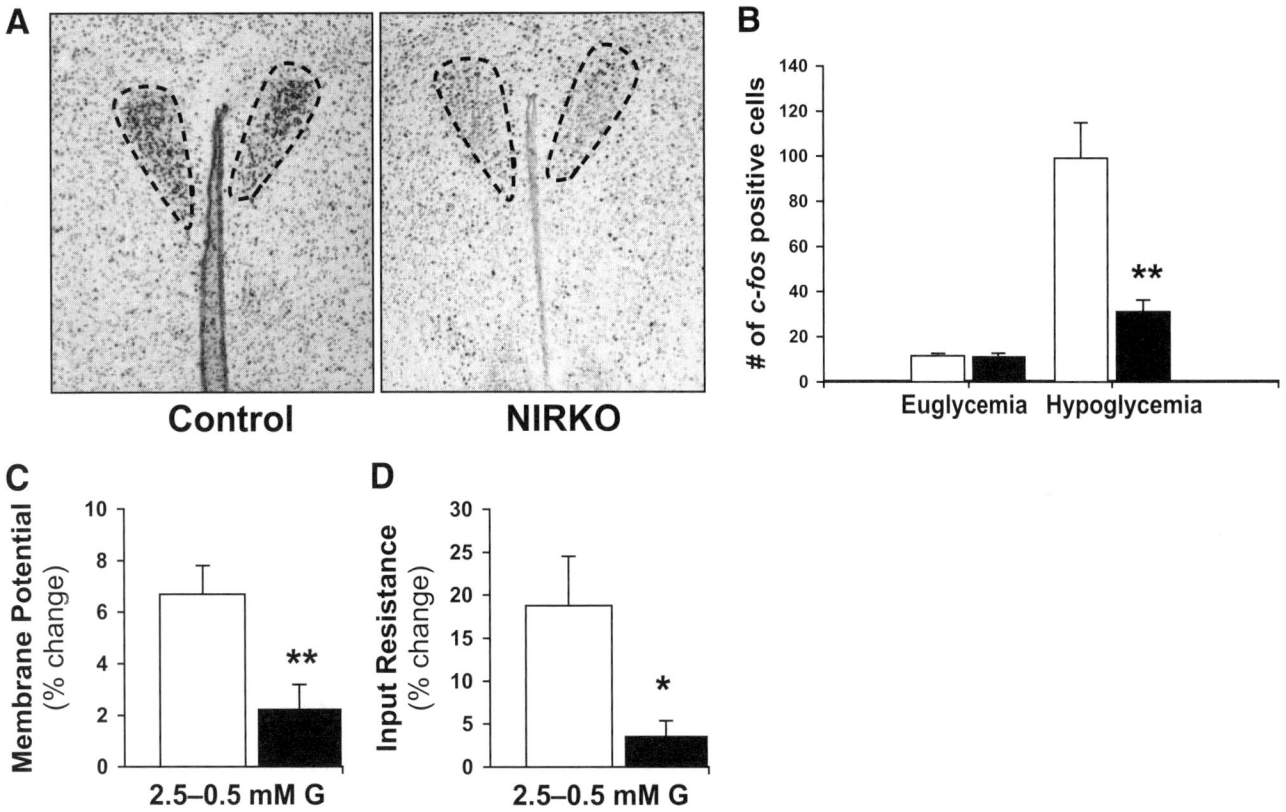

FIG. 4. Blunted neuronal activation and glucose responsiveness in NIRKO glucose-sensing neurons. *A*: After a 2-h hypoglycemic insult, neuronal activity was assessed using the marker *c-fos*. Representative images of matched hypothalamic sections highlighting *c-fos* staining in the PVN in NIRKO (right image) and littermate controls (left image). *B*: The quantity of *c-fos* positive cells located within the PVN was minimally induced in both groups during euglycemia (*n* = 4 mice per group). During matched hypoglycemia, the number of *c-fos* positive cells was significantly less in NIRKO (*n* = 4, closed bars) as compared with littermate control (*n* = 6, open bars) mice. *C* and *D*: Individual glucose-inhibited neurons were identified as those neurons that increased their action potential frequency, membrane potential, and input resistance with decreases in extracellular glucose from 2.5 to 0.1 mmol/l glucose. In response to lowering extracellular glucose levels from 2.5 to 0.5 mmol/l glucose (G), the percentage change in membrane potential (*C*) and input resistance (*D*) of glucose-inhibited neurons was significantly lower in NIRKO (*n* = 7, closed bars) compared with littermate controls (*n* = 6, open bars). **P* < 0.05, ***P* < 0.01. (A high-quality color representation of this figure is available in the online issue.)

groups (Control: 123 ± 4 vs. NIRKO: 129 ± 10, *P* = NS) (Fig. 6*B*).

Abrogated brain insulin action and expression of hypothalamic glucose sensors. To assess whether CNS insulin action regulates GLUTs and glucokinase in the brain, hypothalamic protein and mRNA expression were assessed. GLUT1 and GLUT3 hypothalamic protein expression were threefold higher than either GLUT4 or glucokinase. GLUT1 protein levels in the hypothalamus were similar in control and NIRKO mice (Fig. 7*A* and *B*). Hypothalamic GLUT3 protein levels in NIRKO mice were slightly (80.5 ± 9.8% of control) but not significantly (*P* = 0.08) reduced (Fig. 7*A* and *B*). Glucokinase protein levels were also similar in control and NIRKO mice (Fig. 7*A* and *B*). Glucokinase mRNA expression was preferentially expressed in the VMH and arcuate nucleus, but there was no difference in expression levels between experimental groups (Fig. 7*C*), consistent with the glucokinase protein expression findings. Interestingly, insulin-regulated GLUT, GLUT4, protein levels were significantly reduced (68.5 ± 5.5% of control, *P* < 0.05) in the hypothalamus of NIRKO mice (Fig. 7*A* and *B*). To assess regional localization, immunohistochemistry results demonstrated that GLUT4 protein was highly enriched in the VMH and the ARC of control mice. In NIRKO mice, GLUT4 protein expression was markedly reduced in these regions (Fig. 7*D*). Despite

reductions in GLUT expression in NIRKO mice, regional brain glucose uptake, as assessed during hyperinsulinemic-hypoglycemic clamps, was not different between experimental groups (Fig. 7*E*).

DISCUSSION

Insulin's role in regulating the counterregulatory response to hypoglycemia is an area of active investigation. Insulin has been shown to increase (8–11,18–20), diminish (12,21), and not alter (13–16,22) the sympathoadrenal response to hypoglycemia. In this study, using a model of chronic brain insulin receptor deficiency, it was demonstrated that insulin action in the brain *1*) regulates the glucose sensitivity of glucose-sensing neurons in the VMH, *2*) regulates hypothalamic neuronal activation uniquely due to hypoglycemic stress, and *3*) modulates the sympathoadrenal response to hypoglycemia by altering the glycemic level required to elicit appropriate sympathoadrenal responses.

In these studies, a ~60% rise in corticosterone was observed in response to severe hypoglycemia in NIRKO and control mice (Fig. 2*B*). Although not well characterized in mice, this degree of hypothalamic–pituitary–adrenal induced increment in corticosterone is consistent with other groups (39,40). Contrary to the stimulatory effect of

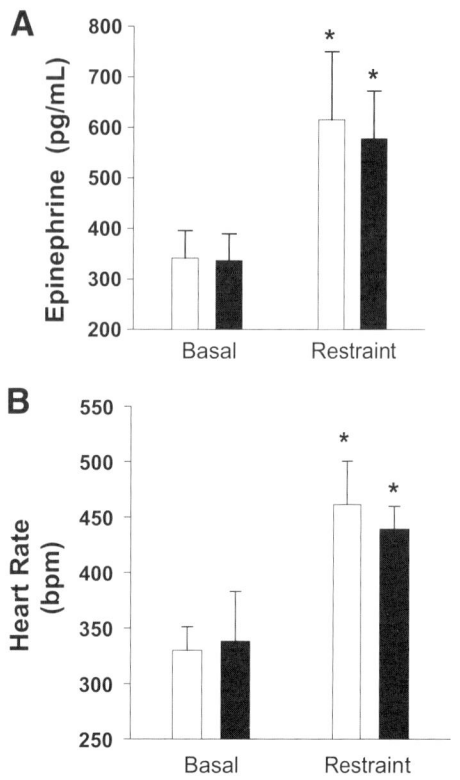

FIG. 5. NIRKO mice have a normal physiological response to restraint stress. NIRKO ($n = 6$, closed bars) and littermate control ($n = 6$, open bars) mice were placed into a confining restraint device for 45 min. A and B: Plasma epinephrine levels (A) and heart rates (B) were elevated in response to restraint stress, but equally in control and NIRKO mice. *$P < 0.05$ vs. basal.

insulin on the cortisol response to hypoglycemia observed in canine models (18,19), these studies in mice demonstrate that the absence of brain insulin action does not impair the hypothalamic–pituitary–adrenal axis response to hypoglycemia.

Reports of insulin action's in the CNS in modulating the glucagon response to hypoglycemia are variable, with studies demonstrating insulin to increase (18,19), decrease (21), or not effect (20) the glucagon response to hypoglycemia. In the current studies, the pancreatic α-cell response to severe hypoglycemia showed a sixfold increase in plasma glucagon levels that was not altered by the absence of CNS insulin receptors in NIRKO mice. Interestingly, although catecholamines stimulate the α-cell, the impaired catecholamine response to hypoglycemia did not diminish the full glucagon response in NIRKO mice (Fig. 2C). These results indicate that factors other than central insulin action and systemic catecholamine responses (perhaps local glycemia, intraislet insulin/zinc, direct innervations, etc.) are more important mediators of the glucagon response to hypoglycemia.

The absence of brain insulin receptors resulted in a significantly impaired epinephrine response in NIRKO mice during moderate (50 mg/dl) and severe (30 mg/dl) hypoglycemia. However, the absence of brain insulin signaling did not result in total deficiency of hypoglycemic counterregulation. An epinephrine response of ~1,500 pg/ml, which was achieved during moderate hypoglycemia (50 mg/dl) in controls, was also elicited at a lower blood glucose level (30 mg/dl) in NIRKO mice (Fig. 3A). Consis-

tent with this finding, the shift in the hypoglycemia–epinephrine response curve (Fig. 3A, inset) indicates that, in the absence of insulin signaling, NIRKO mice needed to reach lower glycemic levels to appropriately activate their adrenomedullary response. While insulin infusion suppressed hepatic glucose production during the clamps, only during severe hypoglycemia (30 mg/dl) was the counterregulatory response of a sufficient magnitude to overcome the suppressive effects of insulin and significantly increase hepatic glucose production. In NIRKO mice, however, the counterregulatory-induced stimulation of hepatic glucose production was significantly blunted during severe hypoglycemia (Fig. 3C), consistent with an impaired sympathoadrenal response. These findings indicate that chronic lack of CNS insulin action alters glucose sensing and/or responsiveness, leading to an impaired sympathoadrenal response and an impaired ability to defend against iatrogenic hypoglycemia.

Because the adrenomedullary response to hypoglycemia was not impaired during mild hypoglycemia in NIRKO mice, it was speculated that mild (restraint) stress, as noted by modest elevations in epinephrine levels (Fig. 5A), might not have been of sufficient magnitude to detect a differential response between control and NIRKO mice. However, by achieving comparable epinephrine levels during severe stress (heat) and severe hypoglycemia (30 mg/dl) and finding a normal catecholamine response to heat stress in NIRKO mice, these findings indicate that absent CNS insulin signaling does not impair the normal adrenomedullary response even to severe nonhypoglycemic stress (Fig. 3A, Fig. 6A).

Increased c-fos expression in the PVN has been used as a marker of transcriptional activity in stress-related neural circuitry (38,41–43). Expression of c-fos was therefore measured to determine whether the impaired sympathoadrenal response in the NIRKO mice was related to impaired activation of hypothalamic sensing neurons. During hypoglycemia, increased c-fos expression was predominantly observed in the PVN and not seen in the VMH, consistent with other studies (44). Hypoglycemia-induced c-fos activation in the PVN may represent direct activation in response to hypoglycemia or indirect activation in response to afferent input from other areas containing glucose-sensing neurons. Thus, the impaired c-fos activation in the PVN of NIRKO mice in response to hypoglycemia could represent reduced glucose sensing of PVN neurons or, given the abundance of insulin receptors in important VMH glucose-sensing neurons, an indirect reduction in afferent inputs from glucose-sensing neurons in the VMH. Whether this defect indicates impaired direct or indirect glucose sensing, the reduced c-fos activation in NIRKO mice was profound and consistent with other models of impaired glucose sensing and impaired counterregulation (43,45). Further, in response to a nonhypoglycemic stressor, heat stress increased c-fos expression to a similar magnitude as observed during severe hypoglycemia (30 mg/dl); however, no difference in heat-induced c-fos expression was noted between control and NIRKO mice (Figs. 4 and 6C and D). These results indicate that NIRKO mice have an intact neuronal circuitry for sensing and responding to nonhypoglycemic stress; therefore, the impaired responses to hypoglycemia in the NIRKO mice appear to be unique to hypoglycemic stress and/or glucose sensing.

Whole-cell current-clamp recordings of spontaneous electrical activity were made in individual glucose-inhib-

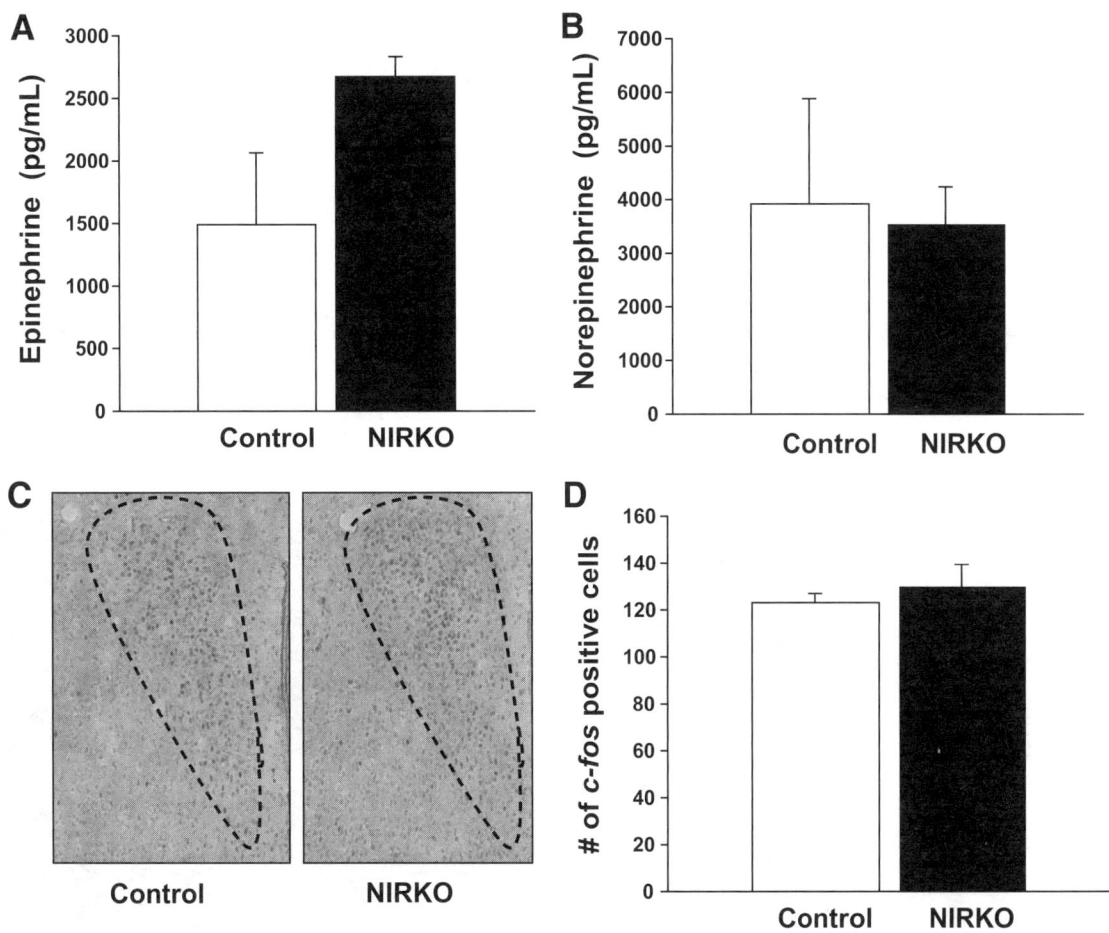

FIG. 6. NIRKO mice display normal physiological responses to heat stress. NIRKO ($n = 6$, closed bars) and littermate controls ($n = 6$, open bars) were subjected to heat stress for 90 min. *A* and *B*: Plasma epinephrine (*A*) and norepinephrine (*B*) levels were not significantly different between NIRKO and control mice. *C*: Representative images of matched hypothalamic sections highlighting heat stress induced *c-fos* staining in the PVN. *D*: The quantity of *c-fos* positive cells was similar between NIRKO and controls. (A high-quality color representation of this figure is available in the online issue.)

ited neurons to assess responses of individual glucose-sensing neurons in the VMH. While a direct relationship between glucose-sensing neurons and sympathoadrenal activation has yet to be definitively established, it is noteworthy that the ability of VMH glucose-inhibited neurons to sense a fall in ambient glucose levels is impaired under several conditions where the sympathoadrenal response to hypoglycemia is also impaired (i.e., rats treated with recurrent hypoglycemia or streptozotocin-induced diabetes) (35,46,47). In NIRKO mice, the observed impaired response of VMH glucose-inhibited neurons to reductions in glucose levels (Fig. 4*C* and *D*) is entirely consistent with the impaired neuronal (*c-fos*) activation (Fig. 4*A*) and the impaired sympathoadrenal activation (Fig. 3*A*). Further, the electrophysiological findings that NIRKO glucose-inhibited neurons respond normally to maximal glucose deprivation (0.1 mmol/l), but impaired responses at 0.5 mmol/l are consistent with a relative, not absolute, impairment in glucose sensing. These results indicate that insulin acts directly in the brain to regulate the glucose-sensing ability of hypothalamic glucose-inhibited neurons that are critically important and functionally linked in mediating the sympathoadrenal response to hypoglycemia. Of particular interest is that glucose-inhibited neurons of NIRKO mice have an impaired ability to

respond to a fall in glucose even in the absence of insulin administration. Combining these in vitro findings to the in vivo findings suggests that it may not solely be a failure of insulin to acutely activate its receptor that leads to impaired glucose sensing and altered neuronal responses; rather, we propose that the chronic lack of insulin signaling in NIRKO mice causes long-term adaptations in gene transcription/transduction (i.e., decrease in GLUT4; see Fig. 7), leading to impaired glucose sensing. Alternatively, because neuronal nitric oxide production is required for glucose-inhibited neurons to sense decreased glucose (48,49) and insulin enhances nitric oxide production in VMH glucose-inhibited neurons (48), the chronic lack of insulin signaling in NIRKO mice may led to impaired glucose sensing by impairing nitric oxide production. It is entirely plausible that the chronic actions of insulin may be mechanistically very different from the acute actions of insulin in regulating neuronal glucose sensing and the counterregulatory response to hypoglycemia.

Similar to its well characterized actions in muscle and fat, insulin-mediated GLUT4 translocation has been demonstrated in neuronal cell lines (50), hippocampus (51), and hypothalamus (52). GLUT4-mediated glucose sensing has been speculated to be important at low glucose concentrations, where insulin-mediated glucose transport

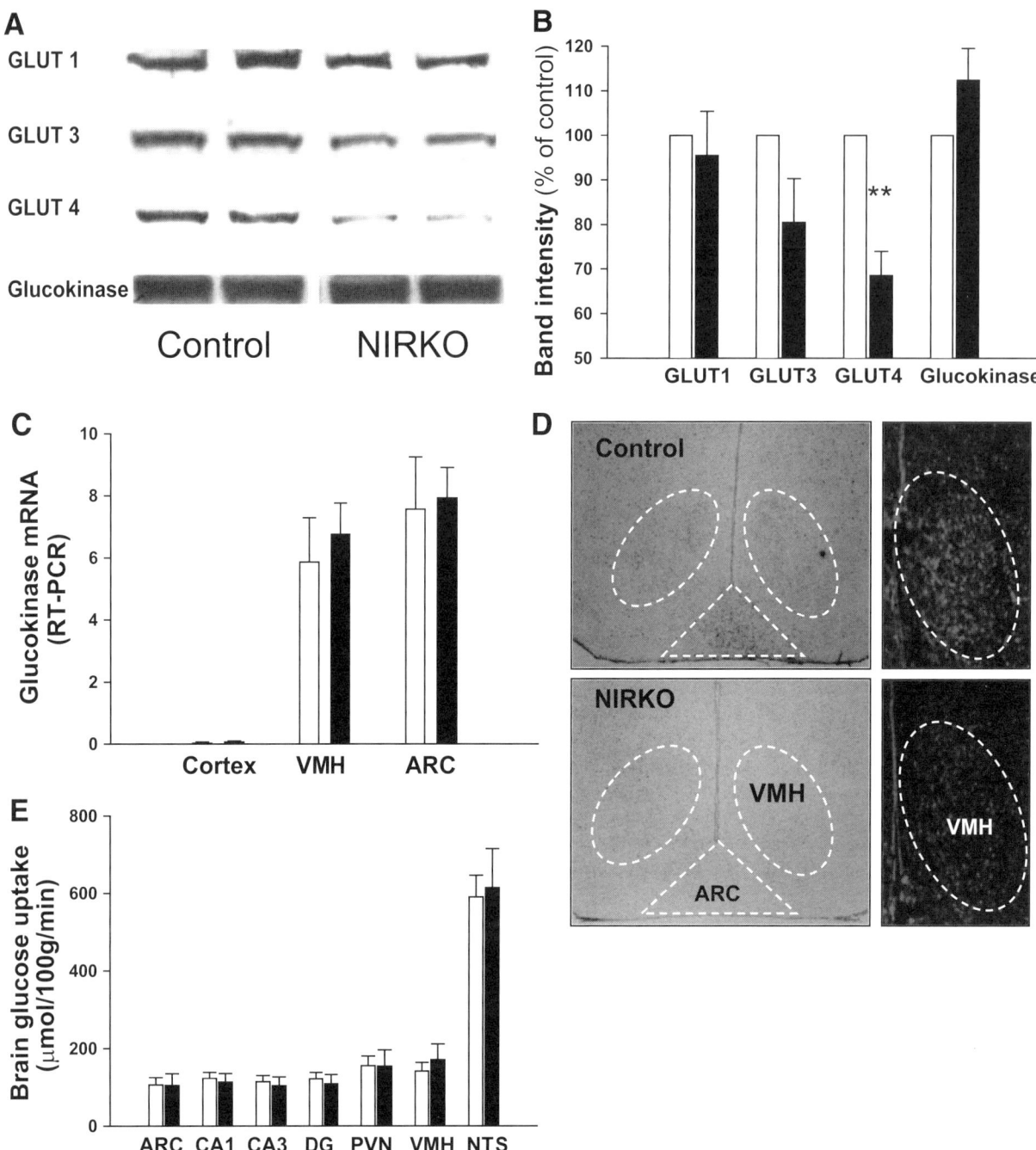

FIG. 7. GLUT 4, not GLUT1, GLUT3, or glucokinase expression, is reduced in NIRKO brains. *A* and *B*: Western blots of whole hypothalamic extracts from NIRKO and littermate controls ($n = 5$–6 mice per group) were performed. Representative images (*A*) and graph (*B*) quantifying protein expression of glucose transporters (GLUT1, GLUT3, and GLUT4) and glucokinase are shown. *C*: Although glucokinase mRNA was highly expressed in the VMH and ARC as compared with the cortex, there was no difference between NIRKO ($n = 7$, closed bars) and controls ($n = 8$, open bars). *D*: Regional localization of GLUT4 protein content, as determined by hypothalamic DAB staining (left) and immunofluorescence (right) of control (above) and NIRKO (below) mice, shows enriched GLUT4 protein content in the VMH (circled) and ARC (triangle) of control mice. GLUT4 protein content was $62 \pm 6\%$ lower in NIRKO mice. *E*: Regional brain glucose uptake was quantified using ^{14}C 2-deoxyglucose during a hyperinsulinemic-hypoglycemic ($\sim$30 mg/dl) clamp. Results show that regional brain glucose uptake in all regions measured [hippocampus (CA1, CA3, DG), hypothalamus (VMH, ARC, PVN), and hindbrain (NTS)] are similar among NIRKO ($n = 6$, closed bars) and controls ($n = 9$, open bars). (A high-quality digital representation of this figure is available in the online issue.)

may act to supplement low intracellular glucose levels in hypothalamic glucose-sensing neurons (24,26). Indeed, supporting a glucose-sensing role for insulin receptors and GLUT4 is their coexpression in up to 75% of glucose-responsive neurons in the VMH (30). Further, neuronal GLUT4 has recently been shown to be an important

mediator of hypoglycemic counterregulation and glucose sensing, as noted in neuronal GLUT4 knockout mice (53). During hypoglycemia, when glucose transport becomes rate-limiting, it was speculated that decreased GLUT4 expression and/or deficient insulin action would result in reduced glucose uptake in critical glucose-sensing regions of NIRKO mice. This study, however, noted equal regional brain glucose uptake during the hyperinsulinemic-hypoglycemic clamp (Fig. 7E), indicating that neither deficient insulin signaling nor the reduced GLUT4 levels altered glucose uptake in these brain areas. Because brain GLUT4 expression is much lower than other glucose transporters, it is likely that glucose uptake was primarily regulated by the more abundant GLUT1 and GLUT3, thus masking any subtle effect caused by decreased GLUT4. While regional brain glucose uptake was not altered in NIRKO mice, an effect of insulin signaling and/or GLUT4 availability on mediating glucose uptake in individual glucose sensing neurons cannot be ruled out.

In summary, it is shown that the chronic lack of insulin receptor signaling in the CNS 1) decreases hypothalamic GLUT4 expression, 2) attenuates individual hypothalamic glucose-inhibited neuronal responses to low glucose, 3) impairs hypothalamic neuronal activation in response to hypoglycemia, and 4) reduces the sympathoadrenal response to hypoglycemia by shifting the glycemic level necessary to elicit appropriate sympathoadrenal responses. These defects are specific for glucose sensing, as the lack of CNS insulin signaling does not restrict neuronal activation or the adrenomedullary response to restraint or heat stress.

It is concluded that insulin acts directly in the brain to regulate both glucose sensing in hypothalamic neurons and the counterregulatory response to hypoglycemia. Because insulin-treated diabetic patients have an impaired ability to sense and appropriately respond to insulin-induced hypoglycemia, the mechanisms by which insulin regulates CNS glucose sensing need to be actively investigated as research scientists endeavor to supplant insulin-induced hypoglycemia as the rate-limiting factor in the glycemic management of diabetes.

ACKNOWLEDGMENTS

We gratefully acknowledge research support from the National Institutes of Health (1F31-DK-084813 [K.A.D.-A.], DK-073683 [S.J.F.], DK-55619 [V.H.R.], DK-081358 [V.H.R.]), Juvenile Diabetes Research Foundation (S.J.F. and V.H.R.), and the core grant support from the Washington University's Diabetes Research and Training Center (DK-020579 [S.J.F.]) and Nutrition Obesity Research Center (P30-DK-056341 [S.J.F.]). No potential conflicts of interest relevant to this article were reported.

K.A.D.-A. wrote the manuscript, researched data, contributed to the discussion, and reviewed/edited the manuscript. X.Z., Z.S., and D.D.-I. researched data. V.H.R. contributed to the discussion and reviewed/edited the manuscript. S.J.F. researched data, contributed to the discussion, and reviewed/edited the manuscript.

Dr. C. R. Kahn graciously supplied the NIRKO mice. Dr. M. Mueckler kindly provided GLUT antibodies, and Dr. B. Levin gratefully provided the glucokinase riboprobe. We thank Dr. P. Cryer and his laboratory for performing the catecholamine assay. We also thank Ron Perez for his technical expertise.

REFERENCES

1. Epidemiology of severe hypoglycemia in the diabetes control and complications trial. The DCCT Research Group. Am J Med 1991;90:450–459
2. Intensive blood-glucose control with sulphonylureas or insulin compared with conventional treatment and risk of complications in patients with type 2 diabetes (UKPDS 33). UK Prospective Diabetes Study (UKPDS) Group. Lancet 1998;352:837–853
3. Laing SP, Swerdlow AJ, Slater SD, Botha JL, Burden AC, Waugh NR, Smith AW, Hill RD, Bingley PJ, Patterson CC, Qiao Z, Keen H. The British Diabetic Association Cohort Study, II. cause-specific mortality in patients with insulin-treated diabetes mellitus. Diabet Med 1999;16:466–471
4. Cryer PE, Davis SN, Shamoon H. Hypoglycemia in diabetes. Diabetes Care 2003;26:1902–1912
5. Jones TW, Davis EA. Hypoglycemia in children with type 1 diabetes: current issues and controversies. Pediatr Diabetes 2003;4:143–150
6. Hirsch BR, Shamoon H. Defective epinephrine and growth hormone responses in type I diabetes are stimulus specific. Diabetes 1987;36:20–26
7. Dagogo-Jack SE, Craft S, Cryer PE. Hypoglycemia-associated autonomic failure in insulin-dependent diabetes mellitus. Recent antecedent hypoglycemia reduces autonomic responses to, symptoms of, and defense against subsequent hypoglycemia. J Clin Invest 1993;91:819–828
8. Davis MR, Mellman M, Shamoon H. Physiologic hyperinsulinemia enhances counterregulatory hormone responses to hypoglycemia in IDDM. J Clin Endocrinol Metab 1993;76:1383–1385
9. Davis SN, Shavers C, Collins L, Cherrington AD, Price L, Hedstrom C. Effects of physiological hyperinsulinemia on counterregulatory response to prolonged hypoglycemia in normal humans. Am J Physiol 1994;267: E402–E410
10. Davis SN, Goldstein RE, Jacobs J, Price L, Wolfe R, Cherrington AD. The effects of differing insulin levels on the hormonal and metabolic response to equivalent hypoglycemia in normal humans. Diabetes 1993;42:263–272
11. Lingenfelser T, Overkamp D, Renn W, Buettner U, Kimmerle K, Schmalfuss A, Jakober B. Insulin-associated modulation of neuroendocrine counterregulation, hypoglycemia perception, and cerebral function in insulin-dependent diabetes mellitus: evidence for an intrinsic effect of insulin on the central nervous system. J Clin Endocrinol Metab 1996;81:1197–1205
12. Diamond MP, Hallarman L, Starick-Zych K, Jones TW, Connolly-Howard M, Tamborlane WV, Sherwin RS. Suppression of counterregulatory hormone response to hypoglycemia by insulin per se. J Clin Endocrinol Metab 1991;72:1388–1390
13. Liu D, Moberg E, Kollind M, Lins PE, Adamson U. A high concentration of circulating insulin suppresses the glucagon response to hypoglycemia in normal man. J Clin Endocrinol Metab 1991;73:1123–1128
14. Mellman MJ, Davis MR, Shamoon H. Effect of physiological hyperinsulinemia on counterregulatory hormone responses during hypoglycemia in humans. J Clin Endocrinol Metab 1992;75:1293–1297
15. Davis SN, Goldstein RE, Price L, Jacobs J, Cherrington AD. The effects of insulin on the counterregulatory response to equivalent hypoglycemia in patients with insulin-dependent diabetes mellitus. J Clin Endocrinol Metab 1993;77:1300–1307
16. Kerr D, Reza M, Smith N, Leatherdale BA. Importance of insulin in subjective, cognitive, and hormonal responses to hypoglycemia in patients with IDDM. Diabetes 1991;40:1057–1062
17. Brüning JC, Gautam D, Burks DJ, Gillette J, Schubert M, Orban PC, Klein R, Krone W, Müller-Wieland D, Kahn CR: Role of brain insulin receptor in control of body weight and reproduction. Science 2000;289:2122–2125
18. Davis SN, Colburn C, Dobbins R, Nadeau S, Neal D, Williams P, Cherrington AD. Evidence that the brain of the conscious dog is insulin sensitive. J Clin Invest 1995;95:593–602
19. Davis SN, Dunham B, Walmsley K, Shavers C, Neal D, Williams P, Cherrington AD. Brain of the conscious dog is sensitive to physiological changes in circulating insulin. Am J Physiol 1997;272:E567–E575
20. Fisher SJ, Brüning JC, Lannon S, Kahn CR. Insulin signaling in the central nervous system is critical for the normal sympathoadrenal response to hypoglycemia. Diabetes 2005;54:1447–1451
21. Paranjape SA, Chan O, Zhu W, Horblitt AM, McNay EC, Cresswell JA, Bogan JS, McCrimmon RJ, Sherwin RS. Influence of insulin in the ventromedial hypothalamus on pancreatic glucagon secretion in vivo. Diabetes 2010;59:1521–1527
22. Ishihara KK, Haywood SC, Daphna-Iken D, Puente EC, Fisher SJ. Brain insulin infusion does not augment the counterregulatory response to hypoglycemia or glucoprivation. Metabolism 2009;58:812–820
23. Yang XJ, Kow LM, Pfaff DW, Mobbs CV. Metabolic pathways that mediate inhibition of hypothalamic neurons by glucose. Diabetes 2004;53:67–73
24. Levin BE, Routh VH, Kang L, Sanders NM, Dunn-Meynell AA. Neuronal glucosensing: what do we know after 50 years? Diabetes 2004;53:2521–2528
25. Spanswick D, Smith MA, Mirshamsi S, Routh VH, Ashford ML. Insulin activates ATP-sensitive K+ channels in hypothalamic neurons of lean, but not obese rats. Nat Neurosci 2000;3:757–758
26. Cotero VE, Routh VH. Insulin blunts the response of glucose-excited neurons in the ventrolateral-ventromedial hypothalamic nucleus to decreased glucose. Am J Physiol Endocrinol Metab 2009;296:E1101–E1109
27. Yang XJ, Kow LM, Funabashi T, Mobbs CV. Hypothalamic glucose sensor:

similarities to and differences from pancreatic beta-cell mechanisms. Diabetes 1999;48:1763–1772

28. Schuit, FC, Huypens, P, Heimberg, H, Pipeleers, DG. Glucose sensing in pancreatic beta-cells: a model for the study of other glucose-regulated cells in gut, pancreas, and hypothalamus. Diabetes 2001;50:1–11

29. Pénicaud L, Leloup C, Lorsignol A, Alquier T, Guillod E. Brain glucose sensing mechanism and glucose homeostasis. Curr Opin Clin Nutr Metab Care 2002;5:539–543

30. Kang L, Routh VH, Kuzhikandathil EV, Gaspers LD, Levin BE. Physiological and molecular characteristics of rat hypothalamic ventromedial nucleus glucosensing neurons. Diabetes 2004;53:549–559

31. Schubert M, Gautam D, Surjo D, Ueki K, Baudler S, Schubert D, Kondo T, Alber J, Galldiks N, Küstermann E, Arndt S, Jacobs AH, Krone W, Kahn CR, Brüning JC. Role for neuronal insulin resistance in neurodegenerative diseases. Proc Natl Acad Sci U S A 2004;101:3100–3105

32. Fisher SJ, Kahn CR. Insulin signaling is required for insulin's direct and indirect action on hepatic glucose production. J Clin Invest 2003;111:463–468

33. Sokoloff L, Reivich M, Kennedy C, Des Rosiers MH, Patlak CS, Pettigrew KD, Sakurada O, Shinohara M. The [^{14}C]deoxyglucose method for the measurement of local cerebral glucose utilization: theory, procedure, and normal values in the conscious and anesthetized albino rat. J Neurochem 1977;28:897–916

34. Song Z, Routh VH. Differential effects of glucose and lactate on glucosensing neurons in the ventromedial hypothalamic nucleus. Diabetes 2005;54:15–22

35. Song Z, Routh VH. Recurrent hypoglycemia reduces the glucose sensitivity of glucose-inhibited neurons in the ventromedial hypothalamic nucleus. Am J Physiol Regul Integr Comp Physiol 2006;291:R1283–R1287

36. Paxinos G, Franklin KBJ. The mouse brain in stereotaxic coordinates. London, Academic Press, 2001

37. Shah SD, Clutter WE, Cryer PE. External and internal standards in the single-isotope derivative (radioenzymatic) measurement of plasma norepinephrine and epinephrine. J Lab Clin Med 1985;106:624–629

38. Kovács KJ. c-Fos as a transcription factor: a stressful (re)view from a functional map. Neurochem Int 1998;33:287–297

39. Inouye K, Shum K, Chan O, Mathoo J, Matthews SG, Vranic M. Effects of recurrent hyperinsulinemia with and without hypoglycemia on counterregulation in diabetic rats. Am J Physiol Endocrinol Metab 2002;282:E1369–E1379

40. Chan O, Chan S, Inouye K, Shum K, Matthews SG, Vranic M. Diabetes impairs hypothalamo-pituitary-adrenal (HPA) responses to hypoglycemia, and insulin treatment normalizes HPA but not epinephrine responses. Diabetes 2002;51:1681–1689

41. Tsay HJ, Li HY, Lin CH, Yang YL, Yeh JY, Lin MT. Heatstroke induces c-fos expression in the rat hypothalamus. Neurosci Lett 1999;262:41–44

42. Harikai N, Tomogane K, Sugawara T, Tashiro S. Differences in hypothalamic Fos expressions between two heat stress conditions in conscious mice. Brain Res Bull 2003;61:617–626

43. Paranjape SA, Briski KP. Recurrent insulin-induced hypoglycemia causes site-specific patterns of habituation or amplification of CNS neuronal genomic activation. Neuroscience 2005;130:957–970

44. Niimi M, Sato M, Tamaki M, Wada Y, Takahara J, Kawanishi K. Induction of Fos protein in the rat hypothalamus elicited by insulin-induced hypoglycemia. Neurosci Res 1995;23:361–364

45. Kale AY, Paranjape SA, Briski KP. I.c.v. administration of the nonsteroidal glucocorticoid receptor antagonist, CP-472555, prevents exacerbated hypoglycemia during repeated insulin administration. Neuroscience 2006;140:555–565

46. Powell AM, Sherwin RS, Shulman GI. Impaired hormonal responses to hypoglycemia in spontaneously diabetic and recurrently hypoglycemic rats. Reversibility and stimulus specificity of the deficits. J Clin Invest 1993;92:2667–2674

47. Canabal DD, Potian JG, Duran RG, McArdle JJ, Routh VH. Hyperglycemia impairs glucose and insulin regulation of nitric oxide production in glucose-inhibited neurons in the ventromedial hypothalamus. Physiol Regul Integr Comp Physiol 2007;293:R592–R600

48. Canabal DD, Song Z, Potian JG, Beuve A, McArdle JJ, Routh VH. Glucose, insulin, and leptin signaling pathways modulate nitric oxide synthesis in glucose-inhibited neurons in the ventromedial hypothalamus. Am J Physiol Regul Integr Comp Physiol 2007;292:R1418–R1428

49. Murphy BA, Fakira KA, Song Z, Beuve A, Routh VH. AMP-activated protein kinase and nitric oxide regulate the glucose sensitivity of ventromedial hypothalamic glucose-inhibited neurons. Am J Physiol Cell Physiol 2009;297:C750–C758

50. Benomar Y, Naour N, Aubourg A, Bailleux V, Gertler A, Djiane J, Guerre-Millo M, Taouis M. Insulin and leptin induce Glut4 plasma membrane translocation and glucose uptake in a human neuronal cell line by a phosphatidylinositol 3-kinase-dependent mechanism. Endocrinology 2006;147:2550–2556

51. Piroli GG, Grillo CA, Reznikov LR, Adams S, McEwen BS, Charron MJ, Reagan LP. Corticosterone impairs insulin-stimulated translocation of GLUT4 in the rat hippocampus. Neuroendocrinology 2007;85:71–80

52. Grillo CA, Tamashiro KL, Piroli GG, Melhorn S, Gass JT, Newsom RJ, Reznikov LR, Smith A, Wilson SP, Sakai RR, Reagan LP. Lentivirus-mediated downregulation of hypothalamic insulin receptor expression. Physiol Behav. 2007;92:691–701

53. Puente E, Daphna-Iken D, Bree A, Suzuki Y, Georgopoulos I, Kahn BB, Fisher S. Impaired counterregulatory response to hypoglycemia and impaired glucose tolerance in brain glucose transporter 4 (GLUT4) knockout mice (Abstract). Diabetes 2009;58:A13

Cognitive Function in Type 1 Diabetic Adults With Early Exposure to Severe Hypoglycemia

A 16-year follow-up study

BJØRN O. ÅSVOLD, MD, PHD[1,2]
TROND SAND, MD, PHD[3,4]

KNUT HESTAD, PHD[5,6,7]
MARIT R. BJØRGAAS, MD, PHD[1,8]

OBJECTIVE — We assessed adulthood cognition in relation to early exposure to severe hypoglycemia (SH).

RESEARCH DESIGN AND METHODS — Sixteen years subsequent to a study of cognitive function in 28 diabetic children and 28 matched control subjects, we reexamined the same subjects with a 96% participation rate. Diabetic subjects were classified as with ($n = 9$) or without ($n = 18$) early (≤ 10 years of age) SH, which was defined as convulsions or loss of consciousness.

RESULTS — Overall, cognitive scores were 0.9 SDs lower in subjects with early SH compared with subjects without early SH ($P = 0.003$). The two diabetic groups particularly differed with respect to problem solving, verbal function, and psychomotor efficiency. Earlier age at first incident of SH was associated with poorer cognition (P for trend = 0.001).

CONCLUSIONS — The findings suggest that early exposure to SH may have lasting and clinically relevant effects on cognition.

Diabetes Care 33:1945–1947, 2010

Early-onset diabetes is associated with reduced cognition (1), possibly due to the effects of severe hypoglycemia (SH) on the developing brain (2–5). Although moderate (1), this cognitive deficit seems to be enduring (5–7). We hypothesized that earlier age at SH occurrence would entail more pronounced effects on cognition. In this 16-year follow-up study of diabetic subjects, we investigated cognitive function in relation to early exposure to SH.

RESEARCH DESIGN AND METHODS

In 1992–1993, we studied cognitive function (8) and quantitative electroencephalograms (9) in diabetic children attending Trondheim University Hospital, the only referral center for childhood diabetes in the region. We included all 15 children who had experienced SH and 13 diabetic children of the same age without previous SH. For each subject, we included a sex- and age-matched control subject, 20 of whom were schoolmates of the diabetic subjects.

In 2008, the participants were invited to participate in a follow-up at mean age 28 years: 27 of 28 diabetic subjects (96%) and all the control subjects participated. The study was approved by the regional ethics committee.

Information on SHs (i.e., episodes with convulsions or loss of consciousness), A1C levels, and comorbidity was obtained from hospital records and personal interviews. Diabetic subjects were classified as with ($n = 9$) or without ($n = 18$) early SH (≤ 10 years of age) (supplementary Table 1, found in the online appendix available at http://care.diabetesjournals.org/cgi/content/full/dc10-0621/DC1).

As in the baseline study (8), neuropsychological tests were grouped into seven cognitive domains (supplementary Table 2). For each domain, we computed a relative score, expressing the difference between diabetic subject and matched control subject, with the SD among control subjects as the unit of measure (e.g., a relative score of -1 implied that the diabetic subjects scored on average 1 SD poorer than the control subjects within that domain). By averaging these relative scores, we obtained an overall relative score as a measure of overall cognition. We estimated mean relative scores for diabetic subjects with and without early SH and examined whether relative scores differed between the diabetic groups.

Using data from the baseline study, we estimated childhood cognitive function and change in cognition from childhood to adulthood. For this analysis, we excluded neuropsychological tests that had no equivalent at baseline.

We studied whether age at first SH (≤ 5 years of age, $n = 4$; 6–10 years of age, $n = 5$; or no early SH, $n = 18$) was associated with overall adulthood cognition (expressed by P value for trend across categories), and we assessed overall cognition in relation to the total number of SHs and lifetime mean A1C (the average A1C since diabetes onset, weighted for the frequency of recordings).

For all analyses, we used the general linear model. As a consequence of the

From the [1]Department of Endocrinology, St. Olavs Hospital, Trondheim University Hospital, Trondheim, Norway; the [2]Department of Public Health, Norwegian University of Science and Technology, Trondheim, Norway; the [3]Department of Neuroscience, Norwegian University of Science and Technology, Trondheim, Norway; the [4]Department of Neurology and Clinical Neurophysiology, St. Olavs Hospital, Trondheim University Hospital, Trondheim, Norway; the [5]Department of Psychology, Norwegian University of Science and Technology, Trondheim, Norway; the [6]Old Age Research Center, Innlandet Hospital Trust, Hamar, Norway; [7]Lillehammer University College, Lillehammer, Norway; and the [8]Department of Cancer Research and Molecular Medicine, Norwegian University of Science and Technology, Trondheim, Norway.
Corresponding author: Bjørn O. Åsvold, bjorn.o.asvold@ntnu.no.
Received 31 March 2010 and accepted 22 June 2010.
DOI: 10.2337/dc10-0621

The costs of publication of this article were defrayed in part by the payment of page charges. This article must therefore be hereby marked "advertisement" in accordance with 18 U.S.C. Section 1734 solely to indicate this fact.

Table 1—*Mean cognitive relative scores* in adulthood and childhood, and change in relative scores from childhood to adulthood† in diabetic subjects with and without early‡ SH*

Cognitive domain	Diabetes with early SH			Diabetes without early SH						
	Relative score	95% CI		Relative score	95% CI		Difference§	95% CI		P‖
Adulthood										
Memory	−0.7	−1.4	0.0	0.1	−0.3	0.6	−0.8	−1.7	0.0	0.06
Motor speed	0.1	−0.6	0.8	−0.3	−0.8	0.2	0.4	−0.5	1.3	0.35
Psychomotor efficiency	−1.1	−2.0	−0.3	0.1	−0.4	0.7	−1.3	−2.3	−0.2	0.02
Attention	−0.3	−1.0	0.3	−0.1	−0.6	0.3	−0.2	−1.0	0.6	0.61
Problem solving	−2.2	−3.0	−1.5	0.0	−0.6	0.5	−2.2	−3.2	−1.2	<0.001
Spatial function	−1.0	−2.0	0.1	−0.1	−0.8	0.6	−0.9	−2.2	0.4	0.18
Verbal function	−1.7	−2.6	−0.8	−0.2	−0.8	0.4	−1.5	−2.6	−0.4	0.01
Overall	−1.0	−1.5	−0.5	−0.1	−0.4	0.2	−0.9	−1.5	−0.3	0.003
Childhood										
Memory	−0.5	−1.3	0.3	0.2	−0.4	0.7	−0.7	−1.7	0.3	0.18
Motor speed	0.1	−0.7	0.9	−0.3	−0.9	0.2	0.4	−0.5	1.4	0.36
Psychomotor efficiency	−0.8	−1.5	0.0	0.2	−0.3	0.7	−1.0	−1.9	−0.1	0.04
Attention	−1.9¶	−3.7	−0.1	0.5	−0.6	1.7	−2.4	−4.7	−0.2	0.04
Problem solving	−0.3	−0.8	0.2	0.0	−0.4	0.3	−0.3	−0.9	0.4	0.41
Spatial function	−0.2	−1.1	0.7	−0.1	−0.7	0.5	−0.1	−1.2	1.0	0.80
Verbal function	−1.0	−1.7	−0.3	0.0	−0.5	0.4	−1.0	−1.8	−0.1	0.03
Overall	−0.7	−1.2	−0.1	0.1	−0.3	0.5	−0.7	−1.5	0.0	0.048
Change from childhood to adulthood										
Memory	−0.1	−0.8	0.6	−0.1	−0.5	0.4	0.0	−0.9	0.8	0.94
Motor speed	0.0	−0.8	0.8	0.0	−0.5	0.6	0.0	−1.0	0.9	0.96
Psychomotor efficiency	−0.4	−1.0	0.3	−0.1	−0.5	0.4	−0.3	−1.1	0.5	0.45
Attention	1.5¶	−0.4	3.4	−0.5	−1.7	0.7	2.0	−0.3	4.3	0.09
Problem solving	−1.9	−2.7	−1.2	0.0	−0.6	0.5	−1.9	−2.9	−0.9	<0.001
Spatial function	−0.8	−1.6	0.0	0.0	−0.6	0.5	−0.8	−1.8	0.3	0.14
Verbal function	−0.7	−1.5	0.1	−0.2	−0.7	0.3	−0.5	−1.5	0.5	0.28
Overall	−0.3	−0.7	0.0	−0.1	−0.4	0.1	−0.2	−0.7	0.2	0.34

*Difference in test scores between diabetic subjects and control subjects with the SD among control subjects as the unit of measure. †Computed as (relative score at follow-up–relative score at baseline). ‡Defined as first SH ≤10 years of age. §Difference in relative score between diabetic subjects with and without early SH. ‖P value for the difference between diabetic subjects with and without early SH. ¶n = 8 (diabetic–matched control subject) pairs.

matched design, the results were controlled for the effects of sex and age. The results were adjusted for parental education and work (8). The data were analyzed using SPSS statistical software, version 14.0, for Windows (SPSS, Chicago, IL).

RESULTS — The characteristics of the participants are given in supplementary Table 1 and the mean neuropsychological test scores in supplementary Table 2. Diabetic adults without early SH had similar cognitive function as control subjects (overall relative score −0.1 SD), whereas subjects with early SH scored on average 1.0 SD lower than control subjects (Table 1). Overall relative score was 0.9 SD lower in subjects with early SH compared with subjects without early SH (P = 0.003). The diabetic groups particularly differed in problem solving, verbal function, and psychomotor efficiency. They also tended

to differ in memory. All results were adjusted for parental education and work at baseline, but even before this adjustment, the overall relative score was 0.9 SD lower in subjects with early SH compared with subjects without early SH.

Subjects with early SH already had reduced cognitive function in childhood (overall relative score −0.7 SD) (Table 1). They also tended to have a less favorable development in cognitive function during follow-up compared with control subjects (overall relative score −0.3 SD). This adverse tendency was driven by a reduced problem–solving ability.

Earlier age at first SH was associated with poorer cognitive function in adulthood (P for trend = 0.001). Overall, diabetic subjects with first SH before 6 years of age scored 1.3 (95% CI [0.7–2.0]) SD lower than control subjects, whereas sub-

jects with first SH 6–10 years of age scored 0.7 (0.1–1.3) SD lower than control subjects. Overall cognition in adulthood was not related to the total number of SHs or to mean lifetime A1C (data not shown).

CONCLUSIONS — In this 16-year follow-up study, diabetes with early SH was associated with ~1 SD poorer cognitive function in adulthood, which is considered a large effect size (3). The deficit was found across several cognitive domains and was most pronounced in subjects exposed to SH before 6 years of age.

Most (1,5,6,8,10,11), but not all (12–14) studies indicate cognitive effects from SH occurring in childhood. Possibly the developing brain is particularly vulnerable to the effects of SH (2,3,5,6,11). Unlike previous long-term studies, we specifically included diabetic subjects with exposure to SH in early childhood. This could explain why our data suggest larger persistent cognitive decline than previously reported in the studies of early-onset diabetes or SH in childhood (5–7).

Our subjects with early SH were younger at diabetes onset than subjects without early SH (average 5 vs. 10 years of age). Even though we did not find an association between lifetime A1C and cognition, we cannot exclude the possibility that hyperglycemia in early childhood, or a synergism between hyperglycemia and the occurrence of SH (15), may underlie the cognitive deficits demonstrated.

We present a nearly complete follow-up of diabetic subjects and matched control subjects from childhood to adulthood. Participants were enrolled in childhood, and any effects from diabetes on cognitive abilities appearing later did not bias the selection. Influence from recall bias is not likely since all early SHs were contemporarily documented in hospital records. Potential confounding by parental cognition is possible; however, adjustment for parental education and work did not change the results. In conclusion, our findings suggest that early exposure to SH may have lasting and clinically relevant effects on cognition.

Acknowledgments— This study was financially supported by the faculty of medicine, Norwegian University of Science and Technology; St. Olavs Hospital, Trondheim University Hospital; the Norwegian Diabetes Association; Unimed Innovation AS; sanofi-aventis Norge A/S; and Novo Nordisk A/S.

No potential conflicts of interest relevant to this article were reported.

B.O.Å. researched the data, contributed to the discussion, and wrote the manuscript. T.S., K.H., and M.R.B. researched the data, contributed to the discussion, and reviewed/edited the manuscript.

Parts of this study were presented in abstract form at the 70th Scientific Sessions of the American Diabetes Association, Orlando, Florida, 25–29 June 2010.

We are indebted to Anne Lisbet Moen, Department of Psychology, Norwegian University of Science and Technology, for conducting the neuropsychological testing and to Sissel Salater, St. Olavs Hospital, for excellent practical assistance.

References

1. Gaudieri PA, Chen R, Greer TF, Holmes CS. Cognitive function in children with type 1 diabetes: a meta-analysis. Diabetes Care 2008;31:1892–1897
2. Ryan C, Gurtunca N, Becker D. Hypoglycemia: a complication of diabetes therapy in children. Pediatr Clin North Am 2005; 52:1705–1733
3. Biessels GJ, Deary IJ, Ryan CM. Cognition and diabetes: a lifespan perspective. Lancet Neurol 2008;7:184–190
4. Perantie DC, Lim A, Wu J, Weaver P, Warren SL, Sadler M, White NH, Hershey T. Effects of prior hypoglycemia and hyperglycemia on cognition in children with type 1 diabetes mellitus. Pediatr Diabetes 2008;9:87–95
5. Lin A, Northam EA, Rankins D, Werther GA, Cameron FJ. Neuropsychological profiles of young people with type 1 diabetes 12 yr after disease onset. Pediatr Diabetes 2010;11:235–243
6. Northam EA, Rankins D, Lin A, Wellard RM, Pell GS, Finch SJ, Werther GA, Cameron FJ. Central nervous system function in youth with type 1 diabetes 12 years after disease onset. Diabetes Care 2009; 32:445–450
7. Ferguson SC, Blane A, Wardlaw J, Frier BM, Perros P, McCrimmon RJ, Deary IJ. Influence of an early-onset age of type 1 diabetes on cerebral structure and cognitive function. Diabetes Care 2005;28: 1431–1437
8. Bjørgaas M, Gimse R, Vik T, Sand T. Cognitive function in type 1 diabetic children with and without episodes of severe hypoglycaemia. Acta Paediatr 1997;86: 148–153
9. Bjørgaas M, Sand T, Gimse R. Quantitative EEG in type 1 diabetic children with and without episodes of severe hypoglycemia: a controlled, blind study. Acta Neurol Scand 1996;93:398–402
10. Rovet JF, Ehrlich RM. The effect of hypoglycemic seizures on cognitive function in children with diabetes: a 7-year prospective study. J Pediatr 1999;134:503–506
11. Hershey T, Perantie DC, Warren SL, Zimmerman EC, Sadler M, White NH. Frequency and timing of severe hypoglycemia affects spatial memory in children with type 1 diabetes. Diabetes Care 2005;28: 2372–2377
12. Schoenle EJ, Schoenle D, Molinari L, Largo RH. Impaired intellectual development in children with type I diabetes: association with HbA(1c), age at diagnosis and sex. Diabetologia 2002;45:108–114
13. Wysocki T, Harris MA, Mauras N, Fox L, Taylor A, Jackson SC, White NH. Absence of adverse effects of severe hypoglycemia on cognitive function in school-aged children with diabetes over 18 months. Diabetes Care 2003;26:1100–1105
14. Strudwick SK, Carne C, Gardiner J, Foster JK, Davis EA, Jones TW. Cognitive functioning in children with early onset type 1 diabetes and severe hypoglycemia. J Pediatr 2005;147:680–685
15. Ryan CM. Why is cognitive dysfunction associated with the development of diabetes early in life? The diathesis hypothesis. Pediatr Diabetes 2006;7:289–297

Novel Use of Glucagon in a Closed-Loop System for Prevention of Hypoglycemia in Type 1 Diabetes

Jessica R. Castle, md[1]
Julia M. Engle, ba[2]
Joseph El Youssef, mbbs[1]
Ryan G. Massoud, bs[2]

Kevin C.J. Yuen, md[1]
Ryland Kagan, bs[2]
W. Kenneth Ward, md[1,2]

OBJECTIVE — To minimize hypoglycemia in subjects with type 1 diabetes by automated glucagon delivery in a closed-loop insulin delivery system.

RESEARCH DESIGN AND METHODS — Adult subjects with type 1 diabetes underwent one closed-loop study with insulin plus placebo and one study with insulin plus glucagon, given at times of impending hypoglycemia. Seven subjects received glucagon using high-gain parameters, and six subjects received glucagon in a more prolonged manner using low-gain parameters. Blood glucose levels were measured every 10 min and insulin and glucagon infusions were adjusted every 5 min. All subjects received a portion of their usual premeal insulin after meal announcement.

RESULTS — Automated glucagon plus insulin delivery, compared with placebo plus insulin, significantly reduced time spent in the hypoglycemic range (15 ± 6 vs. 40 ± 10 min/day, $P = 0.04$). Compared with placebo, high-gain glucagon delivery reduced the frequency of hypoglycemic events (1.0 ± 0.6 vs. 2.1 ± 0.6 events/day, $P = 0.01$) and the need for carbohydrate treatment (1.4 ± 0.8 vs. 4.0 ± 1.4 treatments/day, $P = 0.01$). Glucagon given with low-gain parameters did not significantly reduce hypoglycemic event frequency ($P = NS$) but did reduce frequency of carbohydrate treatment ($P = 0.05$).

CONCLUSIONS — During closed-loop treatment in subjects with type 1 diabetes, high-gain pulses of glucagon decreased the frequency of hypoglycemia. Larger and longer-term studies will be required to assess the effect of ongoing glucagon treatment on overall glycemic control.

Diabetes Care 33:1282–1287, 2010

S evere hypoglycemia is an acute complication of insulin therapy that can lead to seizures, coma, and death (1) and creates a barrier to optimal glycemic control in diabetes management (2). Despite treatment advances such as insulin pump therapy and continuous glucose monitoring, hypoglycemia remains a concern, even when insulin is given in a closed-loop system (3). Here, we report on a novel, automated, sensor-controlled method of insulin delivery accompanied by glu-

cagon delivery at times of impending hypoglycemia.

A closed-loop system consists of a glucose-measuring device, from which data are collected and entered into an algorithm, which in turn controls insulin delivery (4). The difficulty of delivering regular or analog insulin in such a manner is related to its slow onset and prolonged effect when delivered subcutaneously. Until a more rapidly acting insulin preparation is available, discontinuation of subcutaneous insulin during impending

hypoglycemia, with any algorithm, may be insufficient to prevent hypoglycemia.

Glucagon, a hormone secreted from the α-cells of the normal endocrine pancreas, rapidly raises circulating glucose levels within minutes via glycogenolysis, even when given subcutaneously (5). Glucagon is approved for use as a parenteral injection for treatment of severe hypoglycemia. In children, an off-label use has been described using small subcutaneous doses to prevent or treat mild hypoglycemia (6,7).

In 1982, Shichiri et al. (8) published the concept of including glucagon delivery in an automated closed-loop glycemic control system. More recently, such a system has been studied in animals by our group (9) and by the Boston University group (10) with promising results. In this study of subjects with type 1 diabetes, we compared the frequency and duration of hypoglycemia during treatment with insulin plus glucagon to treatment with insulin plus placebo. Delivery of insulin and glucagon was automated and controlled by an amperometric glucose sensor. We hypothesized that when given for impending hypoglycemia, glucagon would decrease the frequency of overt hypoglycemia more than placebo.

RESEARCH DESIGN AND
METHODS — Patients were recruited from the Oregon Health and Science University (OHSU) outpatient clinics in Portland, Oregon. Patients who were pregnant or had cardiovascular, cerebrovascular, kidney, or liver disease or any other uncontrolled chronic medical conditions were excluded. Other exclusion criteria included oral or parenteral corticosteroid use, immunosuppressant use, visual or physical impairments that impede the use of a continuous glucose-monitoring device, insulin or glucagon allergy, hypoglycemia unawareness or hospitalization within the past 2 years for severe hypoglycemia, serum insulin antibody titer >100 μU/ml, or requirement of >200 units insulin/day. The research protocol was approved by the OHSU Institutional Review Board, and all subjects provided written informed consent. Per-

From the [1]Oregon Health and Science University, Department of Medicine, Division of Endocrinology, Portland, Oregon; and [2]Legacy Health, Division of Research, Portland, Oregon.
Corresponding author: Jessica R. Castle, castleje@ohsu.edu.
Received 10 December 2009 and accepted 8 March 2010. Published ahead of print at http://care.diabetesjournals.org on 23 March 2010. DOI: 10.2337/dc09-2254.

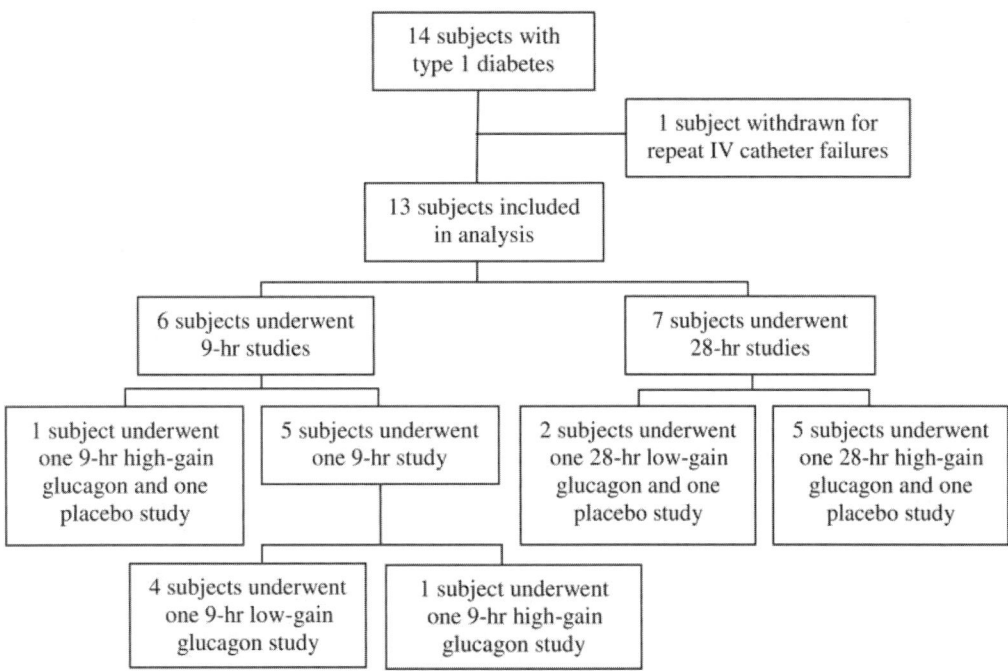

Figure 1—*Study diagram depicting the number of subjects studied under each condition and the study lengths.*

mission to carry out these studies was granted by the U.S. Food and Drug Administration (FDA) (investigational device exemption no. G080130).

A total of 22 closed-loop studies in 14 subjects were performed. Age was 36.7 ± 3.7 years, with a duration of diabetes of 14.1 ± 3.1 years. A1C was 7.6 ± 0.3% and BMI 27.8 ± 1.5 kg/m². The study for one patient was stopped early because of repeated intravenous catheter failures. The data from this study were excluded from the analysis, leaving 21 datasets from 13 subjects.

As requested by the FDA, five subjects participated in single 9-h studies with both insulin and glucagon to assess the safety and effectiveness of the study protocol. Eight subjects underwent one study with insulin and placebo and one with insulin and glucagon (see Fig. 1). Of the 13 studies during which glucagon was given, it was delivered using high-gain parameters in seven studies and using low-gain parameters in six. Low- versus high-gain glucagon is discussed in detail below. The treatment order of each paired study was determined by a randomization scheme. In paired studies, subjects were blinded as to whether they received glucagon or placebo.

Subjects wore two subcutaneous glucose sensors, either DexCom Seven Plus or Medtronic Guardian Real-Time glucose sensors. Sensors were placed 8–24 h

prior to beginning the study. For subjects taking long-acting insulin at night, the dose was reduced by 50% the night prior to the study. The following morning, subjects were admitted to the Oregon Clinical and Translational Research Institute at OHSU. An intravenous catheter was placed in a forearm vein. The forearm was warmed with a heating pad to arterialize the venous blood. Venous glucose was measured every 10 min in duplicate using a HemoCue Glucose 201 Analyzer. Glucose sensor readings were recorded from the receivers every 5 min. For the first 2 h, the insulin and glucagon delivery rates were determined by venous glucose levels. After the first 2 h, the sensed glucose values from the sensor with better accuracy were input into the algorithm every 5 min to determine the hormone delivery rates. If the sensor accuracy became suboptimal, defined as a median absolute relative difference (MARD) exceeding 20% or median absolute difference (MAD) exceeding 20 mg/dl, control was switched to the other sensor. If the accuracy of both sensors was poor, control was switched to venous glucose and the sensors were recalibrated. Sensors were calibrated at a minimum of every 12 h.

The Fading Memory Proportional Derivative (FMPD) algorithm (9,11) was used to determine the insulin and subcutaneous glucagon (or placebo) delivery rates. Aspart insulin (Novo Nordisk) was

delivered subcutaneously via an Animas IR 1000 insulin pump. Glucagon or saline placebo was given through a subcutaneous catheter via a Medfusion 2001 syringe pump. One milligram of glucagon (Novo Nordisk) was mixed with 3 ml of sterile water. The glucagon preparation was freshly reconstituted every 8 h. A study physician was onsite at all times and had the ability to override the hormone infusion rates called for by the FMPD algorithm, which occurred only 1.7% of the time. Either a registered nurse or physician was responsible for adjusting the insulin delivery rate and glucagon delivery rate every 5 min, based on the controller output.

The FMPD algorithm determined the hormone delivery rates based on proportional error, defined as the difference between the current glucose level and the target level, and the derivative error, defined as the rate of change of the glucose. The "fading memory" designation refers to weighting recent errors more heavily than remote errors. This weighting provides an adaptive component to the algorithm, as described previously (9,11). In simple terms, the insulin rate was increased for high or rising glucose levels and glucagon was given for low or falling glucose levels. The basal insulin infusion rate (in units per hour) was given at a rate of 35% of the patient's typical total daily insulin dose, divided by 24.

Determination of insulin delivery
In the FMPD algorithm, the gain factors determined the degree to which proportional or derivative errors led to changes in hormone delivery rates. There were separate gain factors for insulin and glucagon. Positive proportional errors (glucose level above target) and positive derivative errors (rising glucose level) called for an increase in the insulin delivery rate. The overall insulin delivery rate was determined by adding the rates called for by the proportional error (IIR_{pe}), the derivative error (IIR_{de}), and the basal insulin rate.

The proportional error gain factor was $1.2 \times 10^{-3} \pm 0.078 \times 10^{-3}$ units/kg per mg/dl/h for glucagon studies and 1.3×10^{-3} units/kg per mg/dl/h for placebo studies. The derivative error gain factor was $2.0 \times 10^{-3} \pm 0.096 \times 10^{-3}$ units/kg per mg/dl for glucagon studies and was 2.0×10^{-3} units/kg per mg/dl for placebo studies. The mean blood glucose target was 110 ± 1 mg/dl for glucagon studies and 110 mg/dl for placebo studies. There were no significant differences between any of these parameters between the groups. For subjects who underwent two closed-loop studies, the algorithm parameters were identical for both.

Insulin on board, the amount of insulin that had been delivered and was assumed to be active, was continually estimated using a model that we derived from data published by Holmes et al. (12). To minimize hypoglycemia, the insulin infusion was discontinued if the estimated insulin on board reached 15% of the subject's estimated total daily insulin requirement.

Determination of glucagon delivery
The proportional and derivative error gain factors for glucagon were negative, such that negative proportional and derivative errors called for an increase in the glucagon rate. For glucagon, the average weighted proportional error was calculated over a 15 min interval and the average weighted derivative error was calculated over a 10 min interval. There was no basal glucagon infusion rate.

In this project, we tested two closely related algorithms for administering glucagon. Four subjects completed 9-h studies and two subjects completed 28-h studies with low-gain factor settings. In these low-gain glucagon studies, the mean proportional error gain factor was -0.23 ± 0.04 ml/kg per mg/dl/h, the

mean derivative error gain factor was -0.06 ± 0.009 ml/kg per mg/dl, and target glucose for glucagon infusion was 108 ± 3 mg/dl. Two subjects completed 9-h studies and five subjects completed 28-h studies with high-gain factor settings. For all of these high-gain glucagon studies, the proportional error gain factor was -2.70 ml/kg per mg/dl/hour, the derivative gain factor was -0.60 ml/kg per mg/dl, and the target glucose for glucagon infusion was 97 ± 1 mg/dl. To avoid overdelivery of glucagon, when total glucagon delivery over the prior 50 min reached a ceiling of 1.0 μg/kg, the algorithm initiated a refractory period for the subsequent 50 min, during which glucagon could not be delivered. Thus, short pulses of glucagon delivery over 5–10 min were followed by the absence of glucagon delivery for 50 min. The insulin rate was reduced by 75% for 40 min after each maximal glucagon pulse.

Meals
Patients were given two meals during each 9-h study and four meals during each 28-h study. Each meal was announced to the controller and an open loop premeal bolus was given. Aspart insulin was given 0–10 min before meals, depending on the subject's premeal glucose level. For low-gain glucagon studies, $53.3 \pm 7.0\%$ of usual premeal insulin dose was given. The amount of premeal insulin was increased after the first four studies because of a pattern of postprandial hyperglycemia in those studies. For all placebo and high-gain glucagon studies, 75% of the usual premeal insulin dose was given.

Hypoglycemic treatment
Subjects were treated for hypoglycemia if the venous glucose value fell below 70 mg/dl. For glucose levels 60–69 mg/dl, subjects were given 15 g oral carbohydrate, and the treatment repeated as needed every 15 min. For a glucose value <60 mg/dl, 10 g dextrose was given intravenously.

Statistical analysis
Arterialized venous glucose values, not sensed glucose values, were used to compare hypoglycemia and glucose control between groups. Glucose area under the curve (AUC) was calculated as published elsewhere (13). Minutes in the hypoglycemic range, defined as glucose <70 mg/dl, hypoglycemic events, treatments for hypoglycemia, units of insulin delivered,

and micrograms of glucagon delivered were normalized to 24 h for data from both 9- and 28-h studies. Data are expressed as means $\pm$ SE. Sensor accuracy was calculated by comparing sensor glucose to reference glucose values (14). Comparisons were made using paired or unpaired t tests, as appropriate. Calculations were performed using Microsoft Excel 2007 (version 12).

RESULTS — Six women and seven men with type 1 diabetes participated in a total of 21 human closed-loop studies with a duration of 21.5 ± 2.0 h. Seven subjects received glucagon delivered in a brisk fashion (high-gain) and six subjects received glucagon delivered in a slower fashion (low-gain). In both the high- and low-gain glucagon studies, glucagon was typically delivered at times of impending hypoglycemia when glucose was 90–120 mg/dl, depending on the rate of glucose decline (Fig. 2). At these times, insulin delivery was also markedly reduced or discontinued by the insulin algorithm.

The high-gain glucagon results (paired analysis), low-gain glucagon results (unpaired analysis), and combined high- and low-gain glucagon results (unpaired analysis) are presented separately below. One subject who received high-gain glucagon but did not return for a placebo study was included in the combined results but was not included in the paired high-gain analysis.

High-gain glucagon results
In six subjects who underwent both a high-gain glucagon study and a placebo study, there was a 56% reduction in time spent in the hypoglycemic range (18 ± 11 vs. 41 ± 13 min/day, $P = 0.01$). The number of hypoglycemic events, with events lasting >20 min being considered a new event, was also significantly reduced during the high-gain glucagon versus placebo studies (1.0 ± 0.6 vs. 2.1 ± 0.6 events/day, $P = 0.01$), as was the number of oral or intravenous carbohydrate treatments for hypoglycemia (1.4 ± 0.8 vs. 4.0 ± 1.4 treatments/day, $P = 0.01$). There was no significant difference in mean glucose between the high-gain glucagon versus placebo studies (138 ± 17 vs. 131 ± 17 mg/dl, $P = NS$), as shown in Fig. 3A. The mean fasting glucose was also quite similar (123 ± 14 vs. 120 ± 15 mg/dl, $P = NS$). There was a nonsignificant trend toward a higher postprandial glucose in high-gain glucagon versus placebo studies, defined as mean value

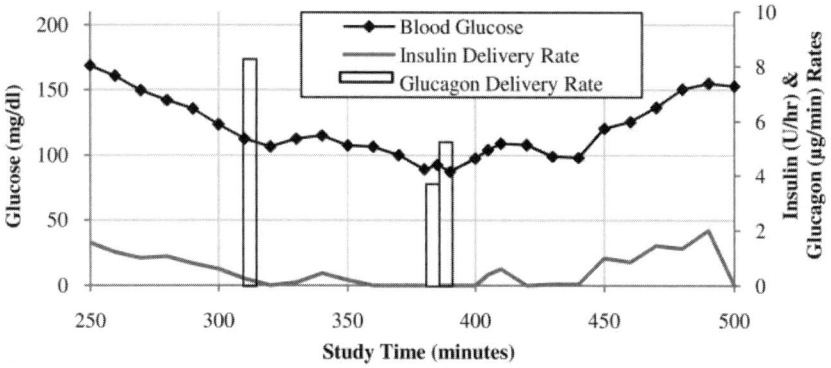

Figure 2—*Example of data taken from a closed-loop study. Venous blood glucose is noted by black diamonds, insulin delivery rate by a gray line, and glucagon delivery rate by rectangles. Note that glucagon is delivered by algorithm in the late postprandial period at times of impending hypoglycemia. Overt hypoglycemia is avoided without the use of carbohydrate supplementation.*

0–180 min after meals (157 ± 18 vs. 144 ± 17 mg/dl, P = NS). The amount of insulin delivered during the high-gain glucagon versus placebo studies was nearly identical (48.9 ± 6.2 vs. 48.3 ± 5.5 units per day, P = NS).

Low-gain glucagon results
In six subjects who received low-gain glucagon compared with the eight subjects who received placebo, there was a nonsignificant reduction in time in the hypoglycemic range (15 ± 8 vs. 40 ± 10 min/day,

P = NS). There was also a trend toward a reduction in the number of hypoglycemic events that did not reach statistical significance (1.4 ± 0.7 vs. 2.3 ± 0.5 events/day, P = NS). There was a reduction in the number of treatments for hypoglycemia in studies with low-gain glucagon of borderline significance (1.0 ± 0.7 vs. 3.9 ± 1.0 treatments/day, P = 0.05). Mean glucose was somewhat higher in low-gain glucagon versus placebo studies (157 ± 24 vs. 135 ± 16 mg/dl, P = 0.04). There was also a trend toward higher fasting glucose in the low-gain glucagon versus placebo studies (137 ± 20 vs. 122 ± 13 mg/dl, P = NS). There was a similar trend, of borderline statistical significance, suggesting a larger elevation in postprandial glucose in the low-gain glucagon versus placebo studies (179 ± 26 vs. 151 ± 18 mg/dl, P = 0.05). There was a nonsignificant difference in insulin delivered in low-gain glucagon versus placebo studies (60.1 ± 14.1 vs. 46.9 ± 5.5 units/day). The mean dose of glucagon delivered during the low-gain glucagon studies was higher than the high-gain glucagon studies but did not reach statistical significance (746 ± 134 vs. 516 ± 108 μg/day, P = NS).

Combined high- and low-gain glucagon results
Glucagon, when given either via high- or low-gain, compared with placebo, led to a 63% reduction of time spent in the hypoglycemic range (15 ± 6 vs. 40 ± 10 min/day, P = 0.04). The number of hypoglycemic events per day was not significantly different between glucagon versus placebo studies (1.1 ± 0.4 vs. 2.3 ± 0.5 events/day, P = NS). The number of treatments for hypoglycemia per day was considerably reduced in the glucagon versus placebo studies (1.1 ± 0.5 vs. 3.9 ± 1.0 treatments/day, P = 0.01). Mean glucose was somewhat higher in the glucagon studies, but this increase did not reach statistical significance (145 ± 14 vs. 135 ± 16 mg/dl, P = NS). Other metrics of glycemic control, including percent of AUC in the target (70–180 mg/dl) and hyperglycemic (>180 mg/dl) ranges and mean amplitude of glycemic excursions were not significantly different between the groups (data not shown).

Sensor accuracy
Overall sensor accuracy was very good, with combined MARD of 8.7 ± 1.5% and MAD of 13.3 ± 1.5 mg/dl. Sensors were calibrated on average every 5.7 ± 0.5 h.

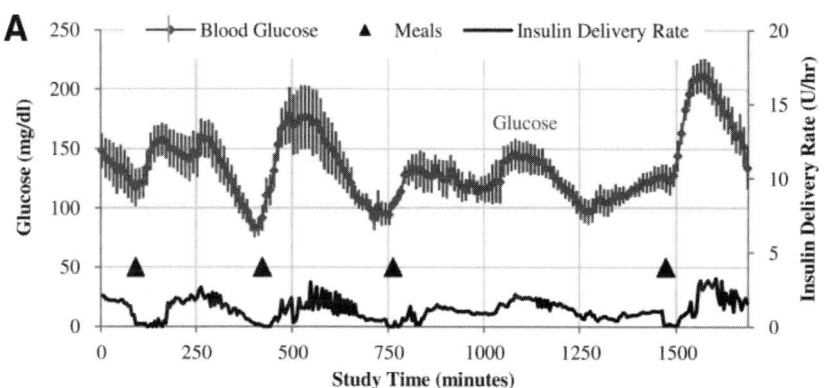

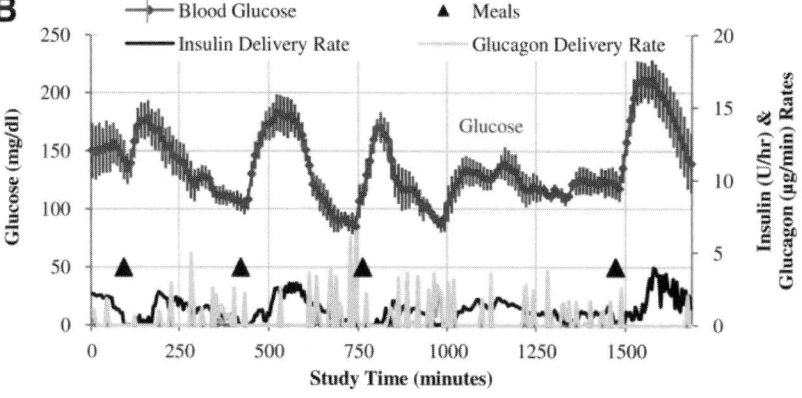

Figure 3—*Summary of glucose levels (means ± SE), insulin delivery rate, and, for glucagon studies, the glucagon delivery rate. Venous blood glucose is noted by gray diamonds, insulin delivery rate by a black line, glucagon delivery rate by a light gray line, and meals by black triangles. A: Composite of eight insulin plus placebo studies. B: Composite of seven insulin plus high-gain glucagon studies. Insulin delivery and overall glycemic control were similar in both conditions.*

In 8.6% of cases, venous blood, rather than sensed, glucose values were sent to the controller due to suboptimal sensor accuracy.

Tolerability

Only one subject developed transient nausea and vomiting after receiving 350 µg glucagon over 175 min during a low-gain glucagon study. No subjects in the high-gain glucagon or placebo studies experienced any side effects.

CONCLUSIONS — In this automated glycemic control system, we compared the effect of subcutaneous glucagon, delivered in small doses at times of impending hypoglycemia, to saline placebo. In both conditions, the algorithm called for a significant reduction or discontinuation of insulin delivery during impending hypoglycemia. We found that compared with placebo, glucagon delivered in pulses using high-gain parameters significantly decreased the time spent in the hypoglycemic range, the number of hypoglycemic events, and the number of treatments needed for hypoglycemia. Only the high-gain, not the low-gain, glucagon delivery system was superior to placebo in reducing all three of these outcomes, despite the fact that a lower amount of glucagon was delivered in the high-gain studies. The high-gain glucagon infusion consisted of a pulse of glucagon typically given over 5–10 min at a time of impending hypoglycemia followed by a 50-min off period. The low-gain glucagon was delivered in a slow, more prolonged manner without a mandatory off period. The high-gain glucagon infusion is arguably more physiologic, as glucagon is secreted rapidly in response to hypoglycemia in humans without diabetes (15).

Minimizing glucagon delivery, as described here, is important to avoid potential side effects, such as acute hyperglycemia and nausea, and more severe effects, such as depletion of liver glycogen. Notably, the mean glucose levels in the high-gain glucagon and placebo studies were very similar. However, larger and longer-term studies will be required to assess the effect of ongoing glucagon treatment on overall glycemic control.

Limitations of this study include the absence of paired studies for some individuals. In addition, the lower amount of premeal insulin in the low-gain glucagon studies compared with the placebo studies may have affected the results, in particular the differences in mean and postprandial glucose levels. In some regards, the need to announce the meal to the controller and the delivery of substantial amounts of premeal insulin might also be considered a limitation. A true closed-loop system without meal announcement using currently available insulin preparations delivered subcutaneously is unlikely to provide optimal blood glucose control.

After reconstitution, glucagon forms fibrils over time (16,17) and is currently approved for use only immediately after reconstitution. Despite the occurrence of fibrils and aggregates, our group (9) and El-Khatib et al. (18) have shown that even when glucagon is aged for 1 week at room or body temperature, large doses retain full hyperglycemic activity in animals. The reason that the aggregated form of glucagon retains its physiologic effect is unclear. It is possible that, after injection, the aggregates dissociate into monomeric form in the subcutaneous space.

There is some evidence that glucagon can be cytotoxic if it is "aged" at very high concentrations (19), but there are no reports of cytotoxicity during aging at concentrations of 1 mg/ml or lower. Further studies are needed to examine the efficacy of glucagon used for several days after reconstitution and to assess potential cytotoxicity at clinically appropriate concentrations. It is possible that aggregation may be overcome using glucagon analogs (20) or novel methods of glucagon preparation (21).

In conclusion, we found that glucagon given to subjects with type 1 diabetes by algorithm during impending hypoglycemia is effective in preventing most cases of hypoglycemia. Glycemic control was good in this study, in part due to open-loop insulin delivery before meals. These results suggest that an automated system of closed-loop glucagon delivery, with a hybrid pattern of insulin delivery including meal announcement, is able to control glycemia safely and effectively in people with type 1 diabetes. There is a need for further research into the issue of glucagon stability and for the development of a fully automated insulin and glucagon delivery device.

Acknowledgments — This work was supported by grants from the Juvenile Diabetes Research Foundation, Good Samaritan Foundation (Portland, OR), and the National Institutes of Health (NIH) (grant T32 DK007674). We also thank the staff and research subjects who carried out these studies at the Oregon Clinical and Translational Research Institute (OCTRI), which is supported by grant no. UL1 RR024140 from the National Center for Research Resources, a component of NIH, and the NIH Roadmap for Medical Research.

No potential conflicts of interest relevant to this article were reported.

We thank Jillian Hansen for her technical support.

References
1. Cryer PE, Davis SN, Shamoon H. Hypoglycemia in diabetes. Diabetes Care 2003; 26:1902–1912
2. Cryer PE. Hypoglycaemia: the limiting factor in the glycaemic management of type I and type II diabetes. Diabetologia 2002;45:937–948
3. Steil GM, Rebrin K, Darwin C, Hariri F, Saad MF. Feasibility of automating insulin delivery for the treatment of type 1 diabetes. Diabetes 2006;55:3344–3350
4. El Youssef JE, Castle J, Ward WK. A review of closed-loop algorithms for glycemic control in the treatment of type 1 diabetes. Algorithms 2009;2:518–532
5. Graf CJ, Woodworth JR, Seger ME, Holcombe JH, Bowsher RR, Lynch R. Pharmacokinetic and glucodynamic comparisons of recombinant and animal-source glucagon after IV, IM, and SC injection in healthy volunteers J Pharm Sci 1999;88:991–995
6. Hartley M, Thomsett MJ, Cotterill AM. Mini-dose glucagon rescue for mild hypoglycaemia in children with type 1 diabetes: the Brisbane experience. J Paediatr Child Health 2006;42:108–111
7. Haymond MW, Schreiner B. Mini-dose glucagon rescue for hypoglycemia in children with type 1 diabetes. Diabetes Care 2001;24:643–645
8. Shichiri M, Kawamori R, Yamasaki Y, Hakui N, Abe H. Wearable artificial endocrine pancreas with needle-type glucose sensor. Lancet 1982;2:1129–1131
9. Ward WK, Engle J, Duman HM, Bergstrom CP, Sonia FK, Federiuk IF. The benefit of subcutaneous glucagon during closed-loop glycemic control in rats with type 1 diabetes. IEEE Sensors J 2008;8:89–96
10. El-Khatib FH, Jiang J, Damiano ER. Adaptive closed-loop control provides blood-glucose regulation using dual subcutaneous insulin and glucagon infusion in diabetic Swine. J Diabetes Sci Technol 2007;1:181–192
11. Gopakumaran B, Duman HM, Overholser DP, Federiuk IF, Quinn MJ, Wood MD, Ward WK. A novel insulin delivery algorithm in rats with type 1 diabetes: the fading memory proportional-derivative method. Artif Organs 2005;29:599–607
12. Holmes G, Galitz L, Hu P, Lyness W. Pharmacokinetics of insulin aspart in obesity, renal impairment, or hepatic impair-

ment. Br J Clin Pharmacol 2005;60:469–476

13. Food and Agriculture Organization. Carbohydrates in human nutrition, Food and Agriculture Organization [article online], 1998. Available from http://www.fao.org/docrep/w8079e/w8079e0a.htm. Accessed 15 April 2010

14. Clinical and Laboratory Standards Institute. Performance metrics for continuous interstitial glucose monitoring: approved guideline, Clinical and Laboratory Standards Institute [article online], 2008. Available from http://www.clsi.org/source/orders/free/poct05-A.pdf. Accessed 15 April 2010

15. Bolli G, De Feo P, Perriello G, De Cosmo S, Compagnucci P, Santeusanio F, Brunetti P, Unger RH. Mechanisms of gluca-gon secretion during insulin-induced hypoglycemia in man: role of the beta cell and arterial hyperinsulinemia J Clin Invest 1984;73:917–922

16. Pedersen JS, Dikov D, Flink JL, Hjuler HA, Christiansen G, Otzen DE. The changing face of glucagon fibrillation: structural polymorphism and conformational imprinting. J Mol Biol 2006;355:501–523

17. De Jong KL, Incledon B, Yip CM, DeFelippis MR. Amyloid fibrils of glucagon characterized by high-resolution atomic force microscopy. Biophys J 2006;91:1905–1914

18. El-Khatib FH, Jiang J, Gerrity RG, Damiano ER. Pharmacodynamics and stability of subcutaneously infused glucagon in a type 1 diabetic Swine model in vivo. Diabetes Technol Ther 2007;9:135–144

19. Onoue S, Ohshima K, Debari K, Koh K, Shioda S, Iwasa S, Kashimoto K, Yajima T. Mishandling of the therapeutic peptide glucagon generates cytotoxic amyloidogenic fibrils. Pharm Res 2004;21:1274–1283

20. Li P, Rogers T, Smiley D, DiMarchi RD, Zhang F. Design, synthesis and crystallization of a novel glucagon analog as a therapeutic agent. Acta Crystallogr Sect F Struct Biol Cryst Commun 2007;63:599–601

21. Matilainen L, Maunu SL, Pajander J, Auriola S, Jaaskelainen I, Larsen KL, Jarvinen T, Jarho P. The stability and dissolution properties of solid glucagon/gamma-cyclodextrin powder. Eur J Pharmacol Sci 2009;36:412–420

OBSERVATIONS

Long-Term Effect of an Education Program (HyPOS) on the Incidence of Severe Hypoglycemia in Patients With Type 1 Diabetes

A new education program for treating diabetic patients with hypoglycemia problems, named HyPOS, was developed and evaluated in a randomized controlled trial. The present study investigated the long-term effect of HyPOS on the prospectively assessed incidence of severe hypoglycemia defined as an episode requiring medical assistance by injection of glucose intravenously or glucagon intramuscularly.

HyPOS comprises five lessons of 90 min each over 5 weeks. The program informs about the vicious cycle of frequent hypoglycemia increasing the risk for future hypoglycemia (1,2). Patients were trained in symptom awareness by using diaries and performing blood glucose estimation. The control group consists of four 90-min sessions over 4 weeks. Both interventions were described in more detail previously (3). After 6 months, patients receiving HyPOS improved hypoglycemia awareness compared with control subjects (3).

The incidence of severe hypoglycemia at a 31-month follow-up was compared with the retrospectively assessed prevalence at baseline in the previous 12 months. Patients were asked about the occurrence of severe hypoglycemia at each visit in the study center. When an episode of severe hypoglycemia was reported, the patients were contacted by telephone to verify the hypoglycemic episode. The telephone interview was conducted by a person who was not aware of the patient's group assignment.

The sample was recruited at 23 outpatient study centers. Of 164 randomized patients, 140 (85.3%) type 1 diabetic patients (aged 46.0 ± 12.5 years, 50% female, A1C 7.3 ± 1.0%, disease duration 21.4 ± 10.9 years, 41% with continuous subcutaneous insulin infusion therapy, 4.9 ± 1.1 injections/day, BMI 25.4 ± 3.7 kg/m^2, and insulin dosage 0.54 ± 0.18 IU/kg) were reassessed after a 31-month follow-up period. At baseline the prevalences of severe hypoglycemia were 0.8 ± 1.5 and 0.7 ± 1.05 episodes/patient-year in the control group and HyPOS, respectively. The incidence of severe hypoglycemia was lower in HyPOS than in the control group (0.1 ± 0.2 vs. 0.2 ± 0.4 episodes/patient-year; $P = 0.04$). The reduction of severe hypoglycemia from baseline to follow-up was 0.5 ± 0.3 events per patient-year in the control group and 0.6 ± 0.3 events per patient-year in HyPOS ($P = 0.042$, adjusted for baseline differences). In the control group, 26.5% of the patients experienced at least one severe hypoglycemic episode compared with 12.5% in HyPOS (odds ratio 0.4 [95% CI 0.2–0.9]; $P = 0.04$). There were no significant differences between the control group and HyPOS with regard to glycemic control (A1C 7.3 ± 1.1 vs. 7.1 ± 0.9%; $P = 0.18$) or treatment factors (insulin dosage, number of injections, use of insulin pump, or use of insulin analogs) at the follow-up measurement. The HyPOS program can contribute to better treatment of diabetic patients who have hypoglycemia problems.

Norbert Hermanns, phd[1]
Bernd Kulzer, phd[1]
Michael Krichbaum, ma[1]
Thomas Kubiak, phd[2]
Thomas Haak, md[1]

From the [1]Research Institute of the Diabetes Academy Mergentheim (Forschungsinstitut der Diabetes Akademie Mergentheim [FIDAM]), Bad Mergentheim, Germany; and the [2]University of Greifswald, Institute of Psychology, Greifswald, Germany.
Corresponding author: Norbert Hermanns, hermanns@diabetes-zentrum.de.
DOI: 10.2337/dc09-1656

Acknowledgments— Berlin-Chemie, Germany, funded the development of HyPOS and supported the evaluation study by a restricted educational grant. N.H., B.K., and T.K. received reimbursement from Berlin-Chemie for organizing and conducting additional training courses related to HyPOS. No other potential conflicts of interest relevant to this article were reported.

● ● ● ● ● ● ● ● ● ● ● ● ● ● ● ● ● ● ● ●

References
1. Cryer PE. Hypoglycemia: the limiting factor in the glycaemic management of type I and type II Diabetes. Diabetologia 2002; 45:937–948
2. Cryer PE, Davis SN, Shamoon H. Hypoglycemia in diabetes. Diabetes Care 2003; 26:1902–1912
3. Hermanns N, Kulzer B, Kubiak T, Krichbaum M, Haak T. The effect of an education programme (HyPOS) to treat hypoglycaemia problems in patients with type 1 diabetes. Diabete Metab Res Rev 2007;23:528–538

The Medial Amygdalar Nucleus: A Novel Glucose-Sensing Region That Modulates the Counterregulatory Response to Hypoglycemia

Ligang Zhou,[1] Nina Podolsky,[2] Zhen Sang,[1] Yuyan Ding,[1] Xiaoning Fan,[1] Qingchun Tong,[3] Barry E. Levin,[2] and Rory J. McCrimmon[1,4]

OBJECTIVE—To determine whether the medial amygdalar nucleus (MAN) represents a novel brain glucose-sensing region involved in the detection of hypoglycemia and generation of a counterregulatory hormone response.

RESEARCH DESIGN AND METHODS—Fura-2 calcium imaging was used to assess glucose responsivity in neurons isolated from the MAN and single-cell real-time reverse transcription PCR used to examine gene expression within glucose-responsive neurons. In vivo studies with local MAN perfusion of the glucoprivic agent, 2-deoxyglucose (2-DG), under normal and hypoglycemic conditions and also after MAN lesioning with ibotenic acid, were used to examine the functional role of MAN glucose sensors. In addition, retrograde neuronal tracer studies were used to examine reciprocal pathways between the MAN and the ventromedial hypothalamus (VMH).

RESULTS—The MAN contains a population of glucose-sensing neurons (13.5%), which express glucokinase, and the selective urocortin 3 (UCN3) receptor CRH-R2, but not UCN3 itself. Lesioning the MAN suppressed, whereas 2-DG infusion amplified, the counterregulatory response to hyperinsulinemic hypoglycemia in vivo. However, 2-DG infusion to the MAN or VMH under normoglycemic conditions had no systemic effect. The VMH is innervated by UCN3 neurons that arise mainly from the MAN, and ~1/3 of MAN UCN3 neurons are active during mild hypoglycemia.

CONCLUSIONS—The MAN represents a novel limbic glucose-sensing region that contains characteristic glucokinase-expressing glucose-sensing neurons that respond directly to manipulations of glucose availability both in vitro and in vivo. Moreover, UCN3 neurons may provide feedback inhibitory regulation of the counterregulatory response through actions within the VMH and the MAN. *Diabetes* **59:2646–2652, 2010**

From the [1]Department of Internal Medicine, Yale University, New Haven, Connecticut; the [2]VA Medical Center, Neurology Service, East Orange, New Jersey; the [3]Department of Internal Medicine, Beth Israel Deaconness Medical Center, Boston, Massachusetts; and the [4]Biomedical Research Institute, University of Dundee, Dundee, Scotland.
Corresponding author: Rory J. McCrimmon, r.mccrimmon@dundee.ac.uk.
Received 7 July 2009 and accepted 5 July 2010. Published ahead of print at http://diabetes.diabetesjournals.org on 13 July 2010. DOI: 10.2337/db09-0995.

In some patients with type 1 (and 2) diabetes, the ability to detect and respond to hypoglycemia is markedly impaired (1). Specialized glucose-sensing neurons exist within discrete regions of the brain and are thought to have a particular role in the regulation of glucose homeostasis. Glucose-excited neurons increase their activity as glucose levels rise, and glucose-inhibited neurons increase their activity as glucose levels fall (2,3). The mechanisms used by glucose-excited neurons to detect a fall in the glucose level to which they are exposed are thought to resemble those used by the classical glucose sensor, the pancreatic β-cell, with in particular roles for glucokinase and the ATP-sensitive potassium channel (K_{ATP}) (1), while glucose-inhibited neurons also use glucokinase, as well as nitric oxide and adenosine 5′-monophosphate-activated protein kinase to modulate their glucose sensing (4–6). Glucose-sensing neurons are located in a number of brain regions, although only those present in the ventromedial (VMH) (7–9), dorsomedial, and paraventricular hypothalamus (10,11) to date have been shown in vivo, in rodent models, to modulate counterregulatory responses during insulin-induced hypoglycemia.

We have recently shown that urocortin 3 (UCN3), a member of the corticotrophin-releasing hormone (CRH) family of neuropeptides, and a selective ligand for the CRH-R2 receptor, may regulate the magnitude of the counterregulatory response to hypoglycemia through actions in the VMH (12,13). UCN3 nerve terminals provide a dense innervation to the shell of the VMH and tubercle area (14). The cell bodies of UCN3 neurons are found predominantly in the medial amygdalar nucleus (MAN), the hypothalamic medial preoptic nucleus, and the rostral perifornical area lateral to the paraventricular hypothalamic nucleus (14). Intriguingly, the pancreatic isoform of glucokinase, the rate-limiting step of glucose oxidation and a key step in the glucose-sensing mechanism (2,6), is also expressed in the MAN (15). This study examined the hypothesis that the MAN may represent a novel central glucose-sensing region and, moreover, that it might be directly linked with the VMH via UCN3 neurons.

RESEARCH DESIGN AND METHODS

Male Sprague-Dawley rats (mean ± SEM wt, 305 ± 4 g) were housed in the local Animal Resource Center with water and chow pellet available ad libitum. The animal care and experimental protocols were reviewed and approved by Yale University Institutional Animal Care and Use Committee and the Institutional Animal Care and Use Committee of the East Orange Veterans Affairs Medical Center.

Animal surgery. The surgical procedures used in this study have been described in detail elsewhere (8,16). In brief, one week prior to each study, all animals were anesthetized with an intraperitoneal injection (1 ml/kg) of a mixture of xyzaline (20 mg/ml; AnaSed, Lloyd Laboratories Inc.) and ketamine (100 mg/ml; Ketaset, Wyeth) at a ratio of 1:2 (vol/vol). Vascular catheters [PE50 tubing with a tip made from silastic laboratory tubing (0.51 mm inner diameter)] were inserted via a neck incision into the internal jugular vein and carotid artery. After catheter implantation, cannula guides were stereotaxically inserted, bilaterally to the MAN (coordinates from bregma, anterior-posterior [AP] = −2.80 mm, medio-lateral [ML] = ±3.3 mm, and dorso-ventral [DV] = 8.9 mm at an angle of 90°) or VMH (coordinates AP = −2.6 mm; ML = ±0.5 mm; DV = 9.4 mm). Guide cannula were designed to reach a point 1 mm proximal to the target nucleus, limiting gliosis in the region where microinjection would take place 7 days after guide catheter insertion.

Lesion study. At the initial surgery, as described above, and instead of guide cannula insertion, each rat received bilateral microinjections to the MAN of 2 pg of ibotenic acid ($n = 6$) using a 1 μl Hamilton syringe (total volume 200 nl over 30 min), after which the skin was closed with wound clips. Sham-lesion rats received the identical surgical procedure but were administered saline rather than ibotenic acid ($n = 9$).

Normoglycemic study. Seven days after surgery, overnight fasted rats had their catheters opened and were allowed to acclimatize over 90 min. Bilateral 26-guage injection needles, designed to extend 1 mm beyond the tip of the guide cannula, were then inserted into each MAN or VMH, and each rat received bilateral microinfusions (1 μl given at a rate of 0.033 μl/min for 30 min) of 10 mmol/l 2-deoxyglucose (2-DG), a nonmetabolizable form of glucose that creates local glucopenia, or artificial extracellular fluid (aECF), depending on the study. Venous samples for measurement of plasma glucose were taken every 10 min and for glucagon and epinephrine preinjection ($t = 0$ min) and at 30 and 60 min after microinjection.

Hyperinsulinemic hypoglycemic study. A modified hyperinsulinemic glucose clamp was used to produce a standardized hypoglycemic stimulus, as described previously (17). Thirty min after bilateral MAN microinfusions of 2-DG ($n = 6$) or artificial aECF ($n = 9$), a constant 20 mU/kg/min infusion of insulin (Human Regular Insulin, Lilly, IL) was started. Both solutions were mixed with 4% wheat germ agglutinin (WGA) to confirm the location of microinjection (supplementary Fig. 1, available in an online appendix at http://diabetes.diabetesjournals.org/cgi/content/full/db09-0995/DC1). The plasma glucose was allowed to fall to 70 mg/dl (∼3.9 mmol/l), where it was maintained for 90 min using 20% dextrose, with the dextrose infusion rate adjusted every 5 min based on plasma glucose determinations. Blood samples for measurement of epinephrine, glucagon, and insulin were taken at 0, 60, and 90 min. Plasma glucose was measured by glucose oxidase method (Glucose Direct; Analox Instruments, Lunenberg, MA). Catecholamine analysis was performed by high-performance liquid chromatography using electrochemical detections (ESA, Acton, MA); plasma insulin and glucagon were measured by radioimmunoassay (Millipore, Temecula, CA).

Retrograde neuronal tracer studies. The retrograde tracing technique has been described previously (18). Briefly, each rat was microinjected bilaterally to the VMH or MAN (coordinates as above) with the retrograde neuronal tracer WGA or 4% fluorogold dissolved in aECF and delivered through a glass micropipette with tip diameter 10–15 μm by passing 2-μA positive current pulse (7 s on/off) for <10 min. The rats were then allowed to recover for 7 days before undergoing a 90-min hyperinsulinemic (20 mU/kg/min) hypoglycemic (70 mg/dl) or hyperinsulinemic euglycemic (120 mg/dl) clamp, as described above.

Immunohistochemistry. The immunohistochemistry protocol used has been described in detail previously (18,19). Briefly, analysis was performed on every six 40-μm-thick frontal sections. Sections were washed in PBS for 10 min and then pretreated in 0.3% H_2O_2 for 1 h to block endogenous peroxidase. They were then incubated overnight at room temperature with 1:1,000 rabbit anti-UCN antibody (1:2000; a gift from Dr. W. Vale) in 0.3% fresh normal donkey serum, goat anti-WGA (1:1,000; Vector) and PBT-azide (0.02% sodium azide and 0.04% Triton X-100 in PBS). The next day, sections were incubated with biotinylated donkey anti-rabbit antibody (Jackson Laboratories; 1:500) for 1 h, followed by incubation with a cocktail of Alexa Fluor 594-conjugated Streptavidin (Molecular Probes, Eugene, OR; 1:1K) and Alexa Fluor 488-conjugated chicken anti-goat antibody (1:400) for 1 h. After mounting on polylysine slides, the sections were cover-slipped with antifade mount medium for fluorescence (Vectashield, Vector, CA). Dual fluorescence images in the MAN from the representative brain were taken with a digital camera. Counting of dual staining for UCN3 and WGA was performed in three brains. All single-labeled UCN3 neurons and dual-labeled neurons for UCN3 and WGA in the MAN were counted. Cytoarchitectonic areas in the amygdala were determined with reference to the atlas of Paxinos and Watson (20). Light-microscope images in the MAN and its adjacent regions from a representative brain were taken with a digital camera. The digital images were arranged in

the software Canvas (Deneba System, Miami, FL). The border of the MAN, its adjacent structures, and distribution of single labeling of UCN3 neurons were drawn using Canvas software. For triple staining, immunofluorescence serial sections from the brains of fluorogold-injected rats were incubated overnight with a mixture of 1 μg/ml anti-Fos goat antibody (1:1K; Santa Cruz) and anti-UCN3 rabbit serum (1:2,000). After a rinse with PBS-X, the sections were incubated for 1 h with 10 g/ml biotinylated anti-rabbit IgG donkey antibody (Jackson) and then for 1 h with a mixture of 1 μg/ml Alexa488-conjugated chicken anti-goat antibody (1:400; Molecular Probes) and 1 μg/ml Alexa594 Streptavidin-conjugated antibody (Molecular Probes). Sections were observed under an epifluorescence microscope Olympus BX-50 with appropriate filter sets for Alexa488 (excitation, 450–490 nm; emission, 514–565 nm); Alexa594 (excitation, 530–585 nm; emission, ≥615 nm) and fluorogold (excitation, 359–371 nm; emission, 397–590 nm). Although Alexa488 fluorescence could be partially seen with the filter set for fluorogold, Fos-immunoreactive neuropil with Alexa488 fluorescence was easily differentiated from retrograde labeled cell bodies with fluorogold fluorescence. The counting of triple staining for UCN3, Fos, and fluorogold was performed in three brains. All single-labeled UCN3 neurons and dual-labeled and triple-labeled neurons in the MAN were counted.

MAN mRNA assays by quantitative real-time PCR. Frozen brains were cut on a cryostat at −12°C and placed in RNAlater (Ambion, Foster City, CA) until being micropunched. Micropunches of the MAN were performed by modifications of the method of Palkovits (21), where brain micropunches are made under microscope guidance from brain slices placed on the base of a stereotaxic frame. Micropunched brain areas were sonicated in a guanidinium thiocyanate solution and purified using magnetic beads (Ambion MagMax-96). Quantitation of mRNA was carried out by real-time quantitative PCR (QPCR) as previously described (22). Primer sets for each mRNA were designed by reference to published sequences, and their specificity was verified using Genebank. Primers and their sequence-specific FAM-labeled probes prepared by Applied Biosystems were sequenced and then quantified with an Applied Biosystems 7,700 real-time PCR system set for 40 PCR cycles. Standard curves were generated from serially diluted pooled samples for each probe and for constitutively expressed mRNA (cyclophilin) to control for differences in amplification efficiency and micropunch size. Results were calculated from the standard curves relative to cyclophilin mRNA levels in the same samples.

Fura-2 calcium imaging to assess glucose-induced changes in intracellular calcium ($[Ca^{2+}]_i$) oscillations. Studies were carried out in 3–4 week old male Sprague-Dawley rats (Charles River). The MAN punched cells were dissociated with papain (2 mg/ml, 30 min, 37°C) and mechanically triturated. Cells were plated onto cover slips and allowed to adhere for 60 min before loading with the Ca^{2+} fluorophore fura-2 acetoxy methyl ester (Molecular Probes) for 20 min in Hank's balanced salt solution buffer containing 2.5 mmol/l glucose, washed twice, and transferred to a microscope chamber held at 37°C. Fura-2 fluorescent images were acquired every 5 s by alternating excitation at 340 and 380 nm using a cooled, charge-coupled device camera at 420–600 nm emission. Changes in glucose were maintained for ∼10 min after addition. Cells were classified as glucose-responsive in >500 neurons by significant ($[Ca^{2+}]_i$) fluctuations (as area under the curve) after changes in glucose concentrations using Origin 7.0 software (OriginLab). Neurons were classified as glucose-excited, glucose-inhibited, and nonglucosensing, as previously described (7). Cytoplasms of individual characterized neurons were then collected for single-cell QPCR (sc-QPCR) as previously described (23); analysis was according to previous standards.

sc-QPCR. After characterization by Ca^{2+} imaging, cytoplasmic mRNA of individually imaged cells was analyzed by sc-QPCR. Cytoplasm from each neuron was aspirated into a micropipette that was prefilled with DEPC-treated water containing 1 μl RN_{ASE} OUT RNase inhibitor (Invitrogen, Carlsbad, CA). Subsequently, synthesis was performed with Superscript II first-strand synthesis kit (Invitrogen) following the manufacturer's directions. The RT reaction was incubated at 42°C for 50 min after heat inactivation at 70°C. cDNA was purified to completely remove inhibitory RT components by slight modification of the methods described by Liss (24). After the purification of single-cell cDNA, QPCR was performed using specific primers. Glial fibrillary acidic protein was used to exclude astrocytes, and β-actin was used as an internal control for constitutively expressed mRNA. Primer sequences were designed using Biology WorkBench Primer design software. Amplification was carried out in a LightCycler (Roche Perkin-Elmer, Foster City, CA), using 40 cycles (95°C, 1 s; 56–63°C, 2 s; and 68°C, 30 s) with Advantage 2 Polymerase Mix (BD Biosciences, Palo Alto, CA). Amplified products were run directly on a 1.5% agarose gel and visualized by ethidium bromide staining. Gels were imaged and photo inverted for presentation. To optimize conditions for primer amplification and standardize for the linearity of the amplification process, hypothalamic cDNA was used.

For glucagon and epinephrine, differences between treatments were assessed via repeated-measures ANOVA and based on hormonal readings

TABLE 1
Glucose-responsive MAN neurons

Neuron	Number	Percentage
GE	32/522	6%
GI	39/522	7.5%
NG	449/522	86.5%

Fura-2 calcium imaging was used to measure changes in $[Ca^{2+}]_i$ oscillations while varying glucose concentrations 2.5 to 0.5 to 2.5 mmol/l glucose in neurons isolated from the MAN. GE, glucose-excited neuron; GI, glucose-inhibited neuron; NG, glucose-unresponsive neuron.

at 0, 60, and 90 min. Post hoc analysis was made using Bonferroni testing. Mean data were compared using a two-tailed Student t test. For all analyses, significance was assigned at the $P \leq 0.05$ level. Data are presented as mean ± SEM.

RESULTS

The MAN contains glucose-sensing neurons. Of 522 individual MAN neurons examined using fura-2 calcium imaging, 13.5% were glucose-sensing (Table 1). Six percent were glucose-excited, and 7.5% were glucose-inhibited (Fig. 1). By sc-QPCR, 54% of glucose-excited, 42% of glucose-inhibited, and 9% of nonglucosensing MAN neurons expressed glucokinase (Table 2). However, UCN3 was isolated from only 2, 16, and 4% of the glucose-excited, glucose-inhibited, and nonglucosensing neurons, respectively.

Glucokinase, CRH-R2, and UCN3 show different spatial relationships within the MAN. Having shown that only a minority of glucose-sensing neurons contained mRNA for UCN3, quantitative real-time PCR was used to examine the spatial distribution of glucokinase, UCN3, and CRH-R2 mRNA expression in MAN micropunches. A rostrocaudal gradient in glucokinase, UCN3, and CRH-R2 gene expression in the MAN was seen. Both glucokinase and CRH-R2 expression showed a similar rostrocaudal distribution, whereas UCN3 showed the opposite rostrocaudal distribution in the MAN (supplementary Fig. 2, available in an online appendix).

Lesioning the MAN results in a suppressed counterregulatory hormonal response to acute hypoglycemia. To examine whether the MAN contributed to the generation of a counterregulatory response during acute hypoglycemia in vivo, the MAN of male Sprague–Dawley rats was lesioned by direct microinjection of ibotenic acid.

TABLE 2
Glucokinase and UCN3 mRNA expression in glucose-excited, glucose-inhibited, and glucose-unresponsive neurons in the MAN identified by Fura-2 calcium imaging, revealed by single-cell RT-PCR

Neuron	Number	Co-expressing with GK	Co-expressing with UCN3
GE	46	54%	2%
GI	45	42%	16%
NG	23	9%	4%

GE, glucose-excited neuron; GI, glucose-inhibited neuron; GK, glucokinase; NG, glucose-unresponsive neuron.

During the subsequent hyperinsulinemic hypoglycemia study, plasma glucose levels did not differ between MAN lesioned and control rats (70 ± 1 vs. 69 ± 1 mg/dl, respectively; Fig. 2A). Glucose infusion rates (GIR) required to maintain the hypoglycemic plateau were ~18% higher in MAN-lesioned rats (mean GIR over 60–90 min, 24.7 ± 1.7 vs. 20.3 ± 1.4 mg/kg/min), although the overall interaction was not significant ($F = 4.0; P = 0.07$; Fig. 2B). However, MAN lesioning did result in significantly impaired plasma epinephrine ($F = 6.0, P < 0.05$) and glucagon ($F = 6.9, P < 0.05$) responses to the hypoglycemic challenge (Fig. 2C and D).

Localized glucoprivation in the MAN and VMH in the fasting state has no effect on glucose counterregulation. To determine whether the MAN might respond directly to a local glucoprivic challenge, the MAN was locally perfused with 2-DG over 30 min. MAN glucoprivation did not result in a significant rise in plasma glucose or change in plasma levels of glucagon and epinephrine (Table 3). Application of 2-DG at an identical concentration and rate to the VMH also failed to elicit a glucoprivic response (Table 3). Additional studies injecting 5-Thioglucose (a more potent glucoprivic agent) into the MAN or VMH also had no significant effect on glucose or counterregulatory hormones (data not shown).

MAN glucoprivation during mild systemic hypoglycemia amplifies the counterregulatory response. In contrast to the lack of effect of local MAN glucoprivation during euglycemia, comparable MAN glucoprivation during mild systemic hypoglycemia did alter the subsequent counterregulatory response. Despite equivalent hypoglycemia [mean (SEM) 60–90 min glucose levels, 70 ± 2

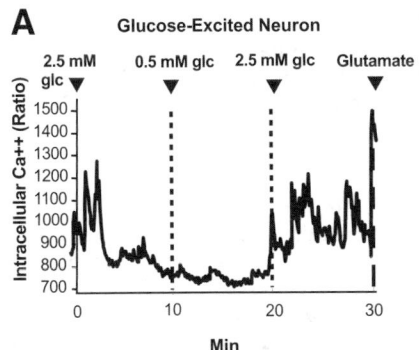
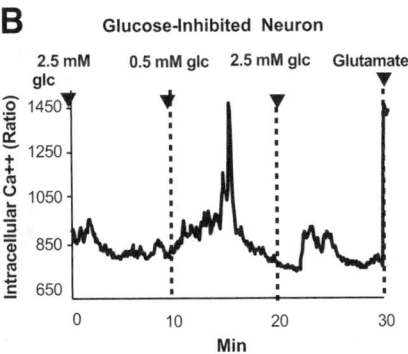
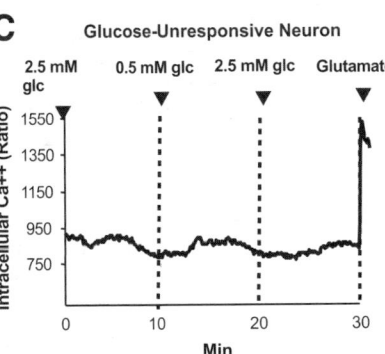

FIG. 1. Representative changes in $[Ca^{2+}]_i$ oscillations after exposure to incremental dose glucose in freshly dissociated medial amygdalar neurons from 3–4-week-old male Sprague–Dawley rats. All recordings were carried out in 2.5 mmol/l glucose (2.5 mmol/l glc) followed by two doses of glucose (0.5 and 2.5 mmol/l), and then tested with glutamate. A: Glucose-excited neuron ($n = 25$) showing increased $[Ca^{2+}]_i$ oscillations at 2.5 mmol/l, decreased $[Ca^{2+}]_i$ oscillations at 5 mmol/l, and a robust response to glutamate. B: Glucose-inhibited neuron ($n = 27$) showing low $[Ca^{2+}]_i$ oscillations at 0.5 mmol/l and substantial response at 2.5 mmol/l. C: Neuron unresponsive to different physiological levels of glucose ($n = 14$).

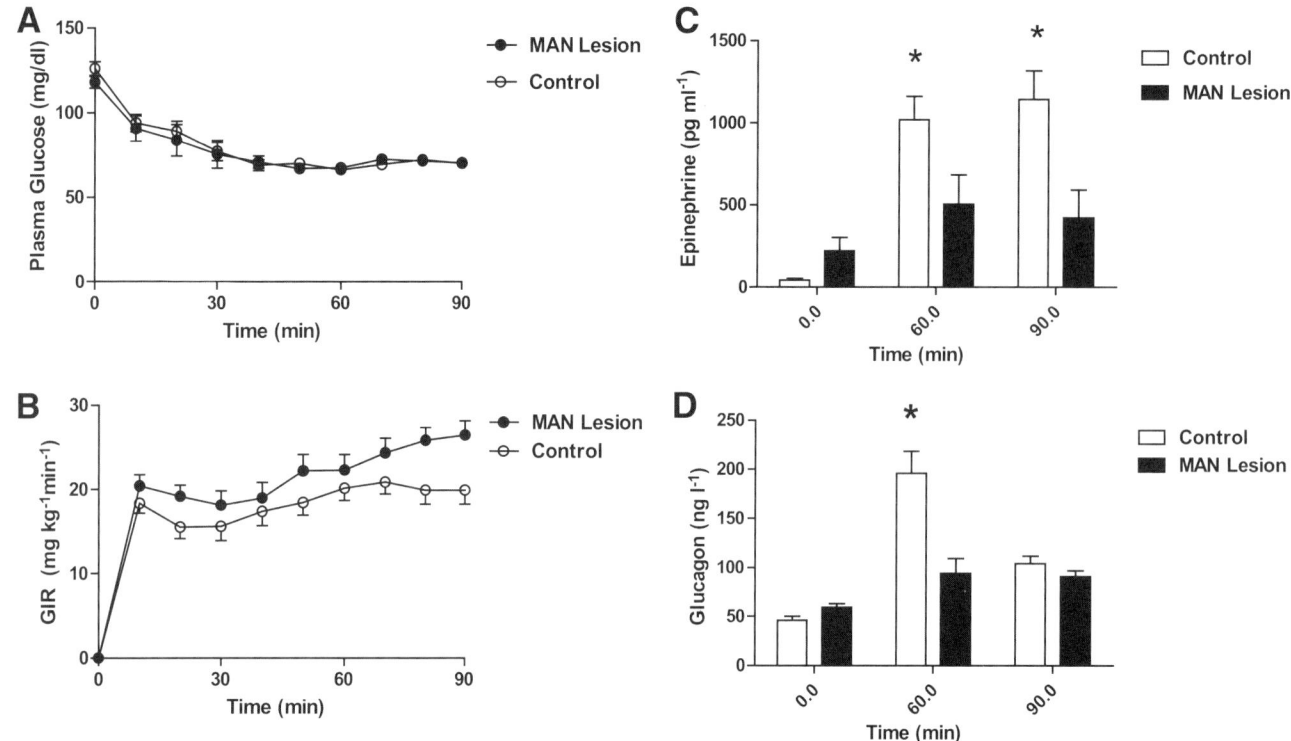

FIG. 2. Lesioning of the MAN leads to suppression of counterregulatory responses to acute hypoglycemia. *A*: Declines in plasma glucose level in response to the hyperinsulinemic clamp (70 mg/dl) did not differ between control (white circle) and MAN lesion (black circle) groups. *B*: Decreased need for exogenous glucose (decreased glucose infusion rate [GIR]) after MAN lesion. *C*: Suppressed epinephrine and (*D*) glucagon secretory responses to hypoglycemia after MAN lesion. Data are expressed as mean ± SE.

versus 69 ± 1 mg/dl (3.9 ± 0.1 vs. 3.9 ± 0.1 mmol/l); Fig. 3*A*], GIR (60–90 min) were threefold lower in the MAN 2-DG infused rats compared with the aECF control group (3.8 ± 1.1 versus12.3 ± 2.2 mg/kg/min, respectively; $F = 24.6$, $P < 0.01$) (Fig. 3*B*). Consistent with the lower GIR, 2-DG microinjection to the MAN significantly amplified the glucagon ($F = 4.8$, $P < 0.05$) and epinephrine ($F = 7.2$, $P < 0.05$) responses during hypoglycemia (Figs. 3*C* and *D*).

UCN3 neurons innervating the VMH arise primarily from the MAN. To determine the origin of UCN3 neurons innervating the VMH, the retrograde neuronal tracer, WGA, was microinjected into the VMH. While UCN3 neurons are present in the medial preoptic nucleus and the rostral perifornical area as expected, by double-label immunohistochemistry, that most of the UCN3 neurons in the MAN project to the VMH (cell bodies positive for [WGA+UCN3]/UCN3 = 492/520). Moreover, microinjection of a retrograde tracer to the MAN demonstrated direct neural pathways in the reciprocal direction from cell bodies in the VMH to nerve terminals in the MAN (supple-

TABLE 3
Microinfusion of the nonmetabolizable glucose analog 2-DG to the VMH and MAN of rats following an overnight fast had no effect on plasma glucose or counterregulatory hormones

	MAN + 2-DG ($n = 6$)		VMH + 2-DG ($n = 4$)	
	0 min	60 min	0 min	60 min
Glucose (mg/dl)	114 ± 6	114 ± 7	124 ± 3	112 ± 4
Glucagon (ng/l)	51 ± 3	81 ± 16	72 ± 9	58 ± 9
Epinephrine (pg/ml)	235 ± 66	249 ± 99	208 ± 56	70 ± 45

mentary Fig. 4). A schematic representation of the location of UCN3 cell bodies innervating the VMH is shown in Fig. 4, whereas microphotographs of cells showing dual labeling of UCN3 and WGA in the MAN are shown in supplementary Fig. 3.

Hypoglycemia activates VMH-projecting MAN UCN-3 neurons. To determine whether the UCN3 cell bodies in the MAN were activated during acute hypoglycemia, rats underwent hyperinsulinemic hypoglycemic (~70 mg/dl) or hyperinsulinemic euglycemic (~120 mg/dl) clamp studies for 120 min as described above. Using triple fluorescence immunostaining for cFOS, UCN3, and the retrograde tracer fluorogold, we found that ~30% (155/520 neurons) of those UCN3 neurons in the MAN that innervate the VMH coexpressed cFOS, a marker of neuronal activation, during acute hyperinsulinemic hypoglycemia when compared with hyperinsulinemic euglycemia (1/655; $P < 0.05$). This suggests that at least one-third of the MAN UCN3 neurons are activated during a mild hypoglycemic stimulus (Fig. 5).

DISCUSSION

The principal finding of the current study is the novel discovery that the MAN contains glucose-sensing neurons that can influence the magnitude of the counterregulatory response to insulin-induced hypoglycemia. The amygdala is a complex structure, containing a number of discrete nuclei involved in a wide range of behavioral and physiological functions. In the rodent, the MAN is strongly connected with the olfactory system, has numerous interconnections with other amygdalar nuclei (enabling it to integrate the neural outputs from these different regions), and, like the VMH, has also been shown to integrate with

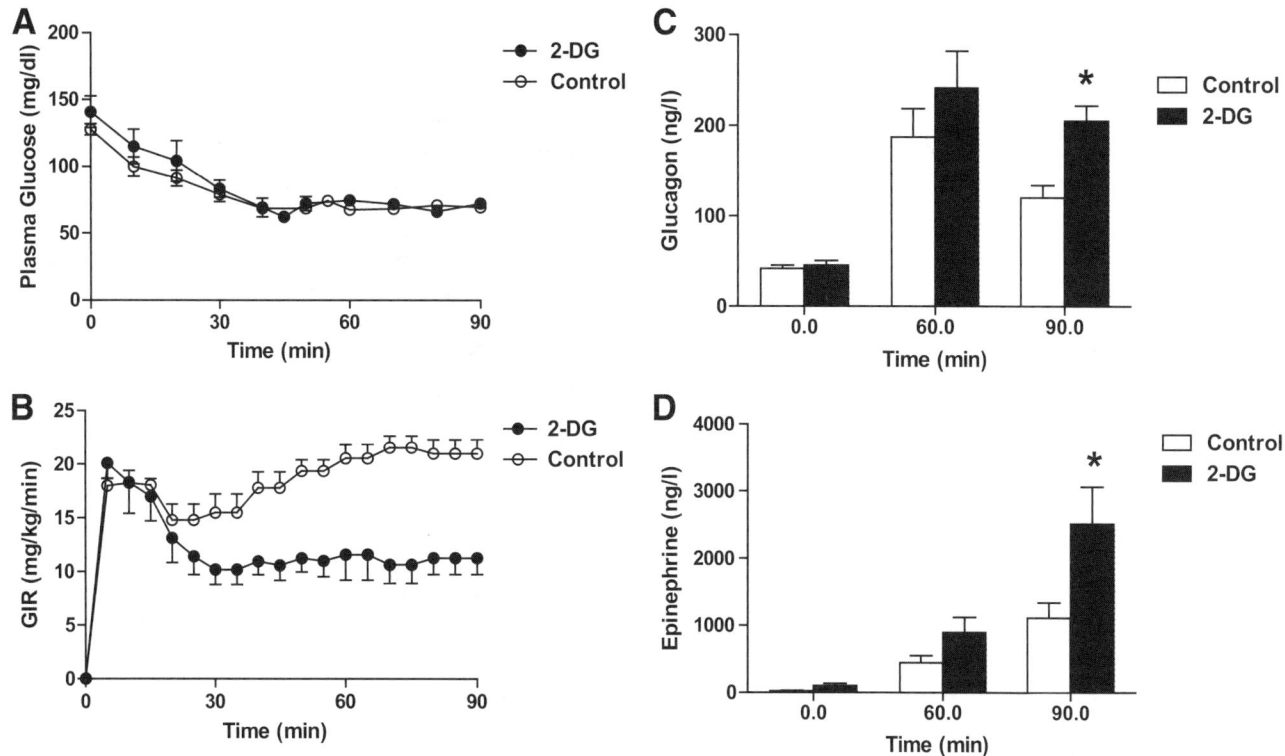

FIG. 3. Provision of an additional glucoprivic stimulus to the MAN amplifies the counterregulatory response to a mild systemic insulin-induced hypoglycemic challenge. *A*: Declines in plasma glucose level in response to the hyperinsulinemic clamp (70 mg/dl) did not differ between control (white circle) and 2-DG (black circle) groups. *B*: Decreased need for exogenous glucose (decreased glucose infusion rate [GIR]) after 2-DG injection into the MAN. *C*: Amplified epinephrine and (*D*) glucagon secretory responses to hypoglycemia in MAN 2-DG injected rats. Data are expressed as mean ± SE.

the neural circuits linked to feeding and body weight control (25,26). Interestingly, a recent study using [18F]-fluorodeoxyglucose positron emission tomography, in 13 men with type 1 diabetes, reported reduced [18F]-fluoro-deoxyglucose uptake in the amygdala during hypoglycemia in those subjects with hypoglycemia unawareness failure, suggesting a potential role for the amygdala in the development of hypoglycemia unawareness (27).

The VMH is integral to glucose-sensing during acute hypoglycemia (for a review, see ref [28]). The VMH contains specialized glucose-sensing neurons (23), and 14–19% of these are glucose-excited, whereas 3–14% are glucose-inhibited in type (29). As in the pancreatic β-cell, glucokinase appears to be a critical regulator of glucose-sensing in VMH neurons (6), where glucokinase is expressed in ~65% of glucose-excited and ~45% of glucose-inhibited neurons (23). In fact, it is most likely that all neurons that express glucokinase are actually glucose-sensing and that the finding of glucokinase mRNA in non-glucose-sensing neurons is due to the stringent criteria used to classify neurons. In the present study, we have been able to show, using fura-2-calcium imaging, that the expression of glucokinase mRNA in the MAN is associated with the presence of specialized glucose-sensing neurons. Of these, ~6% were glucose-excited whereas 7.5% were glucose-inhibited. Moreover, 54% of glucose-excited and 42% of glucose-inhibited, compared with only 9% of non-glucose-sensing neurons, contained mRNA for glucokinase. These findings clearly parallel those of the VMH, providing support for the hypothesis that the MAN may represent a novel glucose-sensing brain region.

To determine whether the MAN plays a functional role

in glucose-sensing, we initially used the selective neuro-toxin, ibotenic acid, to lesion the MAN and then performed a hyperinsulinemic hypoglycemic study. Consistent with a previous study where ibotenic acid was used to lesion the VMH (8), lesioning the MAN was shown to suppress the counterregulatory hormonal response to subsequent hypoglycemia. Subsequently, we sought to determine whether localized glucoprivation in the MAN of euglycemic animals would induce a glucoprivic response, characterized by a rise in plasma glucose and in the counterregulatory hormones glucagon and epinephrine, as previously demonstrated in the VMH (9). However, neither 2-DG nor 5-thioglucose infusions into either the MAN or VMH over 30 min raised plasma glucose, glucagon, or epinephrine levels. We then sought to determine whether combining local MAN glucoprivation during a moderate systemic hypoglycemic stimulus might influence counterregulatory responses to assess whether this additional glucoprivic stimulus might amplify the counterregulatory response. In fact, the combination of local MAN and systemic glucoprivation did have this effect. Taken together, these in vivo studies suggest that the MAN contributes to the counterregulatory response induced by systemic hypoglycemia but that local glucoprivation in the MAN alone is insufficient to generate a counterregulatory hormone response.

A previous study that used unilateral microinjection to localize glucose-sensing brain regions also failed to elicit a glucoprivic response in the majority of hypothalamic regions tested, although it did produce glucoprivic responses with unilateral hindbrain microinjections (30). More recently, bilateral VMH 5-TG microinjections were shown to stimulate food intake; however, no glucose

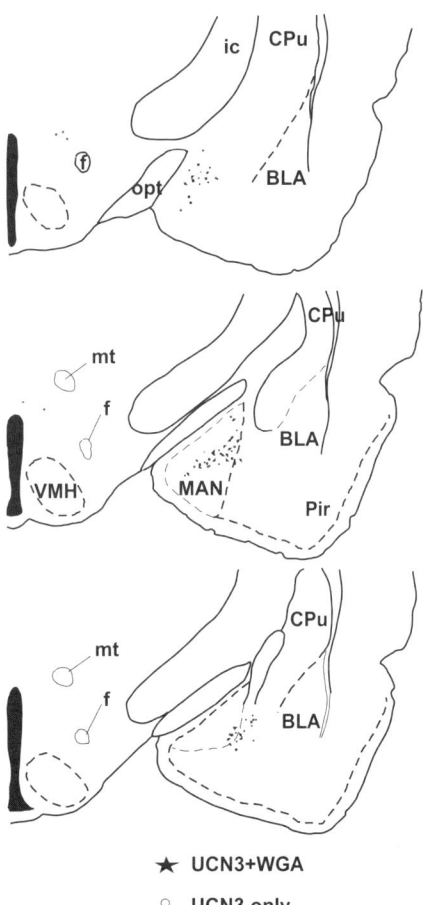

★ UCN3+WGA

○ UCN3 only

FIG. 4. A schematic diagram illustrating the distribution of UCN3 neurons from serial sections through the MAN. Each open circle represents a neuronal cell body staining for UCN3 alone, while the stars show dual staining for UCN3 and WGA. BLA, basolateral amygdalar nucleus; CPu, caudate putamen (Striatum); f, fornix; ic, internal capsule; mt, mammillothalamic tract; opt, optic tract; Pir, Piriform cortex; PH, posterior hypothalamic nucleus.

readings were assessed in this study (31). Food intake was not measured in our study, but we did not find an increase in blood glucose after VMH 5-TG or 2-DG. The reasons for these discrepancies are not clear. Borg et al. (9) used microdialysis to deliver 2-DG locally to the VMH, and it is possible that, under these conditions, the stimulus to glucose-sensing neurons is greater. Interestingly, recurrent glucoprivation impairs hypothalamic but not hindbrain responses to subsequent hypoglycemia (32), suggesting that repeated hypoglycemia restrains hindbrain glucose-sensing via an upstream (hypothalamic and or other brain region) mechanism. On the basis of the present findings and those of Ritter et al. (30), we would speculate that glucose-sensors in the hindbrain may form part of a classical sensory reflex response, whereas glucose-sensors in higher centers are more integrated in their response to a glucoprivation, that is, hypoglycemia might need to be present in a number of glucose-sensing brain and/or peripheral sensors before counterregulation is initiated.

Given the importance of the VMH to the detection of hypoglycemia and our previous studies showing a role for UCN3 in the VMH in modulating the counterregulatory response to hypoglycemia, we then sought to examine

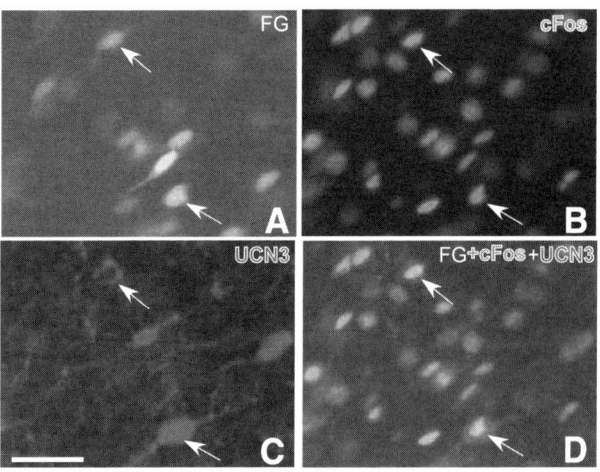

FIG. 5. High magnification image of neuronal cell bodies within MAN. Triple-staining immunohistochemistry was used to indentify UCN3 neurons in the MAN that were activated by hypoglycemia and that directly innervated the VMH. *A*: The retrograde tracer fluorogold (FG) microinjected to the VM and identified as yellow staining within MAN neuronal cell bodies (white arrows). *B*: cFOS immunoreactivity present within MAN neuronal cell bodies during acute hypoglycemia (white arrows). *C*: UCN3 neurons in the MAN (white arrows). *D*: Neuronal cell bodies showing FG (blue), cFOS (green), and UCN3 (red). Triple staining is seen in those neurons identified by white arrows. (A high-quality digital representation of this figure is available in the online issue.)

whether UCN3 might link these two glucose-sensing regions. Previous neuroanatomical studies have shown that the MAN projects topographically to the VMH (25), findings confirmed in our study using retrograde neural tracers to show reciprocal pathways between these two regions. Additionally, we have been able to demonstrate that most of the UCN3 projections to the VMH arise in the MAN. Moreover, using triple-staining immunohistochemistry, we also found that ~1/3 of these activated during acute hypoglycemia. In this context, our previous finding that pharmacological manipulation of CRH-R2 receptors in the VMH markedly altered counterregulatory responses to acute hypoglycemia is very suggestive of a functional role for this neural network (13). It is perhaps counterintuitive that UCN3 activation in the MAN during hypoglycemia might lead to suppression of glucose-sensing neurons in the VMH. However, it is notable that few of the individual MAN glucose-sensing neurons identified by Ca^{2+} imaging also expressed mRNA for UCN3. On the other hand, many did express mRNA for its receptor, CRH-R2. In addition, gene expression analysis from serial MAN micropunches showed that glucokinase and CRH-R2 gene expression had the same rostrocaudal distribution, but the opposite rostrocaudal distribution as UCN3 mRNA. This implies that UCN3 neurons may represent a discrete neuronal population in the MAN that are not in themselves glucose-sensing and, thus, may also directly regulate glucose-sensing neurons locally, as they do in the VMH. This would lead us to speculate that UCN3 neurons may regulate or coordinate the output, in terms of the counterregulatory responses, from these two discrete glucose-sensing regions.

In summary, in the current study we have identified the MAN as a novel limbic glucose-sensing region that contains characteristic glucokinase-expressing glucose-sensing neurons that respond directly to manipulations of glucose availability. In addition, manipulation of the MAN by lesion or through provision of an additional glucoprivic stimulus modulates the counterregulatory response to moderate systemic hypoglycemia. Finally, we have shown that both these glucose-sensing regions are linked by UCN3 neurons, which potentially provides a mechanism for fine-tuning and integrating the stress response during a hypoglycemic challenge.

ACKNOWLEDGMENTS

This work was supported by National Institutes of Health Grants (DK-069831, R.J.M.) and (DK-53181, B.E.L.), the Diabetes and Endocrinology Research Center (DERC) at Yale, and the Juvenile Diabetes Research Foundation (R.J.M.). L.Z. is a Juvenile Diabetes Research Foundation Postdoctoral Research Fellow. B.E.L. is supported by the Research Service of the Veterans Administration.

No potential conflicts of interest relevant to this article were reported.

L.Z. conducted the in vivo studies and performed IHC; N.P. performed the fura-2 calcium imaging and sc-QPCR; Z.S. helped with the in vivo studies and IHC; Y.D. performed rodent surgeries and helped with in vivo studies; X.F. helped with in vivo studies; Q.T. contributed to the discussion; B.E.L. supervised fura-2 calcium imaging and sc-QPCR, helped with manuscript preparation, and contributed to the discussion; R.J.M. wrote the manuscript and designed and supervised the in vivo studies and IHC.

The authors are grateful to Ralph Jacob and Aida Groszmann, Yale University, for their support and assistance. The authors thank Dr. Wylie Vale, Salk Institute, CA, for kindly providing the Urocortin 3 antibody used in these studies, and Dr. Brad Lowell, Beth Israel Deaconness Medical Center, Boston, MA, for his helpful comments.

REFERENCES

1. McCrimmon R. Glucose sensing during hypoglycemia: lessons from the lab. Diabetes Care 2009;32:1357–1363
2. Levin BE, Routh VH, Kang L, Sanders NM, Dunn-Meynell AA. Neuronal glucosensing: what do we know after 50 years? Diabetes 2004;53:2521–2528
3. Routh VH. Glucose-sensing neurons: are they physiologically relevant? Physiol & Behav 2002;76:403–413
4. Canabal DD, Song Z, Potian JG, Beuve A, McArdle JJ, Routh VH. Glucose, insulin, and leptin signaling pathways modulate nitric oxide synthesis in glucose-inhibited neurons in the ventromedial hypothalamus. Am J Physiol Regul Integr Comp Physiol. 2007;292:R1418–1428
5. Fioramonti X, Marsollier N, Song Z, Fakira KA, Patel RM, Brown S, Duparc T, Pica-Mendez A, Sanders NM, Knauf C, Valet P, McCrimmon RJ, Beuve A, Magnan C, Routh VH. Ventromedial hypothalamic nitric oxide production is necessary for hypoglycemia detection and counterregulation. Diabetes 2010;59:519–528
6. Kang L, Dunn-Meynell AA, Routh VH, Gaspers LD, Nagata Y, Nishimura T, Eiki J, Zhang BB, Levin BE. Glucokinase is a critical regulator of ventromedial hypothalamic neuronal glucosensing. Diabetes 2006;55:412–420 [Erratum appears in Diabetes 2006;55(3):862]
7. Borg MA, Sherwin RS, Borg WP, Tamborlane WV, Shulman GI. Local ventromedial hypothalamus glucose perfusion blocks counterregulation during systemic hypoglycemia in awake rats. J Clin Invest 1997;99:361–365
8. Borg WP, During MJ, Sherwin RS, Borg MA, Brines ML, Shulman GI. Ventromedial hypothalamic lesions in rats suppress counterregulatory responses to hypoglycemia. J Clin Invest 1994;93:1677–1682
9. Borg WP, Sherwin RS, During MJ, Borg MA, Shulman GI. Local ventromedial hypothalamus glucopenia triggers counterregulatory hormone release. Diabetes 1995;44:180–184
10. Evans SB, Wilkinson CW, Gronbeck P, Bennett JL, Taborsky GJ, Jr, Figlewicz DP. Inactivation of the PVN during hypoglycemia partially simulates hypoglycemia-associated autonomic failure. Am J Physiol Regul Integr Comp Physiol 2003;284:R57–65
11. Evans SB, Wilkinson CW, Gronbeck P, Bennett JL, Zavosh A, Taborsky GJ, Jr, Figlewicz DP. Inactivation of the DMH selectively inhibits the ACTH and corticosterone responses to hypoglycemia. Am J Physiol Regul Integr Comp Physiol 2004;286:R123–128
12. Cheng H, Zhou L, Zhu W, Wang A, Tang C, Chan O, Sherwin RS, McCrimmon RJ. Type 1 corticotropin-releasing factor receptors in the ventromedial hypothalamus promote hypoglycemia-induced hormonal counterregulation. Am J Physiol Endocrinol Metab 2007;293:E705–712
13. McCrimmon RJ, Song Z, Cheng H, McNay EC, Weikart-Yeckel C, Fan X, Routh VH, Sherwin RS. Corticotrophin-releasing factor receptors within the ventromedial hypothalamus regulate hypoglycemia-induced hormonal counterregulation. J Clin Invest 2006;116:1723–1730
14. Li C, Vaughan J, Sawchenko PE, Vale WW. Urocortin III–immunoreactive projections in rat brain: partial overlap with sites of type 2 corticotrophin-releasing factor receptor expression. Journal of Neuroscience 2002;22:991–1001
15. Lynch RM, Tompkins LS, Brooks HL, Dunn-Meynell AA, Levin BE. Localization of glucokinase gene expression in the rat brain. Diabetes 2000;49:693–700
16. Rossetti L, Shulman GI, Zawalich W, DeFronzo RA. Effect of chronic hyperglycemia on in vivo insulin secretion in partially pancreatectomized rats. J Clin Invest 1987;80:1037–1044
17. Powell AM, Sherwin RS, Shulman GI. Impaired hormonal responses to hypoglycemia in spontaneously diabetic and recurrently hypoglycemic rats. Reversibility and stimulus specificity of the deficits. J Clin Invest 1993;92:2667–2674
18. Zhou L, Furuta T, Kaneko T. Chemical organization of projection neurons in the rat accumbens nucleus and olfactory tubercle. Neuroscience 2003;120:783–798
19. Zhou L, Furuta T, Kaneko T. Neurokinin B-producing projection neurons in the lateral stripe of the striatum and cell clusters of the accumbens nucleus in the rat. J Comp Neurol 2004;480:143–161
20. Paxinos G, Watson C. *The Rat Brain in Stereotaxic Coordinates.* San Diego, CA, Academic Press, 1997
21. Palkovits M. Isolated removal of hypothalamic or other brain nuclei of the rat. Brain Res 1973;59:449–450
22. Levin BE, Dunn-Meynell AA, Ricci MR, Cummings DE. Abnormalities of leptin and ghrelin regulation in obesity-prone juvenile rats. Am J Physiol Endocrinol Metab 2003;285:E949–957
23. Kang L, Routh VH, Kuzhikandathil EV, Gaspers LD, Levin BE. Physiological and molecular characteristics of rat hypothalamic ventromedial nucleus glucosensing neurons. Diabetes 2004;53:549–559
24. Liss B. Improved quantitative real-time RT-PCR for expression profiling of individual cells. Nucleic Acid Res 2002;30:e89
25. Canteras NS, Simerly RB, Swanson LW. Organization of projections from the medial nucleus of the amygdala: a PHAL study in the rat. J Comp Neurol 1995;360:213–245
26. King BM. The rise, fall, and resurrection of the ventromedial hypothalamus in the regulation of feeding behavior and body weight. Physiol Behav 2006;87:221–244
27. Dunn JT, Cranston I, Marsden PK, Amiel SA, Reed LJ. Attenuation of amydgala and frontal cortical responses to low blood glucose concentration in asymptomatic hypoglycemia in type 1 diabetes: a new player in hypoglycemia unawareness? Diabetes 2007;56:2766–2773
28. McCrimmon R. The mechanisms that underlie glucose sensing during hypoglycaemia in diabetes. Diabet Med 2008;25:513–522
29. Dunn-Meynell AA, Routh VH, Kang L, Gaspers L, Levin BE. Glucokinase is the likely mediator of glucosensing in both glucose-excited and glucose-inhibited central neurons. Diabetes 2002;51:2056–2065
30. Ritter S, Dinh TT, Zhang Y. Localization of hindbrain glucoreceptive sites controlling food intake and blood glucose. Brain Res 2000;856:37–47
31. Dunn-Meynell AA, Sanders NM, Compton D, Becker TC, Eiki J, Zhang BB, Levin BE. Relationship among brain and blood glucose levels and spontaneous and glucoprivic feeding. J Neurosci 2009;29:7015–7022
32. Sanders NM, Taborsky GJ, Jr, Wilkinson CW, Daumen W, Figlewicz DP. Antecedent hindbrain glucoprivation does not impair the counterregulatory response to hypoglycemia. Diabetes 2007;56:217–223

Sustained Benefit of Continuous Glucose Monitoring on A1C, Glucose Profiles, and Hypoglycemia in Adults With Type 1 Diabetes

THE JUVENILE DIABETES RESEARCH
FOUNDATION CONTINUOUS GLUCOSE
MONITORING STUDY GROUP*

OBJECTIVE — To evaluate long-term effects of continuous glucose monitoring (CGM) in intensively treated adults with type 1 diabetes.

RESEARCH DESIGN AND METHODS — We studied 83 of 86 individuals ≥25 years of age with type 1 diabetes who used CGM as part of a 6-month randomized clinical trial in a subsequent 6-month extension study.

RESULTS — After 12 months, median CGM use was 6.8 days per week. Mean change in A1C level from baseline to 12 months was $-0.4 \pm 0.6\%$ ($P < 0.001$) in subjects with baseline A1C ≥7.0%. A1C remained stable at 6.4% in those with baseline A1C <7.0%. The incidence rate of severe hypoglycemia was 21.8 and 7.1 events per 100 person-years in the first and last 6 months, respectively. Time per day with glucose levels in the range of 71–180 mg/dl increased significantly ($P = 0.02$) from baseline to 12 months.

CONCLUSIONS — In intensively treated adults with type 1 diabetes, CGM use and benefit can be sustained for 12 months.

Diabetes Care 32:2047–2049, 2009

I n a 6-month randomized trial of intensively treated individuals with type 1 diabetes and baseline A1C ≥7.0%, adults ≥25 years of age benefited from use of continuous glucose monitoring (CGM) compared with adults using conventional blood glucose monitoring (1). In a contemporaneous parallel study of individuals with type 1 diabetes who had A1C levels <7.0%, those in the CGM group had a reduction in biochemical hypoglycemia compared with those in the control group while maintaining A1C levels in the target range (2). This report describes the 12-month follow-up of adult subjects in the two randomized trials' CGM groups.

RESEARCH DESIGN AND METHODS

— The protocol has been described in detail (1–3). We analyzed 12-month follow-up data for 83 of the 86 adults (≥25 years of age) who were initially randomized to the CGM group in either the ≥7.0% ($n = 49$) or <7.0% ($n = 34$) baseline A1C cohorts; 2 subjects discontinued study participation during the first 6 months and one after completion of the 9-month visit. An insulin pump was used by 75 (90%) subjects and multiple daily injections (MDIs) of insulin by 8 (10%). Subjects were provided with either a DexCom SEVEN (DexCom, San Diego, CA), MiniMed Paradigm REAL-Time System (Medtronic MiniMed, Northridge, CA),

or FreeStyle Navigator (Abbott Diabetes Care, Alameda, CA). Follow-up visits during the extension study occurred at 9 and 12 months postrandomization. A1C was measured at the University of Minnesota using the Tosoh A1C 2.2 Plus Glycohemoglobin Analyzer method (4). Severe hypoglycemia was defined as an event that required assistance from another person to administer resuscitative actions (5).

The amount of CGM use was determined from CGM downloads. Statistical testing was performed with a paired t test for measures with an approximate normal distribution and with a signed-rank test for other measures. Changes in glucose variability were evaluated in least squares regression models based on van der Waerden rank normal scores.

RESULTS

— Median CGM use was 7.0 days/week (interquartile range 6.3–7.0) at 6 months and 6.8 days/week (interquartile range 5.8–7.0) at 12 months (see online appendix supplemental Table S1, available at http://care.diabetesjournals.org/cgi/content/full/dc09-0846/DC1). Use at 12 months did not vary with baseline A1C level (Spearman $r = -0.10$; $P = 0.38$).

Among subjects with baseline A1C ≥7.0%, mean change in A1C from baseline to 12 months was $-0.4 \pm 0.6\%$ ($P < 0.001$), similar to the change from baseline to 6 months. The reduction in A1C occurred mainly in the first 8 weeks and then remained relatively stable through the next 44 weeks (supplemental Fig. S1). Among subjects with baseline A1C <7.0%, A1C remained within the target range over the entire 12 months of the study (6.4, 6.3, and 6.4% at baseline, 6 months, and 12 months, respectively; $P = 0.42$ for change from baseline to 12 months).

A severe hypoglycemic event was experienced by 8 (10%) of the 83 subjects (9 events) during the first 6 months and 3 subjects (4%; 3 events) in the second 6 months. The rate of severe hypoglycemic events fell from 21.8 events per 100 person-years during the first 6 months to 7.1 events per 100 person-years (95% CI

Corresponding author: Roy W. Beck, jdrfapp@jaeb.org.
Received 7 May 2009 and accepted 29 July 2009. Published ahead of print at http://care.diabetesjournals.org on 12 August 2009. DOI: 10.2337/dc09-0846. Clinical trial reg. no. NCT00406133, clinicaltrials.gov.
*The members of the Juvenile Diabetes Research Foundation Continuous Glucose Monitoring Study Group are included in the APPENDIX. A complete list of the clinical centers and investigators is available in the online appendix at http://care.diabetesjournals.org/cgi/content/full/dc09-0846/DC1.

Table 1—Clinical features and metabolic control measures

	Overall			Baseline A1C >7.0%			Baseline A1C <7.0%			P*
	Baseline†	Month 6	Month 12	Baseline†	Month 6	Month 12	Baseline†	Month 6	Month 12	
n	83	83	83	49	49	49	34	34	34	
Body weight (kg)	77 ± 15	78 ± 16	79 ± 15	79 ± 16	80 ± 17	81 ± 17	75 ± 13	75 ± 13	76 ± 13	<0.001
Daily insulin dose (U/kg body wt)	0.5 ± 0.1	0.5 ± 0.2	0.5 ± 0.1	0.5 ± 0.2	0.6 ± 0.2	0.6 ± 0.2	0.5 ± 0.1	0.5 ± 0.1	0.5 ± 0.1	0.72
Blood glucose meter tests per day‡	7.0 ± 2.4	6.4 ± 3.1	5.7 ± 2.1	6.5 ± 2.3	5.7 ± 2.3	5.5 ± 2.0	7.6 ± 2.4	7.3 ± 3.9	6.0 ± 2.2	<0.001
A1C (%)	7.1 ± 0.8	6.8 ± 0.6	6.9 ± 0.7	7.6 ± 0.5	7.1 ± 0.5	7.2 ± 0.5	6.4 ± 0.5	6.3 ± 0.5	6.4 ± 0.6	<0.001
CGM glucose measures (n)§	81	81	81	49	49	49	32	32	32	
Mean glucose (mg/dl)	151 ± 25	148 ± 21	148 ± 23	162 ± 24	157 ± 22	158 ± 23	136 ± 18	134 ± 12	133 ± 13	0.22
Glucose level (min/day)										
71–180 mg/dl	983	1,026	1,066	866	962	966	1,151	1,139	1,135	0.02
≤70 mg/dl	62	55	58	53	53	49	82	65	72	0.06
≤60 mg/dl	30	16	19	23	16	14	38	13	25	0.003
≤50 mg/dl	7	4	5	7	3	4	6	6	5	0.002
>180 mg/dl	385	321	293	483	378	422	219	231	211	0.12
>200 mg/dl	246	202	188	335	252	289	133	137	116	0.05
>250 mg/dl	77	48	49	121	61	78	28	33	19	0.02
Summary values										
Hypoglycemia area under the curve‖	0.5	0.3	0.3	0.4	0.3	0.3	0.6	0.3	0.4	0.002
Low blood glucose index¶	1.2	1.0	1.0	0.9	0.9	0.9	1.6	1.3	1.3	0.01
Hyperglycemia area under the curve#	11.6	8.6	8.1	16.0	11.0	12.5	5.4	5.5	4.8	0.05
High blood glucose index¶	5.6	4.8	4.6	6.6	5.5	6.2	3.3	3.7	3.4	0.08
Variability										
Standard deviation (mg/dl)	56	52	52	61	57	55	46	47	45	0.02 (0.03)
Mean amplitude of glycemic excursion (mg/dl)	107	101	97	114	106	107	91	89	93	0.03 (0.04)
Mean absolute rate of change (mg · dl⁻¹ · min⁻¹)	0.63	0.65	0.65	0.69	0.67	0.69	0.57	0.58	0.63	0.11 (0.03)
Coefficient of variation**	0.36	0.35	0.34	0.37	0.37	0.35	0.35	0.33	0.33	0.07 (0.10)

Data are means ± SD or median. *P values for the comparison of baseline vs. month 12 for all subjects pooled. For variability, the unadjusted and adjusted P values are both given: unadjusted (adjusted). †Baseline data are from blinded CGM use for approximately 4–7 days prior to randomization. ‡Self-reported blood glucose meter monitoring. §Subjects required to have at least 24 h of glucose data at all three time points to be included in analysis. One subject with zero use in month 12 and one subject whose CGM use in month 12 was imputed with the self-reported data at the month 12 visit as a result of a missing download data were excluded. ‖Total area under the curve <70 mg/dl reflects both percentage and severity of glucose values in the hypoglycemic range. ¶Blood glucose index (ref. 8). #Total area under the curve above 180 mg/dl. **SD divided by mean glucose.

0–16.7) during the second 6 months ($P = 0.18$). The rate was not associated with baseline A1C (Spearman $r = -0.004$; $P = 0.97$). In subjects with baseline A1C ≥7%, the incidence fell from 20.5 events per 100 person-years in the first 6 months to 12.1 events per 100 person-years in the second 6 months, whereas in the A1C <7% cohort, the incidence fell from 23.6 events per 100 person-years to no events during the second 6 months (supplemental Fig. S2).

The median amount of time per day with glucose in the range of 71–180 mg/dl increased significantly ($P = 0.02$) from baseline to 12 months, reflecting a decrease in both hypoglycemia and hyperglycemia. Similar trends were seen both in subjects with baseline A1C ≥7.0% and in those with baseline A1C <7.0% (Table 1). The increase in time in range was seen during both daytime and nighttime (supplemental Table S2). Variability assessed with the SD of glucose values ($P = 0.02$) and mean amplitude of glycemic excursions ($P = 0.03$) was reduced with CGM use from baseline to 12 months. Body weight, daily insulin dose, and frequency of daily blood glucose meter tests did not change meaningfully during the study.

CONCLUSIONS — In this 6-month extension to a randomized clinical trial, we found that most adults ≥25 years of age continued to use CGM on a daily or near-daily basis and had sustained benefits of improved glucose control noted by A1C levels and the amount of time sensor glucose values were in the target range. These benefits persisted despite less-intensive follow up, designed to approximate usual clinical practice, than that during the 6-month randomized phase of the study.

An additional important observation was the remarkably low rate of severe hypoglycemic events during the extension phase of the study. The rate of severe hypoglycemia in our CGM subjects with a mean A1C of 6.8% during the 6-month extension phase was markedly lower than the rate of severe hypoglycemia in the Diabetes Control and Complications Trial (DCCT) intensive treatment group, which had mean A1C of 7.1% (7 vs. 62 events per 100 person-years) (6). The total absence of severe hypoglycemia during the second 6 months of the study in the subjects who had a baseline A1C <7.0% is particularly striking, especially

because these subjects were able to maintain a mean A1C of 6.4%.

It is possible that the decline in severe hypoglycemic events during the second 6 months of the study resulted from learning from prior experience, including appropriate setting of the low alarms, glucose targets, and titration of basal and bolus insulin doses. It is also intriguing to speculate that the reduction in exposure to biochemical hypoglycemia over the 12 months of the study may have protected subjects from severe hypoglycemic events by enhancing their counterregulatory hormone defense mechanisms against hypoglycemia (7).

Our findings demonstrate that the benefits of CGM can be sustained for at least 12 months in motivated adults with type 1 diabetes practicing intensive diabetes management. In such individuals, CGM provides the ability to achieve target A1C levels much more safely than previously reported.

Acknowledgments — B.B. received consulting fees, honoraria, travel reimbursement, and research funds from Abbott Diabetes Care and Medtronic MiniMed as well as grant support from DexCom. I.H. received consulting fees and travel reimbursement from Abbott Diabetes Care and grant support from Medtronic MiniMed. L.L. received consulting fees from Lifescan, consulting fees and a speaker honorarium from Abbott Diabetes Care, consulting fees and research funding from Medtronic MiniMed, and consulting and speaker fees from Roche. W.V.T. received consulting fees from Abbott Diabetes Care and Lifescan as well as consulting fees, a speaker honorarium, and research funding from Medtronic MiniMed. S.W. received research support, a speaker honorarium, and travel reimbursement from Medtronic MiniMed as well as a speaker honorarium from Animas Corp/Lifescan. H.W. received consulting fees from Abbott Diabetes Care and research funding from Medtronic MiniMed. No other potential conflicts of interest relevant to this article were reported.

The study was designed and conducted by the investigators listed in the online appendix, who collectively wrote the manuscript and vouch for the data. The investigators had complete autonomy to analyze and report the trial results. There were no agreements concerning confidentiality of the data between the Juvenile Diabetes Research Foundation and the authors or their institutions. The Jaeb Center for Health Research had full access to all of the data in the study and takes responsibility for the integrity of the data and the accuracy of the data analysis.

Parts of this study were presented in abstract form at the 69th Scientific Sessions of

the American Diabetes Association, New Orleans, Louisiana, 5–9 June 2009.

The Juvenile Diabetes Research Foundation Continuous Glucose Monitoring Study Group recognizes the efforts of the subjects and their families and thanks them for their participation.

APPENDIX — The Juvenile Diabetes Research Foundation Continuous Glucose Monitoring Study Group writing committee members are as follows: lead authors Bruce Bode, MD, Roy W. Beck, MD, PhD, and Dongyuan Xing, MPH; and additional authors Lisa Gilliam, MD, PhD, Irl Hirsch, MD, Craig Kollman, PhD, Lori Laffel, MD, MPH, Katrina J. Ruedy, MSPH, William V. Tamborlane, MD, Stuart Weinzimer, MD, and Howard Wolpert, MD.

References
1. The Juvenile Diabetes Research Foundation Continuous Glucose Monitoring Study Group. Continuous glucose monitoring and intensive treatment of type 1 diabetes. N Engl J Med 2008359:1464–1476
2. The Juvenile Diabetes Research Foundation Continuous Glucose Monitoring Study Group. The effect of continuous glucose monitoring in well-controlled type 1 diabetes. Diabetes Care 2009;32:1378–1383
3. JDRF CGM Study Group. JDRF randomized clinical trial to assess the efficacy of real-time continuous glucose monitoring in the management of type 1 diabetes: research design and methods. Diabetes Technol Ther 2008;10:310–321
4. Gibb I, Parnham A, Fonfrède M, Lecock F. Multicenter evaluation of Tosoh glycohemoglobin analyzer. Clin Chem 1999;45:1833–1841
5. The Diabetes Control and Complications Trial Research Group. The effect of intensive treatment of diabetes on the development and progression of long-term complications in insulin-dependent diabetes mellitus. N Engl J Med 1993;329:977–986
6. The DCCT Research Group. Epidemiology of severe hypoglycemia in the Diabetes Control and Complications Trial. Am J Med 1991;90:450–459
7. Fanelli CG, Epifano L, Rambotti AM, Pampanelli S, Di Vincenzo A, Modarelli F, Lepore M, Annibale B, Ciofetta M, Bottini P. Meticulous prevention of hypoglycemia normalizes the glycemic thresholds and magnitude of most of neuroendocrine responses to, symptoms of, and cognitive function during hypoglycemia in intensively treated patients with short-term IDDM. Diabetes 1993;42:1683–1689
8. Kovatchev BP, Cox DJ, Gonder-Frederick LA, Clarke W. Symmetrization of the blood glucose measurement scale and its applications. Diabetes Care 1997;20:1655–1658

Medium-Chain Fatty Acids Improve Cognitive Function in Intensively Treated Type 1 Diabetic Patients and Support In Vitro Synaptic Transmission During Acute Hypoglycemia

Kathleen A. Page,[1] Anne Williamson,[2] Namyi Yu,[3] Ewan C. McNay,[4] James Dzuira,[5] Rory J. McCrimmon,[1] and Robert S. Sherwin[1]

OBJECTIVE—We examined whether ingestion of medium-chain triglycerides could improve cognition during hypoglycemia in subjects with intensively treated type 1 diabetes and assessed potential underlying mechanisms by testing the effect of β-hydroxybutyrate and octanoate on rat hippocampal synaptic transmission during exposure to low glucose.

RESEARCH DESIGN AND METHODS—A total of 11 intensively treated type 1 diabetic subjects participated in stepped hyperinsulinemic- ($2 \text{ mU} \cdot \text{kg}^{-1} \cdot \text{min}^{-1}$) euglycemic- (glucose ~5.5 mmol/l) hypoglycemic (glucose ~2.8 mmol/l) clamp studies. During two separate sessions, they randomly received either medium-chain triglycerides or placebo drinks and performed a battery of cognitive tests. In vitro rat hippocampal slice preparations were used to assess the ability of β-hydroxybutyrate and octanoate to support neuronal activity when glucose levels are reduced.

RESULTS—Hypoglycemia impaired cognitive performance in tests of verbal memory, digit symbol coding, digit span backwards, and map searching. Ingestion of medium-chain triglycerides reversed these effects. Medium-chain triglycerides also produced higher free fatty acids and β-hydroxybutyrate levels compared with placebo. However, the increase in catecholamines and symptoms during hypoglycemia was not altered. In hippocampal slices β-hydroxybutyrate supported synaptic transmission under low-glucose conditions, whereas octanoate could not. Nevertheless, octanoate improved the rate of recovery of synaptic function upon restoration of control glucose concentrations.

CONCLUSIONS—Medium-chain triglyceride ingestion improves cognition without adversely affecting adrenergic or symptomatic responses to hypoglycemia in intensively treated type 1 diabetic subjects. Medium-chain triglycerides offer the therapeutic advantage of preserving brain function under hypoglycemic conditions without causing deleterious hyperglycemia. *Diabetes* **58:1237–1244, 2009**

From the [1]Section of Endocrinology, Yale School of Medicine, New Haven, Connecticut; the [2]Department of Neurosurgery, Yale School of Medicine, New Haven, Connecticut; [3]Winthrop University Hospital, Long Island, New York; the [4]Department of Psychology, State University of New York, University at Albany, Albany, New York; and the [5]Yale Center for Clinical Investigation, New Haven, Connecticut.

Corresponding author: Kathleen A. Page, kathleen.page@yale.edu.

Received 10 November 2008 and accepted 4 February 2009.

Published ahead of print at http://diabetes.diabetesjournals.org on 17 February 2009. DOI: 10.2337/db08-1557.

Maintaining plasma glucose (PG) at near-normal levels in individuals with type 1 diabetes reduces the risk for developing long-term microvascular complications (1). However, intensive insulin therapy increases the risk of severe hypoglycemia, which can cause rapid deterioration of cognitive function and often occurs without warning symptoms (1,2). As a result, hypoglycemia limits the ability of patients to achieve target glycemic goals because the immediate fear of hypoglycemia exceeds the fear of long-term complications. Therefore, new strategies to protect the brain from hypoglycemia-induced injury are essential for optimizing the benefits of insulin therapy.

Although the brain relies primarily on glucose, it can use alternative fuels such as monocarboxylic acids, lactate, and ketones to maintain energy homeostasis (3–7). Exposure to prolonged fasting or hypoglycemia causes adaptive changes in the brain, including an enhanced ability to utilize alternative fuels (3,8,9). Thus, patients with intensively managed type 1 diabetes, by virtue of their increased exposure to hypoglycemia, may develop an enhanced ability to use alternate fuels, which, in turn, might provide neuroprotection during hypoglycemia.

Medium-chain triglycerides, constituents of coconut and palm kernel oils, are medium-chain fatty acid esters of glycerol. Medium-chain triglycerides have a favorable safety profile and are used to treat a variety of disorders (10–12). They offer a readily available noncarbohydrate fuel source because they are rapidly absorbed and quickly metabolized into medium-chain fatty acids (10). Medium-chain fatty acids do not require chylomicrons for transport or carnitine for entry into mitochondria (10). As a result, metabolism of medium-chain fatty acids promotes the generation of ketones (10). Furthermore, animal data suggest that medium-chain fatty acids can readily cross the blood-brain barrier (BBB) and be oxidized by the brain (13). Thus, medium-chain fatty acids may provide both a direct and an indirect brain fuel source via the generation of ketones, offering type 1 diabetic patients a prophylactic treatment strategy to preserve brain function during hypoglycemic episodes without raising blood glucose levels.

To explore this possibility, we evaluated whether oral medium-chain triglycerides could improve cognitive performance during acute insulin-induced hypoglycemia in intensively treated type 1 diabetic subjects. In addition, an in vitro hippocampal slice preparation from nondiabetic rats was used to assess the ability of β-hydroxybutyrate

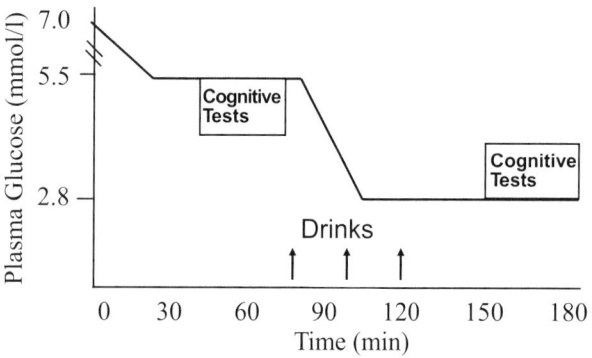

FIG. 1. Variable rate glucose infusion and primed continuous infusion of insulin ($2 \ mU \cdot kg^{-1} \cdot min^{-1}$). Hyperinsulinemic clamps were used to maintain euglycemic conditions for 90 min followed by a 90-min hypoglycemic phase. Cognitive tests were administered during steady-state euglycemia and hypoglycemia. The study drink (medium-chain triglycerides or placebo) was given at time = 75, 100, and 125 min. Upward arrows indicate time of drink administration.

and octanoate to support neuronal activity when the glucose supply is deficient.

RESEARCH DESIGN AND METHODS

A total of 11 individuals (5 men, 6 women, aged [mean ± SD] 34.8 ± 8.9 years, BMI 24.2 ± 3.4 kg/m²) with type 1 diabetes for 15.9 ± 9.5 years participated in the study. Subjects had no medical problems other than type 1 diabetes and had a normal physical exam and electrocardiogram. Blood tests confirmed absent C-peptide levels and normal renal and liver function. Subjects were intensively controlled with insulin (10 with continuous subcutaneous insulin infusion [CSII] and 1 with multiple daily injections), as reflected by a mean A1C of 6.9 ± 0.6 and a history of frequent hypoglycemic episodes, defined as self-reported fingerstick blood glucose <60 mg/dl. The number of hypoglycemic episodes per month was between 1 and 5 in two subjects, between 6 and 10 in two subjects, between 11 and 30 in six subjects, and >30 in one subject. Subjects gave their written informed consent to participate in this study, which was approved by the Yale University human investigation committee.

Experimental protocol. Nine subjects underwent two stepwise hyperinsulinemic-euglycemic-hypoglycemic clamp studies with ingestion of either the medium-chain triglycerides or placebo drink in random order in a crossover design, as described below. Of the 11 subjects, 2 participated in one study session (1 with placebo and 1 with medium-chain triglycerides). Cognitive data from all 11 subjects were included in the analysis as permitted by the mixed model. Paired Student's t tests were used to compare substrate and hormone levels between medium-chain triglycerides and control sessions for the nine subjects who completed both sessions.

Subjects were admitted to the Hospital Research Unit (HRU) of the Yale Center for Clinical Investigation on the evening before the study. Dinner was served at 6:00 P.M., and they were fasted overnight until the end of the study the following day. At approximately 9:00 P.M., an intravenous catheter was inserted into an antecubital vein for infusion of insulin (regular human insulin; Novo Nordisk, Bagsvaerd, Denmark) and dextrose to maintain euglycemia overnight. Subjects who used CSII had the option of being admitted to the HRU on the morning of each session, at which time their CSII infusion was suspended, and an intravenous catheter was inserted in an antecubital vein for insulin and glucose administration. Of the 10 CSII-treated patients, 3 chose this option and were admitted on the morning of each session. These subjects reduced their basal insulin dose by 20% and checked blood glucose at home before bedtime and on awakening. The study was cancelled if blood glucose was <70 mg/dl based on home glucose measurements.

At approximately 7:30 A.M., a second catheter was placed in a retrograde fashion into a dorsal vein of the nondominant hand for blood sampling. The hand was placed in a heated box (~50–55°C) to arterialize venous blood. At time = 0, PG was indistinguishable on the placebo (6.8 ± 0.4 mmol/l) and medium-chain triglyceride days (7.0 ± 0.7 mmol/l). A primed continuous infusion of insulin was then initiated and maintained at a constant rate of 2.0 mU · kg⁻¹ · min⁻¹, and a variable rate of 20% dextrose was infused concomitantly (Fig. 1). At 75 min, subjects ingested over a 5-min period the first of a series of three drinks, each in 50-ml volumes, containing either medium-chain triglycerides or sucralose, a sugar substitute. During the medium-chain triglycerides session, a total of 40 g of medium-chain triglycerides (derived from coconut oil containing 67% octanoate, 27% decanaote, and

6% other fatty acids; Novartis) was ingested at 25-min intervals with front loading of 20 g then 10 g twice. During the control session, cherry-flavored water sweetened with sucralose was ingested at identical time intervals. Drinks were prepared by the HRU. At 5 min after the first drink, PG (mean ± SE) was lowered to 2.8 ± 0.16 mmol/l for the hypoglycemic phase of the clamp. PG was measured in duplicate every 5 min to ensure a stable glucose plateau. Blood samples were collected for glucose, lactate, β-hydroxybutyrate, glycerol, free fatty acids (FFAs), insulin, glucagon, norepinephrine, and epinephrine levels at baseline and at 20-min intervals.

During the euglycemic phase (from 45 to 70 min) and again during the hypoglycemic phase (from 155 to 180 min), subjects completed a battery of cognitive tasks. Tests of nonmemory function included digit symbol substitution, Tests of Everyday Attention, telephone book searching, and map searching in 1 and 2 min. Tests of immediate and delayed verbal memory and verbal memory recognition were adapted from the Wechsler Memory Scale logical memory tests (14). Working memory was assessed by modified versions of the standard Wechsler Memory Scale Digit Span and Letter/Number Sequencing Tests (14). These cognitive tests have been validated in studies of the effect of hypoglycemia on cognition (15,16). Hypoglycemic symptoms were assessed by a self-rating questionnaire during both the euglycemic and hypoglycemic phases. Symptoms of hypoglycemia were classified as autonomic (racing heart, sweating, warmness, trembling, hunger, anxiety) or neuroglycopenic (weakness, tiredness, double vision, difficulty speaking, difficulty concentrating, drowsiness, confusion, blurry vision); the total symptom score was equal to the autonomic plus neuroglycopenic symptom scores.

Measurement of hormones and metabolites. PG and lactate were measured enzymatically using glucose and lactate oxidase, respectively (Yellow Springs Instruments, Yellow Springs, OH). Plasma insulin and glucagon were measured using a double-antibody radioimmunoassay (Millipore, St. Charles, MO), epinephrine and norepinephrine by high-performance liquid chromatography (ESA, Chelmsford, MA), and FFAs using NEFA-HR (Wako Diagnostics, Richmond, VA). Plasma glycerol was measured by an enzymatic end point reaction with a CMA 600 analyzer (CMA Microdialysis, Chelmsford, MA) and β-hydroxybutyrate using an ACE chemical analyzer (Wako Diagnostics, Richmond, VA).

Animal protocol. Standard methods were used for hippocampal slice preparation (17) using adult Sprague-Dawley rats (29 male, 13 female). The standard artificial cerebrospinal fluid (aCSF) contained (in mmol/l): 124 NaCl, 3 KCl, 2 MgSO₄, 1.2 NaH₂PO₄, 26 NaHCO₃, 2.0 CaCl₂, and 10 glucose, pH 7.4. The slices (400 μm) were placed on the stage of an interface recording chamber (Fine Science Tools, Foster City, CA), where they were superfused with aCSF and maintained at 32°C ± 0.5.

Local field potentials were recorded in the cell body layer of CA1 using a low-resistance (3 mol/lΩ) patch pipette filled with aCSF; a twisted bipolar electrode placed in the Schaffer collaterals was used to evoke synaptic responses. The baseline response used for the experiment was 50% of the maximal response recorded in aCSF. The stimulus intensity was not altered for the balance of the experiment. Synaptic responses were studied both at low frequencies (0.1 Hz) and after stimulus trains of 10 Hz for 10 s. At rest, brain slices have lower rates of oxidative phosphorylation than the intact brain. Therefore, to more accurately simulate the increased neural activity and metabolic demand seen during hippocampal memory processing (18) and to model cognitive activation, we used 10-Hz repetitive synaptic stimulation. The protocol will drive oxidative metabolism in slices (17) without causing significant synaptic plasticity (19).

Hypoglycemia was induced by a bath applying aCSF containing 2 mmol/l glucose with 8 mmol/l sucrose added to maintain osmolarity for 30 min. This concentration of bath glucose results in a tissue glucose of ~0.5 mmol/l (20) compared with 5.0 mmol/l with a bath glucose of 10 mmol/l. The synaptic responses were delivered at 0.1 Hz during the wash-on period, and stimulus trains (10 Hz, 10 s) were delivered at 10-min intervals to investigate the relationship between the metabolic load and synaptic responses.

We examined three experimental conditions: 2 mmol/l glucose + 8 mmol/l β-hydroxybutyrate, 2 mmol/l glucose + 8 mmol/l octanoate, and 2 mmol/l glucose + 4 mmol/l β-hydroxybutyrate + 4 mmol/l octanoate. For each condition, the test compound(s) were bath applied for an additional 30 min with one stimulus train midway during the wash-on period. Control aCSF (10 mmol/l glucose) was then washed on to determine the ability of the tissue to recover from hypoglycemia.

Statistical analysis. Data analysis was performed using SAS version 9.2 (Cary, NC). Clamp- and treatment-dependent changes were analyzed independently for each cognitive test using a mixed-model ANOVA. In the mixed-model ANOVA, fixed effects for the treatment order, treatment (medium-chain triglycerides vs. placebo), glucose (euglycemia vs. hypoglycemia), and their interactions were included, and correlation between repeated assessments was modeled using an unstructured covariance pattern (21). Linear contrasts

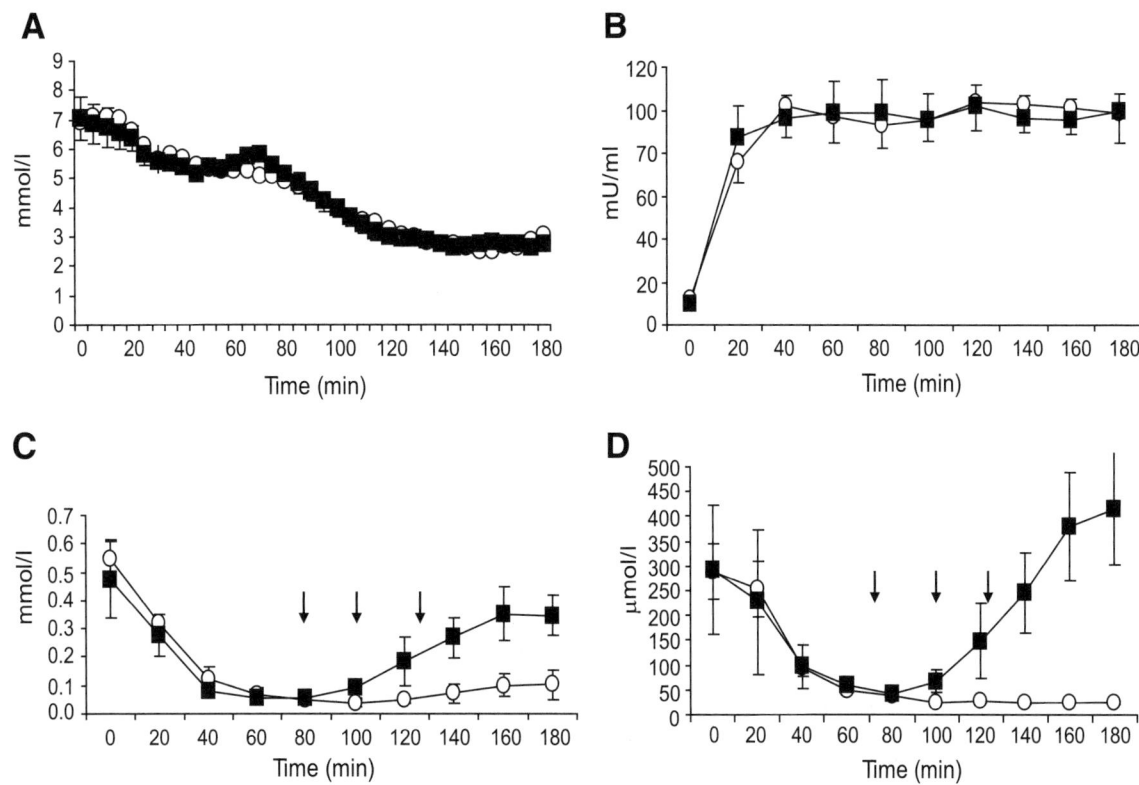

FIG. 2. *A–D*: PG (*A*), plasma insulin (*B*), plasma FFA (*C*), and plasma β-hydroxybutyrate (*D*) profiles during the euglycemic-hypoglycemic clamp studies with medium-chain triglycerides or placebo ingestion. ■, medium-chain triglycerides; ○, placebo. Down arrows indicate drink administration.

were estimated to test differences in euglycemic to hypoglycemic cognitive changes between medium-chain triglycerides and placebo. The level of significance at individual time points was determined by paired Student's *t* tests with a Bonferroni correction for multiple testing. Paired Student's *t* tests were used to compare substrate and hormone levels between medium-chain triglycerides and control sessions during steady-state euglycemia and hypoglycemia. A *P* value <0.05 was considered significant. Except where noted, all data are reported as the means ± SE.

Physiology statistics. The amplitude of the population spike was the primary measure. Paired Student's *t* tests, corrected for multiple comparisons, were used to test for significance at the different points in the experiment.

RESULTS

PG, insulin, and metabolite concentrations. PG profiles were identical throughout medium-chain triglyceride and control sessions (Fig. 2). During steady-state euglycemia (from 30 to 75 min), PG was 5.5 ± 0.07 mmol/l in the medium-chain triglycerides and 5.4 ± 0.1 mmol/l in the control sessions ($P = 0.4$). Similarly, steady-state glucose levels during the final 40 min of the hypoglycemic phase were equivalent during the medium-chain triglyceride (2.74 ± 0.05 mmol/l) and control sessions (2.73 ± 0.06 mmol/l; $P = 0.8$). Plasma insulin also increased comparably in both sessions 99 ± 12 (medium-chain triglycerides) versus 98 ± 11 μU/ml (control; $P = 0.4$).

During the euglycemic phase of both sessions, insulin suppressed plasma FFAs and β-hydroxybutyrate. During hypoglycemia, both metabolites remained suppressed in the control study but rose after administration of medium-chain triglycerides. During the final 40 min of hypoglycemia, plasma FFAs (0.323 ± 0.07 vs. 0.083 ± 0.04 mmol/l, $P = 0.01$) and β-hydroxybutyrate (356 ± 81 vs. 25 ± 1.4 μmol/l, $P < 0.01$) were significantly higher after medium-chain triglycerides compared with placebo. There were no

differences between groups in plasma glycerol (22 ± 7 vs. 31 ± 8 μmol/l, $P = 0.30$) or lactate (0.94 ± 0.16 vs. 1.12 ± 0.17 mmol/l, $P = 0.20$) during hypoglycemia.

Cognitive tests. Acute hypoglycemia impaired cognitive performance in tests of immediate verbal memory ($P < 0.001$), delayed verbal memory ($P = 0.005$), verbal memory recognition ($P < 0.001$), digit symbol coding ($P = 0.03$), digit span backwards ($P = 0.008$), and map searching in 1 min ($P = 0.04$) as assessed by the change in performance from euglycemia to hypoglycemia after placebo ingestion (Fig. 3 and Table 1). When compared with ingestion of the placebo drink, medium-chain triglycerides prevented the decline in cognitive performance during hypoglycemia in tests of immediate verbal memory ($P = 0.009$), delayed verbal memory ($P < 0.001$), and verbal memory recognition ($P = 0.0008$). Medium-chain triglycerides also improved performance during hypoglycemia in digit symbol coding ($P = 0.002$) and total map searching ($P = 0.04$).

Counterregulatory hormones. Hypoglycemia increased plasma epinephrine and norepinephrine levels in both treatment groups (Fig. 4). They were, however, not significantly different during the final 40 min of hypoglycemia (epinephrine 233 ± 102 in control subjects vs. 236 ± 90 pg/ml with medium-chain triglycerides, $P = 0.8$; norepinephrine 239 ± 45 in control subjects vs. 272 ± 69 pg/ml with medium-chain triglycerides, $P = 0.2$). As expected (22), there was no significant glucagon response to hypoglycemia during the control and medium-chain triglycerides sessions (46 ± 7.4 in control subjects vs. 47 ± 8.0 pg/ml with medium-chain triglycerides, $P = 0.75$).

Symptomatic responses. Total hypoglycemic symptom scores were significantly elevated during hypoglycemia

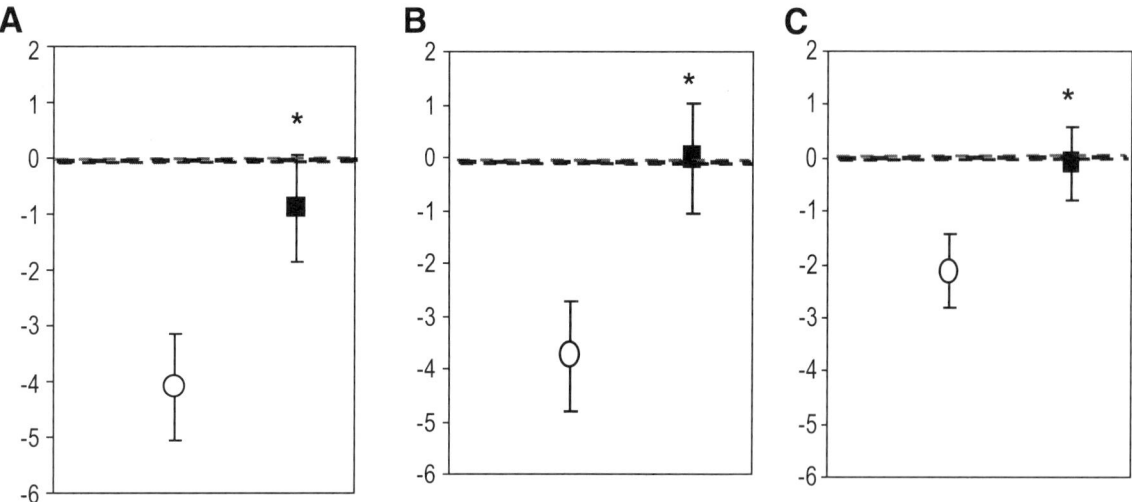

FIG. 3. Medium-chain triglyceride ingestion preserved cognitive performance under hypoglycemic conditions in tests of verbal memory. *A*: Immediate verbal memory. *B*: Delayed verbal memory. *C*: Verbal memory recognition. Figures show change in test scores (euglycemia-hypoglycemia) after medium-chain triglycerides (■) or placebo (○). *$P < 0.01$ medium-chain triglycerides vs. placebo.

compared with euglycemia (control 30.80 ± 3.9 vs. 19.22 ± 1.40, medium-chain triglycerides 35.25 ± 5.8 vs. 21.35 ± 2.3, respectively; $P = 0.002$ for comparison of hypoglycemia to euglycemia). There was no difference in hypoglycemic symptoms after medium-chain triglycerides compared with placebo ingestion (Fig. 4).

Rat hippocampal slice studies. β-Hydroxybutyrate can partially substitute for glucose in vitro. When a 2 mmol/l glucose bath was applied for 30 min with intervening stimulus trains, the field potential amplitude decreased from 7.1 ± 1.2 to 4.1 ± 0.93 mV and then reached steady state. Across the population, this represented a $47.7 \pm 12.3\%$ decrease ($P < 0.05$, $n = 21$). When β-hydroxybutyrate was added iso-osmotically, there was a partial recovery to 5.74 ± 1.03 mV ($83.8 \pm 7.8\%$ of control, $n = 10$). This was significantly ($P < 0.05$) different from the 2 mmol/l glucose values alone, but not different from values in control aCSF. We also assessed whether β-hydroxybutyrate could fully substitute for glucose using a bath applying 8 mmol/l β-hydroxybutyrate in 0 mmol/l added glucose aCSF. In all three slices studied, the synaptic response was lost after the first stimulus train and was only partially recoverable upon washing to 10 mmol/l

glucose, indicating the need for a minimal level of glucose to maintain synaptic transmission under a metabolic load.

β-Hydroxybutyrate in 2 mmol/l glucose was also able to maintain synaptic function during both low- and moderate-frequency stimulation. In control aCSF, there was a modest decrease in the mean population spike amplitude $9.9 \pm 2.5\%$ (first vs. last response) during a 10-Hz train. In contrast, as shown in Fig. 5, the synaptic response was reduced by $80.0 \pm 6.4\%$ of control in 2 mmol/l glucose ($P < 0.05$). When β-hydroxybutyrate was added to the bath, the ability of the tissue to respond to synaptic stimulation was restored to $82.0 \pm 22.4\%$ (18% depression) of control ($n = 10$). It was also notable that β-hydroxybutyrate was able to prevent the initial depression seen in control studies (Fig. 5).

Octanoate does not substitute for glucose in hippocampal slice preparations. In contrast, substitution of octanoate for glucose using the same experimental paradigm produced no recovery of synaptic function in any of the slices tested ($n = 6$). The response only recovered to $49.6 \pm 12.8\%$ of control after washing with 10 mmol/l glucose containing aCSF in three of six cases. Moreover, unlike β-hydroxybutyrate, octanoate did not

TABLE 1
Cognitive test scores during euglycemia and hypoglycemia with medium-chain triglycerides or placebo ingestion

Cognitive test	Medium-chain triglycerides euglycemia (~ 5.5 mmol $\cdot$ l$^{-1} \cdot$ l^{-1})	Medium-chain triglycerides hypoglycemia (~ 2.8 mmol $\cdot$ l$^{-1} \cdot$ l^{-1})	Placebo euglycemia (~ 5.5 mmol $\cdot$ l$^{-1} \cdot$ l^{-1})	Placebo hypoglycemia (~ 2.8 mmol $\cdot$ l$^{-1} \cdot$ l^{-1})
Immediate verbal memory	15.85 ± 0.66	14.97 ± 1.13*	17.36 ± 1.03	13.28 ± 1.04†
Delayed verbal memory	14.82 ± 1.25	14.80 ± 1.31*	15.33 ± 1.40	11.58 ± 0.71†
Verbal memory recognition	13.19 ± 0.53	13.29 ± 0.50*	14.27 ± 0.23	12.14 ± 0.19†
Digit span backwards	0.60 ± 0.05	0.58 ± 0.05	0.64 ± 0.05	0.54 ± 0.05†
Letter/number sequencing	12.04 ± 0.81	10.97 ± 0.76	11.07 ± 0.85	9.92 ± 0.71
Digit symbol coding	72.50 ± 5.27	74.99 ± 4.56*	74.04 ± 4.59	68.56 ± 3.54†
Map search (1 min)	53.11 ± 4.16	48.42 ± 3.19	50.35 ± 3.27	42.94 ± 2.31†
Map search (2 min)	73.30 ± 1.70	75.11 ± 1.51*	75.04 ± 1.92	74.67 ± 1.51
Telephone search	2.86 ± 0.17	3.06 ± 0.20	3.14 ± 0.26	3.46 ± 0.34

Data are least square means $\pm$ SE. *$P < 0.05$ change from euglycemia to hypoglycemia after medium-chain triglycerides vs. placebo; †$P < 0.05$ between euglycemia and hypoglycemia.

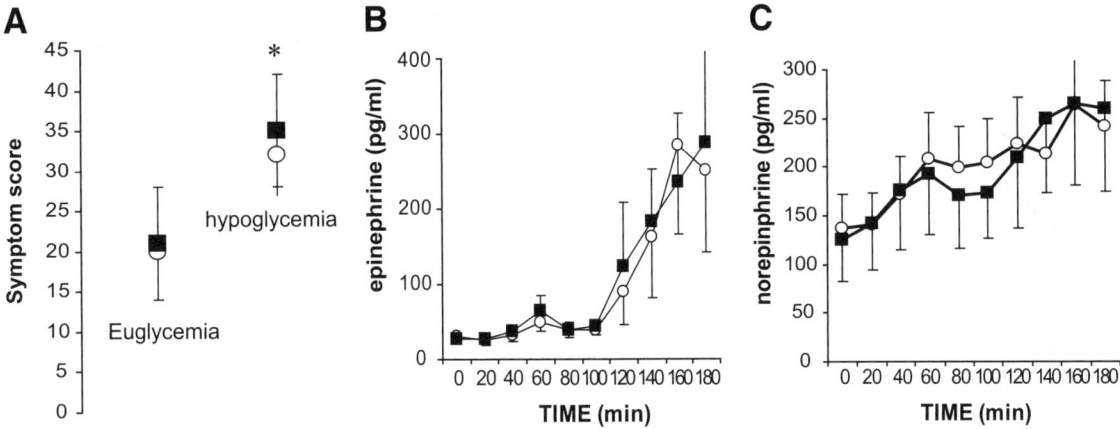

FIG. 4. *A*: Symptoms of hypoglycemia were significantly greater during hypoglycemia compared with euglycemia. *$P < 0.05$. There was no difference in symptoms of hypoglycemia after medium-chain triglyceride ingestion when compared with placebo ingestion. *B* and *C*: Plasma epinephrine (*B*) and plasma norepinephrine (*C*) profiles during euglycemic-hypoglycemic clamp studies with medium-chain triglycerides or placebo ingestion. ■, medium-chain triglycerides; ○, placebo.

preserve population spike amplitude during the stimulus train (Fig. 6).

Octanoate improves recovery after hypoglycemia. To determine whether there was a synergistic effect of β-hydroxybutyrate and octanoate, they were bath-applied together (4 mmol/l each) using the same protocol as above. There was a partial recovery to $75.9 \pm 12.6\%$ of control, an effect not significantly different from that seen with 8 mmol/l β-hydroxybutyrate. However, there was an increase in the speed with which the synaptic response recovered to a stable baseline when washed with control aCSF compared with β-hydroxybutyrate alone (2 mmol/l glucose + 8 mmol/l β-hydroxybutyrate, 31.6 ± 8.7 min, $n = 7$; 2 mmol/l glucose + 4 mmol/l β-hydroxybutyrate + 4 mmol/l octanoate, 21.9 ± 8.2 min, $n = 5$).

DISCUSSION

This study tested the hypothesis that oral medium-chain triglycerides could provide an alternative fuel source to

prevent the deterioration of higher brain function caused by acute hypoglycemia in intensively treated type 1 diabetic subjects. We used a battery of tasks to assess a range of cognitive domains. As expected, hypoglycemia impaired performance in tests of attention, short-term and delayed verbal memory, and working memory. Medium-chain triglyceride ingestion prevented this decline in performance in tests of short-term and delayed verbal memory and tests pertaining to attention. Medium-chain triglycerides' beneficial effect was most notable on tests of verbal memory, which to a large extent involves the hippocampus, a brain region particularly vulnerable to hypoglycemia (18,22–24). From the therapeutic perspective, it is reassuring that the cognitive benefit of medium-chain triglycerides was not associated with an adverse effect on hypoglycemia-induced adrenergic responses or symptoms.

Medium-chain triglycerides, a source of medium-chain fatty acids, have widely used for nutritional support and in patients with malabsorption (10,25). Medium-chain

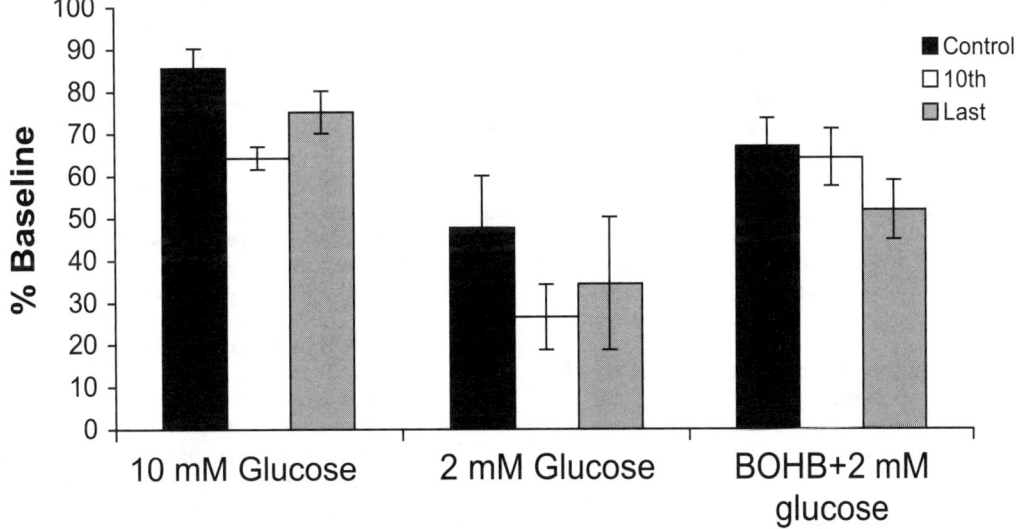

FIG. 5. β-Hydroxybutyrate (BOHB) supports synaptic activity during a stimulus train. Data were taken from the 1st, 10th, and final stimulus during the last of a series of three 10-Hz, 10-s trains delivered under three conditions: control (10 mmol/l glucose), 2 mmol/l glucose, and 2 mmol/l glucose with 8 mmol/l β-hydroxybutyrate. Note that there was a profound decrease in the percent change in the amplitude of the evoked response in 2 mmol/l glucose that was reversed in the presence of 2 mmol/l glucose + 8 mmol/l β-hydroxybutyrate. Also note that β-hydroxybutyrate was able to sustain synaptic activity during the train to a greater degree than 10 mmol/l glucose, as shown by the effect on the 10th stimulus. Data are from a total of 21 slices: β-hydroxybutyrate was applied to 10 of these.

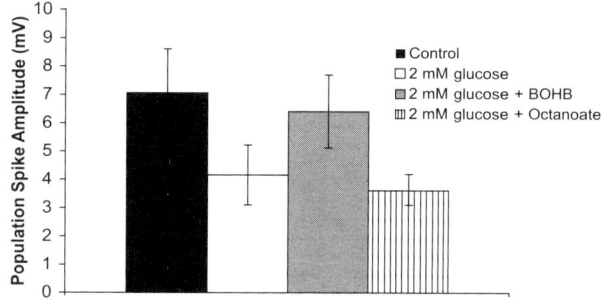

FIG. 6. Octanoate does not support synaptic transmission under hypoglycemic conditions. Graph shows the effect of bath application of 2 mmol/l glucose with or without equimolar substitution of either β-hydroxybutyrate or octanoate. Note that β-hydroxybutyrate was able to substitute for glucose under basal conditions, whereas octanoate had no effect. Data are shown 10 min after the last of three stimulus trains, $n = 10$ β-hydroxybutyrate, $n = 6$ octanoate.

fatty acids are rapidly absorbed and oxidized in the liver. This results in an excess of acetyl-CoA, and in turn the rapid production of ketones (10), an energy source for the brain (3,5,7). Furthermore, medium-chain fatty acids readily cross the BBB and are metabolized by the brain (13). Therefore, medium-chain fatty acids could directly and/or indirectly, via the generation of ketones, act to preserve brain function during hypoglycemia by provision of alternative fuels without raising blood glucose levels in patients with type 1 diabetes.

Medium-chain triglyceride ingestion raised plasma β-hydroxybutyrate and FFA levels during insulin-induced hypoglycemia, and thus both fuels might contribute to the observed effects on cognitive performance. The hippocampal slice data, however, suggest that the predominant impact of medium-chain fatty acids is mediated via the generation of ketones. β-Hydroxybutyrate supported synaptic transmission both at rest and during stimulus trains when glucose supply was deficient, whereas octanoate alone was ineffective. The failure to see an effect of octanoate in the hippocampal slice preparation reflects a time-dependent effect, and longer prior exposure to medium-chain fatty acids might have improved neuronal function. Alternatively, these findings may be explained by differences in brain metabolism of ketones and medium-chain fatty acids. Evidence suggests that octanoate is exclusively metabolized by astrocytes (13,26,27), whereas ketones are oxidized by both neurons and astrocytes (28,29). The finding that octanoate was able to improve the rate of recovery of synaptic function upon restoration of control glucose concentrations, but not the response to hypoglycemia itself, is consistent with the hypothesis that astrocytes may be critical for the restoration of synaptic function after a metabolic challenge such as hypoglycemia.

There is significant literature on the effects of alternative metabolic substrates on synaptic function in brain slice preparations (30–32). However, our studies on β-hydroxybutyrate differ from previous work (30,31) in two important aspects. First, we examined β-hydroxybutyrate in lowered (2 mmol/l) glucose compared with aglycemia, and second, we examined the ability of either β-hydroxybutyrate or octanoate to support synaptic transmission under a metabolic load. In glucose-free medium, β-hydroxybutyrate is able to maintain ATP but neither phosphocreatine levels nor synaptic function in slices prepared from adult rats (30,31). In contrast, our data indicate that β-hydroxy-

butyrate is able to sustain synaptic activity in adult rats only with some glucose present. It is also important to note that β-hydroxybutyrate is comparable to glucose in its ability to support synaptic activity under a metabolic load (Fig. 5). Taken together, these data suggest that there is an absolute requirement for a low concentration of glycolytic substrate to sustain robust synaptic transmission. This possibility is consistent with the data of Kanatani et al. (32); however, other investigators (33) have suggested that lactate can substitute for glucose under most conditions.

Although medium-chain triglyceride ingestion sustained cognitive function during acute hypoglycemia, it did not affect the adrenergic hormonal or symptomatic response to hypoglycemia. This finding might reflect a specific effect of medium-chain fatty acids on brain regions involved in cognition without affecting subcortical regions, such as the ventromedial hypothalamus, that are involved in the detection of hypoglycemia and the initiation of counterregulatory responses. This is consistent with evidence suggesting that there are regional differences in the brain's capacity to use alternative fuels during hypoglycemia (34). Evans et al. (34) demonstrated that intralipid infusion impaired the counterregulatory response to hypoglycemia without affecting cognitive performance, whereas Rossetti et al. (35) recently reported that amino acid ingestion preserved cognitive performance without affecting counterregulatory or symptomatic responses to acute hypoglycemia, much as we observed here.

Some studies, however, suggest that lactate and β-hydroxybutyrate sustain cognitive function while blunting counterregulatory responses during hypoglycemia (4–6). Notably, the β-hydroxybutyrate concentrations in those studies using β-hydroxybutyrate infusions (5,6) were much higher than in this study. Therefore, differences in circulating levels of β-hydroxybutyrate could explain the differences observed. In addition, prior studies (5,6) examined nondiabetic subjects, whereas we focused on intensively treated type 1 diabetic subjects. Pan et al. (8) suggest that it takes up to 72 h for ketones to be metabolized in the brain of nondiabetic individuals, probably because of the time required to increase BBB monocarboxylic acid transporters. In keeping with this view, acute in vitro studies using nondiabetic animals indicate that ketones can be immediately metabolized in the absence of the BBB (30). Moreover, it has been reported that brain acetate transport is increased in type 1 diabetic subjects receiving intensive insulin therapy compared with nondiabetic subjects (9). Thus, adaptive increases in the transport of β-hydroxybutyrate into the brain of intensively managed type 1 diabetic subjects may account for the ability of medium-chain triglycerides to rapidly attenuate hypoglycemic effects on cognitive function, and such adaptations in β-hydroxybutyrate transport may be region specific (36).

A potential limitation of the study is that cognitive performance may decline over time, thereby contributing to the deterioration in performance we observed in the hypoglycemic phase of the study. However, we anticipate that the dominant effect on cognitive decline was hypoglycemia per se, given that both the medium-chain triglycerides and placebo sessions were performed over identical time intervals in random order, making it highly unlikely that the specific benefit of medium-chain triglycerides could be specifically attributed to a time-associated decline in cognitive performance. Of note, all of the type 1 diabetic patients selected for this study were receiving intensive insulin therapy regimens and had a documented history of hypoglycemia. As a result, they had absent glucagon and reduced epinephrine responses during the hypoglycemic clamp. The increase in epinephrine in these patients was less than half that seen in other studies reported by our group in nondiabetic individuals (37). Our aim was to see whether medium-chain triglycerides could maintain brain function in the face of hypoglycemia in such individuals. Whether the prophylactic benefits of medium-chain triglyceride ingestion might differ in patients with and without hypoglycemia unawareness remains to be determined.

It should be emphasized that long-term effects of medium-chain triglycerides on cardiovascular risk factors and glucose metabolism are unknown. Short-term studies of the effects of medium-chain triglyceride ingestion on serum lipoprotein profiles in nondiabetic subjects are conflicting. Some report that medium-chain triglyceride intake causes only minor changes (38–40) or decreases (41) in serum lipid profiles, whereas others suggest it increases serum lipoprotein levels (42). Medium-chain triglycerides are marketed as a weight loss supplement based on reports that they increase energy expenditure and fat oxidation (43–45) and reduce body weight in animals and humans (46,47). Short-term studies of medium-chain triglycerides have also suggested beneficial effects on glucose metabolism in patients with type 2 diabetes (48,49). Whether similar metabolic effects of medium-chain triglycerides are observed in type 1 diabetes will require further investigation.

We conclude that ingestion of medium-chain triglycerides improves cognitive function without affecting the adrenergic hormonal or symptomatic responses to acute hypoglycemia in intensively controlled type 1 diabetic patients. These findings suggest that medium-chain triglycerides could be used as prophylactic therapy for such patients with the goal of preserving brain function during hypoglycemic episodes, such as when driving or sleeping, without producing hyperglycemia.

ACKNOWLEDGMENTS

This study was supported in part by a grant from the Juvenile Diabetes Research Foundation Center for the Study of Hypoglycemia (4-2004-807), the Yale Center of Clinical Investigation supported by a Clinical and Translational Science Awards Grant (UL1 RR024139) from the National Center for Research Resources, and National Institutes of Health grants (R37 DK20495, RO1NA045792, and DK069831).

No potential conflicts of interest relevant to this article were reported.

This study was presented at the American Diabetes Association 68th Scientific Sessions, San Francisco, CA, 6–10 June 2008, abstract no. 15-OR.

We thank Ellen Hintz, Melinda Zgorski, Donna D'eugenio, Osama Abdelghany, Donna Caseria, Mikhail Smolgovsky, Ralph Jacob, Aida Groszmann, and Brenda Wu for their help in executing these studies.

REFERENCES

1. Diabetes Control and Complications Trial Research Group. The effect of intensive treatment of diabetes on the development and progression of long-term complications in insulin-dependent diabetes mellitus. N Engl J Med 1993;329:977–986
2. Diabetes Control and Complications Trial Research Group. Hypoglycemia in the Diabetes Control and Complications Trial. Diabetes 1997;46:271–286
3. Hasselbalch SG, Knudsen GM, Jakobsen J, Hageman LP, Holm S, Paulson OB. Brain metabolism during short-term starvation in humans. J Cereb Blood Flow Metab 1994;14:125–131
4. Maran A, Cranston I, Lomas J, Macdonald I, Amiel SA. Protection by lactate of cerebral function during hypoglycaemia. Lancet 1994;343:16–20
5. Veneman T, Mitrakou A, Mokan M, Cryer P, Gerich J. Effect of hyperketonemia and hyperlacticacidemia on symptoms, cognitive dysfunction, and counterregulatory hormone responses during hypoglycemia in normal humans. Diabetes 1994;43:1311–1317
6. Amiel SA, Archibald HR, Chusney G, Williams AJ, Gale EA. Ketone infusion lowers hormonal responses to hypoglycaemia: evidence for acute cerebral utilization of a non-glucose fuel. Clin Sci (Lond) 1991;81:189–194
7. Hawkins RA, Williamson DH, Krebs HA. Ketone-body utilization by adult and suckling rat brain in vivo. Biochem J 1971;122:13–18
8. Pan JW, Rothman TL, Behar KL, Stein DT, Hetherington HP. Human brain beta-hydroxybutyrate and lactate increase in fasting-induced ketosis. J Cereb Blood Flow Metab 2000;20:1502–1507
9. Mason GF, Petersen KF, Lebon V, Rothman DL, Shulman GI. Increased brain monocarboxylic acid transport and utilization in type 1 diabetes. Diabetes 2006;55:929–934
10. Traul KA, Driedger A, Ingle DL, Nakhasi D. Review of the toxicologic properties of medium-chain triglycerides. Food Chem Toxicol 2000;38: 79–98
11. Craig GB, Darnell BE, Weinsier RL, Saag MS, Epps L, Mullins L, Lapidus WI, Ennis DM, Akrabawi SS, Cornwell PE, Sauberlich HE. Decreased fat and nitrogen losses in patients with AIDS receiving medium-chain-triglyceride-enriched formula vs those receiving long-chain-triglyceride-containing formula. J Am Diet Assoc 1997;97:605–611
12. Gracey M, Burke V, Anderson CM. Medium chain triglycerides in paediatric practice. Arch Dis Child 1970;45:445–452
13. Ebert D, Haller RG, Walton ME. Energy contribution of octanoate to intact rat brain metabolism measured by 13C nuclear magnetic resonance spectroscopy. J Neurosci 2003;23:5928–5935
14. Wechsler D. *Wechsler Memory Scale Revised Manual.* San Antonio, TX, The Psychological Corp., 1987
15. McAulay V, Deary IJ, Sommerfield AJ, Frier BM. Attentional functioning is impaired during acute hypoglycaemia in people with type 1 diabetes. Diabet Med 2006;23:26–31
16. Sommerfield AJ, Deary IJ, McAulay V, Frier BM. Short-term, delayed, and working memory are impaired during hypoglycemia in individuals with type 1 diabetes. Diabetes Care 2003;26:390–396
17. Kann O, Kovacs R, Heinemann U. Metabotropic receptor-mediated Ca2+ signaling elevates mitochondrial Ca2+ and stimulates oxidative metabolism in hippocampal slice cultures. J Neurophysiol 2003;90:613–621
18. McNay EC, Fries TM, Gold PE. Decreases in rat extracellular hippocampal glucose concentration associated with cognitive demand during a spatial task. Proc Natl Acad Sci U S A 2000;97:2881–2885
19. Dericioglu N, Garganta CL, Petroff OA, Mendelsohn D, Williamson A. Blockade of GABA synthesis only affects neural excitability under activated conditions in rat hippocampal slices. Neurochem Int 2008;53:22–32
20. Tekkok SB, Godfraind JM, Krnjevic K. Moderate hypoglycemia aggravates effects of hypoxia in hippocampal slices from diabetic rats. Neuroscience 2002;113:11–21
21. Brown H, Prescott R. *Applied Mixed Models in Medicine.* Chichester, U.K., John Wiley and Sons, 1999
22. McNay EC, Sherwin RS. Effect of recurrent hypoglycemia on spatial cognition and cognitive metabolism in normal and diabetic rats. Diabetes 2004;53:418–425
23. Auer RN, Wieloch T, Olsson Y, Siesjo BK. The distribution of hypoglycemic brain damage. Acta Neuropathol 1984;64:177–191
24. Fujioka M, Okuchi K, Hiramatsu KI, Sakaki T, Sakaguchi S, Ishii Y. Specific changes in human brain after hypoglycemic injury. Stroke 1997;28:584–587
25. Bach AC, Frey A, Lutz O. Clinical and experimental effects of medium-chain-triglyceride-based fat emulsions: a review. Clin Nutr 1989;8:223–235
26. Kuge Y, Yajima K, Kawashima H, Yamazaki H, Hashimoto N, Miyake Y. Brain uptake and metabolism of [1-11C]octanoate in rats: pharmacokinetic basis for its application as a radiopharmaceutical for studying brain fatty acid metabolism. Ann Nucl Med 1995;9:137–142
27. Auestad N, Korsak RA, Morrow JW, Edmond J. Fatty acid oxidation and ketogenesis by astrocytes in primary culture. J Neurochem 1991;56:1376–1386
28. Pan JW, de Graaf RA, Petersen KF, Shulman GI, Hetherington HP, Rothman DL. [2,4-13 C2]-beta-Hydroxybutyrate metabolism in human brain. J Cereb Blood Flow Metab 2002;22:890–898
29. Edmond J, Robbins RA, Bergstrom JD, Cole RA, de Vellis J. Capacity for substrate utilization in oxidative metabolism by neurons, astrocytes, and

oligodendrocytes from developing brain in primary culture. J Neurosci Res 1987;18:551–561

30. Arakawa T, Goto T, Okada Y. Effect of ketone body (D-3-hydroxybutyrate) on neural activity and energy metabolism in hippocampal slices of the adult guinea pig. Neurosci Lett 1991;130:53–56

31. Izumi Y, Ishii K, Katsuki H, Benz AM, Zorumski CF. Beta-hydroxybutyrate fuels synaptic function during development: histological and physiological evidence in rat hippocampal slices. J Clin Invest 1998;101:1121–1132

32. Kanatani T, Mizuno K, Okada Y. Effects of glycolytic metabolites on preservation of high energy phosphate level and synaptic transmission in the granule cells of guinea pig hippocampal slices. Experientia 1995;51:213–216

33. Schurr A. Lactate: the ultimate cerebral oxidative energy substrate? J Cereb Blood Flow Metab 2006;26:142–152

34. Evans ML, Matyka K, Lomas J, Pernet A, Cranston IC, Macdonald I, Amiel SA. Reduced counterregulation during hypoglycemia with raised circulating nonglucose lipid substrates: evidence for regional differences in metabolic capacity in the human brain? J Clin Endocrinol Metab 1998;83:2952–2959

35. Rossetti P, Porcellati F, Busciantella Ricci N, Candeloro P, Cioli P, Nair KS, Santeusanio F, Bolli GB, Fanelli CG. Effect of oral amino acids on counterregulatory responses and cognitive function during insulin-induced hypoglycemia in nondiabetic and type 1 diabetic people. Diabetes 2008;57:1905–1917

36. Hawkins RA, Biebuyck JF. Ketone bodies are selectively used by individual brain regions. Science 1979;205:325–327

37. Goldberg PA, Weiss R, McCrimmon RJ, Hintz EV, Dziura JD, Sherwin RS. Antecedent hypercortisolemia is not primarily responsible for generating hypoglycemia-associated autonomic failure. Diabetes 2006;55:1121–1126

38. Nosaka N, Kasai M, Nakamura M, Takahashi I, Itakura M, Takeuchi H, Aoyama T, Tsuji H, Okazaki M, Kondo K. Effects of dietary medium-chain triacylglycerols on serum lipoproteins and biochemical parameters in healthy men. Biosci Biotechnol Biochem 2002;66:1713–1718

39. Cater NB, Heller HJ, Denke MA. Comparison of the effects of medium-chain triacylglycerols, palm oil, and high oleic acid sunflower oil on plasma triacylglycerol fatty acids and lipid and lipoprotein concentrations in humans. Am J Clin Nutr 1997;65:41–45

40. Hashim SA, Arteaga A, Van Itallie TB. Effect of a saturated medium-chain triglyceride on serum-lipids in man. Lancet 1960;1:1105–1108

41. Kasai M, Maki H, Nosaka N, Aoyama T, Ooyama K, Uto H, Okazaki M, Igarashi O, Kondo K. Effect of medium-chain triglycerides on the postprandial triglyceride concentration in healthy men. Biosci Biotechnol Biochem 2003;67:46–53

42. Tholstrup T, Ehnholm C, Jauhiainen M, Petersen M, Hoy CE, Lund P, Sandstrom B. Effects of medium-chain fatty acids and oleic acid on blood lipids, lipoproteins, glucose, insulin, and lipid transfer protein activities. Am J Clin Nutr 2004;79:564–569

43. Hill JO, Peters JC, Yang D, Sharp T, Kaler M, Abumrad NN, Greene HL. Thermogenesis in humans during overfeeding with medium-chain triglycerides. Metabolism 1989;38:641–648

44. St-Onge MP, Bourque C, Jones PJ, Ross R, Parsons WE. Medium- versus long-chain triglycerides for 27 days increases fat oxidation and energy expenditure without resulting in changes in body composition in overweight women. Int J Obes Relat Metab Disord 2003;27:95–102

45. St-Onge MP, Jones PJ. Physiological effects of medium-chain triglycerides: potential agents in the prevention of obesity. J Nutr 2002;132:329–332

46. Simon E, Fernandez-Quintela A, Del Puy Portillo M, Del Barrio AS. Effects of medium-chain fatty acids on body composition and protein metabolism in overweight rats. J Physiol Biochem 2000;56:337–346

47. Geliebter A, Torbay N, Bracco EF, Hashim SA, Van Itallie TB. Overfeeding with medium-chain triglyceride diet results in diminished deposition of fat. Am J Clin Nutr 1983;37:1–4

48. Han JR, Deng B, Sun J, Chen CG, Corkey BE, Kirkland JL, Ma J, Guo W. Effects of dietary medium-chain triglyceride on weight loss and insulin sensitivity in a group of moderately overweight free-living type 2 diabetic Chinese subjects. Metabolism 2007;56:985–991

49. Eckel RH, Hanson AS, Chen AY, Berman JN, Yost TJ, Brass EP. Dietary substitution of medium-chain triglycerides improves insulin-mediated glucose metabolism in NIDDM subjects. Diabetes 1992;41:641–647